Handbook of Wildlife Chemical Immobilization

Third Edition

Terry J. Kreeger, MS, DVM, PhD

Jon M. Arnemo, DVM, PhD

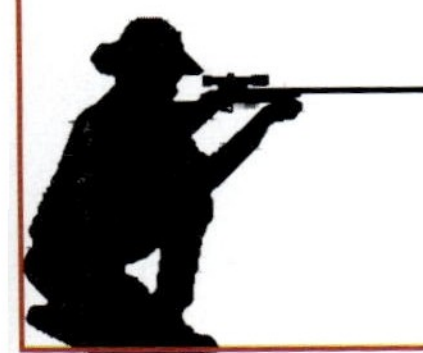

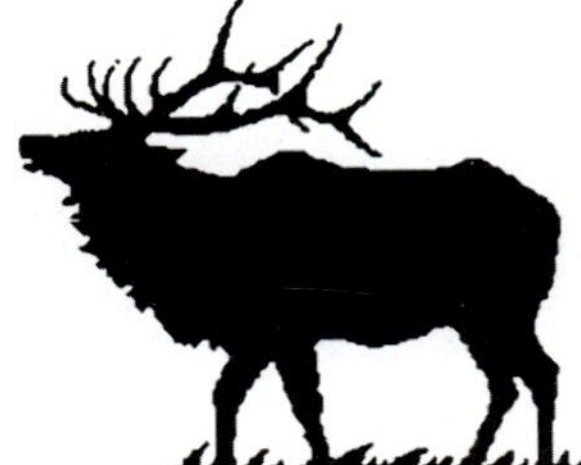

Ordering Information:

For North and South American orders, contact:

Dr. Terry J. Kreeger
E-mail: tkreeger@starband.net

U.S. orders can be placed over the internet via Amazon.com; search for title or authors.

*For European, African, and Asian order*s, contact:

Dr. Jon M. Arnemo, NO-2500 Tynset, Norway
E-mail: jmarnemo@online.no

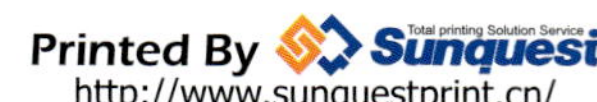

http://www.sunquestprint.cn/

Contents

Drug Possession and Use

Drugs Used for Animal Capture

Equipment Used for Animal Capture

Animal Capture: Putting It All Together

Animal Medical Treatment

Human Medical Treatment

Disclaimer

The recommended drugs and dosages published in this manual are taken from published scientific articles and textbooks, institutional and personal records, and the experience of the authors and their colleagues. Every attempt has been made by the authors and the reviewers to insure accuracy of those recommendations. However despite these efforts, errors in the original sources or in the preparation of this book may have occurred. All users of this manual, therefore, should empirically evaluate all dosages to determine that they are reasonable prior to use. Animal anesthesia is obviously beyond the control of anyone other than the person directly responsible for the immobilization. The vagaries of conditions, weather, age, nutrition, disease, and stress make every immobilization process unique. Because of this, the authors and publisher cannot accept responsibility for mishaps should they unfortunately occur. In addition, the authors and publisher do not endorse specific products, procedures, or dosages reported in this manual. Also, the listing of a drug in this manual does not indicate approval by the Food and Drug Administration or the manufacturer for use on wildlife.

Dedication

This book is dedicated to all those biologists and veterinarians who follow Michael Farady's philosophy:
work, finish, publish.

It is always dangerous to mention names lest you forget someone, but we would be remiss in not recognizing some researchers in this field who published their experiences and findings for all the world to share: A. M. (Toni) Harthoorn, Ulysses S. Seal, Jerry Haigh, Mitch Bush, Murray Fowler, Dave Jessup, E. Young, Hym Ebedes, U. de V. Pienaar, Michael Kock, Richard Burroughs, Marc Cattet, Nigel Caulkett, and Harry Jalanka.

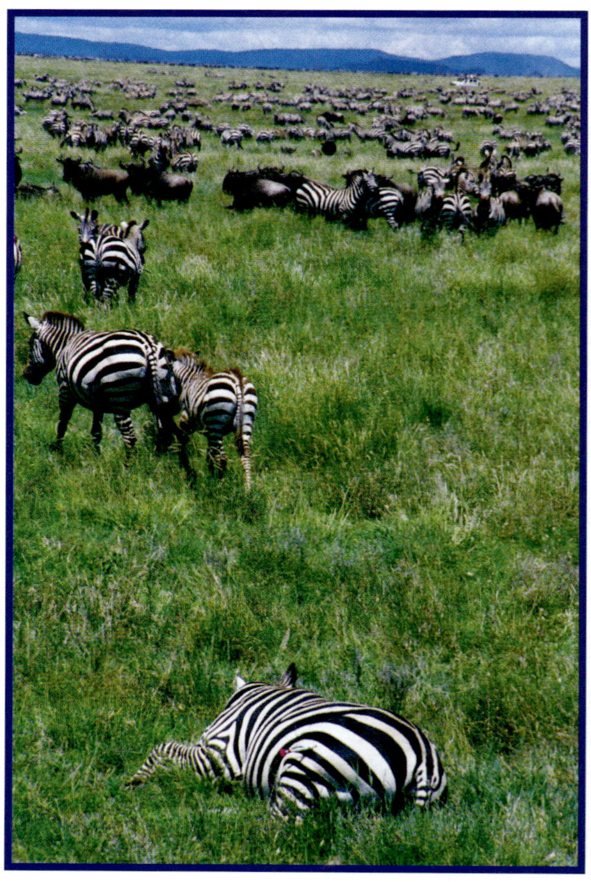

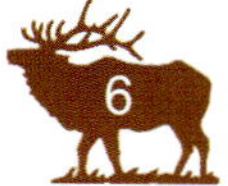

Preface

This is the third edition of the *Handbook of Wildlife Chemical Immobilization.* It is perhaps the largest selling book of its kind, having sold thousands of copies around the world. If the *Handbook* is truly a success, a lot of credit must be given Dr. Ulysses S. Seal who originally had the idea for a comprehensive, but easy-to-use, book for wildlife biologists faced with the challenge of animal capture. The second, or International, edition was published in 2002; five years on, it is time for another edition.

I have asked Dr. Jon Arnemo to join me again in this third effort. I consider Jon a contemporary of mine; one who has an academic as well as practical background in animal capture. Jon has had extensive experience throughout Europe and in Asia and Africa. Between us, we have immobilized literally thousands of animals and have published our works in dozens of scientific publications. Together, we hope to provide a global perspective of animal capture. We also thank Dr. Jacobus Raath for his contributions to the second edition that are retained herein and to Dr. Marno Walters, Artis Zoo Amsterdam, for his contributions to primate anesthesia.

This handbook is intended to provide wildlife biologists, wildlife and zoo veterinarians, game ranchers, animal control personnel, and students with a portable reference for the chemical capture of wild animals. The format is essentially unchanged from the first edition. A few have decried the "cookbook" approach of this format, but their concerns have been overwhelmed by literally hundreds of reports from satisfied readers. We will let this majority dictate the format of this book.

This handbook is designed to accompany the user into the field and should act as a rapid reference source for those faced with the challenge of chemically capturing a wild, and often uncooperative, animal. Its format is intentionally brief, serving to highlight, rather than detail, the salient aspects of each section. Those desiring a more in-depth discussion should seek out the relevant literature offered. Despite the emphasis on brevity, it behooves the novice to be familiar with everything covered in this text. Though designed for rapid access, familiarity with its contents beforehand is just common sense.

The *Drug Dosages* section is designed to rapidly locate the species of interest and select an appropriate immobilizing agent. Many other publications on drug dosages would list the species plus several different drugs, dosage ranges, and combinations - much to the anguish and confusion of the reader who, through inexperience, was overwhelmed to the point of inaction by the choices offered. This handbook should eliminate such quandaries.

We have compiled and analyzed drugs and dosages from published reports or private records and then made a single recommendation for a given species based on our, and others, experience with the drug and species. Other drug choices and appropriate references are also included should you not agree with, or not have available, the recommended drug(s). The primary recommendation does not necessarily mean that the chosen drug(s) is always the best choice under all circumstances. Experience with the various drugs will eventually allow you to make informed choices on your own.

Also included are sections on *Animal* and *Human Medical Treatment*. Again, these are intended to serve as quick reference sources to recognize and treat the most common emergency conditions encountered in the field, but not as a definitive treatise on emergency medicine. These sections have a quick reference guide at the beginning of each section.

In the *Equipment Used for Animal Capture* section, we were not reluctant to point out deficiencies or praise performance. Such praise, however, does not convey endorsement of the product.

Interspersed throughout this book is information that we consider either important to read or that might be a good idea. The important information will be annotated in the margins by the following symbol: (i). Things that we think are ideas which you might find useful are annotated with this symbol:

As always, we would appreciate any comments or criticisms of this handbook. This book was written for you, to make you a better wildlife professional. If it succeeds, then Jon and I have done our jobs.

Terry J. Kreeger, BS, BSVSc, MS, DVM, PhD
Sybille Canyon, Wyoming
January 2007

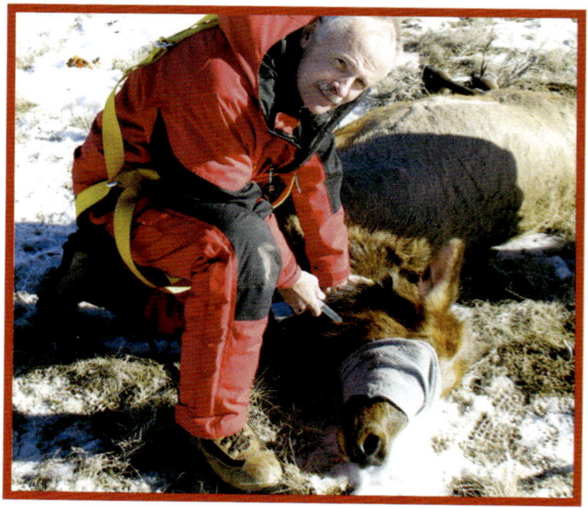

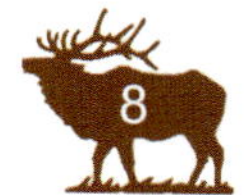

Drug Possession and Use

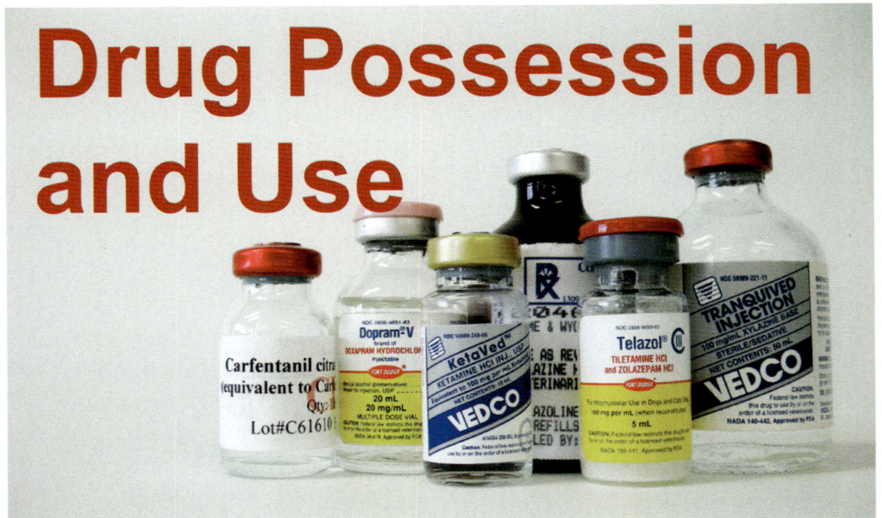

The legalities surrounding the purchase, storage, and dispensation of drugs used for wildlife immobilization vary from country to country. It is beyond the scope of this manual to detail each nation, but a general overview of North America, and Europe is presented below.

United States

Conditions for the use of drugs (pharmaceuticals) to sedate or anesthetize animals are established by the Food and Drug Administration (FDA). The FDA verifies the safety and efficacy of drugs as well as insures manufacturing quality control. Drug manufacturers must undergo a lengthy and expensive process of drug testing to receive FDA approval. Approval by the FDA, when granted, limits the use of the drug to conditions specified on the label, i.e., the intended species, the dosage, conditions of use, withdrawal times, and the like. Only four drugs have been specifically approved by the FDA for use on certain wild animals: carfentanil for use on cervids; xylazine for use on elk and fallow, mule, sika, and white-tailed deer; yohimbine for use on cervids (deer and elk); and ketamine for use on primates. Any use of these or other drugs on any species not identified on the label is termed "extra label" or "off label."

In addition to being prescription drugs, some of the drugs used for wildlife immobilization are termed *controlled* substances. A controlled substance means a drug that is identified in one of five schedules. Federal legislation governing the possession of controlled substances is contained in The Controlled Substances Act (1970). The Drug Enforcement Administration (DEA) is the U.S. federal agency charged with enforcing provisions of this act. Special regulations govern the recording and storage of these drugs. The Controlled Substances Act requires an

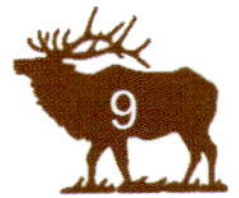

individual to have a special DEA registration number in order to possess controlled substances. Application for this number is made through regional offices of the DEA. If you are unable to determine your regional office, contact the United States Department of Justice, Drug Enforcement Administration, Washington, D.C. 20537 (http://www.deadiversion.usdoj.gov/drugreg/). Holders of professional medical degrees (D.V.M., M.D. etc.) should submit a DEA Form 224 to apply for a registration number. All others should submit a DEA Form 225. Renewal is required every three years. Following is a brief discussion of the five schedules:

Schedule I – This is reserved for experimental and abused drugs such as heroin, marijuana, and lysergic acid diethylamide (LSD). Use of Schedule I drugs requires a separate registration number. Application for Schedule I requires the same forms listed above, but the application should request registration only for Schedule I substances. Schedule I drugs are primarily limited to research use.

Schedule II (IIN) – This includes most of the opioids used for animal immobilization, such as etorphine, fentanyl, and carfentanil and the opioid antagonist, diprenorphine. Phencyclidine and some barbiturates are also in this schedule.

Schedule III (IIIN) – This contains several barbiturates, ketamine, and tiletamine/zolazepam.

Schedule IV – Includes benzodiazepine tranquilizers, such as diazepam and midazolam, and butorphanol.

Schedule V – This covers small, limited quantities of narcotic drugs included in preparations with non-narcotic active medicinal ingredients.

Many biologists have obtained a DEA registration number and have been able to procure drugs through veterinary product distributors. Technically, however, even though they are in *possession* of these drugs, they *cannot use* them on animals without veterinary supervision. Biologists who use veterinary prescription drugs *without the involvement of a licensed veterinarian* should know that they are in violation of federal regulations.

All drugs currently used for the chemical capture of wildlife are *prescription* drugs and must be used *by or on the order of a licensed veterinarian.* Non-veterinarians can legally use drugs if a valid *veterinarian/client/patient* relationship is established. That is, the biologist becomes the "client" and the wild animal becomes the "patient." The biologist consults with the veterinarian on the use of the drug who determines if the dose and application are appropriate. The veterinarian does *not* have to be on site during the immobilization process, but he or she should be involved in the planning process.

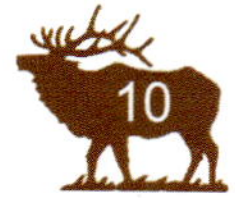

Animal Medicinal Drug Use Clarification Act of 1994

The Animal Medicinal Drug Use Clarification Act of 1994 (AMDUCA; passed into law in 1996) essentially allowed veterinarians to use approved animal and human drugs extra label under certain conditions. The AMDUCA makes a specific distinction between food and non-food animals. Therefore, you must consider the possibility of an animal being harvested and consumed by a human subsequent to your capturing it with drugs (see page 15). Below are listed criteria for extra label drug use in food and non-food animals. There are other restrictions for certain human drugs and drugs specifically prohibited for use in food-producing animals, but such drugs are usually not used for animal capture and will not be discussed here.

Extra label use of animal or human drugs is allowed in *non-food* animals if the drug is: 1) approved by the FDA; 2) used by or on the lawful written or oral order of a licensed veterinarian; and 3) used within the context of a valid veterinarian/client/patient relationship.

Extra label use of FDA-approved animal or human drugs is allowed in *food* animals if there is no approved animal drug labeled for such use or the approved drug is clinically ineffective for its intended use. Prior to extra label use of immobilizing drugs in food animals (e.g., deer, elk, bear, sheep, pronghorn, etc.), the veterinarian must: 1) establish a substantially extended withdrawal time (see pages 16-17); 2) be able to identify the treated animals; and 3) assure that assigned timeframes for withdrawal are met and no illegal residues occur.

To Summarize:

- Wildlife capture drugs can only be used by or on the order of a licensed veterinarian.
- Non-veterinarians can use prescription drugs if they have established a valid veterinarian-client-patient relationship.
- All capture drugs are prescription drugs, but not all of these are controlled drugs.
- The FDA governs the manufacture and use of drugs; the DEA governs the possession of controlled drugs.
- Approved drugs can be used "off label" as long as certain requirements are met.

Canada

An excellent and detailed discussion of drug acquision (Peacock, 2005) can be found in the second edition of *The Chemical Immobilization of Wildlife*, published by the Canadian Association of Zoo and Wildlife Veterinarians (http://www.cazwv.org/).

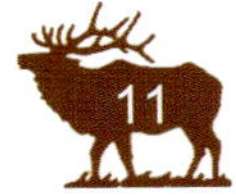

Europe

In most European countries, immobilizing agents are prescription drugs and must be used by or on the order of a licensed veterinarian. Some of these agents are also controlled drugs, i.e. drugs that are capable of being abused, for which specific regulations apply. Non-veterinarians can legally use immobilizing agents if a valid veterinarian/client/patient relationship is established; i.e., the veterinarian should ensure that the animal in question is under his/her care. In some countries, however, the veterinarian is required to be on site during the immobilization process.

Records

Although record requirements differ among countries, an inventory record should be maintained containing at least the following information:

Purchase Inventory:

Type of drug received (e.g., etorphine, carfentanil, etc.)
Amount received
Date received
From where drug received (i.e., manufacturer or distributor)

Use Inventory:

Amount used
Date used
Species used on
Reason for use

Many users of scheduled immobilizing drugs number each bottle and maintain a running inventory of the amount of drug used, opening a new bottle only when the previous bottle is empty. Drug use must be reconciled with drug received. That is, if you received 50 ml of etorphine, you must account for 50 ml used. Reasons for use include not only administration to animals, but also missed darts, accidental spillage, and intentional disposal of unused drug. Records in the U.S. must be maintained for two years and inventories should be taken biannually.

The AMDUCA also has specific record requirements for extra label drug use. The prescribing veterinarian is ultimately responsible for these records, although the end user should also maintain the same information. When drugs are used extra label, the following information should be recorded:

1) Name of drug and active ingredient
2) Condition treated (e.g., capture for translocation)
3) Dosage administered
4) Duration of treatment (usually not applicable for capture)
5) Number of animals treated
6) Specific withdrawal time (for food animals)

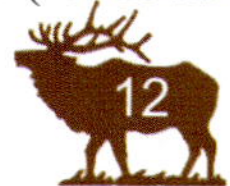

ANIMAL CAPTURE FORM

Date ____________________ Animal number ____________

Name of investigator(s)____

Species _________________________________ Sex (circle) M F UNK

Age ________________ mo yr (estimated or actual)

Weight ______________ lb kg (estimated or actual)

Purpose of capture ____

Location of capture ____

Ambient temperature ______ F° C° Weather conditions __________

Time	Drug	Dose (mg or ml)	Method	Location
_____	__________	____________	______	______
_____	__________	____________	______	______
_____	__________	____________	______	______
_____	__________	____________	______	______
_____	__________	____________	______	______

Time animal immobilized _________ Time animal recovered _______

Vital signs:	Time	Temperature	Pulse	Respiration
	________	_________	_________	_________
	________	_________	_________	_________
	________	_________	_________	_________

Condition of animal - indicate: excellent good fair poor

Injuries or abnormalities noted ________________________________

Sample(s) taken:	Time	Type (indicate blood, tissue, tooth, etc.)
	________	______________________________
	________	______________________________

Radio collar frequency ______________ Radio Signal Checked? ___

Transponder number ________________ Transponder Checked? ___

Ear tag number(s) and color(s) ________________________________

Other Measurements:

Body Length ____________ cm Tail Length ____________ cm

Shoulder Height _________ cm Girth _________________ cm

Comments:

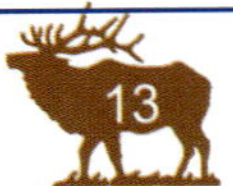

Records for individual animal captures are valuable for reviewing efficacy of the drugs and doses, for keeping track of samples, and for determining reasons for adverse reactions. Record format is as diverse as the individuals designing them; an example of a drug immobilization record is included on Page 13.

It is usually useful to have several blank spaces for drugs administered and vital signs so that you can maintain a running record of the drug and medical history. Below is an example of a record of an animal darted and then given additional drugs. Note that both ketamine and xylazine are listed as being given at 9:00 a.m. indicating that they were administered in the same dart. Also note that in the location column, you can indicate if the injection was IM, IV, or SC, if desired.

Time	Drug	Dose (mg or ml)	Method	Location
0900	Ketamine	400 mg	Dart	L. Hip
0900	Xylazine	100 mg	Dart	L. Hip
0910	Ketamine	200 mg	Pole	Shoulder
1000	Yohimbine	7 mg	Hand	Jugular, IV

Ordering and Storage

All Schedule II controlled substances must be ordered on a DEA form 222 which is preprinted by the DEA and issued to the holder of the DEA registration number. This form must be sent to the manufacturer or distributor. However, before any drug is shipped, the holder must have approved storage facilities for these drugs. Schedule II controlled substances, particularly etorphine and carfentanil, must be stored in a safe or steel cabinet equivalent to a U.S. Government Class 5 security container. This usually means a safe weighing more than 750 lb or a safe that is bolted to the floor with the bolts brazed in such a manner as to prevent tampering. The local DEA office must then physically inspect the storage container and send their recommendations for approval to the DEA in Washington. The DEA will then notify the manufacturer or distributor that the individual is approved. All other controlled substances must be stored in a secure place with limited access. Regulations regarding drug storage are contained in 21 CFR 1301.75d. If you have any questions regarding drug storage, contact your local DEA office or call the DEA Policy Unit in Washington, D.C. (202-307-7297).

Labeling

All approved drugs are labeled by the manufacturer and such labels should not be altered. It is a good idea, however, for lyophilized (freeze dried) drugs to indicate on the label the date on which the drug was reconstituted. Such drugs have a specified shelf life from the date of reconstitution. If for some reason, drugs are transferred to an unlabeled container, be sure to indicate on that container the name and the concentration of the drug as well as its expiration date which appeared on the original container. Never use drugs from an unlabeled container - if in doubt, throw it out!

It also may be advisable to write dosages with a permanent marker on emergency drugs, such as doxapram (a respiratory stimulant), so that valuable time is not lost in looking up the dosage.

Expiration Dates

It has long been presumed that a drug expiration date was the date determined by a drug manufacturer at which the drug retained at least 90% of its potency. This may not be correct. A retired FDA pharmacist said that "manufacturers put expiration dates on for marketing, rather than scientific, reasons" (Cohen, L. P. 2000. The Wall Street Journal, March 28). Although we cannot recommend using drugs after the expiration date, there is evidence that a many drugs remain 100% effective for many years after the expiration date.

According to the package insert, reconstituted Telazol® should be discarded after four days when stored at room temperature or after 14 days when kept refrigerated. Kreeger et al. (1990c), however, tested the shelf life of reconstituted Telazol® and found no clinical difference in wolves immobilized with fresh Telazol® compared to wolves immobilized with solutions stored at room temperature for 30 and 60 days, respectively.

Medetomidine (10 mg/ml), stored in the original packages at room temperature, was tested chemically and then clinically in several mammalian species five years after the expiration date and was found 100% effective (Arnemo, personal observation). Several other immoblizing drugs are probably also stable for years after the official expiration date. In 2006, a batch of etorphine hydrochloride (9.8 mg/ml), stored at room temperature for more than five years past expiration date, was used to immobilize 25 free-ranging moose from a helicopter. No difference in induction times or other clinical effects were seen in these animals compared to 50 moose immobilized with new drugs from the same manufacturer (Arnemo, personal observation). Similar observations have been made with carfentanil (Kreeger, personal observation).

We understand that one may be loathe to discard a vial of drugs which may have cost upwards of US$400 just because it has reached the expiration date. If you choose to use drugs past their expiration date, you may do so at some risk of liability. Animal immobilization is unpredictable and relatively uncontrolled. If an expired drug was used to immobilize an animal and a person was injured or property damaged during the immobilization process, you (or your employer) may be held financially responsible, *even though it was highly unlikely that the expired drug had anything to do with the damage*. You may wish to limit the use of any expired drugs for animals under controlled circumstances, such as captivity.

Human Consumption of Drugged Animals

A "withdrawal time" is a time established by the FDA that specifies the period of time that must expire from the date that a drug was administered to when the

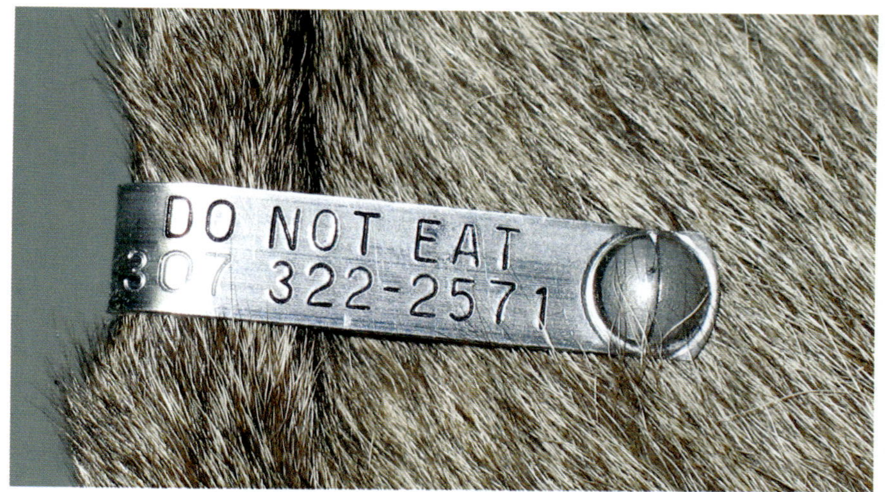

Ear tag advising hunter not to eat previously-drugged animal until contacting agency to determine safety. When contacted, the agency will determine if the withdrawal time has been met.

animal can safely be consumed by humans. In the U.S., many of the animals chemically captured are food-producing animals (e.g., deer, bear) and many are captured just before or during their hunting seasons. Also, many of the animals are captured using drugs extra label (Craigmill et al., 1997).

The FDA has concerns that drug residues may remain in animal tissues, be consumed by humans, and result in an adverse reaction. Thus, the AMDUCA emphasizes the need for establishing withdrawal times for animals that could be consumed by humans. Unfortunately, there are few scientifically-established tissue residue studies (which are used to establish withdrawal times) for any of the drugs used in the U.S. The prescribing veterinarian must therefore use whatever information is available and apply it in a conservative manner to the extra label application. For example, tissue residue studies for ketamine may exist for a certain species of primate. These data may serve as a basis for the withdrawal time for ketamine used in deer.

Semple et al. (2000) published a pharmacokinetic and tissue residue study of Telazol® in polar bears. The authors concluded that it was unlikely that a human consuming polar bear meat from an animal killed more than 24 hours after darting would experience a pharmacological effect from either tiletamine or zolazepam.

For other guidance, we have listed the withdrawal times below for certain drugs used in a theoretical 70-kg deer as established by the Food Animal Residue Avoidance Database (FARAD). When in doubt, a conservative withdrawal time of *at least 30-45 days* should be sufficient for other drugs and other species. You can contact the FARAD "hot line" if you have questions on withdrawal times (888-873-2723) or via the internet (http://www.farad.org/).

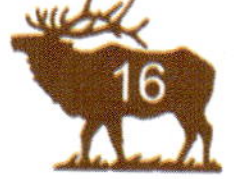

Drug	Dosage	Withdrawal Time (days)
Carfentanil	0.026-0.086 mg/kg	45
Ketamine	5 mg/kg	3
Xylazine	2 mg/kg	10-30[a]
Yohimbine	0.2-0.3 mg/kg	30[a]
Penicillin (procaine G)	30,000 IU/kg	21

[a]FARAD recommends that these drugs not be used in free-ranging cervids within 30 days of hunting season.

Potential food animals should be identified in some manner (ear tag, collar) if there is a possibility that the animal could be killed during the withdrawal period and subsequently eaten by a hunter. This identification probably will have to either: 1) warn the hunter not to consume the meat if harvested before a certain date, or 2) require the hunter to notify the appropriate wildlife management agency who will then determine if the animal can be safely eaten.

Europe

According to the current legislation in force in the European Union (EU), any substance to be used in food producing animals has to be assessed by the European Medicines Evaluation Agency (EMEA) in order to establish Maximum Residue Limits (MRLs). After assessment, substances may be listed in one of four Annexes of Council Regulation (EEC) No 2377/90 of 26 June 1990: Annex I – substances for which a full MRL has been made; Annex II – substances for which an MRL is not required; Annex III – substances for which a provisional MRL has been made; Annex IV – substances for which no MRL can be made. If the animal is a "food producing animal" (i.e. an animal, domestic or wild, captive or free-living, whose flesh or products are intended for human consumption), the veterinarian or the person acting under his/her direction may *only* administer a substance listed in Annex I, II, or III. Substances in Annex IV or substances that do not have an Annex entry (I, II, or III) may *not* be used in food producing animals. As of October 2006, very few of the drugs currently used for wildlife immobilization are authorized for use in food producing animals.

In the EU, a withdrawal period is set during the procedure for granting a marketing authorization, i.e. either by the national authority concerned or, in case of a centrally authorized product, by the EMEA. However, for substances that do not have an Annex entry, no marketing authorization can be granted for use in food producing animals. Further information on MRLs may be found on the EMEA website: http://www.emea.eu.int/

Questions regarding the use of drugs in food producing animals in an EU country should be directed to: EMEA, 7 Westferry Circus, Canary Wharf, London E14 4HB, UK; e-mail: mail@emea.eudra.org; phone: + 44 20 74188400; fax: + 44 74188416.

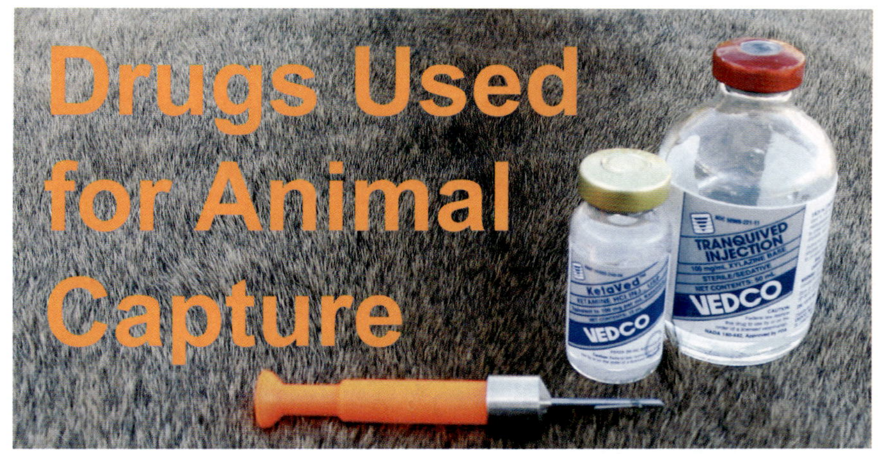

Drugs Used for Animal Capture

Obviously, no perfect capture drug exists; if it did, there would be little need for this book. However, the characteristics of an ideal injectable anesthetic may serve as guide to the evaluation of currently available immobilizing drugs for wildlife. These criteria include both physical and pharmacological properties as well as desirable properties for an immobilizing agent. Many drugs currently in use have several, but not all, of these characteristics. These criteria are as follows with no specific priority implied:

- High therapeutic index (the ratio of the lethal dose in half of the sample to the effective dose in half of the sample)
- Potent (sufficient dose delivered in small volume)
- Fast-acting, smooth onset of action
- Minimum excitement phase (anesthetic induction is rapid)
- Nonirritating following intravenous or intramuscular administration
- Good muscle relaxation
- Minimal depression of cardiovascular or respiratory systems
- Analgesia at subanesthetic levels
- Retention of reflexes, i.e., swallowing
- Causes minimal fear, pain, or distress
- Capable of being antagonized, preferably dose-dependent antagonism
- Rapid, smooth emergence (short elimination half-life) with minimal side effects
- Rapid degradation to inactive, nontoxic metabolites
- Highly water-soluble, stable in solution, and long shelf-life
- Produces an amnestic effect (animal has little or no recollection of event)
- Safe for pregnant animals
- Compatible with other drugs in mixtures
- Compatible with dart material (i.e., no chemical reactions with dart)
- Minimum withdrawal time for safe human/animal consumption
- Low toxicity in humans should accidental exposure occur
- Low potential for human abuse

Calculating Drug Doses

Accurate calculation of drug doses is critical to reduce the problems associated with under- or overdosing. A *dose* is the total amount of drug given an animal; *dosage* is the amount of drug on a per weight basis (e.g., mg/kg). Information required prior to calculating a dose includes:

Animal's Weight

If you lack experience with the average weights by age class of your particular species (male, female, juvenile), either contact someone who has experience or use the information included in this manual on the specific species. Try to train yourself to think of weights in metric units because this is standard scientific notation and it is the measurement system used by most countries. Conversion tables of pounds-to-kilograms are presented in the back of this book (page 418). These tables provide a quick conversion of pounds to kilograms without having to use a calculator.

Concentration of the Drug

Most manufacturers provide concentrations of their products in milligram (mg) of drug per milliliter (ml) of solvent (mg/ml). Some concentrations are expressed as percents, i.e., a "10%" solution. A 100% solution means that there is 1 gram (1 gm = 1,000 mg) of drug dissolved in 1 ml of solvent. Therefore, a 10% solution means that there is 100 mg (0.10 x 1,000 mg) of drug in 1 ml of solvent (i.e., 100 mg/ml).

Some drugs are freeze-dried (lyophilized) and you may only have the weight of the dried preparation. To prepare a solution of known concentration you must calculate backwards from the desired solution to arrive at the volume of solvent to add to the powdered drug. That is, if a drug bottle contains 500 mg of drug and you desire a 100 mg/ml solution, you must add 5 ml of solvent to the bottle.

$$\text{Desired Concentration} = 100 \text{ mg/ml} = \frac{500 \text{ mg drug}}{? \text{ ml of solvent}}$$

$$? \text{ ml of solvent} = \frac{500 \text{ mg drug}}{100 \text{ mg/ml}} = 5 \text{ ml solvent needed}$$

The actual concentration of this dilution, however, will be *less* than 100 mg/ml because the volume of the lyophilized drug is not taken into consideration in the total solution volume. For example, if the lyophilized drug volume was 0.3 cubic centimeters (roughly 0.3 ml), then the total volume in the bottle after adding 5 ml of solvent would be around 5.3 ml (actually somewhat less considering chemical reactions). Thus the *actual* concentration is 94.3 mg/ml (500/5.3). Unfortunately, this error is common in drug formulations and recommended drug doses, although its continued use does maintain consistency if not accuracy.

Dose

Again, the *dose* is the total amount of drug given to an animal. It is derived by multiplying the *dosage* by the animal's weight. In this manual, dosages are mostly given as mg of drug per kilogram (kg) of animal body weight (mg/kg). To convert kg to pounds (lb), multiply kg by 2.2 (e.g., 10 kg = 22 lb). Conversely, to convert lb to kg, multiply lb by 0.45 (e.g., 100 lb = 45 kg). Again, conversion tables of pounds-to-kilograms are presented in the back of this book. Armed with the above data, you can now calculate how much (usually expressed in ml or volume) of a given drug to administer.

Calculating Drug Doses and Volumes

Ultimately, you want to know what volume of drug to administer to the animal. The formula for this is:

$$\text{Volume of Drug Administered} = \frac{\text{Body Weight x Dosage}}{\text{Drug Concentration}}$$

Consider immobilizing an animal that weighs 80 kg (176 lb) with Drug "X". The recommended dosage of Drug X for this animal is 5 mg/kg. Drug X is available in a 100 mg/ml solution. First, calculate the *total mg* (i.e., the *dose*) needed for this animal by multiplying the animal's weight (80 kg) by the recommended drug dosage (5 mg/kg):

mg Drug X needed = 80 kg x 5 mg/kg = 400 mg

Then calculate the *volume* of drug solution to withdraw from the bottle by dividing the dose (i.e., 400 mg) by its concentration (100 mg/ml):

$$\text{ml volume needed} = \frac{\text{400 mg}}{\text{100 mg/ml}} = \text{4 ml of drug solution}$$

Some Points to Remember in Calculating Drug Doses

Never memorize drug dosages.

This is one of the cardinal rules of pharmacology and one we all probably break at one time or another. However, we also all make a mistake at one time or another. It's incredibly easy to mix up dosages when you are in a hurry or otherwise pressured. Also, time has a way of eroding memory, so don't trust it.

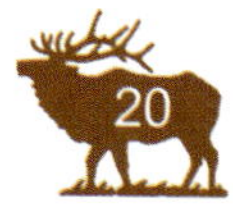

Physically calculate drug doses.

Unless you continually perform mental calculations, take time to use a calculator or paper and pencil to correctly figure doses and volumes.

Calculate the dose at least twice.

Regardless of the method of calculation, it is always a good idea to double check your math.

Look at your answer.

After you have calculated the volume twice, does it seem appropriate for the situation? With drug and animal experience, a drug volume that is miscalculated should trigger a mental alarm.

Drug Combinations

Although drugs are discussed by group or class in this section, they are often employed in combination for wildlife immobilization. "Immobilization" was a term that referred to some of the earliest drugs used to capture animals. These drugs were paralyzing drugs, like nicotine sulfate and succinylcholine. Such drugs, while rendering the animal immobile, did not render the animal unconscious. Today, many drugs used to capture animals are injectable anesthetics. An anesthetic is a drug that causes loss of conciousness. However, some of the most potent drugs that we use today (e.g., opioids) can't really be called anesthetics because they don't appear to render an animal totally unconscious. They seem to be somewhere between an anesthetic and a paralytic, but we will classify opioids as anesthetics for simplicity.

A quick review of the *Dosages* section would reveal that many doses are combinations of two drugs: an anesthetic and a tranquilizer. In most cases the primary anesthetic (e.g., ketamine, carfentanil, etorphine) is sufficient to induce anesthesia on its own. Tranquilizers are often combined with these primary anesthetics because they usually result in improved anesthesia. By themselves, tranquilizers only cause sedation. Such sedation may be profound to the point that the animal may be safely handled (e.g., deer given only xylazine). However, if sufficiently stimulated, a tranquilized animal can arouse and flee (or attack!).

Some common examples of anesthetics/tranquilizers include: ketamine/acepromazine, ketamine/xylazine, ketamine/medetomidine, etorphine/acepromazine, etorphine/xylazine, carfentanil/xylazine, tiletamine/zolazepam, and tiletamine/zolazepam/xylazine.

Advantages of combining drugs include:

- Reduction of doses of all drugs (often reducing total cost of drugs)
- Reduction of total drug volume (thus, smaller darts)
- Reduction of undesirable side effects (convulsions, muscle rigidity, etc.)

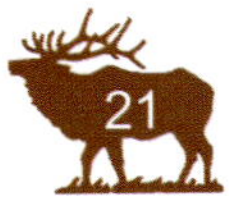

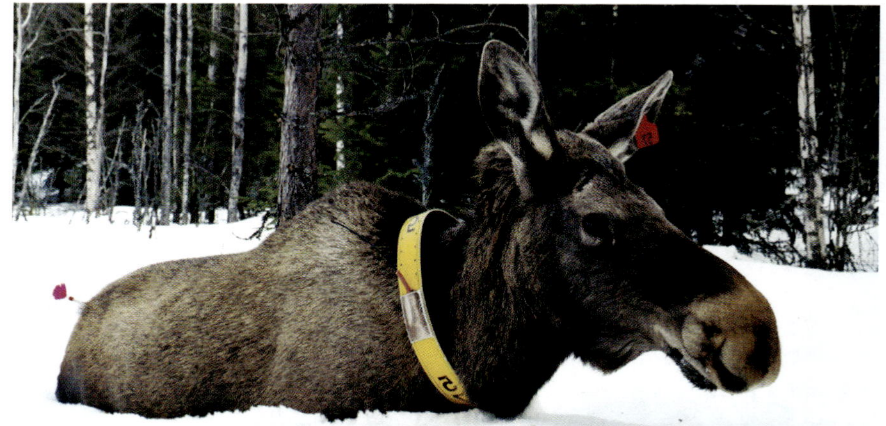

Although it usually advisable to combine tranquilizers with anesthetics, this is contraindicated in moose (Alces alces) *which should not be given a tranquilizer when anesthetized with carfentanil, thiafentanil, or etorphine. The addition of a tranquilizer increases the probability of pneumonia because moose have an increased tendency to roll over and aspirate rumen contents (Kreeger, 2000). Moose given just carfentanil, thiafentanil, or etorphine remain sternal with head upright.*

- Decreased induction time
- Improved recovery (less stumbling, incoordination)

Disadvantages of combining drugs include:

- Difficulty in assessing individual drug effect
- Increased complexity in calculating initial drug doses
- Confusion of appropriate doses if initial combination was insufficient for anesthesia
- Prolonged recovery with some combinations
- Potentiation of adverse effects (e.g., respiratory depression)

Following is a discussion of the properties of paralytics, tranquilizers, anesthetics, and other drugs used for the chemical capture of animals.

Neuromuscular Blocking Drugs

Curare, the South American arrow poison, probably typifies this class of drugs. The neuromuscular blocking (NMB) drugs are some of the first drugs used for the chemical immobilization of wildlife and their use in human clinical situations probably dates back to the 1930's. There are three classes of NMB drugs, which are distinguished by their electrophysiological properties: (1) depolarizing, (2) competitive (or nondepolarizing), and (3) ganglionic.

Depolarizing NMB drugs act by depolarizing postsynaptic membrane receptors, thus mimicking acetylcholine, but with a longer period of activity. Immobiliza-

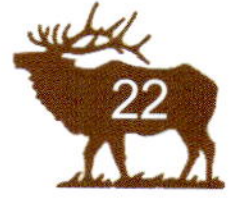

tion with depolarizing NMB drugs is characterized by an initial transient rapid firing of the muscles (muscle fasiculations), which is quickly replaced by general paralysis. The order of paralysis is sequential, starting from the jaw, tail, and face, followed by legs and neck, throat, abdomen, intercostal muscles, and diaphragm. Recovery is in the reverse order.

Competitive NMB drugs occupy postsynaptic cholinergic receptors in skeletal muscle thus preventing their occupancy by the endogenous neurotransmitter, acetylcholine, and they result in flaccid paralysis. The effects of competitive NMB drugs can be antagonized by anticholinesterase drugs which inhibit the enzymatic action of cholinesterase resulting in increased levels of acetylcholine. Acetylcholine has a stronger affinity for the receptor than the NMB drug, thus causing diffusion and diminished rebinding of the NMB drug. Because the antagonist activity of anticholinesterase drugs does not specifically neutralize the NMB drug, the effect of the anticholinesterase drugs may be dissipated before complete elimination or metabolism of the NMB drugs resulting in recycling and renewed paralysis. Also, overdosing resulting in death is possible with anticholinesterase drugs.

Ganglionic NMB drugs exhibit their primary effects via autonomic ganglia stimulation. Nicotine sulfate is the only drug in this class and it was one of the earliest drugs used for wildlife immobilization. Nicotine is a potent ganglionic and central nervous system (CNS) stimulant, the actions of which are mediated by nicotine-specific receptors. Small doses of nicotine cause stimulation of autonomic ganglia; large doses result in blockade of neurotransmission. Because of its low therapeutic index, high animal mortality, and high human toxicity, nicotine is no longer available for animal capture. Nicotine sulfate (Cap-Chur-Sol®), however, is still being found in some old drug kits. Nicotine sulfate should never be used under any circumstances.

Despite their long history of use, NMB drugs are generally inferior to modern drugs. There are two major deficiencies of NMB drugs. One is that NMB drugs have very low therapeutic indices and dosage errors of only 10% can result in either no effect or death (IWVS, 1992). Overdosing results in diaphragmatic paralysis and death by asphyxia. Mortality rates as high as 70% have occurred. The second deficiency is that depolarizing and competitive NMB drugs are virtually devoid of CNS effects because of their inability to cross the blood-brain barrier. Thus, an animal paralyzed with NMB drugs is conscious, aware of its surroundings, fully sensory, and, as such, can feel pain and experience psychogenic stress yet is physically unable to react. Because of these deficiencies, NMB drugs should be used judiciously.

There are, however, certain definite advantages to a few NMB drugs. They are generally very fast-acting (3–5 min) and the duration of effect lasts only for a short while (15–30 min). Succinycholine, the most commonly used drug of this

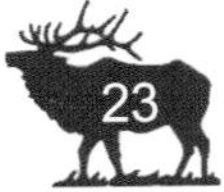

class, is also fairly safe for humans. Unlike some other drugs, the succinycholine dose required to immobilize most animals is much lower than the clinically effective dose for humans. Also, animals that have been given only succinycholine and that have died or been euthanized using physical means (i.e., not other drugs) can be safely eaten by other animals or, in some countries, by humans. Although deer have been intentionally killed with arrows tipped with succinylcholine and then eaten by humans, it must be remembered that succinylcholine has not been approved by the FDA for use on any animal, let alone animals intended for human consumption. And lastly, succinycholine is extraordinarily cheap, perhaps the least expensive immobilizing agent available. This might explain why it is still in widespread use.

Succinylcholine/Suxamethonium

Mechanism of Action: Depolarizing neuromuscular blocking agent.

Elimination: Hydrolyzed by pseudocholinesterases in liver and plasma to succinylmonocholine which is broken down into succinate and choline.

Routes of Administration: IM, IV, IP.

Advantages: Usually rapid induction (3–5 min).

- Usually rapid recovery (15–30 min).
- Low human toxicity at dosages normally used.
- Inexpensive.
- Can be highly concentrated, if needed.

Disadvantages: No effect on consciousness, pain threshold, or cerebration.

- Low therapeutic index requires precise weight estimation; overdose leads to respiratory paralysis and death.
- Can cause bradycardia, tachycardia, or cardiac arrest (due to exacerbation of hyperkalemia in animals having extensive tissue damage or being overly exerted).
- Can cause muscle soreness upon recovery probably caused by potassium release.
- Can release histamine resulting in bronchospasm, hypotension, salivation, and bronchial secretion.
- Can alter packed cell volume, total plasma protein, glucose, aspartate aminotransferase, cortisol, and progestin values.
- Prolonged muscle relaxation can cause hypothermia in small animals.
- Can cause malignant hyperthermia in some species.

Antagonists: None; anticholinesterases will actually prolong effect of depolarizing drugs.

Formulation: 20, 50, or 100 mg/ml solution; 500 and 1,000 mg sterile powder. Keep refrigerated.

Comments: Not controlled substances. Use of succinylcholine is probably best limited to captive situations where problems can be quickly addressed. In white-tailed deer and perhaps other species, the effective dose of succinylcholine can vary with time of year (Jacobsen et al., 1976).

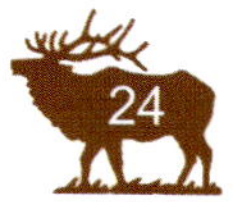

Gallamine, Tubocurarine, Metocurine, Pancuronium, Vecuronium, Atracurium, Alcuronium

Mechanism of Action: Competitive neuromuscular blocking agents.

Elimination: Gallamine, tubocurarine, and metocurine are excreted in urine virtually unchanged; pancuronium, atracurium, and vecuronium undergo various degrees of metabolism. Vecuronium is metabolized the most and thus has the shortest duration of action.

Routes of Administration: IM.

Advantages: Effective immobilization of crocodilians, particularly gallamine.

- Can be antagonized.

Disadvantages: No effect on consciousness, pain threshold, or cerebration.

- Low therapeutic index requires precise weight estimation; overdose leads to respiratory paralysis and death.
- Tubocurarine can release histamine resulting in hypotension, bronchospasm, and secretions.
- Gallamine can cause tachycardia and hypertension because of selective blocking of the cardiac vagus nerve.

Antagonists: Physostigmine, neostigmine, edrophonium, pyridostigmine.

Formulation: Tubocurarine: 3 mg/ml solution.

- Metacurine: 2 mg/ml solution.
- Gallamine: 20 mg/ml solution.
- Pancuronium: 1-2 mg/ml solution.
- Vecuronium: 10 mg vials.
- Atracurium: 10 mg/ml solution.
- Alcuronium: 5 mg/ml solution.

Comments: Not controlled substances. The same caveats for succinylcholine apply to competitive NMB drugs. Competitive NMB drugs should not be used in conjunction with opioids, corticosteroids, inhalation anesthetics, aminoglycoside antibiotics, tetracycline, polymixins A and B, clindamycin, or lincomycin due to significant interactions.

Nicotine

Mechanism of Action: Depolarizing muscle relaxant acting primarily on the autonomic ganglia as opposed to the myoneural junction.

Elimination: Metabolized in the liver, kidney, and lung and excreted by the kidneys.

Routes of Administration: Primarily IM, but nicotine can be absorbed through the skin or mucous membranes (eyes, mouth).

Advantages: None.

Disadvantages: Doses used to immobilize animals are sufficient to *kill* humans should accidental absorption occur.

- Low therapeutic index requires precise weight estimation.
- Nicotine can cause complex and unpredictable physiological reactions including bradycardia, tachycardia, hypertension, convulsions, vomiting, tachypnea.

Antagonists: None.
Comments: Not controlled substance. Immobilization is characterized by an initial transient stimulation followed by a persistent depression of all the autonomic ganglia. This stimulatory phase can be obscured by paralysis, which rapidly develops at the myoneural junction. Although rarely seen today, nicotine should not be used under any circumstances for animal immobilization. It is potentially lethal to both humans and animals and there are many superior drugs readily available.

Tranquilizers and Sedatives

Tranquilizers and sedatives are used primarily in wildlife immobilization as adjuncts to primary anesthetics (opioids, cyclohexanes) to hasten and smooth induction and recovery and to reduce the amount of the primary agent required to achieve anesthesia.

Tranquilizers relieve anxiety with minimal sedation; sedatives relieve anxiety making it easier for the animal to rest or sleep. The differences between tranquilizers and sedatives are not terribly important for your needs. Drugs such as droperidol, fluanison, and zolazepam will be discussed elsewhere as they are generally used only in conjunction with other agents.

Phenothiazines/Butyrophenones

Phenothiazines (promazine, acepromazine) are antipsychotic drugs, formally classified as neuroleptics. They reduce psychomotor agitation, curiosity, and apparent aggressiveness by blocking dopamine-mediated responses in the central bnervous system (Hall et al., 2001). Azaperone is a butyrophenone which has been reported to stimulate respiration in pigs and to counteract narcotic respiratory depression in wild animals (Marsboom, 1969).

Benzodiazepines

Benzodiazepine derivatives are used primarily in wildlife immobilization as an anticonvulsant adjunct to the cyclohexane anesthetics and they are also excellent muscle relaxants. Benzodiazepine antagonists have been developed that could reduce recovery times.

Alpha$_2$ -Adrenoceptor Agonists

The alpha$_2$ adrenoceptor agonists are potent sedatives and can be completely antagonized. They are usually used as adjuncts with opioids or cyclohexanes to hasten and smooth anesthetic induction. By themselves, they are capable of heavily sedating animals, particularly ungulates, to the point of relatively safe handling. However, animals sedated with alpha$_2$-adrenergic agonists generally can be aroused with stimulation and are capable of directed attack. Caution should always be exercised in such animals even though they appear harmless.

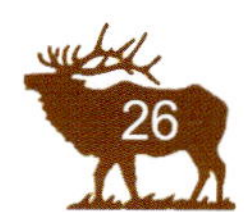

Phenothiazines

Acepromazine, Promazine, Chlopromazine, Propionylpromazine, Methotrimeprazine, Promethazine

Mechanism of Action: Antagonize the neurotransmitter, dopamine, in the basal ganglia and limbic portions of the forebrain.

Elimination: Hepatic oxidation and glucuronic acid conjugation with renal excretion.

Routes of Administration: IM, IV, SC, PO.

Advantages: Smooth anesthetic induction and recovery.

- Potentiates analgesic and anesthetic properties of other drugs.
- Antiemetic (decreases vomiting).
- Protects against adrenaline-induced cardiac fibrillation
- Relatively safe drugs (high therapeutic index).

Disadvantages: Can cause hypotension with reflex tachycardia.

- Can potentiate respiratory and cardiovascular depressant effects of opioids.
- Can cause a precipitous, or even fatal, fall in arterial blood pressure in shocked or hypovolemic animals.
- Can cause hypothermia due to heat loss through dilated cutaneous vessels.
- Can cause temporary or permanent penile prolapse or priapism in horses.
- Can increase glucose levels, increase prolactin secretion, decrease adrenocorticotropin and corticoid secretion, and decrease urinary concentrations of gonadotropins, estrogen, and progesterone.
- Can block ovulation, suppress estrus, and cause infertility.

Antagonists: None.

Formulation: Promazine: 50 mg/ml solution.

- Acepromazine: 10 mg/ml solution or 5, 10, 25 mg tablets.
- Chlorpromazine: 25 mg/ml solution; 10, 25, 50, 100, 200 mg tablets

Comments: Not controlled substances. Acepromazine is more potent than promazine, but promazine has a markedly reduced duration of effect. Clinical effects of acepromazine can last from 4–8 hr and up to 48 hr in older animals.

Butyrophenones

Azaperone

Mechanism of Action: Blocks postsynaptic mesolimbic dopaminergic D_1 and D_2 receptors in the brain; exhibit strong alpha-adrenergic blocking and anticholinergic effect.

Elimination: Hepatic oxidation and glucuronic acid conjugation with renal excretion.

Routes of Administration: IM, IV, SC.

Advantages: Smooth anesthetic induction and recovery.

- May increase respiration.
- Minimal cardiovascular and thermoregulatory effects.
- Relatively safe drug (high therapeutic index).
- Short acting.

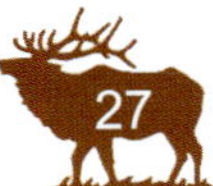

Disadvantages: Could cause excitement in horses at low doses.

- Causes drop in blood pressure upon administration.
- Inhibits ejaculation (do not use for semen collection procedures).

Antagonists: None.
Formulation: 40 mg/ml solution.
Comments: Not controlled substance. May be unavailable in U.S.

Benzodiazepines

Diazepam, Midazolam, Brotizolam, Climazolam

Mechanism of Action: Potentiate inhibitory effects of gamma-aminobutyric acid (GABA) neurotransmitter.
Elimination: Hepatic oxidation and glucuronide conjugation with excretion in urine and feces.
Routes of Administration: IM, IV, SC, PO.
Advantages: Good muscle relaxant.

- Anticonvulsant; particularly useful in decreasing cyclohexane-induced convulsions.
- Minimal respiratory and cardiovascular effects (but see comments).
- Produce retrograde amnesia
- Very safe agents.

Disadvantages: Diazepam is not rapidly absorbed IM.

- Low potency; generally require large volumes when used in combination with immobilizing agents.

Antagonists: Flumazenil (Romazicon®, Anexate®); sarmazenil (Sarmsol®).
Formulation: 5 mg/ml solution; 2, 5, 10 mg tablets.
Comments: Controlled substances (Schedule IV). Diazepam is solubilized in 40% propylene glycol which may produce hypotension, bradycardia, apnea, and cardiac arrest if injected too rapidly IV. Midazolam is in an aqueous base and 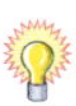 does not cause these cardiovascular reactions. All the benzodiazepines can potentially stimulate appetite and be used to "force" animals to eat novel foods or to induce sick animals to eat (Kreeger et al., 1991; Hall et al., 2001).

Alpha-Adrenoceptor Agonists

Xylazine, Romifidine, Detomidine, Medetomidine

Mechanism of Action: Act on pre- and postsynaptic $alpha_2$-adrenergic receptors in central and peripheral nervous system to inhibit release of norepinephrine.
Elimination: Metabolized in the liver and excreted in urine.
Routes of Administration: IM, IV, SC.
Advantages: Potent sedation.

- Good muscle relaxation.
- Analgesic.
- Can be completely antagonized.
- Compatible with and potentiates other immobilizing agents.

Disadvantages: Respiratory depressants, particularly when used with other

drugs having similar properties.

- Cause hypotension and bradycardia.
- Prolonged effect if not antagonized.
- Can cause ataxia if not antagonized in some species (e.g., pronghorn).
- Cause hyperglycemia and glucosuria (probably not clinically significant).
- Disrupts thermoregulatory capabilities.
- Causes vomiting in canids and felids.
- Decreases gastrointestinal motility, particularly in ruminants.
- Xylazine may cause abortion in late pregnancy

Antagonists: Yohimbine, tolazoline, idazoxan, atipamezole.

Formulation: Xylazine: 20, 100, 300 mg/ml solution; 500 mg powder. Can be lyophylized and reconstituted up to 500 mg/ml (concentrations >250 mg/ml may be difficult to maintain in solution).

- Detomidine: 10 mg/ml solution.
- Medetomidine: 1, 10, 20 mg/ml solution.
- Romifidine: 10 mg/ml solution.

Comments: Not controlled substances. Immobilization or sedation of highly excited animals using alpha-adrenergic agonists alone will be prolonged, if not impossible (Jacobsen, 1983). If a sedated animal is aroused, eliminating the stimulation will usually result in resedation and/or recumbency. Detomidine and medetomidine are much more potent than xylazine and more selective for specific $alpha_2$-adrenergic receptors. The difference in potency between the four $alpha_2$-adrenergic agonists is species dependent and no studies have been done on wildlife. In sheep, the equipotent sedative doses for xylazine, romifidine, detomidine, and medetomidine are 0.15 mg/kg, 0.05 mg/kg, 0.03 mg/kg, and 0.01 mg/kg, respectively (Celly et al., 1997).

Long-acting Tranquilizers

Long-acting tranquilizers (LATs) are used in the transport and holding of wild animals to calm them and reduce aggression. Although used extensively in southern Africa, LATs are generally not available in North America. Readers interested in LATs are referred to Ebedes, 1991; 1992a; 1993; Ebedes and Burroughs, 1992; Holz and Barnett, 1996. See the *Drug Dosages* section for LAT doses and comments as they pertain to individual species.

Long-acting tranquilizers were developed to calm animals subjected to prolonged translocations, new surroundings such as holding pens and quarantine pens, or unnatural activities such as game auctions or experimental projects. Long-acting tranquilizers reduced or eliminated stress, injuries, and mortalities seen when wild animals were forced into these situations. Long-acting tranquilizers relieve anxiety, moderate excitement, and reduce motor activity. They should be administered as soon as possible after capture. Long-acting tranquilizers are formulated so that a single dose gives a therapeutically effective tissue concentration for at least 7 days, but they have a delayed onset of action.

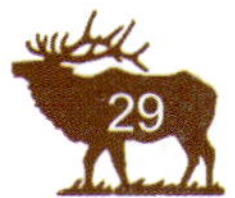

Long-acting tranquilizers consist of fatty acid esters of a basic tranquilizer, which have been dissolved in vegetable or medicinal oils. The prolonged activity derives from the slow release of the esters as they diffuse from the solvent into the tissue fluid and are absorbed into the blood. During this process, the basic tranquilizer molecule is released. The storage depot of the LAT is at the injection site. The duration of effect appears to be dose dependent, but the dose rate seems to be more related to the anxiety level or age of the animal than to body mass.

Administration

Long-acting tranquilizers are always administered in combination with short- and/or intermediate-acting tranquilizers. This insures a constant tranquilization of the animal, because the effect of the short-acting tranquilizer wears off, then the intermediate tranquilizer takes over, and its effect is supplemented and taken over by the LAT.

All animals mixed from different family groups and confined together should be tranquilized, except for aggressive males, which should be confined on their own. When family groups are housed together, it is only necessary to tranquilize the adults, which have a calming effect on the young. It may be necessary to tranquilize young if they become excited or separated from their mothers. Adult and subadult males kept together should all be tranquilized. Individuals, even subadults, which are not tranquilized may become hostile and aggressive and will injure tranquilized animals. All animals at live auctions should be tranquilized. Very young and old animals may react unpredictably to tranquilizers. Long-acting tranquilizers are always given IM and can be added to short-acting tranquilizers in the same syringe, even if they are incompatible and do not mix well.

Adverse Effects

Tranquilizers must always be used with discretion. Overdosing must be avoided because side effects such as deep sedation and extrapyramidal symptoms interfere with feeding and physiological and defensive activities. These side effects are very similar to those seen in humans given these drugs and include dyskinesia with dystonic reactions, such as torticollis, scoliosis, lordosis, opisthotonos, and tardive dyskinesia with uncontrolled movements of the tongue jaw and mouth. This has been seen in red hartebeest, blesbok, springbok, zebra, and buffalo given haloperidol. Catatonia, muscle rigidity, and mental stupor has been seen in red hartebeest, springbok, tsessebe, blesbok, and elephant with haloperidol and in roan antelope and defassa waterbuck with zuclopenthixol. Loss of appetite (anorexia) has been experienced in impala with perphenazine enanthate and kudu with haloperidol decanoate.

Haloperidol

Mechanism of Action: Blocks postsynaptic mesolimbic dopaminergic D_1 and D_2 receptors in the brain; exhibit strong alpha-adrenergic blocking and anticholinergic effect.

Elimination: Hepatic oxidation, conjugation, and renal excretion.
Routes of Administration: IV, IM.
Advantages: Sedation is significant in 15 minutes after IM injection and lasts up to 18 hours depending on the species.

- IV injection results in immediate tranquilization.
- Excellent in smaller game (up to red hartebeest size) as well as in elephants.

Disadvantages: Extrapyramidal symptoms may occur with overdosing.
Antagonists: None.
Formulation: 5, 20, 50, 100 mg/ml.
Comments: Used alone or in combination with longer acting tranquilizers. Extrapyramidal symptoms can be treated with 10-20 mg biperidin (Akineton®), dexetimide (Tremblex®), 5 mg diazepam, or xylazine.

Zuclopenthixol

Mechanism of Action: Enzymatic reactions release the active component zuclopenthixol, which results in an unspecific, transient, dose dependant sedation.
Elimination: Mainly via feces with some degree of urinary excretion.
Routes of Administration: IM.
Advantages: Sedation is significant approximately 2 hours after injection, peaks at approximately 8 hours, and lasts for 2-3 days.

- Single dose injection provides long-term tranquilization.

Disadvantages: Extrapyramidal symptoms may occur with overdosing.
Antagonists: None.
Formulation: 50, 100 mg/ml ampules.
Comments: Give in combination with immediate-acting or shorter-acting tranquilizers. Extrapyramidal symptoms can be treated with 10-20 mg biperidin (Akineton®), dexetimide (Tremblex®), 5 mg diazepam, or xylazine.

Perphenazine

Mechanism of Action: Antagonize the neurotransmitter, dopamine, in the basal ganglia and limbic portions of the forebrain.
Elimination: Hepatic oxidation and glucuronic acid conjugation with renal excretion.
Routes of Administration: IM (never IV).
Advantages: Sedation is significant approximately 12 hours after injection, peaks at approximately 5 days, and lasts for 7-14 days.

- Single dose provides long-term tranquilization

Disadvantages: Extrapyramidal symptoms may occur with overdosing which may include catatonia, dyskinesia, and anorexia.
Antagonists: None.
Formulation: 5 mg/ml solution.
Comments: Give in combination with immediate-acting or shorter-acting tranquilizers. Extrapyramidal symptoms can be treated with 10-20 mg biperidin (Akineton®), dexetimide (Tremblex®), 5 mg diazepam, or xylazine.

Injectable Anesthetics

General anesthesia is usually defined as loss of pain perception (analgesia) combined with loss of consciousness. Although the opioids are included under this heading, they probably are not acting as true anesthetics in that they induce a state of immobilization (as opposed to unconsciousness) characterized by spontaneous movements and responsiveness to external stimuli. The opioids, however, are potent analgesics and minor painful operations (e.g., ear tagging, tooth extraction) should be well toleratedby the animal.

Barbiturates

Although barbiturates have been successfully used to immobilize a variety of wild animals, their use has greatly diminished due to more efficacious and safer drugs. The barbiturates are classified as sedative-hypnotic drugs, but they produce a variety of physiological effects. Depending on chemical substitution of the barbituric acid molecule, the barbiturates may have a long (phenobarbital, barbital), intermediate (amobarbital), short (pentobarbital, secobarbital), or ultrashort (thiamylal, thiopental, methohexital) duration of effect. Barbiturates act throughout the CNS, with the mesencephalic reticular activating system being exquisitely sensitive to the drug. Their site of action can be either presynaptic (cortex, cerebellum, thalamus) or postsynaptic (spinal cord).

Barbiturates act as major respiratory depressants by suppressing the neurogenic drive as well as the hypoxic and chemoreceptor drives. They do not have a major cardiovascular effect other than a fall in blood pressure seen with intravenous administration or high doses. Intravenous administration may also cause cardiac arrhythmias.

A major effect of barbiturate use is their interference with the hepatic cytochrome P-450 system. The barbiturates competitively interfere with the biotransformation of a number of enzyme substrates, including other drugs or steroids. Thus, adverse drug reactions or endocrine imbalances may result from use of these drugs.

Phenobarbital, Pentobarbital, Thiopental, Methohexital

Mechanism of Action: Polysynaptic suppression; facilitation of GABA-ergic inhibition; GABA-mimetic action.

Elimination: Renal excretion and/or hepatic oxidation.

Routes of Administration: PO, IV, IM, IP (caution: most barbiturates, especially thiobarbiturates, should not be given IM because of tissue damage).

Advantages: Produce range of control from sedation to general anesthesia.

- Length of effect can be modulated based on agent used (long 8–12 hr), intermediate (2–6 hr), short (45–90 min), ultrashort (5–15 min).
- Thiobarbiturates are useful for quickly (20–60 sec) inducing general anesthesia which is subsequently maintained by other agents (i.e., gas).

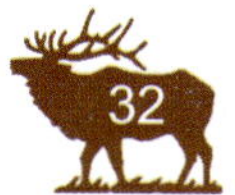

Disadvantages: Generally require large volumes for IM immobilization.

- Major respiratory depressant; also can inhibit fetal respiration without producing anesthesia in mother.
- Can cause laryngospasm, coughing, and sneezing.
- Poor analgesics.
- Poor muscle relaxation.
- Thiobarbiturates given as bolus IV injection or in large doses can cause arrhythmias or cardiac arrest.
- Can cause hyperglycemia, adverse drug interactions, or endocrine alterations.

Antagonists: None.

Formulation: Several solutions or powders available.

Comments: Controlled substances (Schedules II, III). Compared to other immobilizing agents, the barbiturates are generally unsatisfactory for free-ranging wildlife immobilization. Their primary use in veterinary medicine today is to rapidly induce anesthesia which is maintained by inhalation anesthetics. A similar use is appropriate for small, manually-restrained wildlife. Oral barbiturates in bait have been used successfully to capture waterfowl and gamebirds. Barbituates are used for animal euthanasia (see *Animal Capture* section), but the carcasses must either be deeply buried or incinerated to avoid toxicity to scavengers.

Cyclohexanes

Also termed dissociative anesthetics, this group of drugs causes a functional and electrophysiological dissociation between the thalamoneocortical and limbic systems. They are characterized by producing a cataleptic state (a malleable rigidity of the limbs) in which the eyes remain open with intact corneal and light reflexes. When used singly, the cyclohexanes usually cause rough inductions and recoveries, and convulsions are not uncommon. Because of this, they are usually administered concurrently with tranquilizers or sedatives.

The cyclohexanes are also thought to have amnestic properties; that is, humans (and presumably animals) have little or no recollection of the anesthetic event. There is no complete antagonist of the cyclohexanes, although several drugs appear to antagonize some of their effects. Physostigmine, neostigmine, L-amphetamine, 4-aminopyridine, yohimbine, tolazoline, and naloxone may have partial antagonistic properties (Kreeger and Seal, 1986a).

Ketamine and tiletamine are the two cyclohexanes in use today. Both are cogeners of phencyclidine. Phencyclidine was widely used as a wildlife anesthetic until taken off the market due to human abuse. Ketamine is probably one of the most widely used drugs for wildlife anesthesia because of its efficacy and high therapeutic index. It is generally used on small- and medium-sized mammals, but can immobilize species ranging from reptiles to large ungulates.

Tiletamine is unavailable as a single product and it is combined in equal propor-

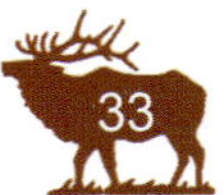

tions with the benzodiazepine, zolazepam. When used alone, tiletamine produces convulsive seizures and clonic muscular reactions while zolazepam alone causes aggressive behavior (in domestic cats). Combining these two drugs (e.g., Telazol®, Zoletil®) results in fewer convulsions, good muscle relaxation, and smoother recoveries. Tiletamine-zolazepam (previously identified as CI-744) is currently approved only for use in dogs and cats, but during its development, it was used on over 200 non-domestic vertebrate species (Gray et al., 1974; Boever et al., 1977b; Schobert, 1987). The relative potencies of phencyclidine, tiletamine, and ketamine is approximately 5:2.5:1, respectively (Beck, 1972).

Ketamine, Tiletamine

Mechanism of Action: Unknown, presumably a complex involving sigma, cholinergic, serotonergic, dopaminergic, and N-methyl-D-aspartic receptors.

Elimination: Metabolized in the liver by N-demethylation via cytochrome P-450 enzymes, conjugated to water-soluble glucuronide derivatives, and excreted in urine.

Routes of Administration: IM, IV, SC, IP, PO.

Advantages: Effective on many species.

- Safe (high therapeutic index).
- Provide peripheral analgesia (visceral pain not abolished).
- Minimal respiratory effects (depressant only at high doses).
- Good cardiovascular support (heart rate and blood pressure increase).
- Synergistic with many tranquilizers and anesthetics.

Disadvantages: Rough inductions and recoveries without tranquilizers.

- Poor muscle relaxation when used without tranquilizers.
- Convulsant, particularly with prolonged administration or high doses (ketamine, phencyclidine).
- Can cause copious salivation.
- Rapid IV administration can cause transient apnea
- Low pH of solution causes burning, irritation upon injection.
- Produce a variety of hematologic, serum chemical, and endocrine alterations.

Antagonists: No complete antagonist (see above).

Formulation: Ketamine: 100 mg/ml (can be lyophilized and reconstituted up to 200 mg/ml).

- Tiletamine: 286 mg tiletamine + 286 mg zolazepam per vial (Telazol®); 250 mg tiletamine + 250 mg zolazepam per vial (Zoletil®)

Comments: Ketamine and Telazol® (Schedule III) are all controlled substances. The eyelids normally remain open during cyclohexane anesthesia and the eyes of animals immobilized outdoors should be protected from drying out and from ultraviolet light. Palpebral and corneal reflexes usually remain intact under cyclohexane anesthesia and shouldn't be used to assess depth of anesthesia. If profound salivation is problematic, it can usually be controlled with atropine (see *Adjuvants*). However, it should be remembered that both cyclohexanes and atropine increase heart rate; the combination of these two drugs may produce unacceptably high heart rates. A tranquilizer/sedative should be used in almost all

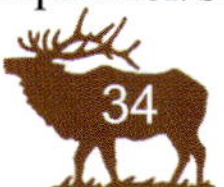

cases with the cyclohexanes to reduce or prevent the untoward effects of these drugs. Cyclohexanes are fairly effective given orally and can be used to spike baits to partially tranquilize animals or sprayed into the mouth of caged/trapped animals rendering them safer to handle.

Cyclohexane Tips

Ketamine-Medetomidine

If you can't find a drug dosage for your species using ketamine and medetomidine, try an initial dosage of 3.0 mg/kg ketamine plus 0.1 mg/kg medetomidine. This dosage is based on the mean of this combination reported in 56 species.

An easy way to "pre-mix" this dosage is to start with 200 mg/ml ketamine (available from veterinary pharmacists) and 20 mg/ml medetomidine (available from Wildlife Pharmaceuticals). For each 20 ml vial of ketamine, remove 5 ml and replace with 5 ml of medetomidine (for 10 ml ketamine vials, remove and replace 2.5 ml). This combination will now provide 150 mg ketamine and 5 mg medetomidine per ml. The standard dosage for most mammals would be *1 ml for every 50 kg body weight* (i.e., the same standard dosage as above). For example, a 100 kg deer would get 2 ml of this mixture (300 mg ketamine plus 10 mg medetomidine total dose).

Tiletamine-Zolazepam

Tiletamine-zolazepam (i.e., Telazol®, Zoletil®) is available worldwide in lyophilized (freeze-dried) form. Zoletil® is produced with 500 mg (250 mg of each drug) per vial. The manufacturer recommends adding 4.4 ml solvent to the vial resulting in a concentration of 100 mg/ml. However, Telazol® is produced with 572 mg (286 mg of each drug) per vial. Manufacturer's instructions call for adding 5 ml sterile water to the vial resulting in an *approximate* concentration of 100 mg/ml. This apparent inconsistency is because when 5 ml of solvent is added, the final volume is actually 5.7 ml due to chemical reactions. Thus, 572 mg in 5.7 ml is approximately 100 mg/ml (Amass and Drew, 2006).

You can increase this concentration by adding less water. Regardless of the amount of water added, figure the final volume will be approximately 0.6–0.7 ml greater (e.g., adding 2 ml will result in about 2.6 ml). You need to keep this total volume in mind because it will affect your calculations. For example when using Telazol®, if you use just 2 ml (2.6 ml final volume), the actual drug concentration will be about 220 mg/ml (572 mg/2.6 ml). You can add as little as 1 ml solvent (1.6 ml final volume), but the solvent must be warm and the solution kept warm or the drug will go back out of solution.

Tiletamine-Zolazepam-Xylazine

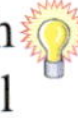

You can also increase the effectiveness of this drug by adding tranquilizers, such as xylazine or medetomidine, instead of water. Adding 2 ml of 100 mg/ml xylazine, for instance, will provide 572 mg tiletamine-zolazepam (for Telazol®)

plus 200 mg xylazine in approximately 2.6 ml solution. One vial of this mixture should immobilize most medium sized mammals (i.e., ≤ 100 kg); two vials should work on larger animals (i.e., 100–250 kg). Alternatively, you can add 1 ml of 100 mg/ml ketamine plus 1 ml of 100 mg/ml xylazine. This is a good combination for carnivores, such as bears. The same doses would apply (i.e., one vial for ≤100 kg bears).

Opioids

Opium is a drug obtained from the juice of the poppy, *Papaver somniferum*, and contains over 20 alkaloids. Opioid immobilizing agents are generally congeners of two of these alkaloids, morphine and thebaine. The opioids have been used for animal immobilization since the 1960s and are the most potent drugs available for this purpose.

The opioids interact with stereospecific and saturable receptors in the CNS. Several opioid receptors have been identified (kappa, delta, mu) which bind natural and synthetic exogenous opioids as well as endogenous opioids (endorphins, enkephalins, dynorphins). Most opioid drugs appear to act preferentially at mu receptors. Opioids either selectively inhibit the release of excitatory neurotransmitters (i.e., dopamine) or act at postsynaptic sites. A major advantage in the use of opioids is the availability of specific antagonists. Some agents (e.g., butorphanol) are classified as agonist-antagonists and have both properties depending on dose.

Although classified herein as anesthetics, opioids more correctly induce *immobilization* as opposed to *anesthesia*. Animals given opioids often respond to noise, touch, and other stimulation which indicates that they are *not* completely unconscious, a characteristic of general anesthesia. Although most opioids are potent analgesics, they do not induce surgical anesthesia and surgical interventions like radiotransmitter implantation should not be done on animals given opioids alone.

The three most commonly used opioids are etorphine, thiafentanil, and carfentanil. Etorphine is an analog of thebaine; thiafentanil and carfentanil are derivatives of fentanyl. In rats, fentanyl is approximately 292 times more potent; etorphine 1,000 times more potent (Dobbs, 1968); and carfentanil 9,441 times more potent (Marsboom, 1985; Meert, 1996) than morphine. In humans, etorphine is 500 times more potent than morphine (Jasinski et al., 1975). In moose for example, we estimate the relative potencies of carfentanil:thiafentanil:etorphine to be 2:1:1.

Sufentanil is another fentanyl congener used primarily in human medicine, but it can be used on wild animals (Kreeger and Seal, 1990). Sufentanil is 4,521 times more potent than morphine and it has a safety margin 2.5 times that of carfentanil (Marsboom, 1985; Meert, 1996).

Thiafentanil (A-3080®) is a synthetic opioid being evaluated in the United States,

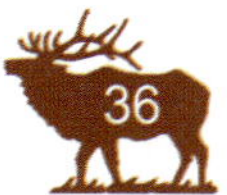

but is available in South Africa upon prescription. In elk (*Cervus elaphus*), thiafentanil appeared to give rapid induction with a shorter duration of action than carfentanil which may be beneficial in reducing resedation (Stanley et al., 1988; Janssen et al., 1991).

Thiafentanil has been shown to be superior to carfentanil for pronghorn capture (Kreeger et al., 2001). In many African species, thiafentanil has a short induction time (< 2 min) and short duration (approx. 30 min) if used alone. Resedation (see below) has not been observed in these African species.

Butorphanol is a morphinan analogue with a potency 3.5–7 times that of morphine. Butorphanol has mixed agonist-antagonist properties. Higher doses (> 0.5 mg/kg) of butorphanol may result in no effect as antagonistic properties tend to dominate. The antagonist potency is about 1/40 that of naloxone, nonetheless high doses can be used to antagonize other opioids. Alone, butorphanol provides only "apathetic sedation." Butorphanol can be combined with other drugs, such as xylazine, medetomidine, or ketamine.

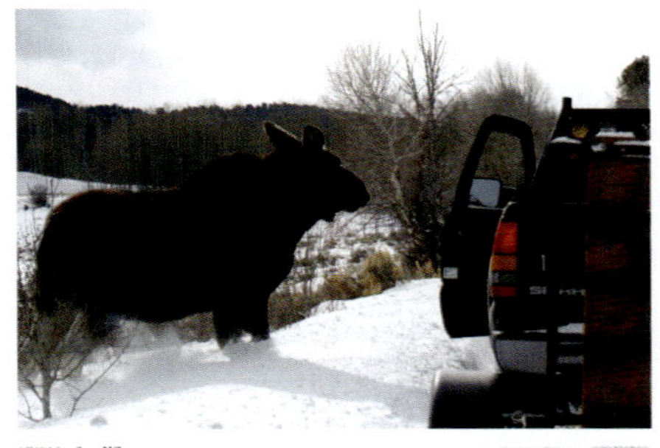

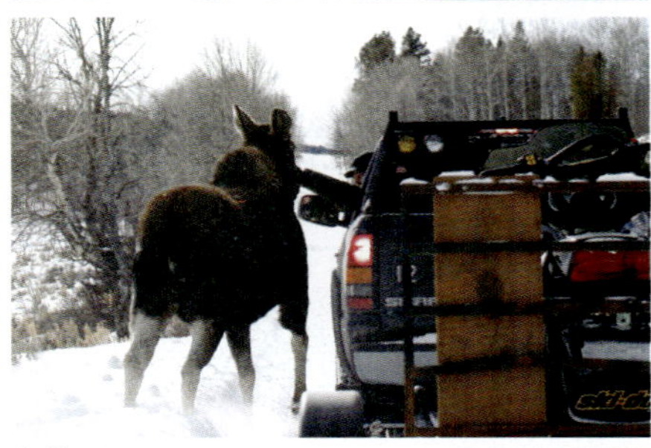

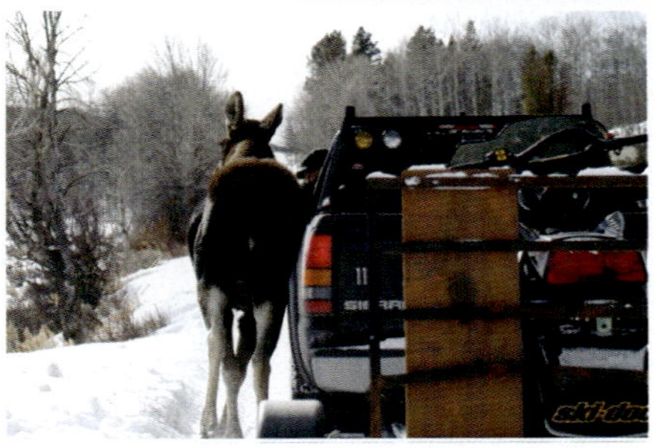

Animals given opioids are often unaware of their surroundings just prior to induction. They can be physically controlled, but do not respond to sights or sounds. This moose was given thiafentanil and was apparently unaware of the truck. It became recumbent moments later.

Resedation

A phenomenon seen with the use of opioids for animal immobilization is "resedation." After antagonism, the animal appears to again come under the influence of the opioid agonist. This can occur relatively quickly or several hours to days after the immobilizing episode. Resedation appears to occur more frequently, but not exclusively, with carfentanil use (Jessup et al., 1984a; Jessup et al., 1985b; Seal et al., 1985b; Kreeger and Seal, 1990). Resedation may be due to (1) the more potent agonists being metabolized slower than the antagonist; (2) the marked lipophilia of opioids resulting in prolonged release from fat depots; or (3) enterohepatic circulation.

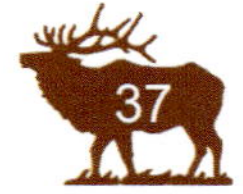

Carfentanil and Opioid Toxicity

The potency of opioids, such as etorphine and carfentanil, is both an advantage and disadvantage. The advantage is that the reduced volume of drug required for anesthesia makes them the only class of drugs capable of remote capture of large animals. The disadvantage is that they are potentially toxic to humans.

The lethal human doses of opioids are unknown. Many people have assumed that the lethal dose of carfentanil, the most potent opioid in use today, was very low. Some have even said that exposure to an almost invisible amount would be fatal. This is probably not true.

There are no data on the effects of carfentanil in humans. Therapeutic indices (ratio of LD_{50} to ED_{50}) for carfentanil range from 16.77 in domestic ferrets (Stanley and McJames, 1986) to 10,600 in rats (Van Bever et al., 1976). The therapeutic index in humans was estimated to be 25-50 (Stanley, pers. comm.). Approximately 0.1 mg carfentanil was given orally to chimpanzees (our closest genetic relative) resulting in clinical effects (respiratory depression) in all chimps (Kearns et al., 1996). This chimp dosage is approximately one drop of carfentanil at the currently available concentration of 3 mg/ml. If the therapeutic index in humans is truly 25-50 and if chimps can be considered good models for humans, then it would take approximately 1 ml (24 drops/ml) of carfentanil taken either IV or IM (absorption through mucous membranes would increase this amount) to kill a human. If these suppositions are true, then the most probable scenerio where a human would die from carfentanil exposure would be if that person was accidentally hit with a dart. This would be a rare event.

We are aware of at least two occasions where people were sprayed in the face with carfentanil with *no effect*. Kreeger (pers. comm.) was exposed when a pre-pressurized dart blew off its needle prior to being placed in a dart gun. Another incident occurred when a dart missed the intended animal and hit the ground, plugging the needle. When retrieved, the dart went off spraying the person in the face. The person could perceive a bitter taste (presumably carfentanil) on his lips.

This is not to say that exposure to some amount of carfentanil, by any route, would result in no effect. One of the authors (TJK) fired a dart containing thiafentanil (approximately one-half as potent as carfentanil) at a female pronghorn which glanced off the animal's neck, discharging its contents. A male pronghorn was approximately 10 m downwind from this discharge. About 15 minutes later, the male pronghorn was seen staggering, down on its hindquarters, circling, vocalizing, and open-mouthed breathing. When approached, the pronghorn could run away, but stumbled and fell in the process. The only logical explanation for this observation was that the mist of the discharged dart traveled downwind and came into contact with the eyes and mouth of the male pronghorn, resulting in narcotization. This is *a priori* evidence that exposure to even a small amount of these drugs can result in clinical, albeit not lethal, effects.

Extra care and concentration is required when working with this drug class. Toxic exposure can be by accidental injection with a syringe or dart, by absorption through the mucous membranes of the mouth, eyes, or nose, or by direct absorption through broken skin. Opioid immobilizing agents should never be used while working alone or without having an antagonist immediately on hand. If you are exposed to these opioids without the availability of an antagonist, by yourself, or even with someone who is ignorant of CPR (cardiopulmonary resuscitation), there is a possibility that you will not survive. Anyone using these agents should read the sections on antagonists and on *Human Medical Treatment* for appropriate responses to opioid overdose. Although opioids are potentially toxic, keep in mind that there have been only two recorded human deaths (due to injection with etorphine) and *no* recorded deaths due to carfentanil or thiafentanil *despite over 20 years of use and tens of thousands of doses given.* 

Fentanyl, Sufentanil, Carfentanil, Etorphine, Thiafentanil

Mechanism of Action: Interact with stereospecific and saturable opioid receptors in the CNS.

Elimination: Metabolized in the liver by glucuronic conjugation or by N-demethylation and excreted in bile or by the kidneys.

Routes of Administration: IM, IV, SC, PO.

Advantages: Potency allows volumes suitable for immobilization of the largest of animals.

- Rapidly antagonized.
- Analgesic.
- No major cardiovascular effects

Disadvantages: Potentially toxic to humans at low doses.

- Major respiratory depressants.
- Can "recycle" after antagonism.
- Can cause prolonged, excitatory state prior to induction.
- Alter thermoregulation.
- Do not interfere with senses of touch, vibration, vision, or hearing (animal responds to such stimulation).
- Poor muscle relaxation in some species (ungulates, equids).
- Increases salivation.
- May cause vomition, defecation, decreased rumen motility, and bloat.
- May induce temporary endocrine changes.

Antagonists: Diprenorphine (M50-50®), naloxone, naltrexone, nalmefene.

Formulation: Wildnil®: 3 mg carfentanil/ml solution.

- Thiafentanil (A-3080): 10 mg/ml solution.
- M99®: 1, 4.9, 9.8, or 10 mg etorphine/ml solution.
- Fentaz®: 10 mg/ml fentanyl + 80 mg/ml azaperone solution.
- Sufenta®: 50 μg/ml sufentanil solution.
- Sublimaze®: 0.05 mg/ml fentanyl solution
- Large Animal Immobilon®: 2.45 mg/ml etorphine + 10 mg/ml acepromazine solution.

- Small Animal Immobilon®: 0.07 mg/ml etorphine + 18 mg/ml methotrimeprazine solution.
- Thalamonal®: 0.05 mg/ml fentanyl + 20 mg/ml droperidol

Comments: Controlled substances (Schedule II). Felids and equids should not be given opioids without tranquilizers/sedatives to avoid excitation upon induction. In general (except for moose, *Alces* spp.), concurrent use of tranquilizers in all species hastens and smoothes induction as well as ameliorates many of the adverse effects of opioids. However, tranquilizers having adverse effects such as respiratory depression or thermoregulation alteration may exacerbate these conditions when used with opioids.

Butorphanol

Mechanism of Action: Kappa opioid receptor agonist; mu receptor antagonist.

Elimination: Metabolized in the liver and excreted by the kidneys.

Routes of Administration: IM, IV.

Advantages: Safe, high therapeutic index.

- Minimal cardiovascular and respiratory effects.
- Can be antagonized.
- Good analgesic.

Disadvantages: Provides only mild sedation when used alone.

- Limited to calm or restrained animals.

Antagonists: Naloxone, naltrexone, nalmefene.

Formulation: 0.5, 1, 2, 10 mg/ml solutions; 1, 5, 10 mg tablets.

Comments: Controlled substances (Schedule IV). Can be combined with xylazine to provide profound sedation to anesthesia (Kreeger et al., 1989a). This combination is best limited to immobilization of calm or restrained animals. Such immobilized animals also tend to be more stimulated by sound or touch than other drug combinations. This combination does have the advantage of being completely and quickly antagonized with opioid and alpha$_2$-adrenergic (yohimbine, idazoxan, atipamezole) antagonists. The human butorphanol product (Stadol®) is a tartrate salt (1 mg tartrate salt = 1 mg base) and dosages should be adjusted accordingly.

Steroid Anesthetics

Steroid anesthetics have been known since the 1940s, but they have found only limited use in wildlife immobilization. They have been used on reptiles (Calderwood and Jacobson, 1979b), birds (Cooper and Frank, 1973), raccoons (Clutton and Duggan, 1986), and cheetahs (Button et al., 1981). The only currently-available product (althesin; Saffan®) is a mixture of two pregnanediones, alphaxalone and alphadolone acetate, in a solution of saline and polyoxyethylated castor oil. Althesin induces a short-acting (5–10 min), dose-dependent anesthesia with good muscle relaxation. Althesin can be administered either IV or IM, but volumes tend to be high when used on larger animals. It can be used in

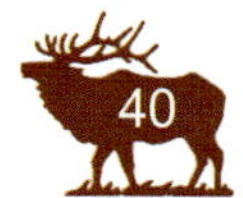

combination with most gas anesthetics and neuromuscular blockers, but it cannot be used with barbiturates. Althesin has been approved for use on humans in Canada and the U.K., but has not been approved for use in the U.S.

Althesin

Mechanism of Action: Unknown.

Elimination: Biotransformation in the liver to polar metabolites and excreted in the bile.

Routes of Administration: IM, IV.

Advantages: Produces general anesthesia of short duration.

- Wide safety margin.
- Minimal respiratory depression.
- Good muscle relaxation.

Disadvantages: Large volumes required.

- Can cause histamine release (see comments).
- Recovery can be rough.
- Can cause necrotic lesions in the extremities in cats (rare).
- Can cause salivation in some primates.

Antagonists: None.

Formulation: 12 mg/ml solution comprised of 9 mg/ml alphaxalone and 3 mg/ml alphadolone.

Comments: Althesin is contraindicated for use in domestic dogs (and presumably wild canids) because the polyoxyethylated castor oil can cause release of histamine resulting in cardiovascular collapse. If given IV, althesin should be given slowly in all species to avoid respiratory depression. Also, althesin cannot be used with barbiturates.

Propofol

Propofol is an injectable anesthetic chemically unrelated to other intravenous anesthetics. The compound comes as an 1% (10 mg/ml) emulsion in oil. It has a milky appearance and it is easily contaminated with bacteria and mold unless strict sterile withdrawal technique is observed. Propofol when given IV in a rapid bolus (6.6 mg/kg) produces general anesthesia of short duration (Mandelker, 1993). Following induction, respiration is often depressed, sometimes to the point of apnea, but this effect lasts only for approximately 30 seconds. Due to its rapid elimination, recovery from propofol can lead to disorientation and paddling of the limbs. The addition of diazepam (0.4 mg/kg) is often helpful in providing muscle relaxation and smoothing recovery. Low doses of acepromazine (0.1 mg/kg) given as a preanesthetic can lower the propofol dose by one-half (Mandelker, 1993). Propofol can be used like the barbiturates to induce anesthesia that will be maintained by gas. Propofol has found some limited use in wild ruminants and camelids (Jalanka and Teräväinen, 1992), but for the time, its use appears restricted to small animals that can be safely restrained.

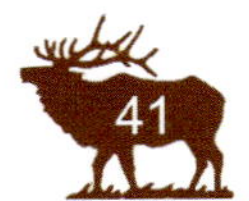

Inhalation Anesthetics

Comprehensive instruction on inhalation (gas) anesthesia is beyond the scope of this handbook. Unless you are dealing with the simplest of gas systems, do not attempt to anesthetize animals without hands-on instruction from a veterinarian or an experienced veterinary technician. In the simplest of terms, gas anesthesia is the delivery of vaporized drugs that are breathed directly into the lungs, taken up by the blood, and delivered to the brain resulting in general anesthesia. Elimination of the drug is mostly by a reversal of this same route.

Inhalation anesthesia sees limited application in field immobilizations. However, it can be used effectively for small mammals and birds or for maintaining anesthesia in larger animals initially anesthetized with injectable drugs (Mathews et al., 2002; Lewis, 2004). Its primary use is in zoos and research facilities. Below we present an overview of inhalation anesthesia to familiarize you with this technology, but reiterate the need for instruction by qualified personnel.

Delivering vaporized drug to the brain is, understandably, not a straight forward task. Unlike directly injecting a drug into the tissue where it is picked up by circulating blood and delivered to the brain, inhalation anesthetics must first be vaporized, then delivered to the lungs, then cross the alveoli into the circulation, and finally cross the blood-brain barrier to interact with appropriate CNS receptors. In most modern inhalation drug delivery systems, the drug is vaporized by flowing oxygen through it in a metal vaporizer. This mixture of vaporized drug and oxygen is then delivered to the patient's lungs.

The vapor pressure of the drug determines its volatility and, thus, maximum concentration of the drug in the gaseous mixture. Vapor pressure can be affected by temperature and flow rate. When the drug/oxygen mixture reaches the lungs, it must achieve sufficient partial pressure within the alveoli to cross into the blood. This partial pressure is a function of the inspired concentration of drug, which can be determined by the vaporizer setting (see below and Table 1). In general, the greater the ventilation (i.e., breathing) the quicker gas concentration will rise in the alveoli. Thus, it will take longer to achieve general anesthesia if breathing is slow or shallow (decreased tidal volume).

The ability of the drug molecule in the gaseous phase to cross the alveoli into the blood is determined its solubility which is expressed as a *partition coefficient* (Table 1). The greater the blood-gas partition coefficient, the longer it will take to achieve induction and recovery and vice versa. Thus drugs, such as isoflurane and sevoflurane, are preferred today because they have low partition coefficients (Table 1), which provide rapid induction and (just as important) rapid recovery from anesthesia. Keep in mind that any disease state which causes pathologic changes in the alveoli (e.g., fibrosis, emphysema, exudates) will impair diffusion and slow drug uptake.

Assuming cardiac output and blood flow are normal, drug uptake by the brain is relatively rapid because of its rich blood supply. Tissues with poorer blood supply, such as fat, absorb drug much more slowly. Fat also has a high tissue solubility for inhalation anesthetics and will have a greater and more prolonged capacity to absorb anesthetic. This will have little effect on induction, however, because of fat's low blood flow. Conversely, once drug crosses into fat tissues, it is diffuses out just as slowly. Thus, patients with lots of fat stores (e.g., bears) that undergo extended anesthesia (> 3 hr) will have a prolonged recovery due to the release of the drug back into the circulation (Muir et al., 2000).

Elimination of inhalation anesthetics is just the opposite of uptake. Once drug is eliminated from the alveoli (by turning off the vaporizer), arterial blood tension (i.e., the partial pressure of gas dissolved in the blood) falls, followed by a fall in tissue tension. Because of the high blood flow to the brain, anesthetic tension falls rapidly resulting in the fairly quick anesthetic recovery with agents such as isoflurane and sevoflurane.

Chloroform

This is an obsolete agent that has been replaced by safer and more effective compounds. Chloroform is both hepatotoxic and nephrotoxic.

Diethyl Ether

Ether is a versatile anesthetic that can be administered with the simplest of equipment. It is little used today, however, because of its high inflammability (it forms an explosive mixture with air or oxygen). It is a potent analgesic and good muscle relaxant, producing gradual suppression of reflexes. Induction and recovery are relatively slow. Ether irritates the respiratory passages, producing salivation and tracheal and bronchial secretions. Cardiac output is unaltered or slightly increased; arrhythmias are rare. Nausea and vomiting may occur during induction. Ether is neither hepatotoxic or nephrotoxic. It causes hyperglycemia as a result of mobilization of liver glycogen, as well as increasing levels of antidiuretic hor-

Table 1. Physical properties of inhalation agents (after Muir et al., 2000).

Drug	Maximum Concentration of Vapor Delivered by Saturation Vaporizer at 20 °C (%)	Ranges of Concentration: Induction (%)	Ranges of Concentration: Maintenance (%)	Blood-Gas Partition Coefficient
Ether	58	10-40	3.0-12.0	15.20
Desflurane	87.4	8-15	5.0-9.0	0.42
Sevoflurane	22	4-5	2.0-3.5	0.69
Isofurane	33	2-6	1.0-3.0	1.41
Halothane	32	1-4	0.5-2.0	2.36
Enflurane	24	3-7	1.0-3.0	1.91
Methoxyflurane	3	<3	0.25-1.0	13.00

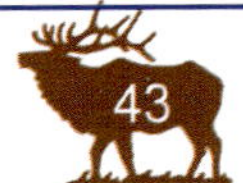

mone, hydrocortisone, thyroxine, and norepinephrine. The majority of ether (85-90%) is eliminated through the lungs, with the remainder lost through the skin, mucous membranes, and liver biodegradation.

Nitrous Oxide

This is used primarily as an adjunct to other gas anesthetics. By itself, it produces only mild anesthesia and analgesia. When combined with a more potent gas, nitrous oxide decreases the amount of gas required for complete anesthesia. Nitrous oxide does not appear to have deleterious effects on the liver, kidneys, or gastrointestinal tract. Nitrous oxide should be used with a minimum of 30% oxygen in the total gas flow to prevent hypoxia.

Halothane

The predecessor of most of the inhalation anesthetics used today, halothane is a potent anesthetic, producing a rapid and smooth loss of consciousness. Halothane produces a hypotension related to the depth of anesthesia. It directly causes vasodilation and decreases cardiac output. Thus, monitoring arterial blood pressure provides the best information about the depth of anesthesia. Halothane also depresses respiration at all levels of anesthesia, decreases gut motility, depresses temperature regulating centers, and only moderately relaxes muscles. Although it is not nephrotoxic, "halothane hepatitis" occurs in 1 out of 10,000 uses in humans. The incidence of such hepatotoxicity in other species is unknown. The majority of halothane is eliminated unchanged in exhaled gas. The remainder undergoes either biotransformation or elimination unchanged by other routes.

Enflurane

Enflurane provides a smooth and fairly rapid induction and emergence from anesthesia. Depth of anesthesia can be adjusted relatively quickly. Enflurane decreases blood pressure to about the same degree as halothane, but bradycardia and arrhythmias are lessened. Enflurane provides good muscle relaxation and analgesia, but depresses respiration as its concentration increases. It is not nephrotoxic, but hepatic necrosis has been reported associated with repeated administration. The majority of enflurane is expired, with small amounts being biotransformed. Tranquilizers should be used to smooth induction and to avoid emergence delirium.

Sevoflurane

Sevoflurane provides more rapid induction, recovery, and change in depth than isoflurane. It produces good muscle relaxation and analgesia. Sevoflurane causes respiratory depression like isoflurane, but less myocardial depression. Sevoflurane rapidly crosses the placenta, causing fetal depression. Sevoflurane causes higher inorganic flouride (F^-) concentrations than isoflurane, but this has not resulted in nephrotoxicity in the few species studied. Sevoflurane also elevates concentrations of Compound A (pentafluorisopropenyl fluoromethyl ether) which is formed

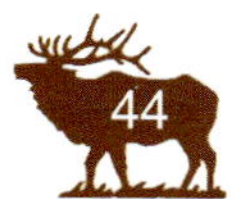

when sevoflurane interacts with carbon dioxide in rebreathing (closed) systems. These concentrations (30-40 ppm) are significantly lower than concentrations associated with renal toxicity and death in rats (Gaynor et al., 1997). When using rebreathing systems, a minimum oxygen flow rate of 2 L/min is recommended. Although the toxicity of Compound A in almost all nondomestic species is unknown, the use of nonrebreathing systems may be prudent.

Isoflurane

This is an isomer of enflurane that provides rapid and smooth induction and emergence from general anesthesia. Anesthetic depth can be changed more rapidly than with most of the previously-mentioned gases. Blood pressure decreases progressively with increasing depth of anesthesia as a result of decreased vascular resistance. However, cardiac output is maintained because of increased heart rate. Arrhythmias are rare, except perhaps in birds. Isoflurane causes a more profound respiratory depression than either halothane or enflurane. It is an excellent muscle relaxant and is neither nephrotoxic nor hepatotoxic. Only a fraction of isoflurane is metabolized. Isoflurane is an excellent inhalation anesthetic when used with a calibrated vaporizer, but its cost may be prohibitive.

Desflurane

Desflurane is identical in structure to isoflurane, except that flourine is substituted for chlorine. Desflurane causes extremely rapid induction and recovery, but it is pungent, causing irritation, coughing, or breath holding. Desflurane requires a special, electrically-heated vaporizer and it is more expensive than most other gases.

Delivery Systems

For details of different delivery systems, we refer you to Chapter 14 in Muir et al. (2000). The simplest method to deliver inhalation drugs is an *open* system. This can be a jar with ether-soaked cotton balls in which you place a small mammal until it loses consciousness or a cone with drug-soaked cotton that is placed over the muzzle of a larger animal. Open systems provide an acceptable means to anesthetize rodents and other small mammals. Cones can be used to maintain anesthesia in animals that have been initially anesthetized in a chamber but then removed for further handling. Open systems waste a lot of anesthetic through uncontrolled vaporization. This vaporization also exposes the human to potentially toxic fumes. There is little control of depth of anesthesia with

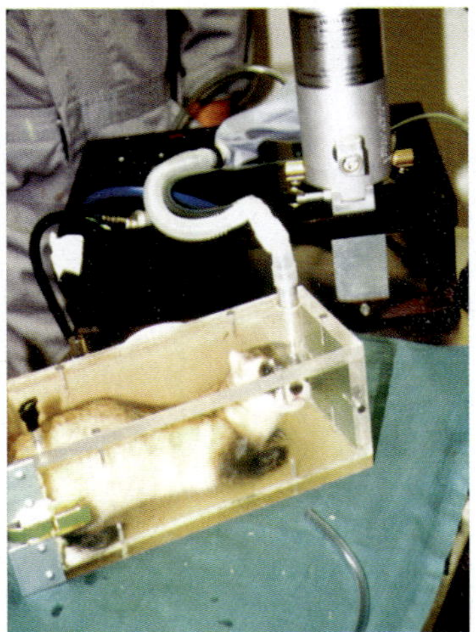

Black-footed ferret in portable sevoflurane anesthesia machine.

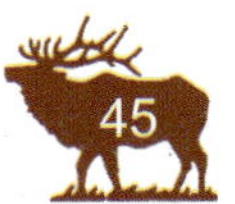

open systems. You must closely observe the depth of anesthesia (Table 2) and remove the animal for awhile to breathe ambient air when needed.

Non-rebreathing systems require the input of a pressurized oxygen to vaporize and deliver the drug to the lungs. The gas must be delivered at relatively high rates (e.g., 50-150 ml/ kg/min) to both deliver the drug and remove carbon dioxide. Non-re-breathing systems can be thought of as one-way systems where the anesthetic gas is delivered by a cone over the muzzle or an endotracheal tube. When the animal exhales, the expired mixture of gases is "forced" along a route different than the incoming anesthetic gas. This alternate route can be by a "Y" or "T" tube where anesthetic goes in one arm of the "Y" or "T" and exhaled gases go out the other arm (e.g., Ayre's T piece system). Other systems have a "tube within a tube" (Bain or Lack system) where the inspired anesthetic gas is delivered to the animal in the outer tube and exhaled gases are delivered to the exterior by a smaller tube within.

Rebreathing systems are the best systems for delivering inhalation anesthetics. They are, of course, the most expensive and the most complex. Rebreathing systems use low gas flow rates to deliver the drug (e.g., 1–5 ml/kg/min) and do not cause abrupt fluctuations in anesthetic depth. Rebreathing systems start with compressed oxygen which passes through a flowmeter to monitor and adjust oxygen flow rate. The oxygen then passes through an adjustable vaporizer where the anesthetic is vaporized and swept along the hose by the oxygen and delivered to the animal's lungs through a one-way valve. Expired gases are forced by the one-way valve along another tube which passes through a carbon dioxide absorbent canister. This canister scavenges the carbon dioxide from the expired gas mixture. This absorbent changes color (usually blue) when saturated and then it should be replaced. Regardless of color change, absorbent should be changed after 6-8 hours of use. This scavenged gas, which contains oxygen and unabsorbed anesthetic, then continues back through the vaporizer to be essentially "reused." Rebreathing systems can employ a secondary gas, such as nitrous oxide, to increase the efficiency of the anesthetic. Such systems also employ rebreathing bags and pop-off valves that assist the animal's breathing and system pressure, respectively. Precision vaporizers are gas specific; for example, isoflurane requires an isoflurane vaporizer. Also, rebreathing systems generally cannot be used for small mammals (i.e., < 2–3 kg) because of their small lung volumes.

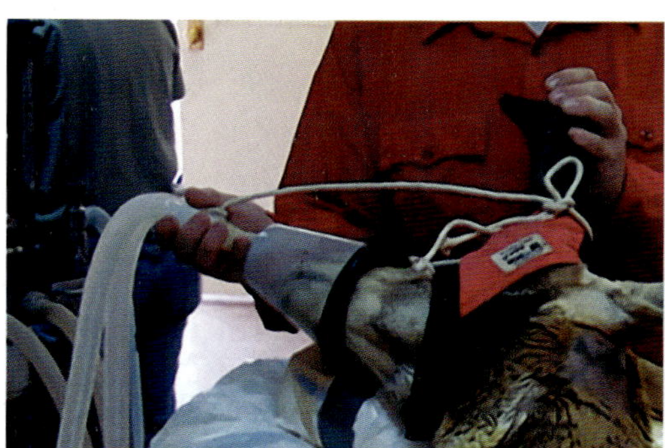

Large animals can be initially anesthetized with injectable drugs (thiafentanil in the case of this pronghorn) and maintained on gas anesthesia (isoflurane).

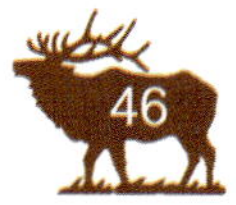

A hypothetical process for using inhalation anesthetics is as follows: fill the vaporizer with anesthetic (let's use isoflurane in this example) and fill the carbon dioxide canister with fresh absorbent. Confirm correct operation of unidirectional valves. Check oxygen cylinder pressure; turn on oxygen and check flowmeter function (repeat for nitrous oxide if so equipped). Make sure all connections are tight and pop-off valve and scavenging system are working. Bring in the patient only when these steps have been completed. Attach the system to animal either via a cone or endotracheal tube. Turn the oxygen on to 3 L/min. Turn the vaporizer to 4% to induce anesthesia. Monitor the patient and assess depth of anesthesia. When general anesthesia is achieved, turn the oxygen down to 2 L/min and vaporizer down to 2%. If the patient starts to arouse, increase the vaporizer percent. If the patient becomes hypoxic (tongue or lips become bluish-gray), increase the oxygen flow. If the patient becomes too deep, reduce the vaporizer setting or turn off completely. Remember, the preceding was just a hypothetical example. Each species will have different settings as will every individual.

You must *constantly* monitor the patient when using gas anesthesia. Unlike injectable anesthetics where the patient is usually quite stable a few minutes after induction, patients on gas anesthesia require continual monitoring. The biggest mistake novices make with gas anesthesia is to become distracted with other tasks (e.g., blood sampling, measurements, ultrasound) and ignore the depth of anesthesia. In a very short period of time, animals can go from an acceptable level of anesthesia (e.g., Stage III, Plane 2; Table 2) to medullary paralysis and death. If you are going to use gas anesthesia, you *must* have a person dedicated to monitoring the patient.

Antagonists

Some of the more notable pharmacological developments relative to wild animal immobilization have been specific, long-lasting opioid and alpha2-adrenergic antagonists. The ability to antagonize anesthesia and return the animal more quickly to physiological normalcy offers many advantages including:

- Alleviation of problems associated with prolonged recumbency such as nerve and muscle damage, bloat, and hypothermia.
- Reduced probability of injury or death after recovery due to accident or predation because there is no residual impairment from the immobilizing drugs such as sedation or ataxia.
- Decreased probability of rejection or interspecific strife due to quicker return to parent, herd, pack, etc.
- Decreased personnel and equipment time dedicated to monitoring the recovery process.

In general, opioid and alpha2-adrenergic antagonists are safe, causing adverse effects only at higher doses. It should be remembered that antagonists act on the animal and not on the agonist. Thus, it does not necessarily follow that the more

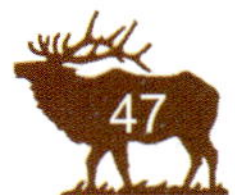

Table 2. Classical stages of anesthesia as defined for ether anesthesia.

I Stage of Analgesia
- disorientation
- increased heart and respiratory rate
- excessive salivation
- urine and feces may be voided

II Stage of Delirium or Excitement
- delirium, excitement, struggling
- loss of voluntary control
- tachycardia, possible cardiac arrhythmias
- irregular respiration, possible apnea
- dilated pupils
- reflex vomition, defecation, urination
- loss of consciousness

III Stage of Surgical Anesthesia

Plane I
- increased depth and rate of respiration
- reflexes present
- normal pulse and blood pressure
- pupils constricted

Plane II
- regular depth and rate of respiration
- loss of reflexes
- normal pulse and blood pressure
- pupils normal; fixed eye movement

Plane III
- increased abdominal respiration as intercostal muscles become paralyzed
- rapid pulse; blood pressure falls
- pupils slightly dilated

Plane IV
- paralysis of intercostal muscles, abdominal respiration only
- pulse rapid; blood pressure continues to fall; impaired cardiac function

IV Stage of Medullary Paralysis
- respiratory arrest leading to circulatory collapse
- pulse, blood pressure weak then absent
- eyes fixed and dilated
- death within 1–5 minutes

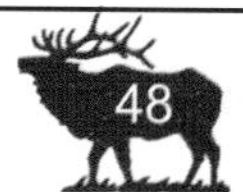

potent the agonist, the more amount of antagonist needs to be administered. Increasing the dose of an antagonist usually does *not* decrease recovery times (Kreeger et al., 1987a), but higher doses could prolong antagonism by maintaining serum concentrations at higher levels. When given a choice, one should select an antagonist that is the most specific for the receptors affected and has the longest biological life in the animal.

Intravenous injection of antagonists provides the most rapid recovery (1–2 min), although such quick recoveries may be less smooth compared to other routes of administration. A slower (app. 5–10 min) recovery occurs with IM injection (Wallingford et al., 1996). A common practice is to give equal doses of the antagonist both IV and IM or SC, or IM and SC. The IM or SC dose theoretically provides a slower release and thus a longer period for the antagonist to prevent recycling of the agonist; however, research on domestic goats does not support this theory (Mutlow et al., 2004).

Opioid Antagonists

Opioid antagonists have been in use for over 40 years and their use in combination with potent opioid agonists made them powerful tools for wildlife capture. Today, they are used extensively to antagonize the effects of such opioid agonists as fentanyl, etorphine, thiafentanil, and carfentanil. Early antagonists included nalorphine, levallorphan, pentazocine, nalbuphine, and diprenorphine. Some of these antagonists (diprenorphine, nalorphine, levallorphan) act antagonistically at the mu receptor while exhibiting agonistic properties at the two remaining opiate receptor sites. Thus, at higher doses, they cause agonistic effects such as respiratory depression. Naloxone, nalmefene, and naltrexone are termed pure antagonists because they exhibit only antagonistic properties at all three opioid receptors.

Naloxone

Naloxone is a synthetic compound of oxymorphone, a thebaine derivative. Naloxone acts by displacing opioid agonists at the receptor because it binds to the receptor with greater affinity without causing activation (Bryson, 1989). However, because the duration of action of naloxone is generally shorter ($T_{1/2}$ = 30–40 min) than the opioid agonists, the opioid effects may recur as the naloxone wear off (Ngai et al., 1976).

Nalmefene

Nalmefene is structurally similar to naloxone and it has a high therapeutic index (5,000). Depending on the species, nalmefene is from 16–28 times more potent and has a much longer duration of action than naloxone (Dixon et al., 1986). Although nalmefene has been used as an opioid antagonist in wildlife (Kreeger et al., 1987b) and is a superior antagonist relative to naloxone, its use will probably be limited because of the development of an even better antagonist, naltrexone.

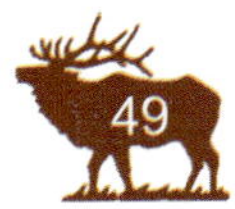

Naltrexone

Naltrexone is a synthetic structural analog of thebaine. Naltrexone appears to have an antagonistic activity 2–9 times greater than that of naloxone (Bryson, 1989). Besides being more potent, naltrexone has a much longer duration of action than naloxone and therein lies its advantage for wildlife use. The reason for this is that naltrexone, like naloxone, undergoes extensive first pass hepatic metabolism, but whereas naloxone's metabolites have little or no antagonistic properties, naltrexone's major metabolite, 6-β-naltrexol, is also a pure antagonist and contributes to opioid receptor blockade. The half-lives ($T_{1/2}$) of naltrexone and 6-β-naltrexol are 4 hours and 13 hours, respectively. An example of the significance of this is that 50 mg of naltrexone will block the pharmacological effects of morphine in humans for up to 24 hours; doubling the dose of naltrexone provides blockade for 48 hours; and tripling the dose provides blockade for about 72 hours (Bryson, 1989). Thus high doses of naltrexone have been shown to be the most effective tool in not only antagonizing the effects of the potent opioid, carfentanil, but also in having the capability of reducing or preventing recycling or renarcotization (Schmitt and Dalton, 1987; Haigh, 1991). Pure opioid antagonists also have advantages over other antagonists such as diprenorphine, nalorphine, and levallorphan in that they have high therapeutic indexes and they are the antagonists of choice for accidental human exposure to the opioid agonists (see *Human Medical Treatment*).

Nalbuphine

An advantage of the less-potent opioid antagonists, such as nalbuphine, is that it can be used to only partially antagonize the opioid effect. Thus, a dose-dependent, graded reversal of opioid anesthesia can be achieved. This has been found useful in Africa for the capture and transport of large, difficult animals like the rhinoceros. Rhinos are initially anesthetized with etorphine and their head and legs secured with ropes. Nalbuphine is then administered at low doses to achieve partial recovery. The rhino becomes ambulatory but somewhat stupefied and seemingly unaware of people or circumstances. It can then be guided or "walked" by the handlers into a transport crate on a truck. The animal is often given no more antagonist so that it can complete the journey in what is equivalent to a tranquilized state (Kock, 2001).

Diprenorphine, Levallorphan, Naloxone, Naltrexone, Nalmefene, Nalbuphine

Mechanism of Action: Competitive opioid antagonists at receptors on synaptic membranes of the amygdala, hypothalamus, and thalamus; primarily act at mu receptors, but may have kappa- and delta-opioid receptor activities.

Elimination: Metabolized by the liver and excreted.

Routes of Administration: IV, IM, SC.

Advantages: Provide rapid and complete opioid antagonism.

- Safe, generally have high therapeutic indices.

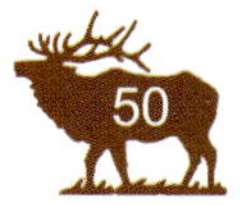

- Can be prepared in high concentrations having long shelf life.
- May be used to attenuate hypotensive shock (not diprenorphine).

Disadvantages: At high doses can cause excitement, incoordination, vomiting, and respiratory depression.

- May affect endocrine systems temporarily.

Formulation: Diprenorphine: 2, 3, and 12 mg/ml solutions.

- Levallorphan: 1 mg/ml solution.
- Naloxone: 0.02, 0.4, 1 mg/ml solution.
- Naltrexone: 50 mg/ml solution.

Comments: Only diprenorphine is a controlled substance (Schedule II). Naloxone, naltrexone, or nalmefene are preferred over diprenorphine. Also, these three antagonists are the only ones suitable for human opioid overdose since they do not possess any opioid agonistic properties.

Alpha-adrenergic Antagonists

Alpha-adrenergic antagonists are used to antagonize tranquilizers such as xylazine, detomidine, and medetomidine. The 1980s saw an explosion of scientific reports when yohimbine, a long-known plant alkaloid, and tolazoline were "rediscovered" as antagonists to xylazine used primarily in the immobilization of ungulates (Jessup et al., 1983; Hsu and Shulaw, 1984; Jacobsen and Kollias, 1984; Allen 1986a; 1986b; Kreeger et al., 1986a), but also of carnivores (Kreeger et al., 1987a).

Yohimbine, Tolazoline

Neither yohimbine nor tolazoline are specific adrenergic antagonists. In addition to adrenergic activity, yohimbine may also have cholinergic, serotonergic, and dopaminergic receptor activity and tolazoline has histaminergic activity. Because of this broad activity, these agents may cause undesirable side effects. On the other hand, tolazoline appears to restore rumen motility faster than yohimbine. For unknown reasons, tolazoline also appears to be more effective than yohimbine in some ungulate species.

Atipamezole

Although effective, both yohimbine and tolazoline will probably be replaced by newer, more specific antagonists. Atipamezole is more potent and more selective than either yohimbine or idazoxan. For example, the $alpha_2/alpha_1$ selectivity ratio for atipamezole is 8,526 compared to 27 for idazoxan and 40 for yohimbine. Atipamezole effectively antagonizes the behavioral, cardiovascular, gastrointestinal, neurochemical, and hypothermic effects of medetomidine (Virtanen and MacDonald, 1987).

Although atipamezole is used for the antagonism of xylazine, detomidine, and medetomidine, only atipamezole should be used to antagonize the effects of medetomidine because medetomidine is a more potent and specific agonist and yohimbine or idazoxan may result in incomplete antagonism.

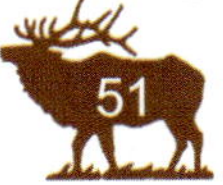

Atipamezole has been used to antagonize the effects of medetomidine in dozens of species and it is generally administered at a dose 5 times higher than medetomidine on weight/weight basis. For example, if medetomidine was given at a dose of 0.01 mg/kg, atipamezole would be given at 0.05 mg/kg. This ratio holds even if medetomidine is used in conjunction with another drug, such as ketamine. Often, the total dose is split with one-half administered IV and the other half given either IM or SC. Atipamezole effectively antagonizes xylazine at a ratio of 1 mg atipamezole for every 10 mg xylazine used (Jalanka and Roeken, 1990).

Yohimbine used with Ketamine Combinations

Early on, many investigators claimed that yohimbine could antagonize ketamine-xylazine anesthesia. However, yohimbine primarily antagonizes only the xylazine component of this combination. Carnivores immobilized with ketamine-xylazine appear to have a residual ketamine effect after yohimbine administration (Kreeger and Seal, 1986b) and yohimbine failed to completely antagonize ketamine-only immobilization of rhesus monkeys (Lynch and Line, 1985) and gray wolves (Kreeger and Seal, 1986b). Because yohimbine does not fully antagonize ketamine, it should not be administered in animals anesthetized with xylazine-ketamine combinations until *at least 30 minutes* have elapsed since the *last ketamine* injection. This is to allow further metabolism of the ketamine component of the combination. If yohimbine (or any adrenergic antagonist) is given when ketamine serum concentrations are still high, the xylazine component will be antagonized resulting in an anesthetic recovery from what is essentially pure ketamine. Such recoveries are characterized by uncontrolled, often violent, body movements and/or severe hyperthermia which can cause injury or death to the animal (Kreeger et al., 1990a).

Yohimbine, Tolazoline, Atipamezole

Mechanism of Action: Displaces adrenergic agonists on pre-synaptic alpha$_2$-adrenergic receptors to allow the release of norepinephrine.

Elimination: Excreted unchanged by the kidneys.

Routes of Administration: IV, IM, SC.

Advantages: Antagonizes effects of alpha$_2$-adrenergic agonists such as xylazine, detomidine, and medetomidine.

- Minimal agonist recycling after their use.

Disadvantages: May be more effective in some species than others.

- High doses may cause tachycardia, hypo- or hypertension, anxiety, tremors, or convulsions.

Formulation: Yohimbine: 1.25, 3, 5, 6.25 mg/ml solutions.

- Tolazoline: 25 and 100 mg/ml solution.
- Atipamezole: 5 mg/ml solution.

Comments: Not controlled substances. High doses (> 0.15 mg/kg) of yohimbine in animals given ketamine may result in an extreme tachycardia and hy-

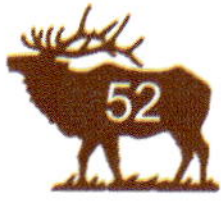

potension due to the synergistic cardioacceleratory properties of both drugs. Tolazoline is also a histaminergic agonist which could result in tachycardia, defecation, vomition, salivation, and edema. Tolazoline appears to provide more consistent antagonism of xylazine sedation than yohimbine in sheep and other ruminants. Bovids in particular do not appear to respond reliably to yohimbine (Klein and Klide, 1989). When using drug combinations consisting of a cyclohexane plus an alpha2-adrenergic agonist, do not administer the alpha2-adrenergic antagonist for at least *30 min after* the last dose of the cyclohexane was given. This is to minimize the residual effects of the cyclohexane which is not affected by the antagonist. Waiting to administer the antagonist hastens and smoothes the recovery process. When cyclohexanes are used, do not expect the animal to quickly return to normal after the alpha2-adrenergic antagonist was given because the animal will usually be ataxic for some time (up to 30 min) due to residual effects of the cyclohexane.

Benzodiazepine Antagonists

Flumazenil and sarmazenil are potent and specific benzodiazepine antagonists that can be used for reversal of the central sedative actions of benzodiazepine agonists (Walzer and Huber, 2002). Benzodiazepine antagonists may be useful in felids (but not in canids) anesthetized with tiletamine-zolazepam because the elimination time of tiletamine in cats is shorter than that of zolazepam (vice versa in dogs). The disadvantage of both antagonists is that resedation tends to occur because they have a shorter half-life than most agonists.

Flumazenil, Sarmazenil

Mechanism of Action: Competitive antagonists with minimal activity at benzodiazepine receptors.
Elimination: Metabolized in the liver and rapidly cleared from plasma.
Routes of Administration: IV, IM, SC.
Advantages: May be used to partially antagonize effects of tiletamine/zolazepam mixtures.
Disadvantages: Has shorter half-life than many benzodiazepine agonists resulting in resedation.
Formulation: 0.1 mg/ml solution.

Non-specific Antagonists

There are two drugs that appear to have some antagonist action against some anesthetics. They are not pure antagonists in that they do not operate on the same receptors as do the agonists. Nonetheless, upon administration a heightened level of arousal is often noted. Although incapable of effecting complete recovery in the anesthetized animal, their use can help diminish some adverse effects of the anesthetic by increasing respiration or cardiovascular function.
4-aminopyridine has been used to antagonize a variety of chemical immobilizing agents. It can be used alone or as an adjunct to other antagonists, such as yohim-

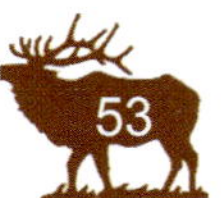

bine. 4-aminopyridine plus yohimbine has been shown to antagonize xylazine immobilization of moose, white-tailed deer, and black-tailed deer (Renecker and Olsen, 1985) as well some domestic species.

Doxapram has been used to "antagonize" xylazine sedation and to shorten barbiturate anesthesia in dogs. Its primary use is to stimulate respiration by affecting the carotid and aortic chemoreceptors and the medullary respiratory centers. It can reverse hypoventilation or apnea caused by several injectable anesthetics other than barbiturates including ketamine, ketamine-xylazine, and ketamine-promazine (Kreeger, unpubl. data) and opioids such as carfentanil (Allen et al., 1991).

4-aminopyridine/fampridine

Mechanism of Action: Antagonizes neuromuscular blockade by increasing release of acetylcholine or other neurotransmitters from presynaptic sites.
Routes of Administration: IV, IM.
Advantages: May partially antagonize effects of $alpha_2$-adrenergic agonists.
Disadvantages: Can cause convulsions, residual sedation and ataxia, muscle tremors and spasms, muscle rigidity, and behavioral alterations.
- Not as efficacious as the more specific $alpha_2$-adrenergic antagonists.

Comments: Because of the specificity, efficacy and fewer side effects of other $alpha_2$-adrenergic antagonists, the use of 4-aminopyridine for the antagonism of $alpha_2$-adrenergic agonists is generally not recommended.

Doxapram

Mechanism of Action: Enhances excitation at all levels of cerebrospinal axis.
Routes of Administration: IV, IC.

Summary of Antagonists

Agonist	Antagonist
Opioids:	
Fentanyl, etorphine, sufentanil, thiafentanil, carfentanil	Naloxone, nalmefene, naltrexone, diprenorphine, nalorphine, nalbuphine
Tranquilizers:	
Xylazine, detomidine, medetomidine	Yohimbine, tolazoline, idazoxan, atipamezole
Diazepam, midazolam	Flumazenil, sarmazenil

All other drugs not listed do *not* have an antagonist.

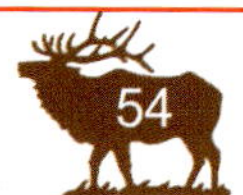

Advantages: Stimulates respiration depressed by several anesthetics.

- May be used to partially antagonize effects of xylazine, cyclohexanes, or barbiturates.

Disadvantages: None when used at recommended doses.

Antagonists: None

Formulation: 20 mg/ml solution.

Comments: Can stimulate respiration for hypoventilation or apnea caused by several injectable anesthetics, including opioids. The duration of respiratory stimulation is brief (5–10 min); doses may be repeated every 15 minutes. Maintenance of respiration should always be done by physical means. Dose at 0.5–2 mg/kg for cyclohexane/opioid respiratory depression; up to 11 mg/kg for barbiturates.

Adjuvants

Adjuvants are substances added to drugs which affect the action of the active ingredient in a predictable way. They may be added to the immobilizing drug "cocktail" to decrease undesirable effects or to heighten desirable effects. Adjuvants should be used conservatively, however, as they are capable of producing undesirable effects of their own if used incorrectly.

Atropine and hyoscine butylbromide are often used to decrease salivation caused by cyclohexanes or increase heart rate depressed by alpha-adrenergic agonists. Hyoscine butylbromide (scopolamine butylbromide) is used more frequently in Africa where it is used on antelope and rhinoceros. Hyoscine is more potent than atropine and affects the CNS more readily. Although high doses of atropine have a sedative effect, hyoscine produces sedation with less side effects. Hyoscine induces a state of catalepsy, photophobia, and mydriasis which facilitates the loading of rhinos in crates after the immobilizing drug has been antagonized (Swan, 1993).

Hyaluronidase is an enzyme that is sometimes mixed with the immobilizing agent in order to increase the absorption rate of the drug. It is most often used on large species, such as elephants and rhinos.

Atropine, Glycopyrrolate, Hyoscine (Scopolamine)

Mechanism of Action: Competitive antagonist of acetylcholine.

Elimination: Excreted unchanged in urine.

Routes of Administration: IV, IM.

Advantages: Decreases salivation caused by cyclohexane drugs.

- Inhibits bradycardia caused by $alpha_2$-adrenergic agonists (e.g., xylazine).

Disadvantages: Higher doses cause tachycardia, mydriasis, bronchodilation, reduction of gastric secretion and motility, and death.

Antagonists: Physostigmine (see comments).

Formulation: 0.2, 0.5, 2, 15 mg/ml solutions.

Comments: Atropine is usually administered as a premedication or immedi-

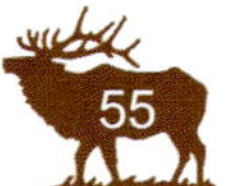

ately following immobilization. The standard dose is 0.04 mg/kg. Atropine and hyoscine use should be carefully justified when used on animals to be released in the wild because these drugs cause prolonged mydriasis (dilation of the pupil) and cycloplegia (paralysis of the pupil) which cause temporary blindness and discomfort. Animals given these drugs should be protected from direct sunlight. Caution should be also used with atropine given to animals immobilized with a cyclohexane–alpha2-agonist mixture (e.g., ketamine-xylazine) then given an alpha2-agonist (e.g., yohimbine). Ketamine, yohimbine, and atropine will all increase heart rate; the synergistic effect of all three drugs may cause extreme tachycardia with a concomitant fall in blood pressure because the heart is beating too rapidly to allow adequate filling and compression (Kreeger et al., 1987a). Glycopyrrolate's anti-sialagogue (salivation) activity is about five times more potent than atropine. It also appears to have little cardiac or ocular effects. Physostigmine antagonism should only be used when atropine overdosage is life-threatening or the animal exhibits extreme agitation and is at risk of injuring itself. Give 0.02 mg/kg IV slowly; if no response, repeat dose every 15 min.

Hyaluronidase

Mechanism of Action: An enzyme that randomly cleaves b-N-acetyl-hexosamine-[1-4] glycosidic bonds in hyaluronic acid, chondroitin, and chondroitin sulfates.

Elimination: Excreted unchanged in urine.

Routes of Administration: SC, IM.

Advantages: Increases absorption rate of other drugs.

Disadvantages: Higher doses can cause tissue damage.

Antagonists: None.

Formulation: Several formulations; most are lyophilized powders from bovine or sheep testes. Available in 300–15,000 units/mg.

Comments: Hyaluronidase acts as a spreading agent to promote diffusion. It has been used to increase drug absorption and thus decrease induction time when used with succinylcholine and opioids in species such as white-tailed deer, moose, and elephants (Morton and Kock, 1991; Kock et al., 1993). Must be kept refrigerated until ready for use. The suggested dose rate is 5,000 IU per 2 ml dart. The dose is a factor of dart volume and irrespective of the type of drugs used. If the dart is not used in 6 hours, either replace the hyaluronidase or discard the dart.

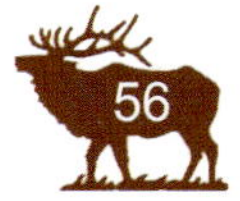

Equipment Used for Animal Capture

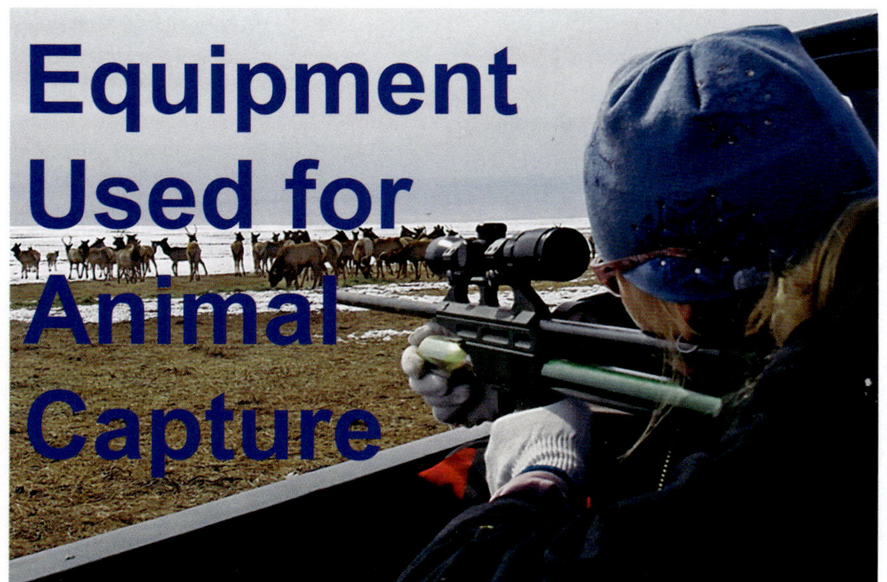

This section discusses the equipment for delivering drugs to animals and for monitoring the effect of those drugs. All of the drug delivery equipment described herein can effectively be used to immobilize animals – given the appropriate conditions. That is, there isn't one type of system that can be used on all animals at all times. This fact is sometimes difficult to accept, particularly when buying decisions are limited by fiscal constraints. You possibly can get by with only a 13-mm (0.50-caliber) dart rifle having variable power settings. The well-equipped professional, however, will have multiple dart guns (pistol, CO_2 and .22 cal. rifles), pole syringe, and blow pipe (or powered blow pipe).

Another mistake (in our opinion) commonly made in the selection of equipment is a reluctance to spend money on it. There are many ways to make your own darts from syringes, blow pipes from conduit, dart guns from modified shotguns, etc. In all probability, none of this equipment is as good as what is commercially manufactured. Manufacturers have spent years and significant amounts of money in the development of their products. The result of their efforts is good quality equipment that performs as expected, is fairly rugged and dependable, and is backed by a knowledgeable service department. This is not an advertisement for the manufacturers listed in this section; this is experience. We've tried all the "cheap" ways of making our own equipment and we don't use any of it anymore. Professionals use professional equipment.

Syringes and Needles

Hand syringes and needles are the basis for any drug delivery system. Not only are they used to administer drugs directly to restrained animals, they are also

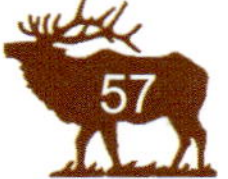

used for measuring and loading immobilization drugs into other delivery devices such as darts. Syringes and needles are also required for taking blood samples and administering antibiotics and other drugs. Most syringes and all needles are sterilized and disposable, and they are intended to be used once and discarded. Some syringes are designed for multiple uses, but these are not commonly used for animal immobilizations.

You can never have enough syringes in your kit, because you will consume them rapidly. For example, a syringe used to measure or administer an anesthetic shouldn't be used to administer any antagonist (there could be residual anesthetic in the syringe). Also, any syringe that is used for an intravenous injection in one animal should not be used on another animal because it will be contaminated with blood.

In some cases, however, syringes may be used more than once if they are intended to be used to withdraw the same drugs needed for filling darts. Such syringes should be labeled with permanent marker identifying the drug (e.g., "carfentanil"). Syringes are available in an assortment of sizes, but 1 ml, 3 ml, 5–6 ml, and 10–12 ml are the most commonly used. Larger sizes ($\geq$ 20 ml) are useful for taking blood samples from large animals when required for multiple assays.

Likewise, you can't have too many needles on hand. Needles should be used to withdraw and/or administer only one type of drug; not be used on more than one animal; and should *not* be reused for any reason. The basic philosophy here is to avoid cross-contamination of either drugs or animal fluids.

Needles also come in a variety of gauges (inside diameter measurement) and lengths. The *larger* the gauge, the *smaller* the inside diameter. For example, a 25-gauge needle is much smaller than a 16-gauge. Needle lengths can vary from 15.9 mm to >75 mm. Needle sizes that you will find most useful are 20 (or 21) gauge by 25 mm (1 inch), 18 gauge by 25 mm or 38 mm (1 or 1.5 inches), and 16 gauge by 25 mm or 38 mm (1 or 1.5 inches).

Manufacturers: Several worldwide
Specifications: Syringes: 1–60 ml, plastic, sterile, disposable or reusable.
• Needles: 27 to 12 gauge, sterile, disposable. The *smaller* the gauge, the *larger* the inside diameter of the needle. Needles come in various lengths, the most common being 25 mm or 38 mm (1 or 1.5 inches).
Range: Arm's length.
Operation: Insert a needle (without syringe) into the space at the top of the drug vial to equalize air pressure. This may be particularly important when vials have been at different altitudes. Be careful that a pressurized vial does not eject drug uncontrollably. Attach syringe to needle or use a new needle.
• Attach a new needle to the syringe by pushing then twisting to assure a secure fit so that the needle does not remain in the animal after injection. Re-

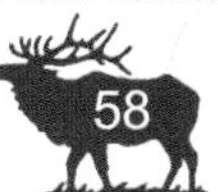

move the protective needle cap by pulling straight away from the syringe (do not pull and twist, or the needle will come off also).

- To avoid developing a vacuum within the vial, withdraw the syringe plunger to a point equal to the desired drug volume. Insert the needle into the drug bottle and inject the air from the syringe into the bottle, but do not over-pressurize. This step may not be necessary when withdrawing small volumes (< 5 ml). Hold the bottle upside down and withdraw the appropriate drug volume as indicated on the syringe barrel gradations. Before withdrawing the syringe and needle, turn the bottle upright. This will avoid fluid contact with the rubber stopper, which may leak after several punctures. It is not uncommon to get a droplet of drug on the rubber after withdrawing the needle if the bottle is kept upside down, which could be hazardous to the handler. After withdrawing the needle from the bottle, carefully expel any air from syringe to obtain an accurate amount of the drug, but avoid spraying the drug and perhaps causing accidental human exposure.
- For intramuscular (IM) injections, use a large-bore needle (16–18 gauge) on large (≥ 30 kg) animals and smaller needles (20–25 gauge) on smaller animals. Inject the drug into the muscle mass quickly and withdraw. However, if animal restraint permits, first withdraw the plunger slightly to verify that the needle is not in a vein (blood will appear in the syringe), and then inject the drug. Be sure to avoid major nerves and bone – know your animal's anatomy!
- For intravascular (IV) injections, use smaller needles (18–21 gauge) as appropriate for the size of the animal. Common veins for IV injection are the

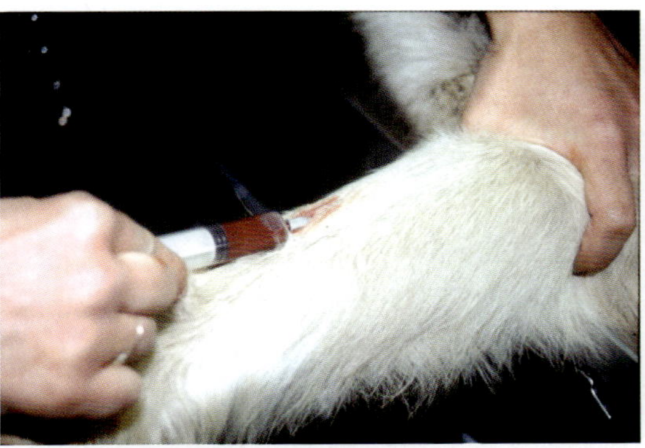

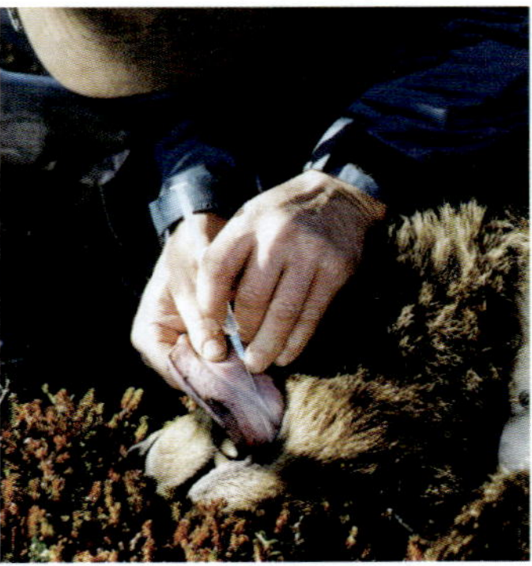

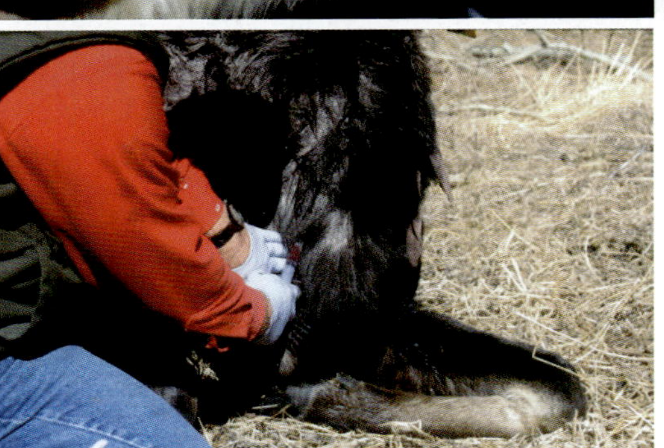

Syringes are used for many purposes, such as administering drugs and taking blood samples. Upper left: withdrawing blood from the saphenous vein of a wolf. Upper right: administering drugs via the sublingual vein in a bear. Lower left: intravenous drug administration via the jugular vein in a moose.

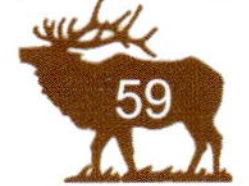

cephalic and jugular. Other veins accessible in larger animals are the femoral, running along the inside of the thigh, and the saphenous, located along the outside of the hock.

- Compress the vein with your fingers or hand so that blood is blocked from returning to the heart. Then insert the needle into the turgid vein on the side of the compression away from the heart.
- For superficial veins, such as the cephalic, insert the syringe at approximately a 10–20° angle to the surface of the animal; for deeper veins, such as the jugular or proximal femoral veins, increase the angle of penetration. For superficial veins, the bevel of the needle should be facing up toward the surface of the animal so that the needle opening does not become occluded by the walls of the vein.
- When the needle slips into the vein, pull back the plunger slightly to withdraw blood to verify that the needle is in the vein, release the proximal vein, inject the drug (or withdraw blood for a sample), and then remove the needle.
- Lastly, compress or rub the injection site to hasten coagulation.

Comments: Keep the protective cap on the needle until just before you intend to inject the drug – syringes with exposed needles just look for a place to inject themselves! Also when replacing the needle cap, it is good practice to brace both hands to steady them. This is particularly true when using potent drugs. Poking oneself with a needle is the number one cause of accidental human exposure (Petrini et al., 1993).

Pole Syringes

Pole syringes are exactly that – a syringe on the end of a pole. These are very useful tools with broad applications, such as administering drugs to trapped or caged animals or safely giving additional drugs to animals not completely immobilized, but approachable. Pole syringes are usually limited to administering ≤10 ml of drug because the animal will usually not hold still long enough to give larger volumes. Homemade pole syringes can be easily and cheaply constructed, but none seem to work as well as the manufactured versions.

Manufacturers: Dan-Inject, Advanced Injection Systems, Paxarms, Zoolu
Specifications: Syringe volumes range from 2.5–20 ml. The syringe portion can vary from disposable to heavy-duty reusable syringe barrels. Needles are usually conventional needles designed for hand syringes. Shafts can be constructed of aluminum, steel, or composites and they usually are capable of adding extensions to increase pole length.
Range: 0.5–3 m, depending on shaft length
Operation: It is usually preferable to withdraw drugs with a conventional hand syringe and then using that syringe to transfer the drug into the pole syringe. Drugs may also be withdrawn directly from a vial using the pole syringe if care is taken and accurate drug volumes can be assured.

- Use a large-bore needle (16–18 gauge) on large (≥ 30 kg) animals and smaller needles (20–25 gauge) on smaller animals. Inject the contents IM rapidly and

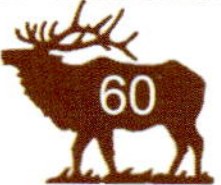

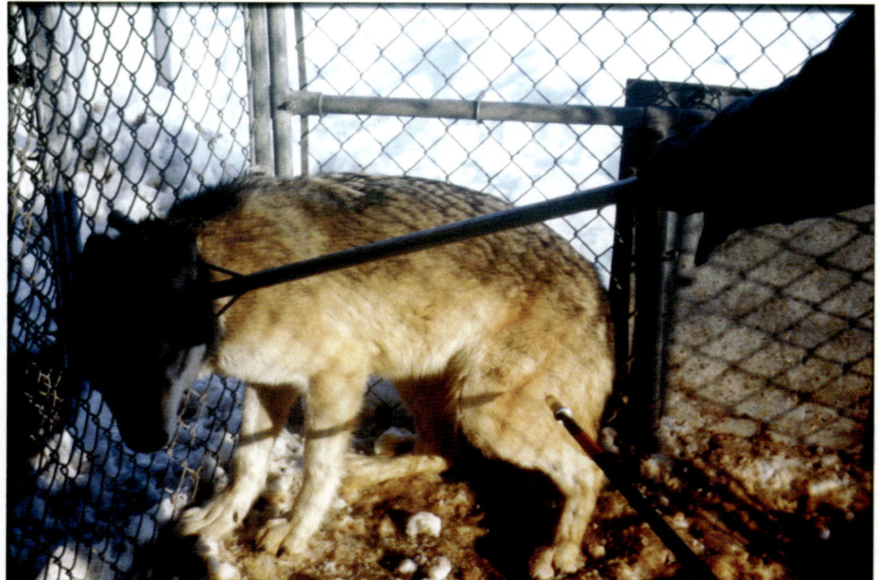

Pole syringe used to administer immobilizing drugs into hip of captive wolf being restrained by forked stick; even wild wolves can be handled in this manner.

firmly and withdraw before the animal can bite or kick the pole. The muscle masses of the hindquarters are the preferred sight for injection, but the shoulder muscles of larger animals can also be used.

Comments: Long pole syringes (≥ 3 m) are too difficult to aim accurately (your arm movements are greatly magnified) and are best used on larger animals with their larger target areas. Try to make the first "stab" count. Many animals quickly learn what you are trying to do and are very adept at grabbing the pole out of your hand (e.g., bears in culvert traps, elephants in trucks). To avoid double dosing captive animals that are moving around, mark them by adding a piece of foam rubber to the needle on the pole syringe. This foam should be about the same diameter as the syringe and the same length as the needle. Dip and saturate the foam with gentian violet. The animal will thus be marked when injected.

Remote Delivery Systems

Most animal immobilizations are done “remotely,” that is, there is no direct contact between you and the animal. Darts, propelled by a variety of means, are the usual means of delivering drugs remotely to animals. Systems capable of propelling darts are termed *remote delivery systems* (RDS) and they are defined as “mechanical devices capable of administering a single dose to an unrestrained animal, usually by means of a ballistic projectile.”

Remote drug delivery dates to pre-Columbian times when aboriginal natives of Africa and South America dipped arrows, spears and blow darts in preparations of muscle-paralyzing drugs derived from plant and animal sources (Bush, 1992).

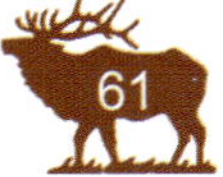

Modern delivery systems have their genesis in the 1950's when the first projectile dart capable of delivering a liquid drug was reported (Crockford et al., 1957). This dart became the predecessor of darts still used today. Many types of delivery systems were developed since then, but only a few proved reliable and versatile enough to survive competition in a limited market. There are both advantages and disadvantages of RDS used to administer drugs.

Advantages of RDS

Specific animals can be targeted.

As opposed to baiting or trapping, animals can be selected and captured based on sex, size, age, or status.

Drugs can be administered on a body weight basis.

Biologists familiar with a species can often estimate body weights of free-ranging animals quite accurately. Fairly precise doses can then be administered under field conditions if necessary for research purposes or efficacy.

A wide range of volumes can be delivered.

Depending on the projectile type and volume, liquid doses ranging from a few μl to as much as 25 ml can be delivered.

Some RDS can treat, mark, or biopsy individual animals.

Some projectiles can be equipped with marking dyes and others can deliver electronic identification devices along with the drug. Biopsy darts take a skin and underlying tissue sample, then fall out. These darts are used for DNA analyses.

Disadvantages of RDS

The target animal must be first located and then approached closely.

Under most circumstances, animals must be to within 75 m or less for projectile to be effective. Many species are secretive and extremely difficult to locate, let alone approach closely.

Many RDS can only be used on larger animals.

RDS using projectiles are not terribly accurate and the preferred target area on smaller animals may only be a few square centimeters. The shot could either be misplaced, causing injury or death, or it could miss the animal entirely. Even if placed correctly, the impact energy or penetration depth could be injurious or lethal to smaller animals. As a general working rule, only animals weighing > 15 kg (33 lb) should be targeted when powered (e.g., CO_2 or .22-cal. systems) RDS are used. If possible, use blow pipes for smaller animals.

RDS are inherently complex.

There are many system variables that can fail or affect successful delivery. A good rule is: *everything that can possibly go wrong with RDS, eventually will!*

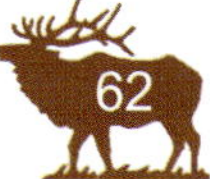

Many RDS are noisy.

Some RDS may spook other animals after the first shot is fired rendering subsequent shots at other animals difficult or impossible.

Training and experience is necessary.

RDS should not be used without some degree of formal instruction by experienced practitioners of remote delivery techniques, and RDS should never be used without fairly intense practice by the user in order to assess the performance of the device prior to using it on an animal.

Blow Pipes

Blow pipes, or blow guns, are useful devices for delivering small volumes of drugs at short to medium ranges. They operate by propelling a dart through a pipe or tube either by rapid expulsion of one's breath, by compressed air, or by CO_2. Blow pipes using compressed air or CO_2 are usually referred to as *powered blow pipes* and they are capable of greater ranges than conventional pipes using lung power.

Conventional (lung-powered) blow pipes consist of one- or two-piece aluminum tubes measuring up to 2 m. Most propel 10 mm-diameter darts having a maximum capacity of 3 ml. Their effective range is limited (< 20 m). Blow pipes are quiet and they usually cause little trauma to the animal because the dart neither

Adjustable CO_2-powered blow pipes are versatile, low-impact devices for darting animals under a variety of conditions up to ranges of 30 m.

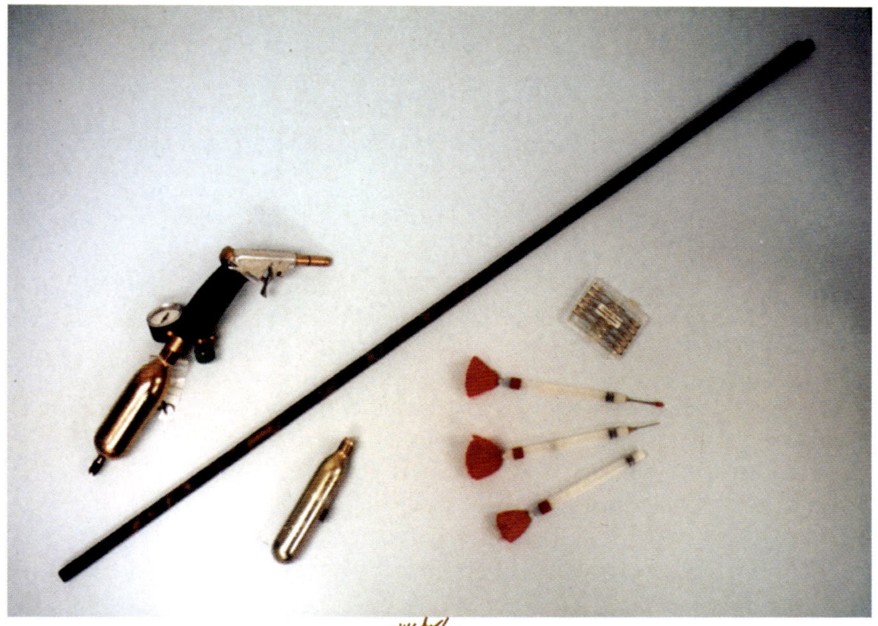

strikes the animal with much velocity nor does the method of dart operation cause injury (see later); animals as small as 3 kg (6.6 lb) can be safely treated. Blow pipes are used primarily on captive animals, but they can be used effectively on free-ranging animals under the right circumstances, such as treed animals or animals approached closely by vehicle (Brockelman and Kobayashi, 1971; Haigh and Hopf, 1976).

Powered blow pipes consist of an aluminum tube connected to a pistol grip containing a metering device and reservoir. Air is compressed by a foot pump connected by a hose to the pistol grip. After the desired pressure has been built up in the reservoir, the hose can be disconnected. When the trigger is pulled, the compressed air is released, propelling the dart. Similarly, some powered blow pipes use CO_2 cartridges that feed into a reservoir that can be adjusted to either increase or decrease the amount of pressure. These devices have a wide effective range from 1–30 m because the dart flight distance is proportional to the pressure built up in the reservoir. Powered blow pipes propel the same type of lightweight darts (10–11 mm diameter; 1–3 ml volume) as do conventional blow pipes and they are preferred for delivering larger volumes at longer distances.

Manufacturers: Dan-Inject, Pneu-Dart, Telinject
Specifications: Dart volumes usually range from 1–5 ml.
Range: Up to 30 m for powered pipes.
Operation: For lung-powered pipes, sight over the end of the pipe at the intended muscle mass, inhale through nose (don't swallow the dart!), insure tight seal between lips and mouthpiece, expel air sharply but not explosively (excessive force causes dart to bounce off animal).
- For powered blow pipes, aim like a pistol. Squeeze the trigger quickly (slow trigger pull may prevent the air/gas from being released in a burst).

Comments: The longer the blow pipe the greater the potential distance the dart can be propelled; however, long pipes are unwieldy and more difficult to aim.
- Use of blow pipes to deliver potent drugs should be avoided to prevent accidental human exposure.
- Blow pipe use in some states and countries, such as Canada, is prohibited without a special permit. If in doubt, check it out.

Longbows/Crossbows

Arrows or crossbow bolts can be modified to administer a liquid product up to 5 ml upon impact (Anderson, 1961; Short and King, 1964; Hawkins et al., 1967). Longbows and crossbows, though, have generally fallen out of favor because of impact trauma. If used at all, they are usually limited to larger animals.
Manufacturers: Palmer (arrow adapters)
Specifications: Syringe capacity probably limited to < 5 ml
Range: Potentially 100 m, but accuracy usually limits range to < 50 m
Application: Should be limited to IM injection of large (> 100 kg) animals

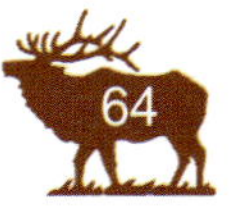

Operation: A dart is attached to end of arrow using an adapter. The dart contents are expelled by powder charge upon impact (also see *Darts*). Aiming is similar to a bow or crossbow, but practice is necessary to determine range and accuracy.
Comments: Bows are seldom used now since dart guns are more accurate and less traumatic. Due to the velocity, weight, and inaccuracy of arrows, mortalities with longbows can be as high as 33% (Hawkins et al., 1967).

Dart Guns

The most widely used RDS are dart-shooting guns. Some dart guns have been constructed by modifying existing shotguns, rifles, pistols, pellet rifles, or pellet pistols; other guns are almost entirely custom-designed and manufactured for this purpose. Dart guns propel darts by either the gas generated from a .22 caliber blank cartridge, compressed CO_2, or compressed atmospheric air. Dart-firing guns are the most versatile of the RDS. Effective ranges can be as far as 75 m and possibly up to 100 m for larger animals having larger target areas. Dart volumes can be as much as 25 ml, although these larger, heavier darts drop rapidly after leaving the barrel making long-range, accurate shots difficult.

All darts, of course, begin falling as soon as they leave the barrel, but small darts (1–2 ml) traveling at higher velocities shoot "flatter" and farther than do large darts. Guns can be equipped with a variety of sights including adjustable open sights, rifle scopes, dot sights, laser aiming devices, and light-intensifying scopes (so-called "night scopes" or "starlight scopes").

Open sights are preferred by many professionals, especially those who dart animals from helicopters. Rifle scopes make aiming easier, unless the animal is at close range where the magnification of the scope makes it difficult to identify where on the animal you are aiming. Also, by closing the opposite eye when aiming through a rifle scope, other animals can easily walk undetected into your shot.

Each of the three types of dart gun propulsion systems have advantages and disadvantages (Table 3). These properties are listed to help first-time users decide on an appropriate gun. In our opinion, there is no one perfect dart gun for all circumstances. If finances limit your arsenal, choose a .22 caliber-powered gun having a range-adjusting device. Even then, the final choice of a dart gun is much like the choice of a conventional firearm; it is a highly personal decision comprising a mix of objective analysis and emotional attraction all tempered by fiscal reality! The criteria analyzed for each system include:

Maximum Effective Range

This is the maximum distance at which the dart can be safely and effectively delivered. The range of most guns can be decreased from this maximum either through the use of a built-in metering device which directs little to all of the gas

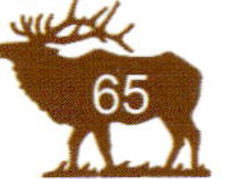

to the dart; by using different strengths of propellant (e.g., .22 blanks); or by pushing the dart further down the barrel to reduce its velocity and thus its range. This criterion does not include dart pistols which have ranges of < 20 m.

Dart Volume

Dart volumes range from 1–25 ml, however, not all guns are capable of delivering this full range of dart sizes.

Availability of Propellant

This category rates the ease of obtaining the propellant from local suppliers.

Temperature Sensitivity

The vapor pressure of some gases (e.g., CO_2) is temperature dependent. Darts may travel less far due to decreased vapor pressure when cold. In extremely cold conditions, some guns may barely function without warming the gas.

Impact Injury

The impact energy (kinetic energy or KE) of the dart striking the animal is a function of its mass and velocity ($KE = 1/2\ MV^2$). It is a common misconception that light darts always cause less impact, and thus injury, to the animal than heavy darts; light darts fired at high velocities actually strike the animal harder (Table 4). All darts that use an explosive charge to inject the drug cause hemorrhage and hematoma. Misplaced shots can break bones or even kill the animal (Thomas and Marburger, 1964).

Report

Muzzle report can cause problems in darting either captive or free-ranging animals. For some animals, this noise can be more disturbing then getting struck with a dart. Disturbed animals are then more difficult to approach for another shot or the entire group of animals may run away.

Maintenance

Some guns need to be cleaned frequently in order to remain operable.

Performance Reliability

Guns are classified regarding consistency of shot-to-shot performance.

Ease of Use

Guns are classified relative to their simplicity of operation or ease of use under field conditions.

Overall Versatility

The above categories are evaluated to arrive at a subjective opinion on the overall versatility of the propulsion system.

Table 3. Characteristics of powered dart guns.

Category	.22-cal.	CO_2	Compressed Air[a]
Maximum Effective Range (m)	90	75	40
Dart Volume (ml)	1–25	1–10	1–10
Availability of Propellant	High	Medium[b]	n/a
Temperature Sensitivity	None	Medium	None
Impact Injury	High[c]	Medium	Med-Low
Report	Med-High	Med-High	Med-Low
Maintenance	High	Low	Low
Performance Reliability	Medium	High[d]	High
Ease of Use	High	High	Med
Overall Versatility	High	High[e]	Med

[a]Compressed air in this context refers to rifles that are pumped by hand or foot to fill a reservoir. The advantage of compressed air systems is that no additional propellant is required (i.e., CO_2 cylinders, .22 blanks), so that you never run out of power. The main disadvantage is that compressed air does not develop the propulsive force, and thus distance, comparable to the other systems.

[b]There are two general types of CO_2 cylinders: threaded and unthreaded. Most sporting goods stores carry the smaller, unthreaded CO_2 cylinder, but the larger, threaded CO_2 cylinder may be very difficult, if not impossible, to procure when working in rural areas. Most rifles accepting the threaded cylinder also have adapters for the unthreaded cylinders.

[c].22 blanks come in a variety of strengths. Charge strengths are coded by different colors, usually brown, green, yellow, red with red being the most powerful. Darts propelled with either the yellow or red charges are capable of causing significant injury or death, but all charges can cause injury if fired at too short of a range or at too small an animal.

[d]CO_2 cartridges generally provide consistent performance except when the propellant runs low. There is only a subtle drop in performance between the last acceptable shot and the next shot where the dart drops precipitously due to a rapid drop in pressure. Experienced shooters often only allow a fixed number of shots per cartridge before changing cartridges even though some shots remain. This is usually not a problem with CO_2 guns equipped with pressure gauges. The gauge indicates how much pressure is in the reservoir. If the gauge needle does not reach the desired level, then there is inadequate pressure to propel the dart the desired distance.

[e]Distance-adjustable CO_2 guns are probably the most versatile (and most expensive) RDS.

Table 4. Kinetic energy produced by darts traveling at different velocities

Weight (lb)	Velocity (ft/sec)	Kinetic Energy (ft-lb)
0.022	200	13.7
0.033	200	20.6
0.022	300	30.8

Kinetic energy calculated by KE =1/2 MV^2. Non-metric values are reported in order to compare with other ballistic data.

Manufacturers: Dan-Inject, Gerwig, Palmer, Paxarms, Peter Ott Co., Pneu-Dart , Telinject, Zoolu Arms.

Specifications: Darts propelled by compressed air, CO_2, or .22 caliber blank cartridge.

Range: 1–90 m (but see comments), depending on dart size (1–25 ml) and propellant charge.

Operation: Choose dart and needle sizes based on amount of drug required and size of animal.

- Follow manufacturer's directions for loading darts (also see Darts below).
- Check that dart is not bent or deformed by inserting into the end of barrel. The dart should slide back and forth easily. If the dart sticks, discard it and reload another dart. Tight-fitting darts tend to leave the barrel at much higher velocities and could cause injury to the animal.
- Load dart into breech; be sure safety is on (treat these guns like firearms!).
- Select powder charge (brown, green, yellow, red) and/or adjust variable range device.
- Aim at large muscle masses.

Comments: Regardless of system used, always practice with the anticipated dart size at the anticipated ranges. Use darts loaded with water as opposed to empty darts in order to mimic actual weight and thus flight characteristics. Make a chart of dart sizes, distances, and pressure settings. Attach this chart to the dart gun; this will save a lot of guessing in the field.

An example of a lightweight dart travelling at high velocity. This wolf was killed when a dart penetrated the thorax and struck the heart.

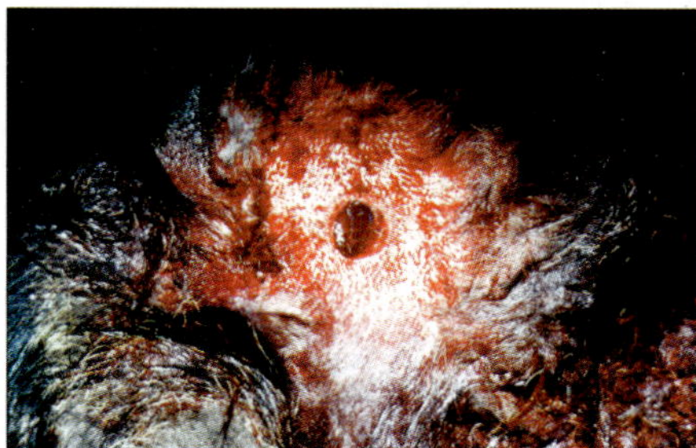

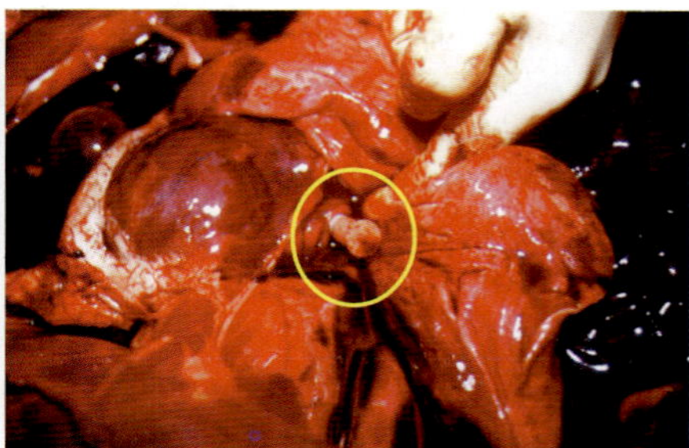

- The trajectory of most darts is characterized by a rapid drop during the final one third of the flight path and you should familiarize yourself with this phenomena prior to field use. Also, despite manufacturer's claims, the realistic maximum effective range is around 50 m.
- In .22-caliber guns, "green" charges are the most commonly used; "brown" charges may be too weak and the "red" charges are potentially too damaging to the animal regardless of range.
- Do not use blanks with wads in Pneu-Dart® guns because the wads will obstruct the gas ports. The .22-caliber guns should not be used at ranges < 10 m unless they are equipped with devices that meter the amount of gas delivered to the dart.
- Cold temperatures (< 0° C/32° F) can decrease the effectiveness of CO_2-powered guns.
- Darts fired at high velocities can imbed in muscle, break bones, or kill the animal (Thomas and Marburger, 1964) – a word to the wise.
- Never leave an unused dart inside the gun. Remove the dart and release the gas pressure or unload the .22 blank. Darts left in the gun not only can be accidently discharged, but they can corrode the barrel if they leak drugs.
- The tip of the dart needle can be bent over the center line of the bevel to reduce plugging (Henwood and Keep, 1989).

Darts

Darts can be thought of as "flying syringes," consisting essentially of a needle, body, plunger, and tailpiece. They differ in the manner in which the plunger is pushed forward to inject the dart's contents and in the materials of construction. Darts discharge their contents either by expanding gas from an explosive powder charge, compressed air, butane, or chemical reaction (acid-base). The mechanisms which enable the darts to discharge their contents upon impact range from moderately simple systems having few parts to complex systems of intricate design and operation. Dart bodies can be made of aluminum or synthetic polymer (polypropylene, polycarbonate, etc.). Dart tail designs range from elaborate fins molded from synthetic polymers to simple strands of yarn stuffed into the back of the dart.

Dart needles can be as long as 75 mm with a 2.16 mm inside diameter. Darts using explosive charges expel their contents in < 0.001 sec and thus require large-bore needles to allow the rapid expulsion of liquid. Needles are designed to either expel contents from the standard front opening (end port) or through a side port with the front opening occluded. End-port needles expel their contents more rapidly than do side-port needles, but large-bore needles can become plugged with a core of tissue when they penetrate hide and muscle (Henwood and Keep, 1989).

Needle shafts can either be smooth or be equipped with a variety of barbs or

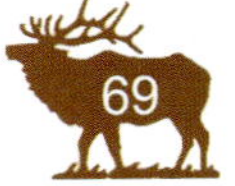

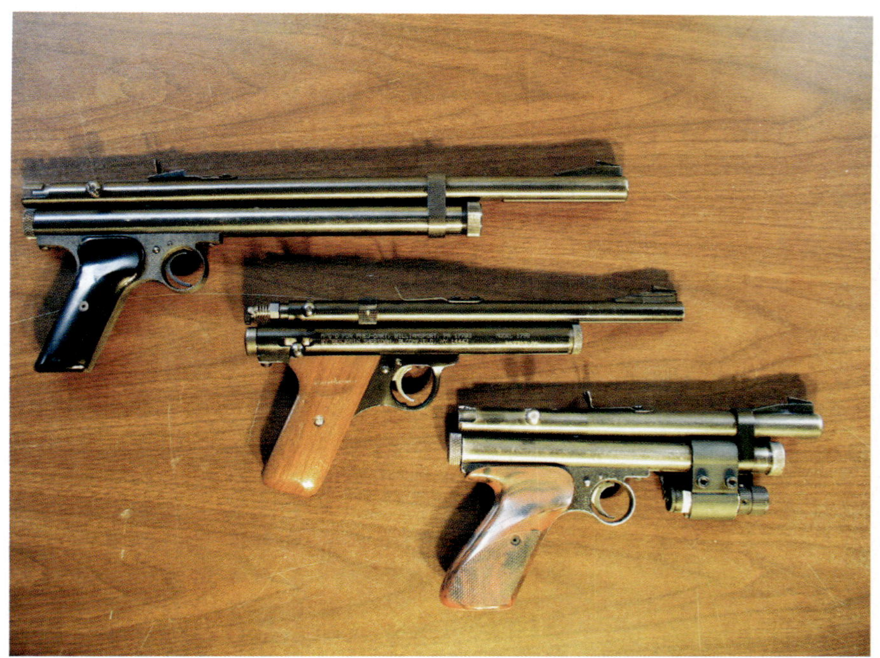

CO_2-powered pistols are very useful for short-range (< 25 m) or restricted (e.g., bear dens) situations. All the above pistols can be adjusted, to a certain degree, for distance and fire 13 mm (0.50 cal.) darts. From top: Cap-Chur Mid Range Projector; Pneu-Dart model 179B; Cap-Chur Short-range Projector (fitted with laser sight).

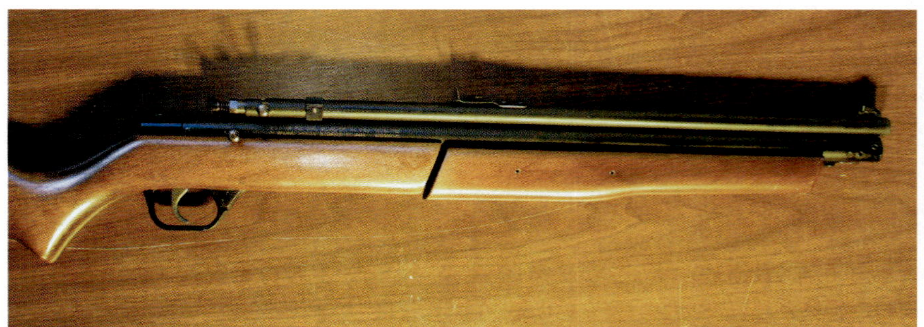

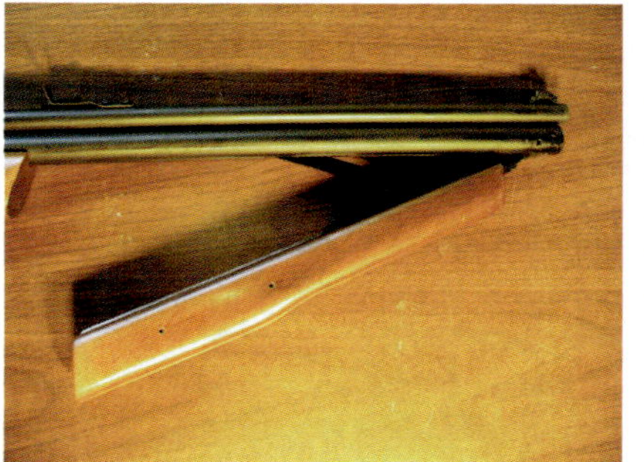

An often overlooked, but still quite useful, dart rifle is the Pneu-Dart model 178B. Propulsion is by air being compressed via a forearm pump (left); the more pumps, the further the dart flies. Distance for most 13 mm (0.50 cal.) darts is < 30 m. The rifle is short, lightweight, and totally self-contained. That is, there are no external propulsion devices (such as CO_2 cylinders or .22 blanks) to lose, forget, or deplete.

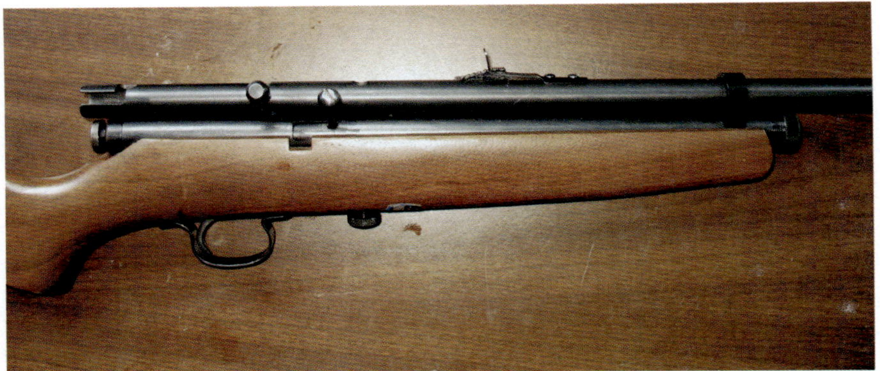

The Cap-Chur Long Range Projector is a CO_2-powered dart rifle that is inexpensive, but rugged and reliable. It is capable of projecting small-volume (e.g., < 3 ml) 13 mm (0.50 cal.) darts up to 40 m. It has two power settings.

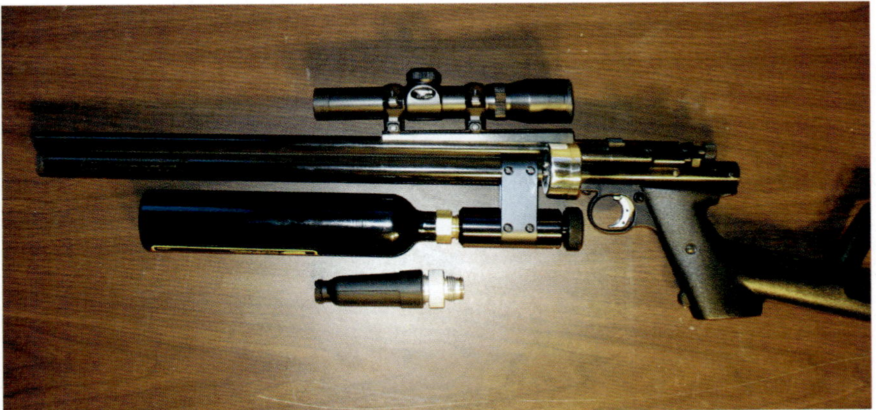

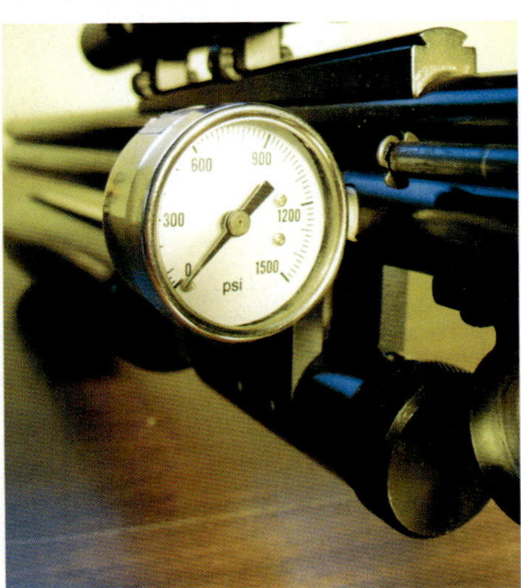

The Pneu-Dart Oplus-XT is perhaps the least expensive CO_2-powered rifle/pistol capable of full power adjustability. Theoretically, once a power setting has been made, the gun will automatically recharge to that same setting after the dart has fired. This rarely happens, however, and the the power has to be "fine-tuned" for the subsequent shot. It does have the advantage of accepting large, rechargeable CO_2 tanks, such as those used with paintball guns, as well as the more common, smaller CO_2 cylinders. It is equipped with Pneu-Dart's Airflow Control Port which serves to eliminate the "tail kick" of darts exiting the barrel to increase accuracy. In our experience, this has been a surprisingly accurate rifle for its lightness and small size.

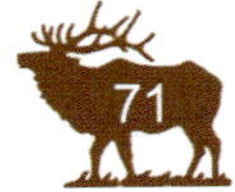

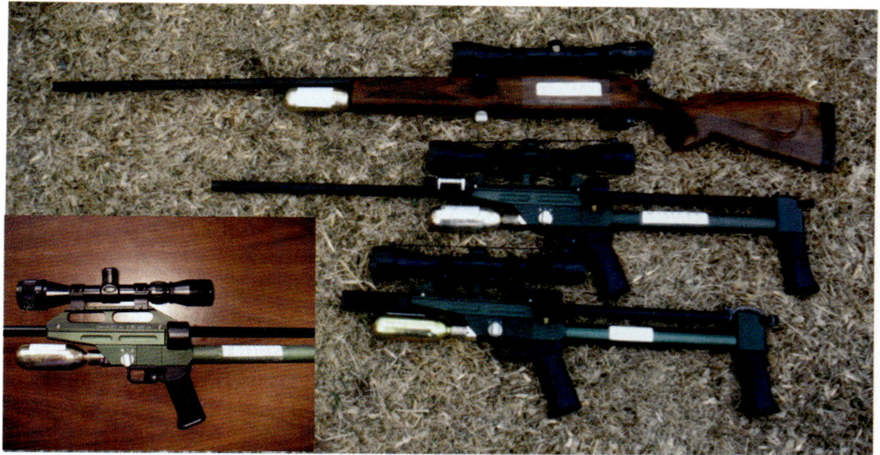

Dan-Inject produces a line of high quality CO_2-powered dart rifles. The three models are (from top): IM, JM, and JM Special. The JM Special can be fitted with a longer barrel so it functions more like the JM model. All the rifles are fully adjustable for distance with a knob (inset, A) that both increases and decreases pressure indicated on a gauge (inset, B). Rifles come with 11 mm barrels which fire compressed-air darts, but 13 mm (0.50 cal.) barrels can be ordered which can fire darts made by other manufacturers. For example, one of the authors (TK) almost exclusively fires 13 mm Pneu-Darts from Dan-Inject rifles, which he has found to be highly accurate and consistent. Between the two authors of this manual, they have fired virtually thousands of darts through Dan-Injects without a problem. None of the models have fixed sights, which may be a disadvantage to those who don't like rifle scopes. While the JM and JM Special models are somewhat clumsy to point, the IM model is a pure joy.

Pneu-Dart recently introduced its response to high-end adjustable CO_2-powered dart rifles with the X-Caliber below. The X-Caliber incorporates many features new to the field. Darts are loaded from a rear, pivoting breech (inset, upper right) and power is adjusted by an acorn-type knob in front of the receiver (inset, lower left). The location of this knob allows power adjustment without having to lower the gun and, thus, taking your eyes off the target. Other features included interchangeable 11- and 13-mm barrels, protective gauge housing, and ability to be powered by a variety of CO_2 or nitrogen gas tanks.

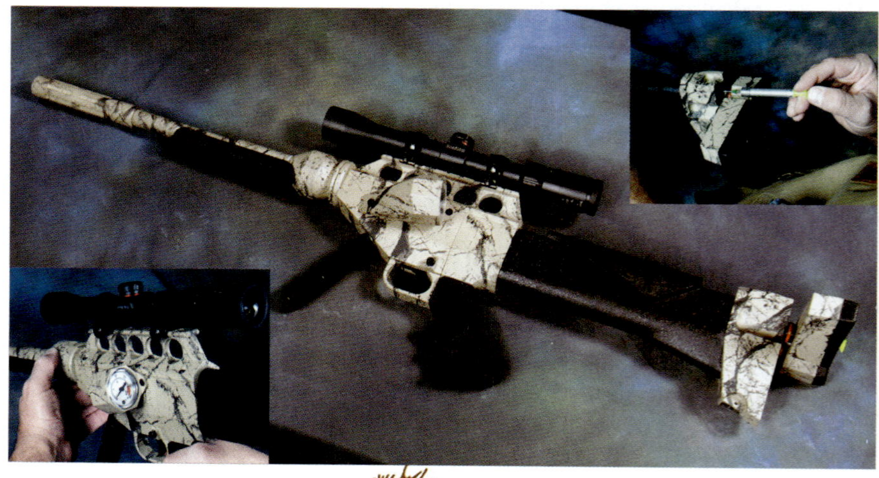

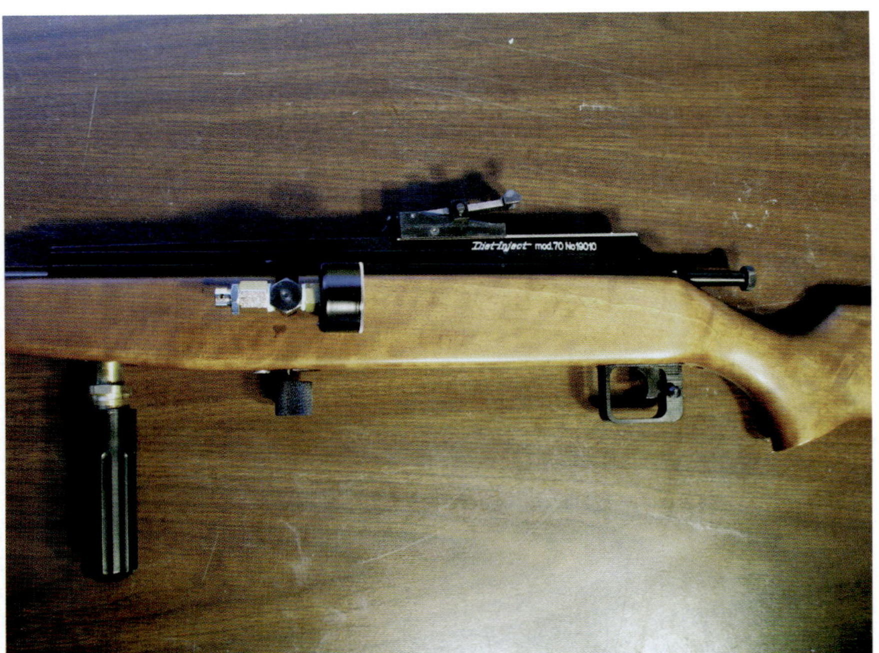

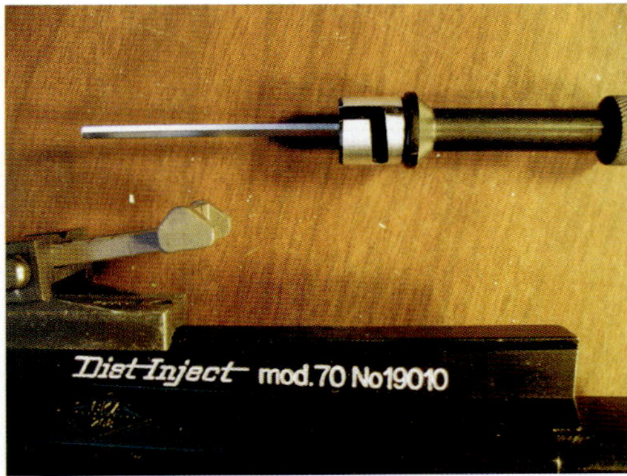

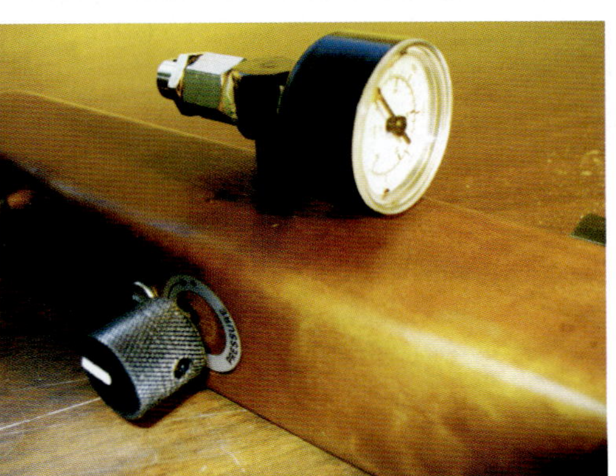

Another high quality, fully adjustable CO_2-powered rifle is the Dist-Inject model 70. It can be equipped with 11 and 13 mm (0.50 cal.) barrels, which can quickly and easily be changed using an allen wrench tool cleverly incorporated into the breech plug (left). The Dist-Inject is a bit more versatile than the Dan-Inject because it comes equipped with adjustable open sights, but can be equipped with a variety of optical sights as well. Subjectively, it also seems to shoot more quietly and "softer" than the Dan-Inject. Its biggest drawback, however, is the adjusting knob (lower left) which is maddeningly difficult to precisely select the desired pressure on the gauge. Dist-Inject can supply an eccentric knob which improves precision, but it is still not as quick and easy to adjust as other manufacturers of high-end CO_2-powered rifles.

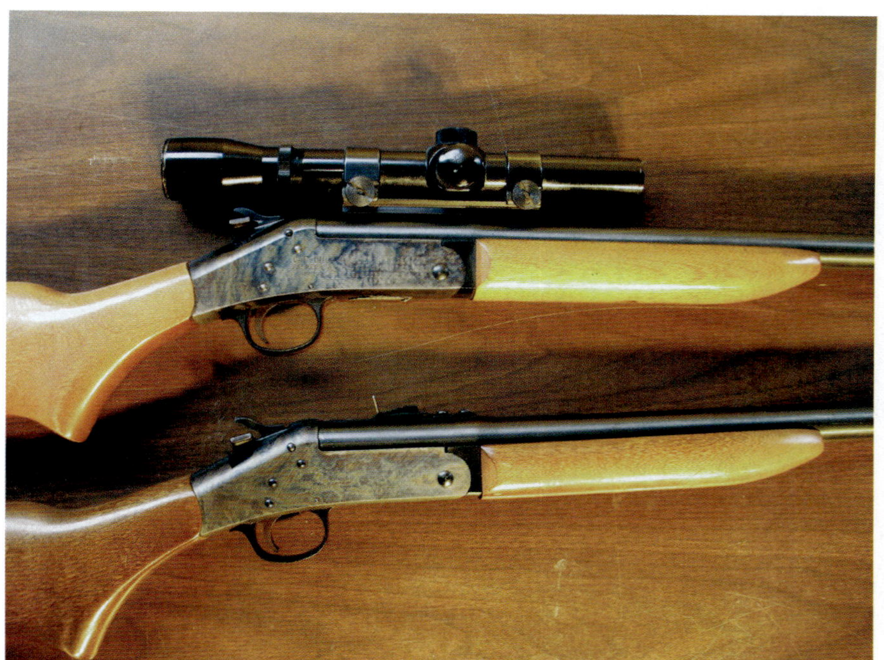

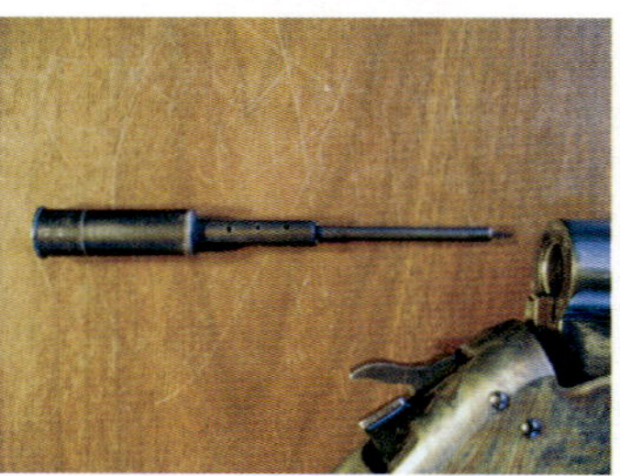

The Cap-Chur Extra Long Range Projectors above were the first dart rifles made. Using .22 blanks to propel 13 mm (0.50 cal.) darts, these rifles are simple, extremely rugged, and inexpensive. They are excellent for helicopter darting. Their biggest drawback is the lack of adjustability, other than to use different .22 blanks. There are at least five different power levels of .22 blanks available from different manufacturers, so there is some flexibility. Always carry extra charge adapters (right) because they are easy to drop, never to be found.

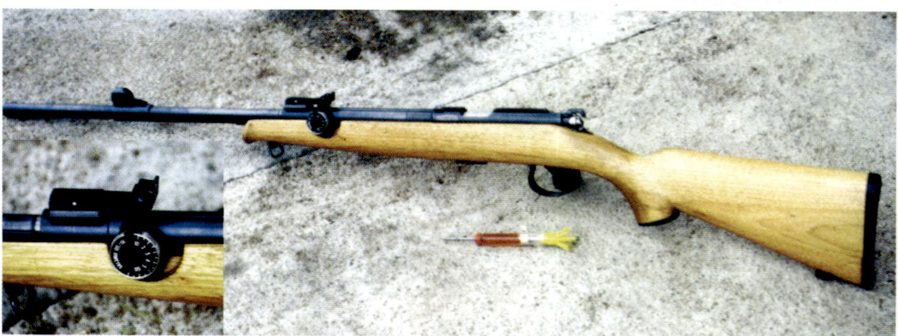

The Paxarms is another .22 blank-powered dart rifle made in New Zealand. It is well made, but ridiculously expensive compared to other .22 rifles. It has multiple power settings and different diameter barrels are available. When turning the adjusting knob to the desired power setting, the rear sight also raises or lowers (inset), improving accuracy. This is a very accurate rifle when using the lightweight Paxarms dart. The Paxarms dart, unfortunately, is expensive, complex, and slow to prepare for use.

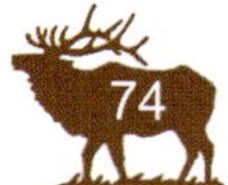

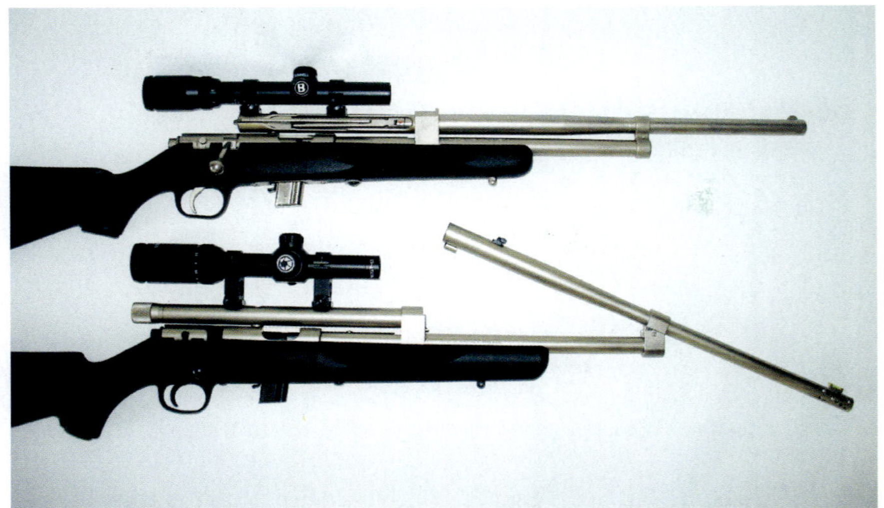

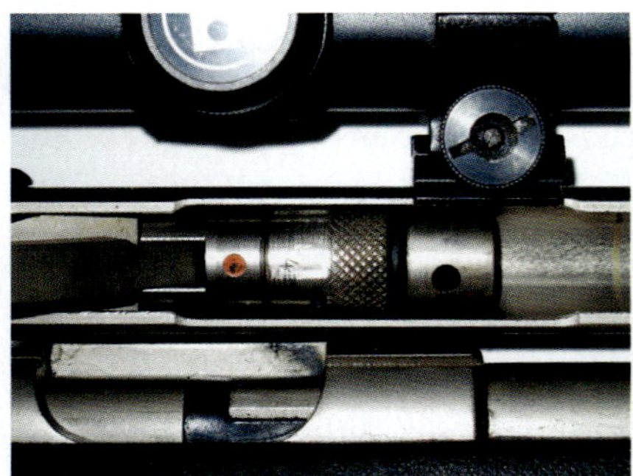

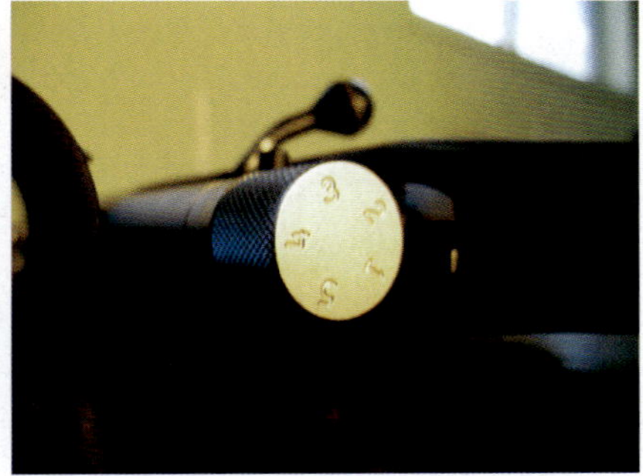

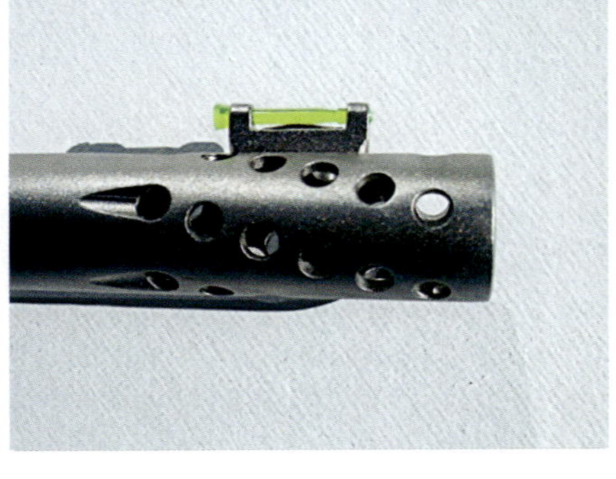

The Pneu-Dart models 193 and 389 (top) are two relatively inexpensive, high quality .22 blank-powered dart guns. Both have five power settings. These power settings, combined with the different-powered .22 blanks, plus varying dart sizes offer a great deal of flexibility. Such flexibility, however, can be confusing because there can be at least 275 combinations of charge, setting, and dart size! Most users of these rifles stick with one charge size (e.g., green) and only one or two dart sizes and learn how the rifle performs at the different power settings. The power setting for the model 193 is incorporated into the bolt face (upper left), which can be slow to adjust and difficult to see. The newer model 389 has the adjustment knob at the rear of the barrel (upper right), making it much easier to see and to change. The model 193 loads from the breech which limits dart sizes somewhat. However, unfired darts can be easily retrieved by opening the bolt and tilting the gun upwards. The model 389 has a break open barrel allowing insertion of the largest darts. The 389 also incorporates Pneu-Dart's Airflow Control Port (below right) which serves to eliminate the "tail kick" of darts exiting the barrel to increase accuracy.

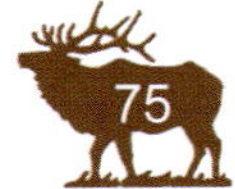

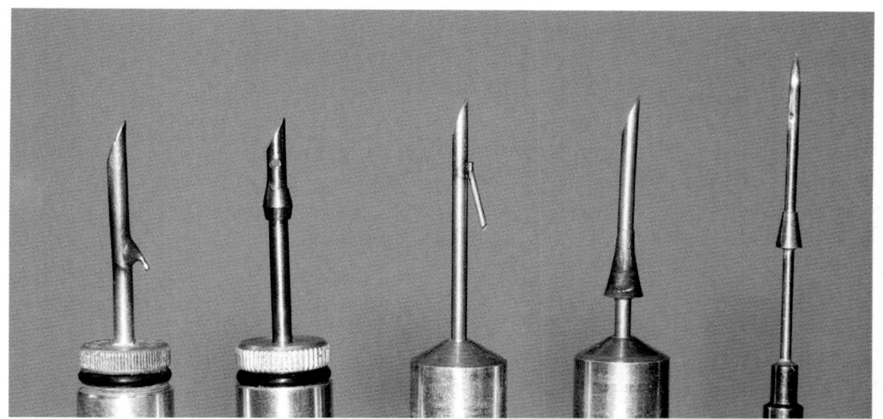

Examples of dart barbs. From left: short soldered wire, collar, long soldered wire, biodegradable, machined.

collars to retain the dart in the animal. Smooth-shafted needles are used to deliver the drug and then fall out on their own, eliminating the need to capture the animal to remove the dart. Such darts are commonly used to remotely treat or vaccinate, but not necessarily to capture, animals. If the dart contents are under high pressure, however, smooth-shafted needles can "rocket" back out of the animal due to the expulsion of the liquid and therefore not inject any or all of the substance.

Some needles are equipped with small collars that barely secure the dart in the animal, but will eventually fall out on their own. One company (Pneu-Dart) manufactures a gelatin collar that is rigid when dry, but dissolves when it comes into contact with tissue fluids. This dart stays in the animal long enough to insure complete expulsion of the contents, but it will eventually fall out on its own.

To securely retain the dart in the animal, either wire barbs or metal collars are used. These darts require manual removal from the animal. Experimentation with retractable barbs has been successfully accomplished, but these are not commercially available (Van Rooyen and De Beer, 1973; Smuts, 1973). Barbs probably should be used when the dart contains opioids because barbed darts will stay in the animal which will allow recovery of the dart as opposed to it falling out somewhere. Most wildlife agencies prefer to recover opioid-containing darts, even when discharged. Although some recommend using a scalpel to remove barbed darts, keep in mind that the larger, cleaner wound created by the scalpel will bleed more and actually may take longer to heal than if you simply yank the dart out. Regardless, all darted animals should receive antibiotics.

Darts have been devised that mark as well as treat the animals that they hit. Darts can be equipped with dye-filled bladders fixed to the base of the needle which burst upon impact to mark the treated animal (Bush, 1992). These bladders also

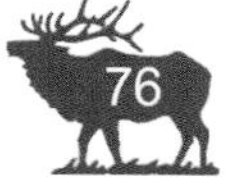

serve as cushions to decrease the impact trauma of the dart. Another dart (Pneu-Dart) utilizes a "piggy-back" tailpiece containing the dye or paint that breaks loose from the dart body upon impact to spray the target area.

Darts have can also be equipped with small radio transmitters enabling location of animals that have run off after being darted with immobilizing drugs (Nielsen, 1982; Lawson and Melton, 1989). The effective transmitter range of these darts is usually < 300 m, but the growing technology of small transmitters that can withstand impact energy holds promise of extended ranges.

There are advantages and disadvantages of each dart injection system. Below, we discuss some dart characteristics and the relative merits of the different systems.

Injection Speed

All darts which use a powder-based injection system will inject their contents explosively (e.g., < 0.001 sec). All compressed air or butane gas injection systems inject their contents in approximately 0.5–1 second. If injection speed is rapid, the underlying tissue will always be injured (e.g., hemorrhage). However, if injection speed is slow, some animals (e.g., carnivores, primates) may have time to remove the dart before all the contents have injected.

Weight

Lightweight darts may cause less impact when they strike the animal (but see Table 4), however, they may be more subject to wind drift or prop wash from helicopters. The compressed air or butane gas injection darts are the lightest, but the plastic, small-volume (≤ 1.5 ml), explosive-charged Pneu-Darts are almost as light.

Volume

Dart volumes of the compressed air or butane gas injection systems range from 1–10 ml whereas explosive-charged darts can hold up to 20 ml (e.g., Cap-Chur®).

Reliability

Reliability, as applied to darts, is defined as the probability of the dart functioning correctly by injecting the drug into the animal. Darts which use a powder-based injection system tend to be fairly reliable thesedays (this wasn't always the case!). Compressed air or butane gas injection systems may lose pressure through leakage before hitting the animal.

Contents Under Pressure

The contents of some darts are pressurized by compressing air or injecting butane into them when they are initially loaded. This type of dart is more prone to leaking or spraying its contents than darts which do not develop any expulsion pressure until they strike the animal (e.g., powder). *Few people use these pressurized darts with opioids.* Some of our most adrenal gland-stimulating mo-

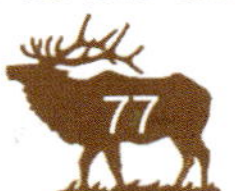

ments have occurred while pressurizing darts containing opioids and having the needle come off, spraying several people in the vicinity!

Manufacturers: Dan-Inject, Palmer, Paxarms, Pneu-Dart, Dist-Inject, Telinject
Specifications: Darts expel contents by compressed air or powder charge. Dart bodies constructed primarily of plastic or aluminum.
Operation: *Powder Charge Darts (Cap-Chur®)* – Check that the aluminum dart body is not distorted from previous firings by inserting it into the end of the dart gun barrel and insuring that the entire dart body moves freely back and forth.

- Be sure that the inside of the dart body is clean. Lubricate the plunger with a good quality, water-resistant lubricant such as silicone. Move the plunger back and forth within the dart body to lubricate the body walls. Position the plunger with its open end all the way to the rear of the dart body.
- Insert the powder charge into the plunger base making sure that the movable striker in the charge *faces towards the rear* of the dart. The striker end of the powder charge can be determined by poking it slightly with a pen (or other pointed object) which causes the striker to move. Be sure that the powder charge matches the volume of dart body (i.e., 1–3 ml, 4–10 ml, etc.).
- Screw in the tail piece into the dart body which moves the plunger and its charge forward.
- Load the front of the dart with the desired volume of drug. The drug level should just reach the bottom of the screw threads at the front of the dart body; if the drug volume does not reach this point, top off with sterile water.
- Screw in the appropriate-sized needle for the target animal; the larger the animal, the larger the needle length (but use good sense and knowledge of your animal's anatomy for exceptions to this rule).
- Although the vacuum formed by the fluid in the dart body should prevent any drug from leaking out of the needle (even when held upside down), jarring the

Components of a Palmer Cap-Chur dart. From left: tail piece, explosive charge, plunger, dart body, needle. Inset: internal components of explosive charge. Explosive powder is contained in the front of the charge. When the dart strikes the target, the brass plunger moves forward, igniting the powder. The expanding gases resulting from the explosion rapidly discharge the dart's contents.

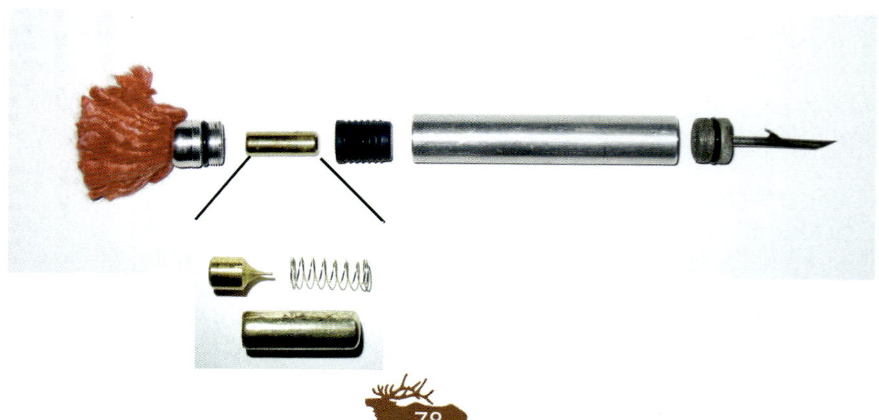

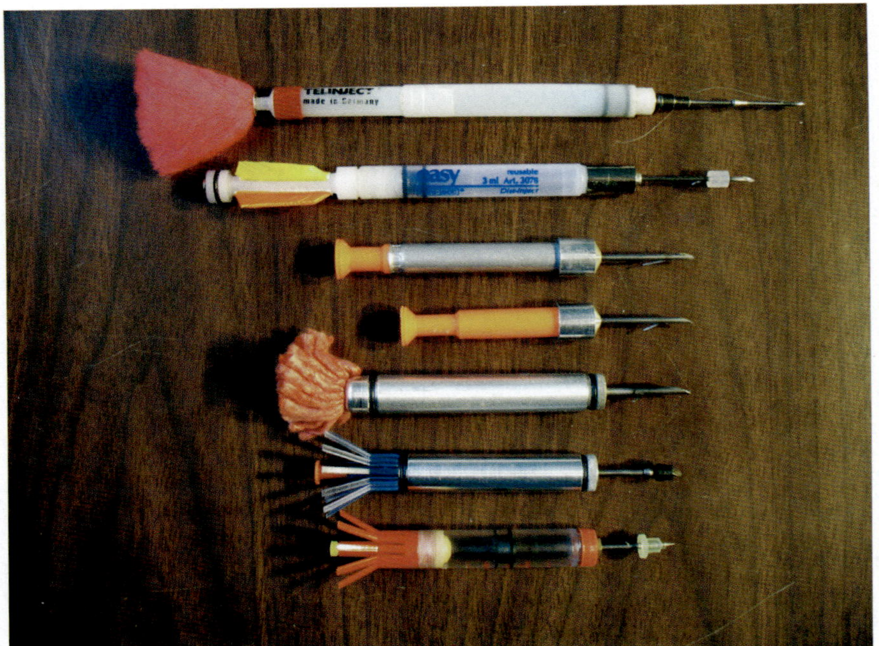

Examples of darts with method of discharge in parentheses. From top: Telinject (compressed air), Dist-Inject (butane gas), aluminum Pneu-Dart (powder), plastic Pneu-Dart (powder), Cap-Chur (powder), Cap-Chur (compressed air), Paxarms (compressed air). Although the compressed air/butane darts tend to weigh the least, the plastic Pneu-Darts are almost as light.

dart has been known to spill drug. If this could be a problem, seal the needle opening with petroleum jelly.

Pneu-Dart ®Darts – These darts are single-use darts using either a powder charge or an acid-base mixture to expel the dart's contents. The acid-base darts mix only after the dart strikes the animal and they have a slower injection time than do the powder charged darts. In either case, these darts are loaded through the needle since the darts are of one-piece construction.

- Withdraw the desired drug volume in a syringe. It is important to load these darts *using a needle that is longer than the dart needle*. This loading needle must be small enough to fit within the inside diameter of the dart needle; usually a 38-51 mm (1.5–2.0 inch), 18-gauge needle works fine for this. If the loading needle is shorter that the dart needle, drug will be expelled back out of the dart needle.
- Using the loading syringe, slowly push the drug into the dart body. Again, if the drug volume is less than the dart volume, top off with sterile water.
- The needle can be plugged with petroleum jelly to prevent leakage.
- Older Pneu-Dart® darts had a safety wire wrapped around the tailpiece. This wire *must be removed* prior to loading into the dart gun or else the dart will not discharge its contents upon impact.

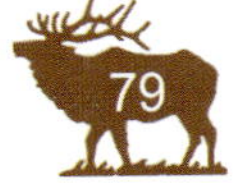

Compressed Air Darts (Dan-Inject, Dist-Inject, Telinject) – These darts can be thought of as two syringes joined at their bases. Each half has a plunger; one that moves readily and another that seals against the syringe walls and is used to deliver the drug. The half with the freely movable plunger is the rear portion.

- If the plunger in the front chamber is all the way forward, hold the dart upside down so that the movable plunger in the rear chamber falls forward and inject air into the front end of the dart using an empty syringe fitted with a coupling device. The injected air moves the front plunger into the appropriate position for the amount of drug being delivered. For example, you can push the plunger to the 2-ml mark in a 3-ml dart.
- Load the front portion of the dart with the desired drug volume, insuring that the drug fills the chamber (again, use sterile water to top off).
- *Firmly* attach the dart needle so that it doesn't come off under pressure.
- Occlude either the end of the needle or its side port, as appropriate, with the needle plug supplied.
- Insert the front of the dart into a container, such as a test tube, to contain any accidental spraying of drug when the dart is being charged.
- Holding the dart with the needle pointing up, insure that the movable plunger falls to the bottom of the rear chamber.
- Pull back the plunger on an empty 10–20 ml syringe fitted with the coupling device and attach this syringe to the rear of the dart.
- Compress the syringe's air into the dart; the movable plunger will seal the rear opening of the dart as air pressure builds up in the rear chamber.
- When there is firm resistance on the plunger of the syringe loaded with air, quickly remove the syringe from the dart.
- Attach the dart's tailpiece.
- Carefully check the needle and plug for any sign of leakage.
- Oftentimes, there is a little air bubble in the front drug chamber which will compress or disappear when the dart has been properly charged, thus providing a handy visual cue as to the dart's readiness.
- Keep the dart stored in a tube until just prior to use.

Compressed air dart and syringe with coupling device attached used to pressurize dart: a. tailpiece; b. air chamber; c. drug chamber; d. needle; e. silicone needle plug.

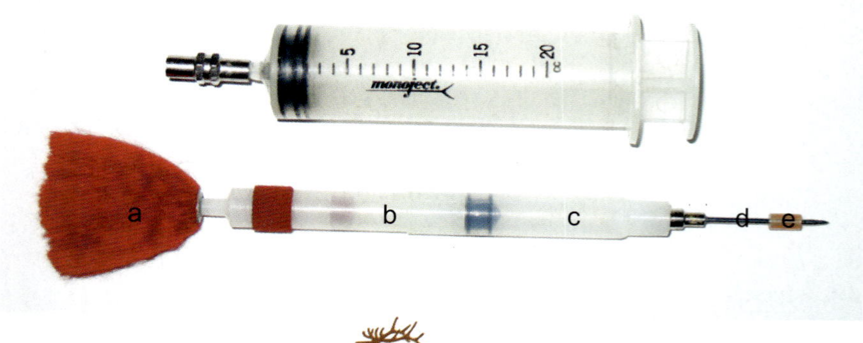

Comments: Some dart needles discharge from the end and others from the side port. End-port needles discharge rapidly but they must strike the animal almost perpendicularly in order to stick. This is due to the end being capped by a silicone plug, which acts as a "bumper" should the dart strike at an angle. Side-port needles slide the silicone plug up the shaft to cover the opening, thus exposing the sharp needle tip and increasing the probability of the dart penetrating, even when striking at an angle. Side-port units inject their contents more slowly than end-port needles.

- Use sterilized dart needles (store in alcohol or commercial solution or autoclave and securely wrap).
- Darts which employ a powder charge to expel dart contents do so very rapidly (< 0.001 sec) often resulting in severe underlying tissue damage.
- If possible, flush injection site with diluted povidone-iodine (10%) or chlorhexidine diacetate (0.05%) solution. Antibiotic "teat tubes" used to treat mastitis in dairy cows can be useful for treating dart wounds since they are equipped with a rounded, plastic "needle" that can be safely inserted into the dart hole. Regardless if the dart wound can be treated or not, all animals being struck by a dart should be given an appropriate dose of antibiotic, such as penicillinase-resistant penicillins, cephalosporins, tetracyclines, or trimethoprim-sulfadiazine.
- When loading multiple darts, use a test tube rack or wooden block with drilled holes to support the darts.
- Be careful when removing darts not only from the animal, but also from the ground, trees, etc. Pressure may still remain inside the dart causing drug to be sprayed uncontrollably when removed (we all know this from personal experience!).
- Place used darts in safe containers, such as cigar tubes, sharps containers, or the plastic packages in which they were sent from the manufacturer.
- Clean reusable darts by submersing them in cold water while disassembling them, which dilutes any residual drugs; be sure to wear gloves when doing this.
- Despite many opinions and unsubstantiated claims, there does not appear to be any difference in induction times among the different dart type injection methods (Kreeger, 2002).

Range Finders

Range finders that utilize the principle of reflected laser beams to accurately measure distance are essential items of equipment when using dart guns. Inaccurate range estimation is probably the single major cause of missed shots. Range finders are accurate to within ± 1 m. We never use dart guns now without the concurrent use of a range finder. The combination of a laser range finder and a highly-adjustable CO_2 dart gun dramatically reduces missed shots. We highly recommend calibrating dart guns with known ranges and different dart sizes before the capture event. That is, set up a target range with measured distances of 10, 20, 30, 40, and 50 m (or farther). Fire the darts that you most commonly use (e.g., 1, 2, 3 ml) at each range. Write down the power settings for each dart size and each

range where the dart is accurately and consistently hitting the target. Prepare a chart from this information and attach it to your dart gun. In the field, all you have to do is quickly get a range from the range finder, look at the chart, and set your gun for the appropriate distance.

A word of advice; once you go through all the trouble of calibrating the dart gun to distance and settings, *believe* these data when in the field! It seems to be human nature to rely more on one's own estimation of distance and dart trajectory than real data. For example, the range finder says the animal is 30 m away; your calibration chart for a 2-ml dart indicates that the gun should be set at 5 bars on the gauge; you look at the animal; you think that maybe it is really 32 m away; you increase the power setting to 5.5 bars; and the dart flies over the top of the animal! Also, be aware that drastic changes in altitude will affect the dart's point of impact. A gun sighted in at 2,000 m will shoot low at sea level (0 m) and high at 4,000 m.

Manufacturers: Several world-wide (Bushnell, Leupold, Nikon).
Specifications: Distance measured by reflected laser beam. Accurate to within ± 1 m.
Range: 10–1,000 m (see comments)
Operation: Locate target through viewfinder.
- Place crosshairs in viewfinder on target.
- Press power button until a distance reading is obtained.
- Read distance and adjust dart gun accordingly.

Comments: Although dart guns are rarely employed at distances greater than 75 m, there is some opinion that range finders capable of measuring distances up to 1,000 m operate more accurately and quickly than less powerful range finders

All adjustable dart guns should be calibrated for various dart sizes and ranges. Make a chart of these data and attach it to the rifle. This chart, combined with a range finder, will reduce misplaced as well as missed shots.

Yards	15	20	25	30	35	40
1 ml	4	5	6.5	7	8	9
1.5 ml	4	5	7	7.5	8.5	10
2 ml	5	6	7.5	8	9.5	11

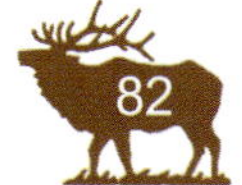

(i.e., 400-m range finders). Whether this is true or not remains to be determined. The capability of reflecting the laser beam depends upon the reflectivity of the target. In general, most animals reflect the beam well. If you cannot get a good reading on the animal itself, try aiming the device at an object close to the animal.

Laser Sights

There are variety of laser sights manufactured for firearms that can be adapted to dart guns. Once sighted in, all you have to do is place the beam of the laser on the desired target and pull the trigger; you don't even have to aim. Unfortunately, laser sights are only effective in low light or dark conditions. They can be very useful for darting bears or wolves in dens when attached to a dart pistol. There are several manufacturers worldwide.

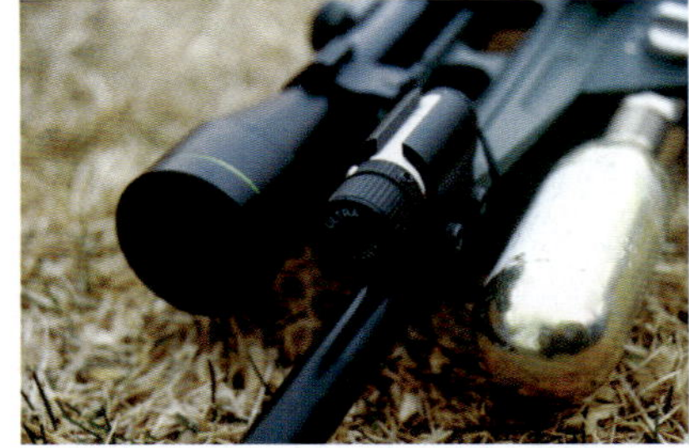

Dot Sights

Dot sights are electronic pointing devices that project a dot or circle on a glass viewing lens, but do not magnify the target and no beam is projected onto the target. They are designed to be used with both eyes open with the dot becoming part of the field of vision and superimposed on the desired target. They are quite effective for short ranges, helicopter darting, or at night, but may not work as well as telescopic sights for longer ranges. Dot sights can hardly be seen on very bright days, especially with snow cover. There are several manufacturers and styles.

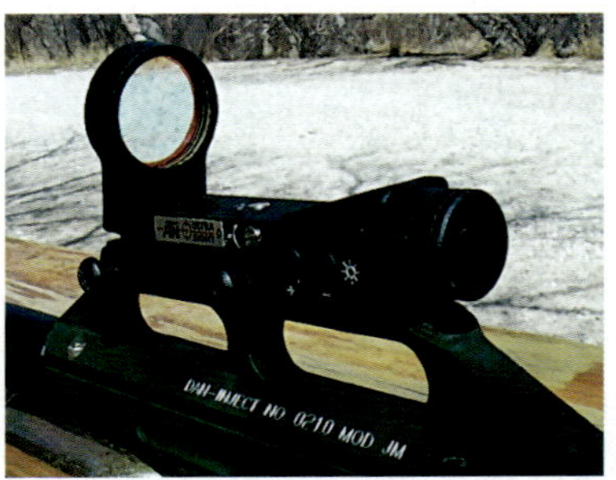

Monitoring Equipment

Thermometer

Many immobilizing agents disrupt an animal's thermoregulatory capability. Additionally, the physical exertion of being chased or restrained prior to immobilization often results in elevated body temperatures. Either hyper- or hypothermia can kill an animal. Thus, monitoring rectal temperatures is important. The glass mercury thermometer is basic equipment, although readings are slow to develop and they are prone to breakage. Inexpensive, electronic thermometers sold in human drug stores are

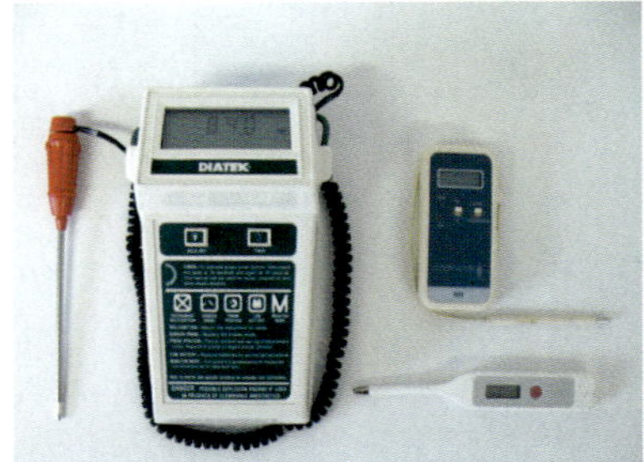

rapid and accurate, but batteries have a habit of expiring at the most inopportune moments. They are generally not moisture resistant. Some types have a long, flexible temperature probe (pictured) which allows greater probe insertion for large animals, which is essential to obtain accurate temperatures, or protection of the electronics box by placing it away from the animal.

Pulse Oximeter

Pulse oximeters are electronic devices that measure the percent oxygen saturation of hemoglobin in the blood (SpO_2). They provide information on the respiratory function of the animal which can be useful because many immobilizing drugs depress respiration. Many oximeters can be used in the field.

Oximeters use a clip that can be attached to the tongue or other thin, non-pigmented tissue or a rectal probe to measure SpO_2. The SpO_2 is determined by passing two wavelengths of light, one red and one infrared, through body tissue to a photodetector. The oximeter processes these signals, separating the time invariant parameters (tissue thickness, skin color, light intensity, and venous blood) from the time variant parameters (arterial blood and SpO_2). Because oxygen-saturated blood predictably absorbs less red light than oxygen-depleted blood, oxygen saturation (as well as the pulse) can be calculated.

In human medicine, patients are monitored with oximeters while anesthetized and they are usually given supplemental oxygen when the SpO_2 falls below 90% in order to insure adequate oxygenation of tissue (particularly of the central nervous system). This "90%" rule is usually employed for anesthetized animals

Pulse oximeter measuring oxygen saturation on a European lynx. The upper reading (86) is the percent oxygen saturation and the lower reading (84) is the pulse.

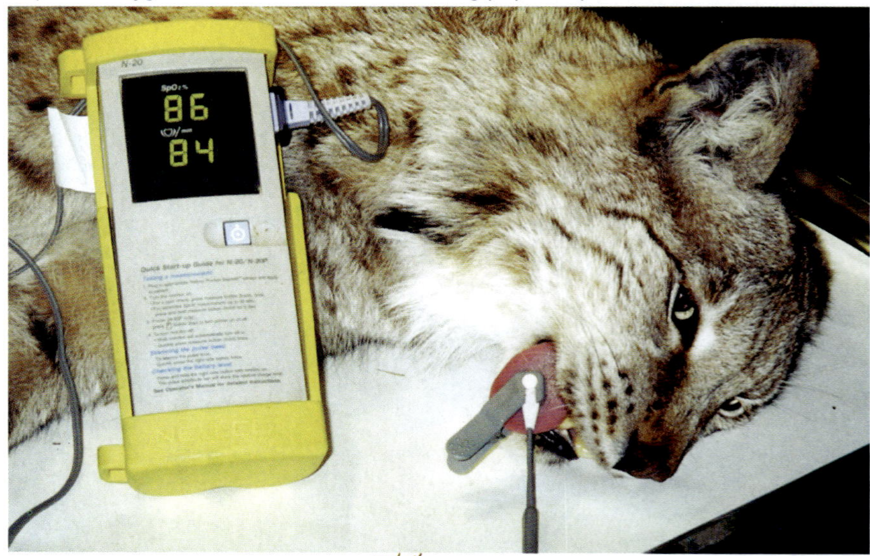

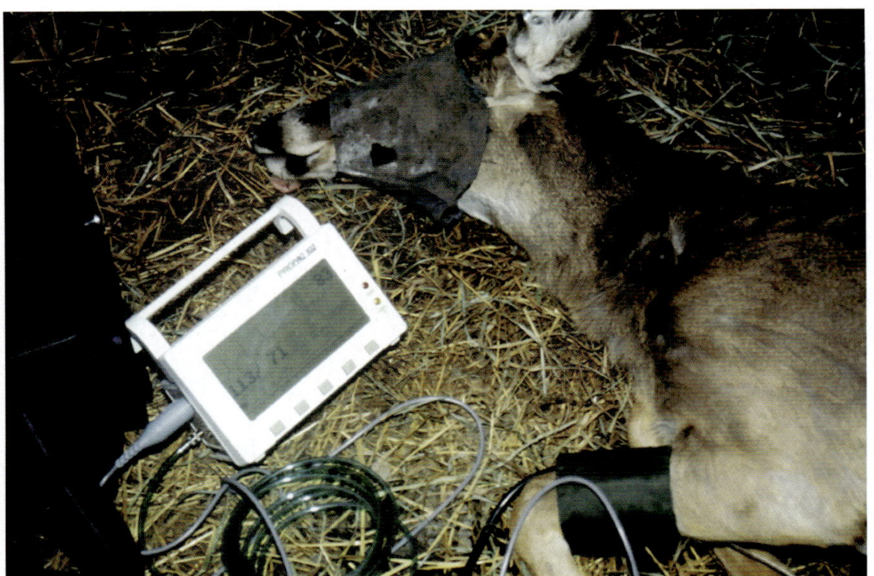

Vital signs monitor measuring electrocardiogram, blood pressure, and rectal temperature on a white-tailed deer.

when oxygen supplementation is available; however, many times oxygen is simply not available.

It is not uncommon for animals anesthetized with potent narcotics or alpha$_2$-adrenergic agonists to have SpO_2 values that fall markedly below 90%. However, there currently are no data on the pathological effects, if any, of depressed SpO_2 values in wild animals and we are left to speculate if absolute SpO_2 values have any biological significance to the immobilized animal.

Nonetheless, the *trend* of SpO_2 values do have value. That is, if the SpO_2 steadily decreases, it can be presumed that the animal is in some sort of respiratory crisis. Such downward trends have been used to detect severely compromised respiration due to pneumothorax in a wolf, bloat in an elk, and isoflurane overdose in a black-footed ferret (Kreeger, unpubl. data).

Vital Signs Monitor

In unusual situations or when immobilizing particularly critical animals, monitoring cardiac function may be required. Additionally, such information may be useful when evaluating a new drug. Portable, rechargeable, vital signs monitors, primarily designed for human emergency use, have been successfully adapted for use on a variety of birds and mammals. Some of these units can simultaneously display electrocardiogram (ECG), systolic/diastolic/mean arterial blood pressure, as well as temperature.

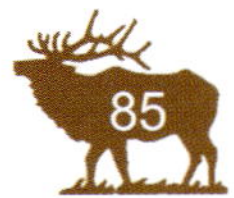

Equipment and Supply Checklist

- Dart guns
  - .22 charges (brown, green, yellow, red)
  - CO_2 propellant
  - Extra batteries for electronic sights, range finder
- Re-usable Powder Charge Darts
  - Dart bodies (1, 2, 3, 5, 7 ml)
  - Dart charges (1–3, 4–10 ml; keep dry)
  - Dart needles
  - Dart plungers
  - Dart tailpieces
  - Silicone lubricant (for dart plungers)
  - Rod for pushing plunger through dart to lube
  - Extra .22 adapters for Cap-Chur® guns
- Disposable Darts (1, 2, 3, 5 ml)
  - Loading needle (must be longer than dart needle)
- Compressed Air Darts
  - Darts (2, 3, 5 ml)
  - Dart needles
  - Dart needle sleeves or caps
  - Tailpieces
  - Coupler
  - 20 ml syringe
  - Plunger rod (for discharging reservoir)
- Pole Syringe
  - Extra syringe barrels, parts
- Petroleum Jelly
- Marking pen, pencil
- Needles (16–25 ga)
- Syringes (1, 3, 5–6, 10–12, 20 ml)
- Blood collection tubes (with and without anticoagulant)
- Multi-tool (knife blade, screwdrivers, etc.)
- Pliers
- Cigar tubes (or other device to safely store loaded darts until used)
- Sterile water (for topping off darts)
- Scalpel blades (for removing barbed darts)
- Flashlight (plus extra bulb and batteries)
- Range finder
- Gun cleaning materials
  - Shotgun cleaning rod (also use to remove stuck or unused darts)
  - Solvent
  - Swabs

List of Manufacturers and Major Distributors

To save space and for simplicity, only internet addresses are listed. Many manufacturers have distributors throughout the world; their main web sites should list contact information for each.

Animal Care Equipment and Services, Inc.
www.animal-care.com
(Dart guns, darts, blow pipes, other animal capture equipment)

Dan-Inject
www.dan-inject.com
(Dart guns, darts, blow pipes)

Dist-Inject
www.allosite.com/distinject
(Dart guns, darts, blow pipes)

Palmer Chemical & Equipment Co., Inc.
www.palmercap-chur.com
(Dart guns, darts)

Paxarms
www.paxarms.net
(Dart guns, darts, pole syringes)

Pneu Dart, Inc.
www.pneudart.com
(Dart guns, darts, blow pipes)

Telinject USA, Inc.
www.telinject.com
(Dart guns, darts, blow pipes)

Wildlife Pharmaceuticals, Inc.
www.wildpharm.com
(North American supplier of capture drugs)

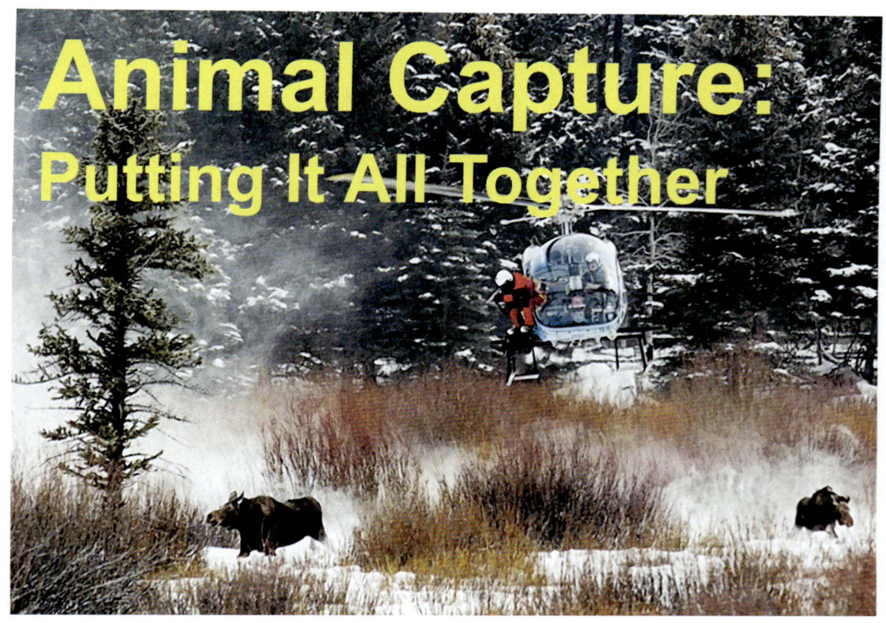

Animal Capture:
Putting It All Together

At this point, you should be familiar with the drugs and the equipment used capture animals. This section will now put this information together. The following "rules" have been developed through years of experience and they should always be recalled prior to any capture operation.

Most of the effort involved in the handling and treatment of a wild animal will be attributed to the capture process.

Until you get some experience under your belt, you won't believe how much time it takes to locate, get close to, dart, and finally capture a wild animal. Thus, allow plenty of time to both capture the animal and monitor its recovery. To accomplish this, most captures should be conducted in the early morning so that you will have ample daylight for the operation.

Always plan ahead and be prepared for any contingency.

Whatever can go wrong, probably will (particularly when someone important is watching!). Most cases of animal loss can be attributed to human error, so think twice and act once. Before you set out to capture an animal, take a few minutes and mentally walk through the process. Try to imagine for each step what equipment is required and what can go wrong. Then make sure you have the appropriate supplies, drugs, etc. to respond to each event that you visualized.

When in doubt, dose high!

This rule may cause a great deal of angst for some readers, but in our experience, more "wrecks" have occured when an animal was underdosed than when it was

overdosed. Your job is to capture the animal. An underdosed animal can injure itself or die from residual drug effects or infection if it escapes altogether. Most capture drugs have high therapeutic indices and high dosages rarely cause life-threatening sequelae. Any medical complications that arise from overdosing can be addressed when you get your hands on the animal. If you are trying to capture a highly stressed animal, increase your dosage by 20–25%. If you are not sure about an animal's weight, estimate it on the heavier side. Remember, the goal of remote capture is: *one dart, one animal down!*

A captured animal becomes a valuable animal - both intrinsically and economically.

The loss of any animal is regrettable; the loss of an endangered species is tragic. Also, a great deal of personnel and equipment costs are usually invested in an immobilization; thus, care and treatment of the animal should not be trivialized.

Keep records.

Good records are essential references for future captures, research, and analyzing disasters(!). Refer to the sample record presented on page 13.

Considerations Prior to Animal Capture

The species, purpose, and circumstances of the capture must be considered prior to undertaking the drugging of any animal. Reasons for drugging animals include capture, translocation, sampling, marking, instrumentation, treatment, and removal from a trap. One should ascertain if the capture is really necessary and whether the *risk of killing the animal justifies the planned gains*. If committed to the capture, there are factors to consider prior to, during, and after the process.

Species

Drug choice, drug doses, and animal response change between species and may vary within species. Adhering to an inflexible drugging protocol can easily end in disaster. Know the species in terms of body weight range, basic feeding habits, seasonal reproductive and condition cycles, habitat, and response to available drugs. Be prepared to adapt to conditions.

Free-ranging Versus Captive

Free-ranging animals usually require higher doses than do captive animals. Free-ranging individuals are usually highly excited and stressed in a capture situation (e.g., chased by a helicopter or trapped in a snare), while captive animals tend to be more docile and used to human activity and handling. Effective doses for free-ranging animals can be twice that for captive individuals of the same species. The dosages listed in the *Drug Dosages* chapter are mostly intended for free-ranging animals. These dosages can be reduced for captive animals, if desired, but the free-ranging dosages can still be used *safely* and *effectively* on captive animals.

Injection Method

The method of drug administration will influence the dose required to induce immobilization. Hand injection with syringes almost always results in faster inductions using less drug than injections by darts. In reindeer, for example, the effective doses for medetomidine and ketamine were 50% higher using darts compared to hand injection (Ryeng et al., 2001a, b). The dosages listed in the *Drug Dosages* chapter are mostly based on effective remote injections via darts. However, these same dosages can still be *safely* and *effectively* administered by hand-held syringes (the animal may simply be down for a longer time).

Sex

There is evidence that the sex of the animal can influence drug dose response (Berrie, 1972; King et al., 1977; Kreeger and Seal, 1986b). If this is known for your intended species, be prepared to adjust your doses accordingly.

Age

Young (not neonates) animals require *more* and older animals usually require *less* drug per unit body weight than do prime-age adult animals. Neonates usually require lower dosages. There is higher risk of complications developing with older animals.

Weight

Most current drug dosage literature is based on milligram of drug per kilogram of body weight. Weight estimates accurate to ±20% are easy to make with experience and doses based on such estimates should be safe. More accurate estimates (±10%) are necessary when using drugs that have low therapeutic indices. Keeping records of animal weight estimates coupled with actual weights after the animal is captured are useful reference sources. Animal weights may change with seasons or conditions (e.g., winter, drought).

Season

For certain drugs, such as succinylcholine, the time of year may have a profound effect on the amount of drug required to immobilize an animal. For instance, white-tailed deer require 61% more succinylcholine in fall than during winter (Jacobsen et al., 1976).

Physical Condition

A sick, exhausted, or malnourished animal will usually require less drug than a healthy, well-fed animal. Such compromised animals are high-risk candidates for anesthesia and frequently die after capture despite everything being done correctly.

Pregnancy

Animals in late stage pregnancy may require more drugs for immobilization, but may experience more respiratory distress once immobilized because the large uterus may impinge on the diaphragm. Although anesthetics may depress fetal respiration, there has been no evidence that immobilization during pregnancy results in fetal loss (DelGiudice et al., 1986). We have immobilized wolves with ketamine and xylazine throughout pregnancy, up to and including the day of whelping, with no loss of pups (Kreeger, unpubl. data).

Psychological Condition

As the excitement level of the animal increases, the chances of a successful capture decrease. The calmer the animal, the safer and smoother will be the procedure. An excited animal usually will require a higher drug dose. Failure to consider this phenomenon usually results in underdosing, which leads to even more excitement, increased chances of injury, trauma, hyperthermia, and capture myopathy. When in doubt, *dose high*!

Weather

Adverse weather conditions, ambient temperature, and relative humidity must be considered when immobilizing an animal. During extremes of temperature (below -15 ºC/5 ºF and above 33 ºC/91 ºF), equipment or facilities should be available to prevent and treat hypo- or hyperthermia. The physiological effects of the chosen drug on an animal's thermoregulation should be understood so that its response may be anticipated.

Hazards

The physical environment must be considered both before and after the capture. A drugged animal cannot choose where it finally becomes anesthetized. Water (including *water bowls*) presents a constant drowning hazard. Falls from rocks, ledges, and steep slopes can injure a semiconscious or ataxic animal. If predation or intraspecific aggression is possible, the animal should be protected or monitored until it recovers.

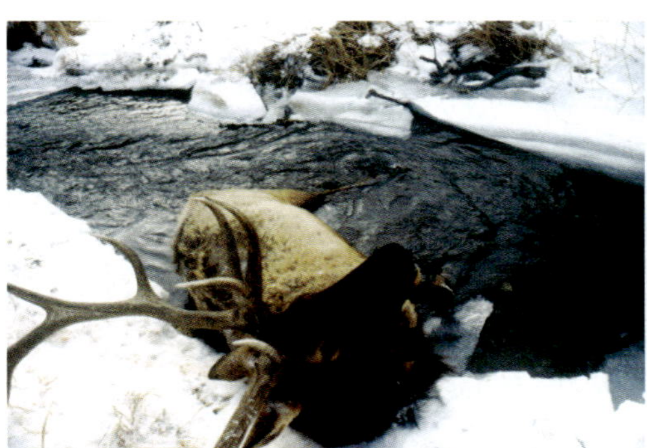

A dual hazard: drowning and hypothermia! If this elk could not be physically removed from the water, your best course of action may be to antagonize the drugs, let the elk extricate itself, and call it a day.

Drugs

Proper selection of the capture drug is critical. The best drug available that will provide the desired result should be selected. Compared to all other factors, drug costs are the least significant. If you can't afford the proper drug, then the capture probably can't be justified. Remember that immobilization does not always imply a surgical plane of anesthesia. Use of painful or stressful manipulations to an immobilized, but sensory aware, animal is inhumane and unjustified.

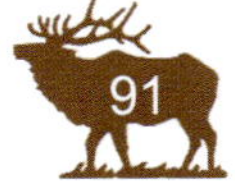

Preparation

Have everything that you need with you.

Before you begin the capture procedure, be sure that you have all drugs and equipment that you may need. These include additional capture drugs and darts should boosters be required (or if you miss with the first dart!), antagonists for both animals and humans in case of accident, monitoring equipment such as stethoscope and thermometer, blindfolds and hobbles, antibiotics, etc. Fishing tackle boxes usually make good receptacles for all this and they come in a variety of sizes and shapes to suit almost all tastes. Vests with multiple pockets, such as a fly fishing or photographer's vest, can be used to carry most items and they free the hands to carry such things as dart guns and pole syringes.

Prepare dart(s) beforehand.

Have one or more darts loaded before you begin your approach. You will usually expend more darts than you would think possible; darts miss, bounce out, fail to discharge, and generally exist to frustrate your life. For example, during the Yellowstone wolf reintroduction, an average of 5.5 darts was expended for each wolf captured! Be sure that all loaded darts are safely stored so as to prevent accidental injection; plastic test tubes or cigar holders make good holding devices. If you are working in freezing weather, be sure to keep the extra darts warm. It is generally best to load darts under controlled conditions, such as inside a heated building where you can lay everything out and reduce the chance for drug or volume error. Unless absolutely necessary, do not load darts in a moving vehicle or helicopter. When loading multiple darts, do one step at a time for all darts to avoid mix-ups.

Check darts and gun before using.

Always inspect your dart gun prior to use to insure that it is unloaded and the barrel clean and clear. If you are using any form of electronic sights, be sure that they are working (and *always* carry spare batteries!). If you are using reusable aluminum darts, place both ends of the dart body into the gun barrel to be sure that they have not distorted from previous firings. If both ends of the dart do not fit smoothly into the barrel, do not use it. For CO_2 guns, carry extra gas cylinders and "O" rings.

Don't load gun until ready to approach the animal.

Until you are actually in a position to approach and dart an animal, it is generally unnecessary to load your dart gun. Remember dart guns are exactly that – guns! At close ranges, dart guns can be lethal and they should always be treated like their bullet-firing counterparts. Keep the safety on or the gun uncocked until just before you shoot. Also never load a dart gun in a helicopter until you are in position to dart the animal. Before loading, point the barrel outside of the aircraft and keep it there. We'll leave it up to your imagination as to what an accidentally-discharged dart can do inside the cockpit.

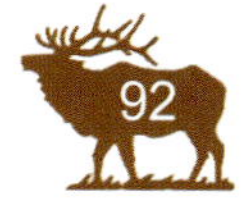

Approach

Approach captive animals quietly and calmly.

Even if you are working with captive animals that are restrained in a chute or a trapped wild animal, you should approach it quietly and calmly. Do not make rapid or exaggerated movements that will panic the animal. Captive animals will often pace or run back and forth if they see you approach too closely which makes accurate shot placement difficult. If your approach cannot be hidden, don't "focus" too much on your intended target. Animals seem to know when you are interested specifically in them and they become increasingly nervous. If captive animals are used to a routine such as feeding or cleaning, try to mimic that activity (at the same time of day) to allow a closer approach.

Use devices to approach free-ranging animals.

Approaching a free-ranging or captive animal close enough so that you can get a suitable shot with a dart gun can be frustrating. Free-ranging animals, if shot from the ground, are best shot from a blind overlooking a feeding station or some other device that draws the animal into range. If this is not available, be prepared to use all of your hunting skills when on foot, such as wearing camouflage clothing, watching wind direction and scent, and no noise. Wild animals can often be approached quite closely with a vehicle, but you must remain inside the vehicle even when taking a shot. Darting from horseback has proven to be very successful, especially on ranches where horses are used for work or patrols and wildlife are used to them. If using a vehicle or helicopter to pursue and dart animals, try to limit the length of the chase. Many ungulates have evolved for quick bursts of running only and are physiologically ill-equipped for long-distance pursuits. Such species, if run too hard, will survive the immobilization process only to die several hours or even weeks later due to capture myopathy or stress-related diseases.

Helicopters are often used to dart animals under a variety of conditions. Animals as small as wolverines can be darted from the air (if you are a good shot!). Usually shot distances are short (< 20 m), but if the animal is standing still, longer shots can be taken. For example, animals may run into trees and stop, thinking

Using devices to approach animals for darting: left: feedground elk approached by truck; right: Indian rhino approached by elephant.

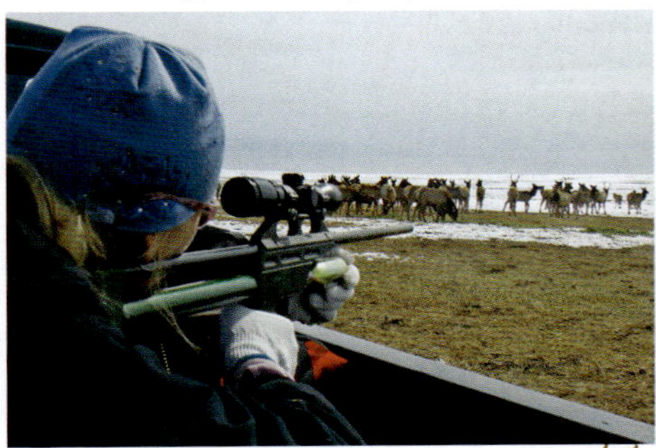

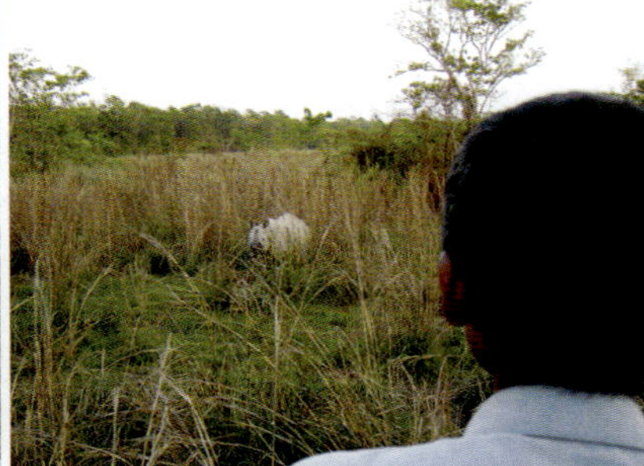

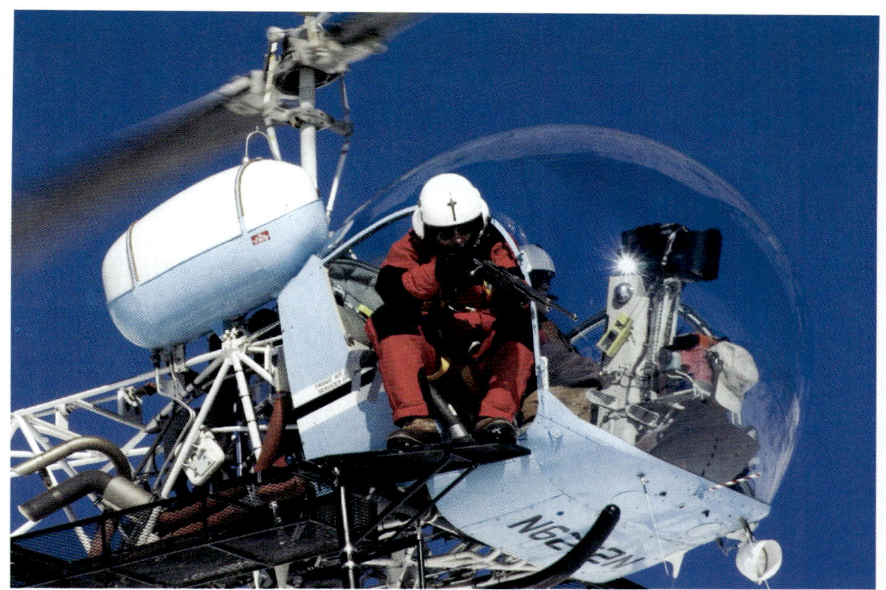

Darting from a helicopter requires an experienced pilot, training in safety and survival, and proper equipment such as helmet, fire-resistant flight suit, and windproof outer garments. Most shooters prefer .22-caliber dart guns with open sights, but other gun types and sights can be used successfully.

that they are safe from pursuit. With the helicopter hovering straight above, a long shot can be taken straight down through the trees. Darting equipment is mostly a matter of personal preference as most dart gun and dart types can be used from helicopters. In general, the target animal is spotted from some distance before it is aware of your intentions. The dart gun remains unloaded until the decision is made to pursue the animal. Once the gun is loaded and the shooter is in position (usually outside of the helicopter with safety harness attached), the approach is made. Although it is not always possible, try to limit the chase to less than two minutes. This may sound short, but many chases actually last less than 30 seconds. Once the animals is darted, notify the pilot and then pull the ship as far from the animal as possible while still maintaining visual contact. When the animal is down, either notify a ground crew of its location (GPS coordinates) or land as close as possible. If you are leaving the ship to process the animal, have everything that you need with you, usually in a backpack. If you are in deep snow country, don't leave the ship without snowshoes (if you forget them, it will take you forever to get to the animal and you will be exhausted when you do!). Needless to say, helicopter darting is *extremely* dangerous. A good discussion on helicopter safety can be reviewed in Nielsen (1999) and Kock, M. et al. (2006).

Estimate distance and wind.

Many dart guns can be adjusted to deliver more or less propellant to the dart. Additionally, .22-cal.-powered dart guns can use different power loads for different ranges. If possible, estimate the probable shooting distance that you expect to

encounter and adjust the metering device and use the power load appropriate for the distance and dart weight. However, be prepared to adjust these factors at the last moment; if in doubt, it is better not to shoot. Overpowered darts can cause severe wounds or death; underpowered darts can miss altogether (thus spooking the animal) or strike the lower legs resulting in injury or poor drug absorption and prolonged induction times. We have found that laser range finders are virtually indispensable for determining distances. They are particularly effective when combined with finely-adjustable CO_2 dart rifles.

Also be sure to consider wind speed, particularly with crosswinds, when using lightweight darts or shooting at long distances (>15 m). Increasing your power settings can help ameliorate wind drift, but this step should not be taken when darting small or thin-skinned animals. The change in wind conditions experienced at the outer edge of the downdraft caused by helicopter rotors can change the angle of flight of lightweight darts; heavier darts tend to overcome this deflection.

Adjust for altitude.

A dart gun that is sighted in at one altitude may perform quite differently at another. For example, a gun sighted in at an altitude of 2,000 m will shoot high at 4,000 m and low at sea level (0 m).

Administration Sites

Intramuscular Injection

Immobilizing drugs are almost always administered intramuscularly (IM). The usual injection sites are the large muscle masses of the proximal hindlimb and forelimb, with the former being the most commonly used. Hindlimb injections preferably should be placed towards the rear so as to avoid the femur; forelimb shots should be placed towards the front. Although anatomically small, a surprising number of darts strike the spine of the scapula. Also, the posterior portion of the scapula is not well muscled and long-needled darts (> 3 cm) can lodge in the bone, even in an animal the size of an elk. Darts striking the bone are painful, can cause fractures, and may not inject the drug due to blockage of the dart needle. There is some evidence that intramuscular absorption rates can differ depending on site; absorption being most rapid from the neck, then the shoulder, then the

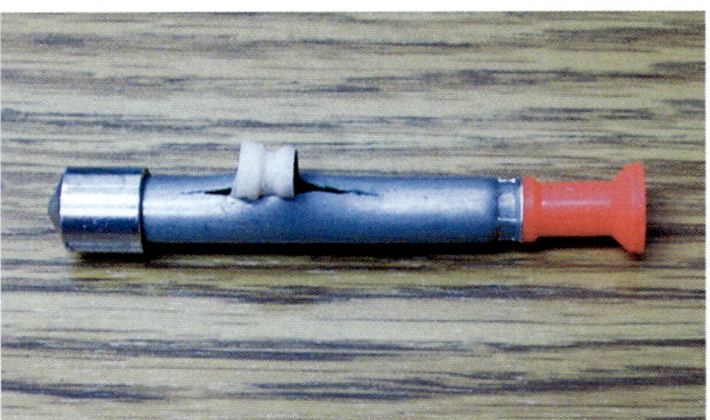

Misplaced darts using an explosive charge that hit bone will most likely not inject any drug into the animal, explode loudly scaring the animal and others, and usually cannot be extricated without the use of pliers. The same kind of malfunction can occur if the drug in the needle freezes. When the dart's charge explodes, the resulting pressure will result in the dart coming apart.

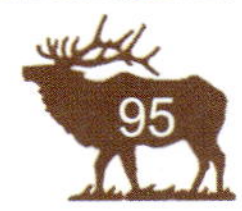

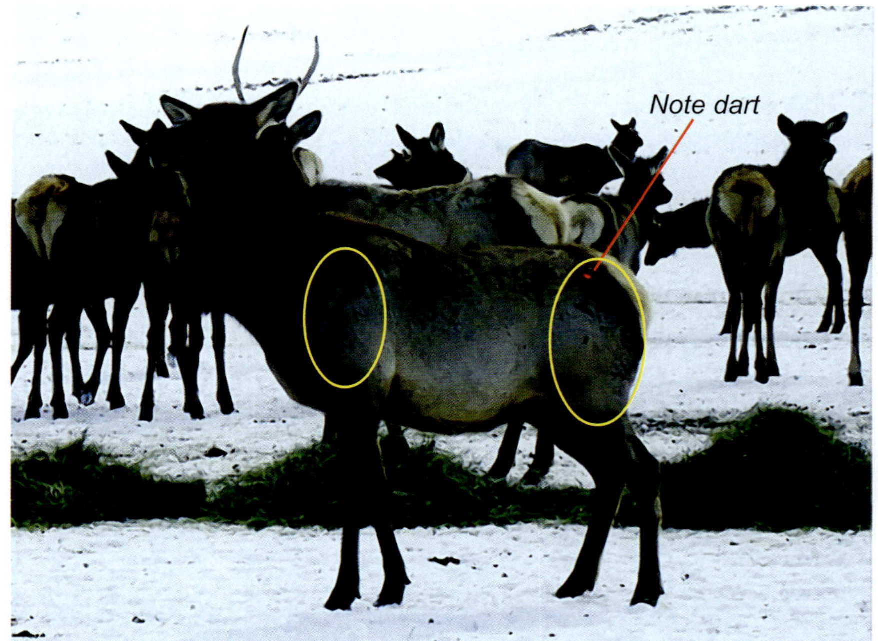

Intramuscular injection sites in an elk. The preferred area is the large muscle mass of the hindquarters. In elk and many other ungulates, the region where the light hair meets the dark hair is a good aiming point.

hip (Berrie, 1972). Areas of large fat deposits should also be avoided as absorption from these sites is slow and unpredictable. For example, bears should be injected in the lower regions of the hindlimbs to avoid the fat deposits around the rump or the shoulder. Some drugs, such as the barbiturates, have historically been given intraperitoneally (Erickson, 1957). However, this can result in slow absorption as well as possibly causing peritonitis. For helicopter darting, the hindlimb muscles or the back muscles running along the rear one-third of the animal are suitable sights. No "leading" of the animal is necessary if the helicopter is matching the animal's speed; otherwise, lead the animal if it is running faster than the helicopter, or slightly behind the desired target site if the helicopter is overtaking the animal.

Intravascular Injection

Intravascular (IV) administration is usually reserved for antagonists. Intravenous administration of anesthetics should be done with caution, because the onset of action is often quite rapid and, in some cases, respiratory depression or arrest can occur. Any drug containing propylene glycol (i.e., diazepam) should be given slowly IV, because a bolus can cause cardiac arrest. Intravenous administration of antagonists could result in very rapid recovery; be sure that you have a cleared escape route in mind and that all hobbles and blindfolds have been removed. For example, elk heavily sedated with medetomidine recover quickly and are fully

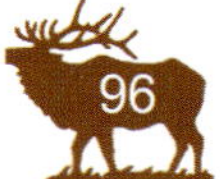

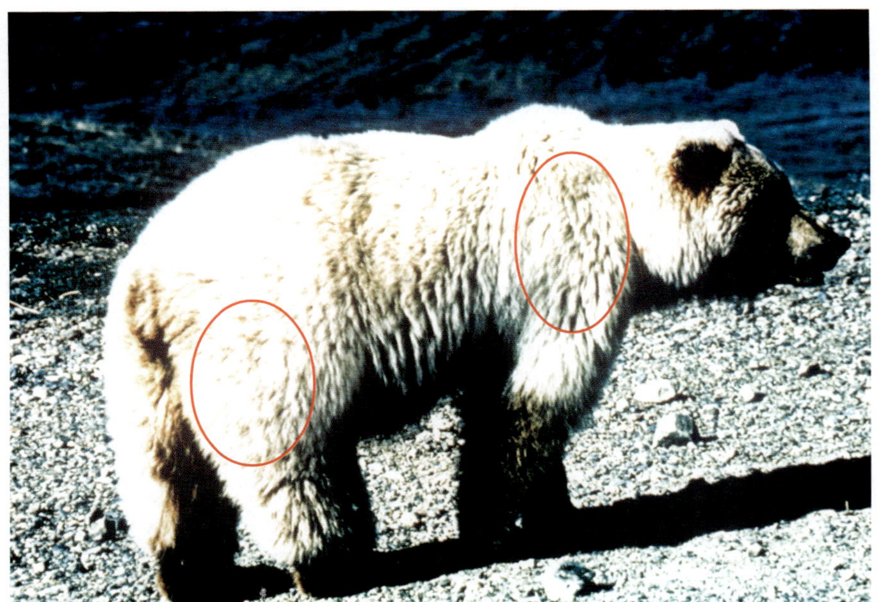

Because of their large subcutaneous fat deposits which absorb drugs poorly, bears should be injected in their shoulders or lower rear legs.

sensate after antagonism with atipamezole. If you are too close to this animal upon recovery, it may strike out at you rather than running away. Similarly, IV antagonism of thiafentanil with naltrexone can result in the animal standing in as little as 20 seconds (J. Raath, unpubl. data).

Oral Administration

Oral administration is not often used in wildlife capture primarily because of the difficulty in predicting the dose that the animal receives. Also, drugs taken orally have variable absorption rates, resulting in prolonged and erratic induction and recovery times. Drugs can be placed in tabs that are attached to traps so that when a captured animal chews on the trap, it ingests the drug (e.g., diazepam for foxes and coyotes). Drugs can also be placed in food baits, but it is particularly difficult to predict the administered dose with this method (Ratcliffe, 1962; Montgomery and Hawkins, 1967). Gray wolves have been heavily sedated by placing concentrated tiletamine-zolazepam into bait (Kreeger et al., unpubl. data). Midazolam in bait has been used to sedate nervous free-ranging lions prior to darting (J. Raath, unpubl. data). If other methods of administering drugs fail, one can spray drug into the mouth of the animal.

Immobilization Signs

Although some drugs do not cause true anesthesia (loss of consciousness and analgesia), many of the commonly used drugs or drug combinations do. The classic stages of anesthesia were initially defined for rats given ether (Table 2)

and they are applicable to the more modern agents only in the broadest terms. However, it is important to remember that Stage II of anesthesia (Delirium or Excitement) is often applicable to many modern drugs, particularly the opioids. During this stage, the animal loses voluntary control and may stumble or fall, particularly if the animal was *underdosed.* It is critical that the immobilizing dose be *sufficient to minimize the duration of Stage II* in order to drive the animal quickly through Stage II and into Stage III (Surgical Anesthesia) which is the desired stage. The ideal level of anesthesia is Stage III, Plane II. If the animal is *overdosed*, it will progress through the planes of Stage III with increasing physiologic impairment until it finally enters Stage IV (Medullary Paralysis) where death is imminent unless counteractive measures are taken (antagonist, CPR).

Familiarity with the signs of anesthesia is essential – not knowing the depth of anesthesia can be lethal for both the animal and you! You can assess drug effect through changes in behavior (Table 5), but to determine such effects, it is critical to be familiar with the target species. Know what is normal and look for the abnormal.

Table 5. Sequential signs of chemical immobilization of animals given an injectable anesthetic. Not all signs are applicable to all species or all drugs.

- Slight behavioral changes
- Licking
- Lowering of eyelids
- Standing (not moving or not keeping up with herd)
- Moving away from other animals
- Lowered head, standing
- Increased salivation
- Abnormal behavior
- Aimless walking
- Agitated walking and running
- Straddle-legged stance
- Down but able to rise on own
- Down but able to rise if stimulated
- Down but unable to rise—head up
- Down but unable to rise—head down
- Lateral recumbency
- Spontaneous movements present
- Loss of ear twitch reflex (touch inside of ear, ear twitches)
- Loss of pedal reflex (pinch toe, limb withdraws)
- Loss of swallowing reflex (pull tongue, release, animal swallows)
- Loss of palpebral reflex (touch eyelashes, animal blinks)
- Loss of corneal reflex (touch cornea, animal blinks)

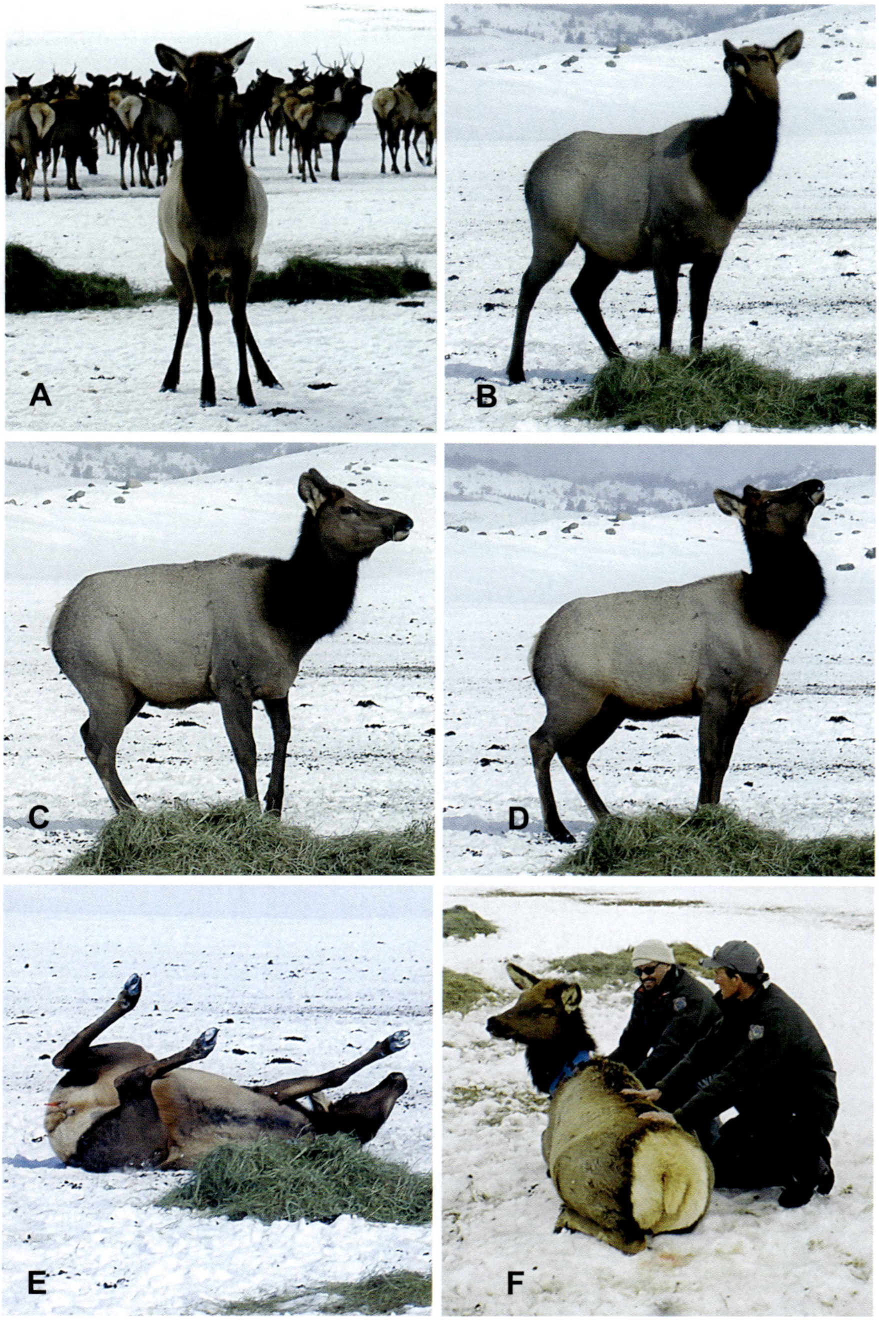

Immobilization of an elk: A. Straddle-legged stance; B. Slight behavioral changes (elk not moving); C. Animal starts to become unsteady; D. Lowering of hindquarters, head starts to tilt upwards; E. Down, but probably able to get up if approached - wait 1-2 minutes before approaching; F. Animal should be placed on sternum when possible.

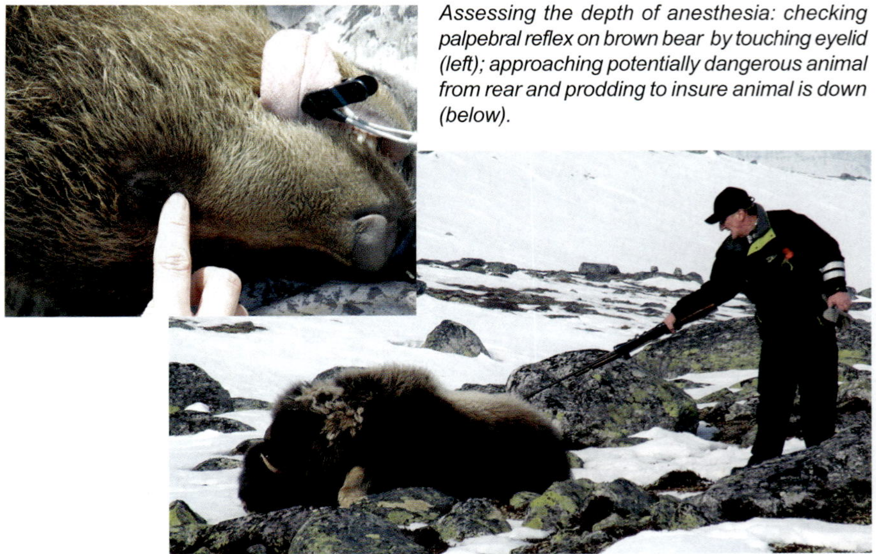

Assessing the depth of anesthesia: checking palpebral reflex on brown bear by touching eyelid (left); approaching potentially dangerous animal from rear and prodding to insure animal is down (below).

Once the animal is down, you need to assess the depth of anesthesia. Always exercise caution when checking a downed animal. Approach the animal slowly and quietly; approach dangerous animals from the rear and be sure that you have an escape route. Initially observe for spontaneous, *non*-repetitive movements and, if present, you can usually assume that the animal is not fully immobilized. Repetitive, stereotypical movements are often seen with opioid agents. Such animals are effectively immobilized, but can still deliver a crippling kick under these conditions!

If the animal appears unconscious, check for ear twitch (touch inside of ear, ear twitches), pedal reflex (pinch toe, limb withdraws), swallowing reflex (pull tongue, release, animal swallows), palpebral reflex (touch eyelashes, animal blinks), and corneal reflex (touch cornea, animal blinks). If the animal has lost the ear twitch, it is probably at an appropriate stage of anesthesia for most field procedures. The cyclohexanes often do not abolish the blinking reflexes, even when the animal is quite anesthetized.

Incomplete Immobilization

If the animal has been hit with the dart and either the animal is showing no signs of the drugs or is not fully immobilized, you should assess the situation carefully by determining:

Did the animal receive all the drugs administered.

For example, there may have been partial dart-hits where all of the drug may not have gone into the animal. If your dart hit the animal, but bounced out almost immediately and the animal shows some signs of drug effect, chances are good

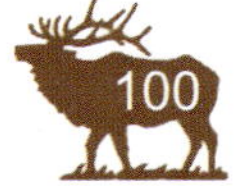

that it only received a portion of the drug. If you are using carfentanil or thiafentanil and even though the dart bounced out upon impact, many of these animals will still become immobilized although they probably did not receive the full dose.

The animal's psychological state.

Was the animal was highly excited during the drugging episode? Highly excited animals can absorb a frightening amount of some drugs (particularly xylazine or ketamine/xylazine) before they finally can be approached. When dealing with highly-excited animals, such as deer, you may have to *increase the suggested dose by as much as 50%*. Only experience will help you deal with these situations. Although down, the animals still might be conscious – exercise caution!

The pharmacology of the drug and its therapeutic index.

Does the drug(s) have a sufficiently high therapeutic index that would allow you to safely give the animal more? Drugs such as ketamine can usually be administered at 2-3 times the recommended dose and still not cause problems. On the other hand, drugs such as succinylcholine have low indices and booster doses can easily result in overdose and respiratory arrest.

What the animal is "telling" you.

Remember the signs of immobilization (Table 5). Is the animal showing any of these signs? That is, what is it "telling" you regarding its response to the first dart? In general, we are talking about administering booster doses via a dart because the animal is either not down or goes down but continues to get up and run away.

What to do if the animal received some drug

If at all possible, get a the time when the first dart hit the animal. A stopwatch works very well for this. Allow 10-15 minutes (but *never more* than 15 minutes) to elapse after the first dart before giving booster doses. If the animal is showing signs of receiving some of the drug, administer 50% of the original dose. If you used a combination of a primary anesthetic (e.g., carfentanil, ketamine, etc.) plus a tranquilizer (e.g., xylazine, medetomidine), you probably only need to booster with a half dose of the anesthetic and no more tranquilizer. However, it is still perfectly safe to administer half of the tranquilizer as well.

For example, you used 500 mg ketamine and 100 mg of xylazine to immobilize a deer. The dart bounced out almost immediately and 10 minutes later the deer was stumbling about or even lying down, but it would get up or walk away when you tried to approach it. A safe and effective booster dose in this case would be 250 mg ketamine and no more xylazine (but 50 mg of xylazine could be safely added, if you wished to do so).

When an animal is showing some drug effect, but is not down, try to minimize further chasing or stress. If an animal gets up when approached, retreat immedi-

ately and continue observing. Watch the time and prepare another dart. Oftentimes, a partially drugged animal will go down again after getting up, offering another opportunity for darting. Do not approach the animal too closely (< 25 m) or it will get up again. The more times it gets up, the more drug is metabolized, and the more difficult it will be to dart it again.

What to do if the animal received no drug

If *no* sign of drug effect is apparent after 10 minutes, you can assume that the animal probably received little or none of the original dose. If you are confident that the drug(s) and dose(s) that you originally selected were appropriate, then give the animal the same drug(s) and dose(s) again.

Only when these factors have been considered can you make an informed decision on whether to administer additional drugs or abandon the immobilization attempt. Animals can be kept immobilized for extended periods (several hours) with supplemental boosters of 33-50% of the initial immobilizing dose. This is particularly true when using ketamine. Where ketamine was given initially in combination with another agent, such as xylazine, usually only the ketamine needs to be given to maintain immobilization, particularly with carnivores.

If the animal is down and can be handled, but it continues to struggle and is generally making your life difficult, a low dose of a potent tranquilizer, such as medetomidine (e.g., 1 mg), often calms the animal enough to allow safer and easier handling. This technique should be used with extreme caution when handling dangerous animals such as bears and large cats. These animals can awake suddenly when the alpha-adrenergic tranquilizers are used.

If the Animal Doesn't Go Down

Under most circumstances, animals will show definite signs of being drugged within 5 minutes of IM injection.

Note the time. Allow 10-15 (but no more than 15) minutes to elapse from the time of injection. If the animal shows some drug effect, but is not down, re-administer 50% of the original dose of the anesthetic, with or without a tranquilizer.

If the animal shows *no* drug effect after 10-15 minutes, re-administer the entire original dose.

Remember: the goal for free-ranging animals is to achieve immobilization with a *single dose*. If in doubt about the correct initial dose, it is better to administer *more*, rather than less, drug.

Handling the Immobilized Animal

When an animal is finally "down" and can be safely handled, there are several immediate steps that need be taken before you embark on whatever action prompted the immobilization in the first place. This section lists those steps; their order is not absolute as obvious emergencies might take precedence. Specific emergency treatments are discussed in the section, *Animal Medical Treatment*.

Position body.

- Insure that nothing impinges on breathing, i.e., neck straight, nose/trunk clear.
- Position ruminants sternally if at all possible. Most other animals can be placed on either side or sternally *except* for elephants which *must* be placed on their sides. The head should preferably be higher than the thorax with the nose pointing down to avoid aspiration of fluids.
- Try to keep the animal on relatively flat ground to avoid occlusion of the trachea, pressure neuropathy, or circulatory impairment.
- Some animals, such as rhinos, may require acute emergency care once immobilized. For these species, it may be prudent to establish an IV drip line.
- For lengthy immobilizations, roll the animal on its other side or sternally at least every 60 min. Massage the "down" legs to restore circulation. It is preferable to roll ungulates across the sternum as opposed to across the back.

Cover eyes.

Covering the eyes protects them from harmful ultraviolet light from the sun, reduces drying, and prevents dirt and debris from entering them. Coating the eyes with a lubricant further prevents drying, however, some feel that eye oint-

Ruminants should be positioned on their sternum, if possible.

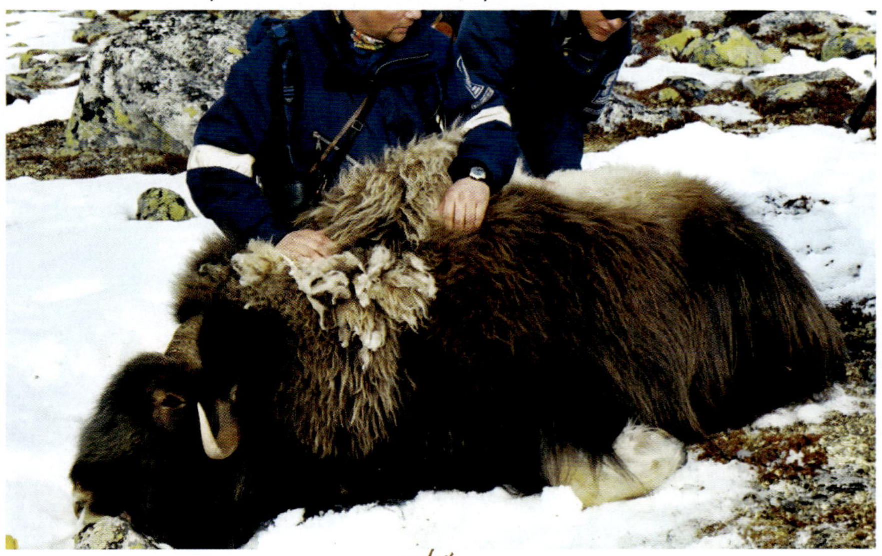

ments result in dirt and grit sticking to the eye. A saline wash (e.g., contact lens saline) can also be used. Covering the eyes also appears to further calm the animal even when effectively anesthetized.

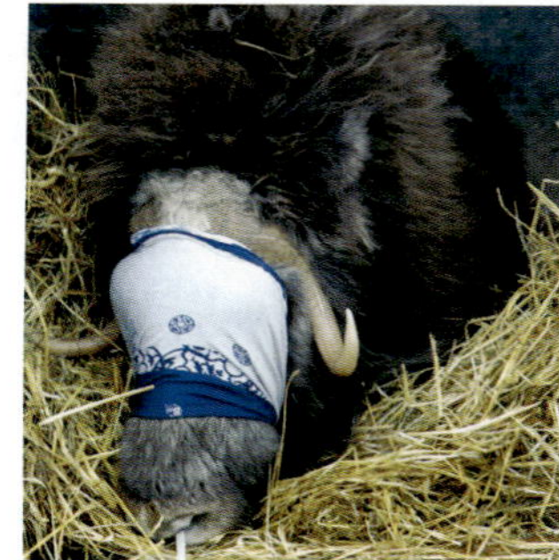
A blindfold not only protects the eyes, but often appears to calm the animal as well.

You may wish to plug the animal's ears with cotton or cloth to avoid response to sounds which can happen with animals given opioids. If you do this, attach the plugs to each other and/or mark with a bright string or ribbon so *you don't forget to remove them!*

Hobble the legs.

This is particularly necessary with ungulates to avoid spontaneous kicking which may injure someone. Hobbles also prevent human injuries or possible escape should the animal partially or spontaneously recover. Hobbles can be made from leather, but leather can rot and weaken over time. The best hobbles are made from a "bioplastic" material, a laminate of fabric and plastic. They are extraordinarily strong, flexible, and waterproof. Horse tack shops can make such hobbles. Have them made about a meter long with holes punched every 2 cm or so. Heavy duty snaps by the buckle can be used to connect front and back hobbled legs together. The key to securing hobbles on ungulates is to get them as tight as you can - and then tighten one more notch! Loose hobbles are as dangerous as no hobbles at all because they give you a false sense of security. Animals appear to sense when hobbles are loose and they increase their struggling as a result.

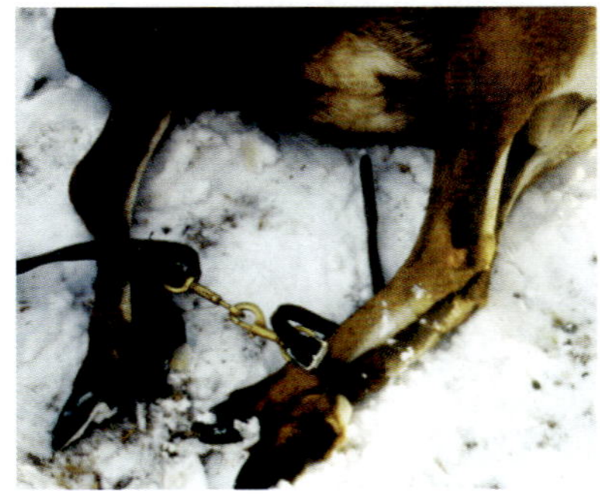

Check vital signs.

Respiration

Once assured that the animal's body position will not affect breathing, you should check its respiratory rate (RR). Regardless of claims, there are really very few scientifically-proven normal resting RRs of undrugged, wild animals. Experience with a given species and capture process is your best guide. Respirations can be seen (watch the abdomen or chest), felt (place hand in front of nostrils), or heard (place ear by nostrils – a very sensitive technique).

Slowed RRs are most likely drug-induced, but they can be caused by hypothermia. In cases of respiratory arrest or poor oxygenation, respiration can be supported mechanically or pharmacologically. Rapid RRs could indicate hyperther-

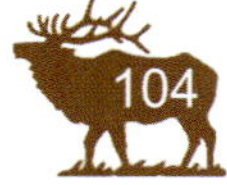

mia, bloat, aspiration, pulmonary edema, or shock. Use other parameters (i.e., temperature, capillary refill time) to differentiate the causes of a rapid RR and treat accordingly. If you have a stethoscope (and you should), listen for abnormal chest sounds such as gurgling which may indicate pulmonary edema. If the animal's gums (or other mucous membranes) are pinkish (as opposed to blue, gray, or muddy), tissues are probably adequately oxygenated, even if the RR is 5-6/min.

Depth of respiration is as important as rate. An adequate rate with a shallow depth may result in a low volume of air being moved resulting in an increase in CO_2 in the blood. You should also be familiar with respiratory rhythms. Roan antelope under opioid anesthesia, for instance, often take a single deep breath, followed by 5-6 shallow ones, followed by a brief period of apnea. This rhythm is maintained throughout anesthesia.

Portable pulse oximeters are the best means for assessing respiratory efficiency because they measure oxygen saturation of hemoglobin. The trend of oxygen saturation is usually more informative than absolute percents. That is, if the percent oxygen saturation falls from 90% to, say, 70%, then you need to determine the cause. In general, oxygen saturation above 90% is desirable, but anesthetized animals often have oxygen saturations of 70-80% with no apparent harm.

Temperature

Always carry a thermometer and *use* it continually throughout the immobiliza-

Immobilized bear being monitored with pulse oximeter. Note the organization and ready availability of sampling supplies and other items.

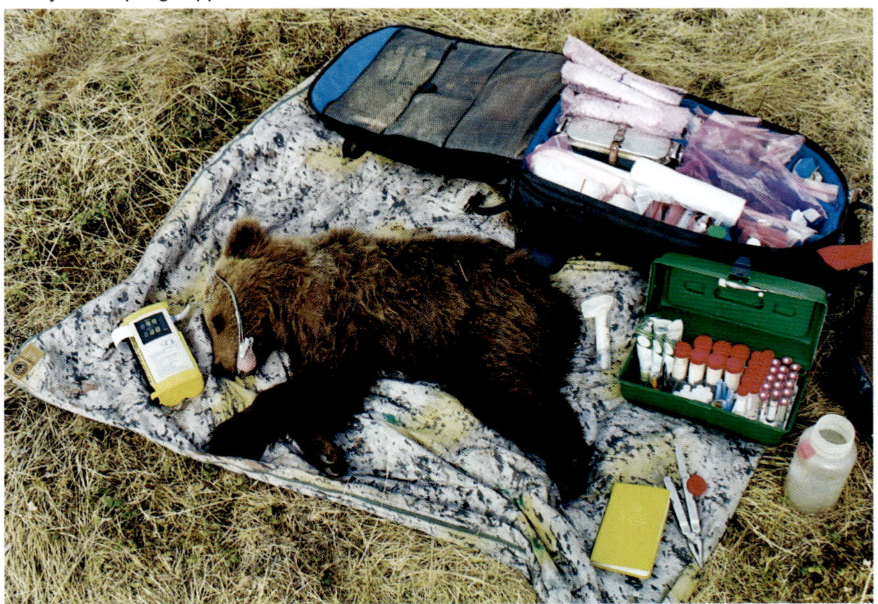

tion period. Normal mammalian rectal temperatures range from 37.5–40° C (99.5–104° F). Cell damage may begin when oxygen demand exceeds supply at temperatures > 40° C (104° F). You should probably take action to lower an animal's temperature if it is > 40° C (104° F); such action is mandatory at temperatures > 41.1° C (106° F); survival without residual impairment is questionable at temperatures > 42.2° C (108° F); survival itself is doubtful at temperatures ≥ 43.3° C (110° F). Although not as common, don't forget about *hypo*thermia!

Conventional large animal glass thermometers are sufficient, but readings are slow to develop and they easily break. If using glass thermometers, tie a bright string to it and have a clip attached to the free end. When using the thermometer, clip the string to upper side of the animal so that you can see the string. This serves as a reminder to remove the thermometer before you release the animal! Electronic digital thermometers, particularly those with a probe, are preferable. These devices are inexpensive, fairly rugged (saltwater is death to them, however), and rapid. Insert the probe into the rectum and place the unit on the upper side of the animal where it can be checked periodically by simply pushing a button.

Pulse

Again, there are very few proven, normal resting heart rates of wild animals, so let experience be your best reference. Smaller animals generally have higher heart rates than larger animals. Heart rates can be detected: 1) with a stethoscope (usually best detected on the "down" side of the animal, between the fourth to sixth ribs or behind the point of the elbow); 2) by feeling the heart beat directly by compressing the chest slightly; 3) by locating an arterial pulse; or 4) by using a pulse oximeter or electrocardiogram.

A very fast heart rate could be a function of drugs (e.g., ketamine), physiological responses (i.e., stress, excitement), hyperthermia, or shock. Use other parameters to differentiate the causes of tachycardia. An abnormally slow heart rate could be a function of drugs (e.g., xylazine), hypothermia, or metabolic disorders (e.g., hyperkalemia, hypercalcemia). Generally, if the capillary refill time is < 2 sec, adequate perfusion is assumed and no action is required in the absence of other signs.

Check for wounds, injuries, and general condition.

Start from the nose and work toward the tail. Look for blood, swelling, hair loss, and abnormal body configuration (e.g., fractures or luxations).

- Nose: check for blood, excess fluid, dirt, foreign objects.
- Mouth: check for jammed sticks (particularly with trapped carnivores), broken teeth, lacerated tongue, dirt, food, etc.
- Eyes: clear of dirt, lubricate, and cover.
- Ears: blood could indicate concussion, but could be due to ectoparasites.
- Chest: listen for gurgling, moist sounds, rasping (think edema, pneumonia).

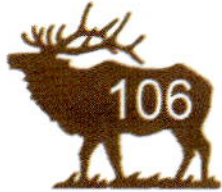

- Abdomen: watch for signs of bloat.
- Limbs: check for lacerations, fractures.
- Feet: check for lacerations, fractures of toes, imbedded sticks, burrs etc.
- Anus: check for bleeding (think hyperthermia), diarrhea.
- Skin: check for lacerations, abrasions. Also check for dehydration by pinching loose skin (e.g., back of neck) to form a "tent." Upon release, the "tent" should collapse within 1 second. If the pinched skin remains raised or resumes its normal configuration slowly, the animal is probably dehydrated Also check for ectoparasites (ticks, mites, lice). Treatment for a heavy parasite infection may not be feasible, but a high parasite load may indicate an animal in marginal condition which could have impact on its recovery from anesthesia or long-term survival.

Do not make loud or sharp noises.

Animals that have been anesthetized with opioid agents often spontaneously respond to loud or sharp noises, such as a slammed truck door. The response is usually a kick, but such animals may try to stand. We *do not* recommend the use of ear plugs (as others have); invariably there will come a time when you will forget to remove them and most animals cannot dislodge ear plugs on their own. Animals anesthetized with cyclohexane agents are usually less responsive to sound. Do not try to be overly quiet around such animals, because some noise may serve to partially stimulate the animal resulting in an "early warning" of recovery.

Transport of the Immobilized Animal

Moving animals for short distances, as from the capture site to a truck, can be aided by the use of a heavy tarp. Tarps can be made from heavy-duty canvas or synthetic material with multiple hand-holds attached to the edges. Animals weighing as much as 400 kg can be handled by 4–6 people. Tarps, toboggans, sleds, or plywood sheets can be used to skid even the largest of animals over the snow.

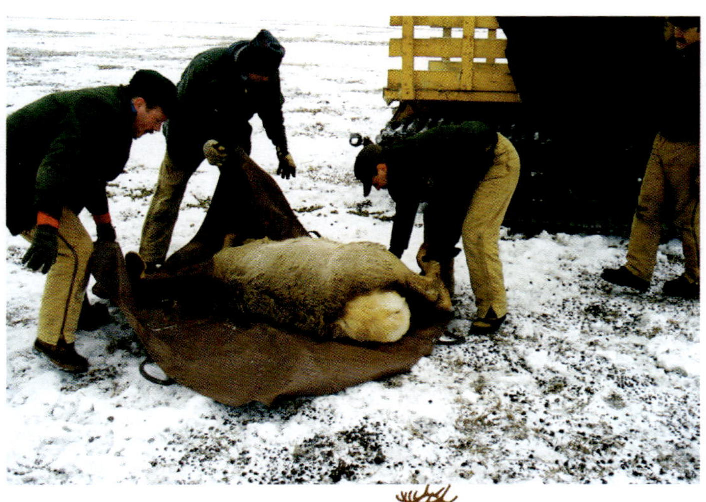

A tarp can be used to move heavy animals by just a few people or serve as a clean ground cloth when processing animals in the field.

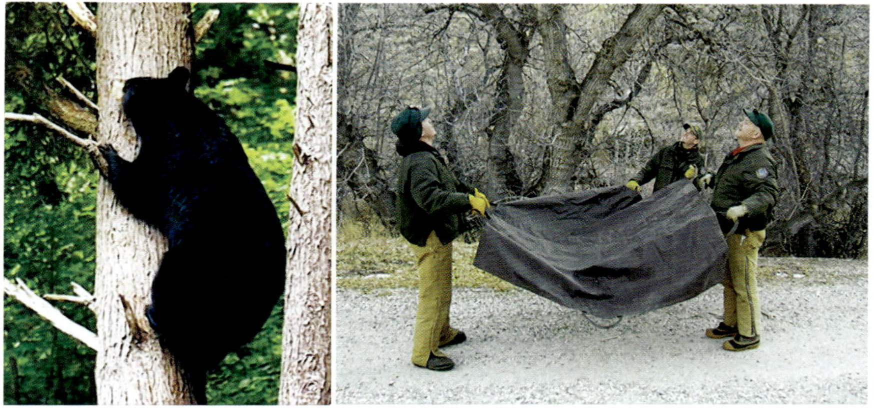

A tarp can be used to break the fall of an animal in a tree. This is recommended because, if for nothing else, it is acceptable to the public. The physics of a large animal falling some distance, however, argues against the true efficacy of this procedure!

The same tarps can be used to catch bears or mountain lions which have climbed trees where they were immobilized but remained in the branches. Preferably, climb the tree, place a rope around the animal (use a bowline knot so it doesn't tighten), and lower it to the ground. If this is not possible, a tarp can be used to break the fall of the animal as it is pushed or falls from the tree.

The efficacy of a tarp to truly absorb the animal's fall is debatable. A 200-lb bear falling from a 30-ft tree generates over 3,000 foot-pounds of energy! So the benefit of a tarp may be more perception than reality. Nonetheless, if the press or public are observing this operation, you would be very wise to use a tarp even if unconvinced of its efficacy. It is almost a guarantee that you will see yourself on the "6 o'clock news" if the bears falls from the tree, crashes to the ground, and bounces uncontrollably if you make no attempt to break its fall.

Helicopters are necessary for moving animals out of remote areas. Animals are best moved while hobbled and blindfolded in either cargo nets or bags especially designed to hold the species. The animal should be kept sternal with the head upright if at all possible. Be sure that the neck is not bent to avoid strangulation. Many ungulates have been transported by helicopter while hung upside down by their four legs. Although animals apparently survive such handling without harm, this should never be done with an anesthetized animal which may regurgitate and aspirate stomach contents.

There is much discussion on the appropriate method of transporting animals over long distances i.e., should animals be moved while anesthetized or while awake? Anesthetized animals may stop breathing or overheat in transit because they are not continually monitored. On the other hand, awake animals may pace continuously, jump, kick, trample one another, overheat, or develop capture myopathy.

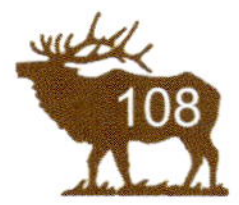

Each species and situation is different. If the species is fairly calm, such as moose, then transport in an awake, revived condition is best. If the animal is hyperactive, such as deer or pronghorn, then moving it while anesthetized (if the animal is stable) might be best. The males of many ungulate species should have either their horns removed, covered with piping or tubes, transported in individual crates, or one male (with horns removed or protected) with a group of females.

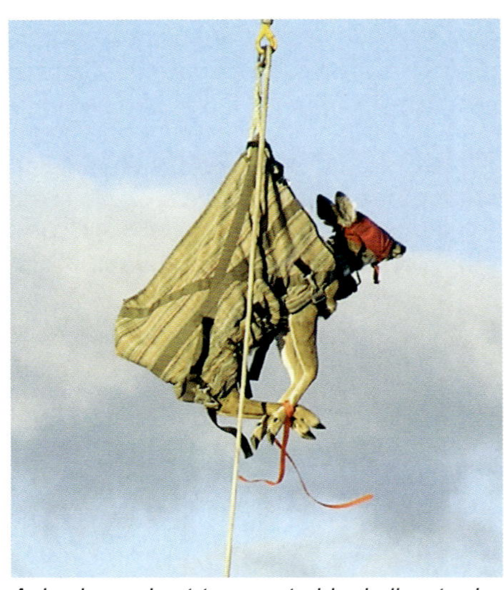

Animals are best transported by helicopter in bags specifically designed for the species. Awake animals can be transported if hobbled and blindfolded; anesthetized animals can also be transported if their heads are kept upright to avoid regurgitation.

Tranquilizers are often used to calm excitable animals; this is particularly true of long-acting tranquilizers (LATs). Other tranquilizers, such as diazepam (5–10 mg total dose for adult ungulate), can also effectively take the edge off an awake animal.

Transport trailers should be dark, but not so enclosed as to preclude adequate air circulation. Animals crowded in a closed trailer can quickly overheat, even at sub-freezing temperatures. It is more important to allow for good air circulation then it is to have a darkened trailer. Many North American ungulates have been transported safely in unmodified, standard stock or horse trailers.

In general, movement should be fairly restricted when transporting awake animals by placing as many as reasonable into a given space. This will prevent excessive movement and the potential for developing capture myopathy or hyperthermia. When shipping several ungulates together, keep them the same approximate size (to prevent trampling of smaller animals) and avoid mixing males and females. If feasible, male ungulates should have their antlers removed prior to transport to avoid their injuring other animals from displaced aggression.

Individual crates can also be used to restrict movement of ungulates. Ungulate crates should be constructed with doors at both ends (easier to load and unload the animal) and with plenty of air holes. Handles should be placed on the sides to allow lifting. Crates should be wide enough to allow the animal to lie sternally, but not allow the animal to turn around. It should be tall enough for the animal to barely stand, but not so tall as to allow the animal to flip over backward.

Carnivores should be crated and shipped separately. Carnivore crates can be

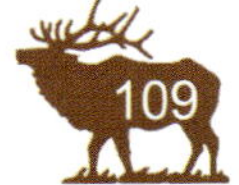

relatively larger than ungulate crates because excessive movement and capture myopathy are less of a concern. Carnivores often lay down throughout the journey. Blocks of ice in a pan can provide needed moisture while preventing spills.

Recovery from Immobilization

An animal recovering from anesthesia should not be left unattended. Ideally, you should remain with the animal until it can walk in a relatively coordinated manner (i.e., respond appropriately to objects, people, other animals) whether an antagonist was administered or not. At the minimum, you should stay with the animal until it can at least raise itself to a sternal position. Keep the animal cool or warm, depending on weather conditions (i.e., out of the sun in summer, in the sun during winter), dry, and free from inter- or intraspecific harassment or aggression.

Look around the recovery area for possible hazards such as sharp rocks, ledges, or water. Either relocate the animal or stay with it through recovery so as to direct it away from such hazards. Animals recovering while on a slope will usually travel downhill. And what is often at the bottom of a hill? Water. More often than not, a recovering animal will stumble downhill right into a lake or stream. Be prepared to take heroic actions if this happens!

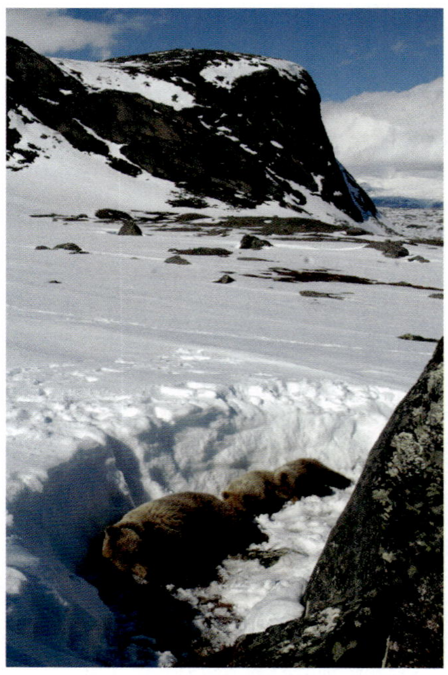

Bears recovering from anesthesia placed in the sun and protected from the wind for warmth and away from cliffs or other hazards.

When releasing animals that have been transported in a trailer, be sure that the release area is free of obstacles in the immediate area. Many ungulates simply walk out of the trailer when the door is opened, but some leap out and run in a panic. Enough clear area should be available to allow the animal to quickly orient itself and avoid obstacles. For these same reasons, try to never release animals at night. The sound of bodies crashing into trees in the dark is not soon forgotten!

Some species may benefit from being released in a temporary enclosure containing food and water. Subsequent release from this site, hours or days later, may result in the group staying together instead of fragmenting as well as their staying closer to the original site.

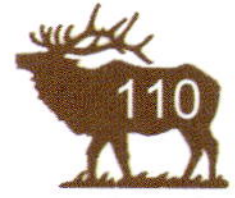

Recovery of Lost Darts

A common concern when capturing animals in areas frequented by humans is the recovery of darts that have missed or did not stay imbedded in the animal. Darts containing potent opioids probably are the most worrisome. There is the fear that a person finding the dart may somehow become exposed to the drug and have an adverse reaction. However, drugs do appear to deteriorate over time when stored in aluminum darts. Elk that were given carfentanil stored in aluminum darts for 14 days did *not* become immobilized, indicating significant loss of potency (Kreeger, 2002). Thus, lost aluminum darts containing carfentanil may become less hazardous over time. 

There are different methods for retrieving darts that have missed their target. It is always a good idea to have a "spotter" looking over the shoulder of the person firing the dart. The spotter's job is to visually follow the dart and nothing else. The spotter has the best opportunity of following the dart's path and approximating where it may have gone should it miss the target. If a dart misses the animal, the general area where the dart was thought to have landed should be marked with a flag, stake, or other device. If enough people are involved in the capture effort, someone can be deployed to locate the dart immediately. Otherwise, continue pursuit of the animal and return to the lost dart site later. Search for the dart by walking increasingly larger circles around the marker. Be slow and methodical; darts often get buried under grass and leaves and can be very difficult to locate. A metal detector can aid in the search for darts containing metal.

There are two types of darts that contain devices to aid location. The first type contains a tiny radio transmitter operating in the 148-174 MHz bands. A radio receiver equipped with a directional antenna is used to locate the dart. The transmitter weighs less than 3 grams and fits in the back of the dart.

The theoretical maximum range of the transmitter is 1,500 m under optimal conditions (flat terrain without significant vegetation), but can be less than 100 m in mountainous, heavily forested terrain or if the animal is lying on the dart. Al-

Left: an effective darting team using a person to determine range as well as follow the dart's path. Right: looking for a missed dart with a metal detector. A flag (circle) was used to mark the approximate spot where the dart was seen hitting the ground.

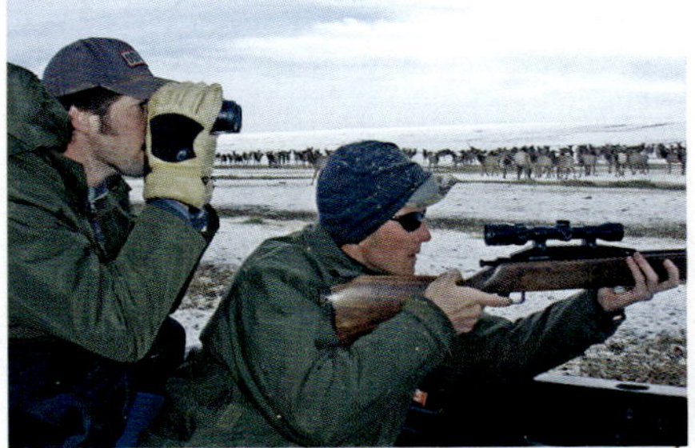

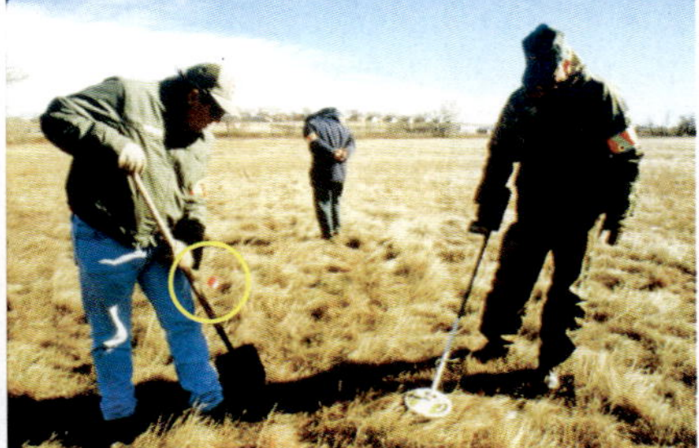

though these transmitter darts can be expensive (US$200), they are reusable. Transmitter darts are available from Palmer and Pneu-Dart in North America and Wildlife Pharmaceuticals in South Africa and Wildpharm in the U.K.

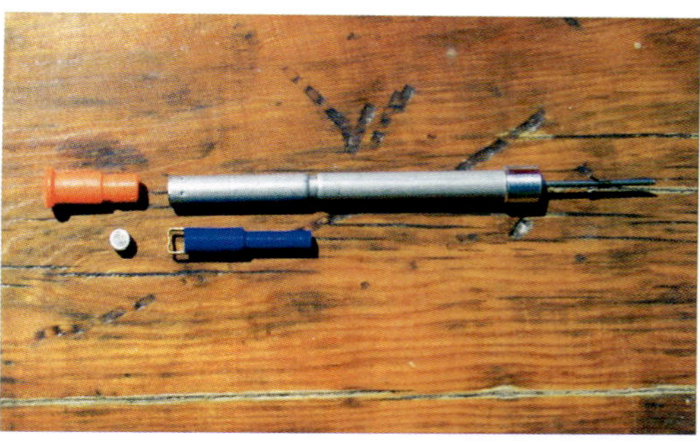

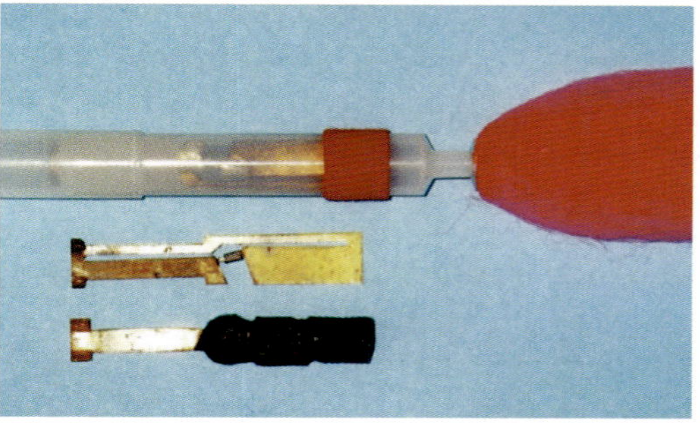

Top: Radio transmitter and battery which is inserted into the rear of a Pneu-Dart dart. Bottom: Recco reflector components and Dan-Inject dart.

The second type operates on the frequency doubling principle. The dart contains a lightweight (2 gram) reflector inserted in the air chamber of a Dan-Inject® plastic dart. A directional signal is transmitted from a hand-held detector, which strikes the reflector in the dart. The frequency of the reflected signal is doubled and sent back to the scanning antenna and receiver of the detector. The receiver detects this signal and a tone is heard via headphones. The maximum search distance is 20-25 m when the angle between the signal and reflector is optimal. However under most conditions, the range is less than 10 m. Although this range may seem limiting when compared to radio transmitter darts, 99.6% of darts equipped with reflectors were located in moose capture operations in Norway (Arnemo, unpubl. data). Darts equipped with reflectors are much cheaper than radio transmitter darts, but the detector used in this system is much more expensive than a radio receiver. The reflector system is available from Recco in Sweden (www.recco.com). Also, reflective tape can be attached to regular darts to aid in their nighttime recovery or to help follow darted animals in the dark with the use of a spotlight.

Euthanasia

Invariably, there will come a time when an animal must be euthanized either because it has been critically injured or it is terminally ill. If an animal needs to be euthanized, it should be done safely and effectively with some consideration for the dignity of the animal and the sensitivities of the public. Many methods of euthanasia, such as shooting and stunning, are effective and medically acceptable but are reprehensible to the public (or even other biologists!). Chemical euthanasia is generally the preferred method because it is safe, effective, and aesthetically acceptable. Listed below are the various methods of euthanasia that are generally employed for wildlife. Other methods, such as carbon dioxide and inhalant anesthesia, are not listed only because they are not practical for field application. A

detailed discussion of euthanasia methods appears in the Journal of the American Veterinary Medical Association, Vol. 218, No. 5, 1 March 2001, entitled, *2000 Report of the AVMA Panel on Euthanasia.*

Note: It should be remembered that no animal that has been chemically captured and then euthanized by physical methods or one that has been directly euthanized with drugs can be used for human or animal food consumption (but see Carcass Disposal).

Cervical Dislocation

Cervical dislocation can be used to euthanize birds, small rodents, and rabbits. For mice and rats, the thumb and index finger are placed on either side of the neck at the base of the skull. With the other hand, the hind limbs are quickly pulled, causing separation of the cervical vertebrae from the skull. For small rabbits, the head is held in one hand and the hind limbs in the other. The animal is stretched and the neck is hyperextended and dorsally twisted to separate the first cervical vertebra from the skull. For birds of poultry size or smaller, cervical dislocation is accomplished by stretching and twisting.

Decapitation

Decapitation is generally not acceptable due to animal (and public) distress.

Exsanguination

Exsanguination (bleeding to death) is acceptable *only* if the animal has been rendered unconscious by drugs or stunning. It is often a slow, messy, and unsightly process. Bilateral sectioning of the jugular or femoral veins can be effective, but often the blood flow slows after awhile. If possible, try to severe the major arteries leading from the heart by inserting a long-bladed knife into the junction of base of the neck and shoulder and slicing inwards and downwards.

Stunning

Stunning by a sharp blow to the head with a hard object can be used for smaller animals (< 5 kg). Stunning by a penetrating captive bolt can be used on larger animals including the largest hoofstock. The disadvantage of any method of stunning is that it may not cause death, so you must check that the animal is dead by monitoring heart rate, respiration, or pupillary reflex. If you are not sure that the animal has expired, it is wise to insure death by exsanguination. *Note: non*penetrating captive bolts are *not* recommended as a method of euthanasia.

Gunshot

Gunshot is often the most practical, if not only, means of euthanizing wild animals. Ideally, the animal is under some sort of physical or chemical control so that carefully-placed shots can be made. If the animal is *not* controlled, heart or lung shots are preferable to head or neck shots.

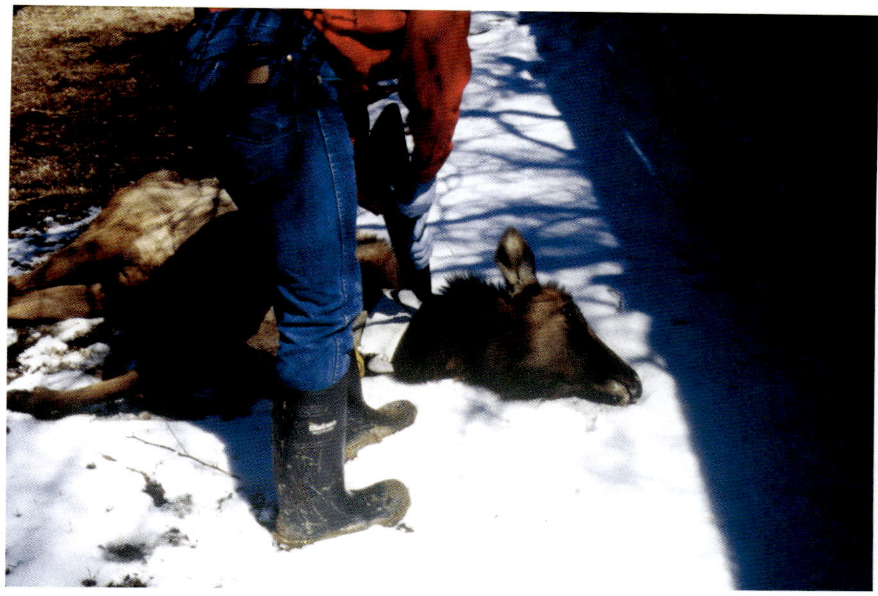

Immobilized elk being euthanized by shotgun with slugs. A neck shot was required to preserve the head for disease analysis. The cervical vertebrae are first located by feel (don't guess where they are at) and the muzzle placed appropriately.

If the animal is under physical control or chemically immobilized, the best target for shooting is at the intersection of two imaginary lines connecting the ears with the contralateral eyes. Large, heavy, slow-moving bullets (e.g., shotgun slugs) are more effective and safer than high-power rifle bullets. Be sure that all personnel stand behind the shooter; bullets hitting bone can take off at unexpected angles. Place the muzzle of the gun as close to the animal as feasible and aim at juncture of the "X" connecting the ears and eyes. On large animals, or animals with heavy skulls, you may want to shoot at a point slightly off center of this imaginary intersection. Try to insure that the shot is placed as perpendicular to the skull as possible; bullets fired at a shallow angle may bounce off thick skulls. For accurate bullet placement, it usually preferable to place the barrel of the gun right on the skull or neck.

Although head shots are the most sure and humane method, sometimes the head must be preserved for disease diagnoses (e.g., rabies, chronic wasting disease). In these cases, the neck is the next preferred site. Again, shotgun slugs are most effective for such shots. If you don't have slugs, shotgun shells loaded with bird shot will suffice since, at these close ranges, the shot leaves the barrel virtually as an intact unit. Although euthanasia by gunshot (or penetrating captive bolt) is usually instantaneous, the animal may thrash and convulse for several seconds after the shot. Large ungulates can deliver bone-breaking kicks during this period, so wait several seconds after cessation of thrashing to handle the animal.

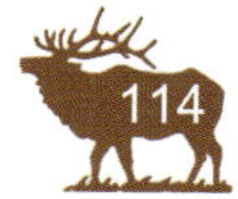

T-61®

T-61® is an injectable nonbarbiturate, non-narcotic mixture of embutramide (a general anesthetic), mebezonium iodide (a neuromuscular blocker), and tetracaine hydrochloride (a local anesthetic) dissolved in dimethylformamide. These drugs provide a combination of general anesthesia, curariform, and local anesthetic actions. T-61® is no longer available in the U.S., but it is in Canada. It must be administered intravenously.

Barbiturates

Several euthanasia products are formulated to include a barbituric acid derivative (usually sodium pentobarbital) with added local anesthetic agents (e.g., Beuthanasia®-D Special; FP-3®). These drugs are Schedule III controlled substances. Barbiturates are generally the preferred method to euthanize domestic animals and they are acceptable for almost all species and sizes of animals. However, the effective volume needed to euthanize large ungulates (>300 kg) is surprisingly high (>100 ml). An entire bottle of commercial euthanasia solution can be insufficient cause death, so have enough on hand to complete the task. Intravenous injection is the preferred route, although intraperitoneal (IP) and intrathoracic injections can be given to small animals and birds.

Potassium Chloride

Another method of euthanasia that is available to anyone is IV injection of potassium chloride. Increasing the concentration of circulating potassium (hyperkalemia) in the blood directly influences electrical activity of the heart resulting in cardiotoxicity and arrest. Potassium chloride can be inexpensively obtained from chemical suppliers. Potassium chloride is also available in grocery stores as "light salt," which is a substitute for sodium chloride.

A saturated solution can be made by adding about 300 mg of potassium chloride per ml of solvent (sterile water, physiological saline, distilled water, or even tap water). Shake vigorously and immediately draw into a syringe as the potassium chloride will settle out quickly of this saturated solution. This solution *must* be given IV *quickly* (slow, drawn out administration will not be effective). Administer at a dosage of at least 50 mg potassium chloride per kg body weight. The animal should be anesthetized before potassium chloride is administered.

Cardiac arrest is quite rapid (<30 sec) and should be verified by listening for heartbeat or feeling for a pulse. Animals euthanized with potassium chloride will often have clonic muscle spasms (arching of neck, twitching) for a few minutes following administration.

Carcass Disposal

In the U.S., animals euthanized with barbiturate solutions must be cremated or deeply buried by federal law. This is to prevent pass-along toxicity to scavengers.

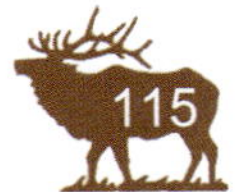

Animals that have been immobilized with the opioids (carfentanil, thiafentanil, etorphine) and have died shortly after immobilization (i.e., < 60 min) should also be buried or removed from the field. Felids, in particular, are very sensitive to opioid toxicity and have been documented to have adverse reactions after consuming freshly-killed carcasses containing opioids (Wolfe and Miller, 2005; Kreeger, unpubl. data). Animals that have received *only* succinylchloride or potassium chloride, however, can be safely eaten by birds or mammals.

Mountain lion showing effects (dilated eyes, ataxia) of consuming freshly-killed carcass of a pronghorn that had been immobilized with thiafentanil. Animals that have been immobilized with the opioids (carfentanil, thiafentanil, etorphine) and have died shortly after immobilization (i.e., < 60 min) should be buried, covered, or removed from the field.

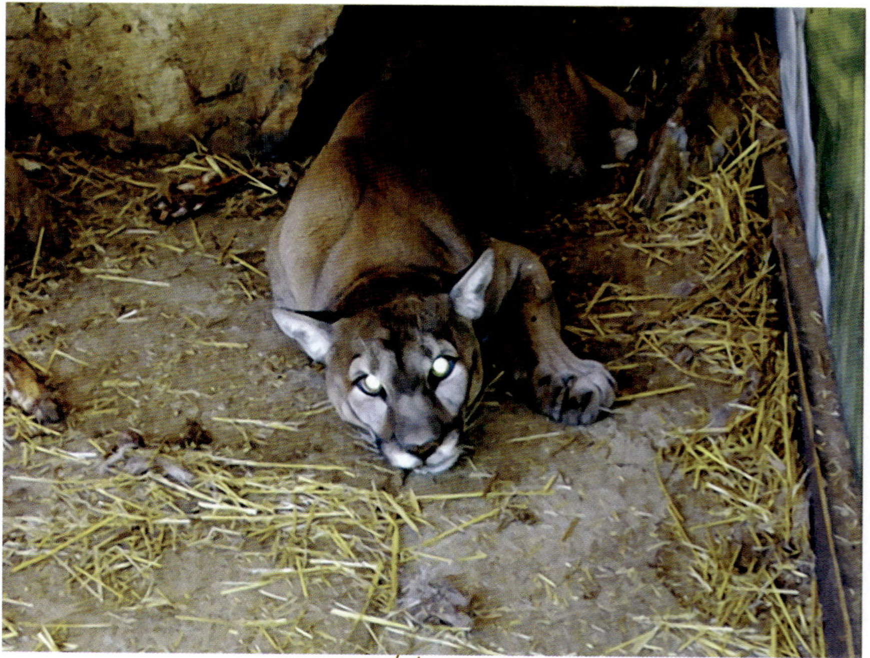

Animal Medical Treatment

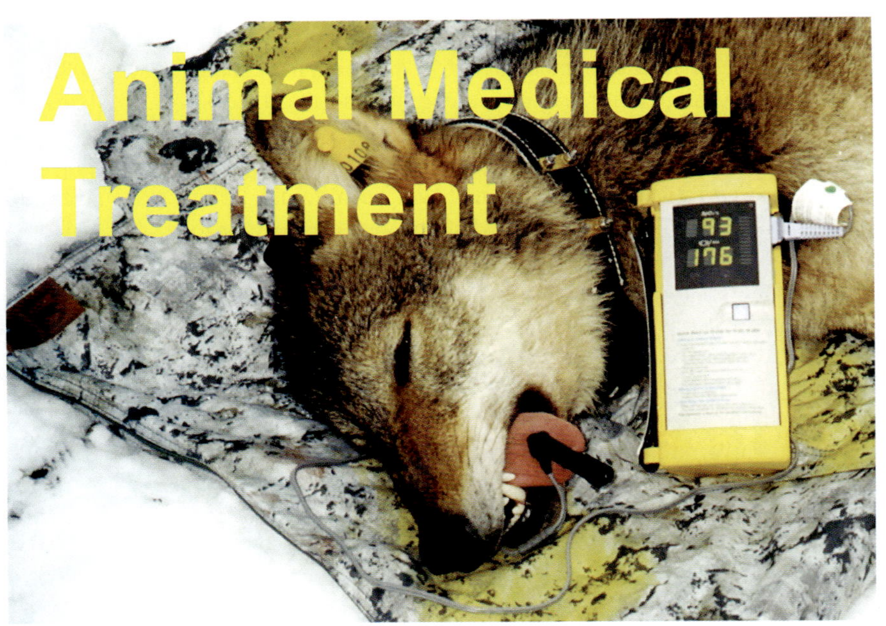

Quick Reference Guide to Animal Emergencies

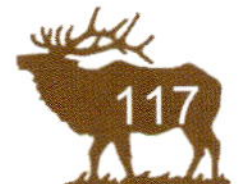

This section is not intended to be a comprehensive course on veterinary emergency medicine. Rather it is intended to familiarize you with the most common medical emergencies encountered in the chemical capture of wild animals. The list of possible complications is lengthy, but the majority of problems are concerned with TPR - Temperature, Pulse, Respiration. This chapter is also written with the assumption that many captures are conducted in the field where monitoring and emergency equipment will be minimal. Thus, your ability to assess problems will be limited to what you can see, hear, or feel.

This manual cannot teach techniques, such as inserting an endotracheal tube. Although such techniques may be recommended, you should receive training from an experienced individual if you are unfamiliar with them. The below order is based on the probability of occurrence as well as necessity for immediate action. Contents of a minimal veterinary first aid kit are included at the end of this section for your information and to aid in selection of emergency equipment and supplies.

Respiratory Depression or Arrest

Definition:

Tissue hypoxia resulting in cell death or damage caused by inadequate oxygenation of blood hemoglobin.

Causes:

- Drug-induced depression of respiratory center
- Airway obstruction
    - nose, trunk occluded
    - trachea occluded (neck draped over log, neck twisted, etc.)
    - vomitus blocking airway
    - edema blocking airway
- Pressure on the diaphragm
    - bloat
    - intestinal, uterine (fetus) contents

Signs:

- Few, shallow, or no respirations
- Cyanosis - gums blue, gray, or "muddy"
- Noisy breathing, wheezing, rattling
- Oxygen saturation (measured via pulse oximeter) $< 70\%$ for more than 2 minutes or oxygen saturation trend is continually downwards.

Treatment:

1. *Cease all further administration of immobilizing drugs.*

2. *Establish patent airway.*

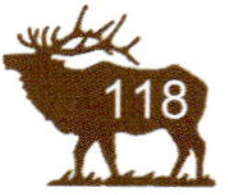

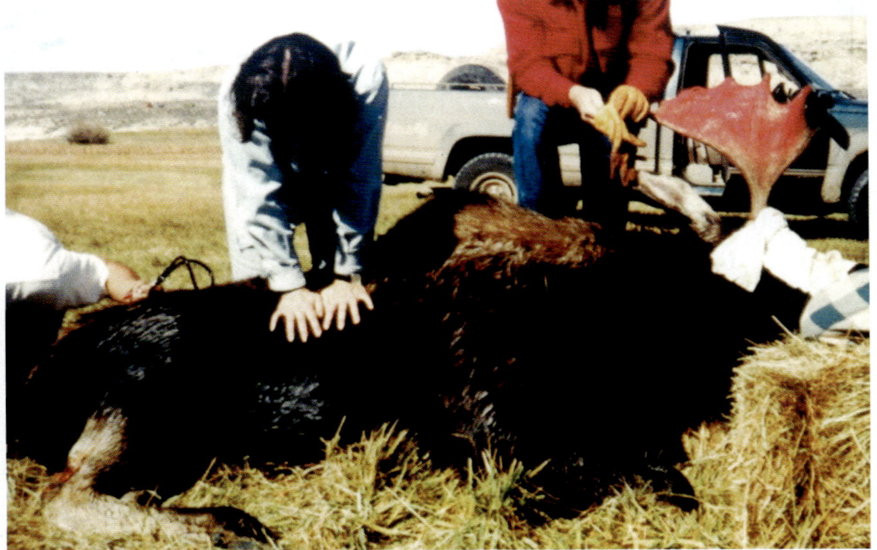

Artificial rescuscitation via manual chest compressions can increase oxygenation even in large animals, such as this moose.

Insure that neck is straight, tongue pulled out, trachea clear of vomitus, foreign objects, etc. Position animal correctly; ruminants should be placed on their sternums; elephants should *always* be on their sides; carnivores can be sternal or lateral.

3. Begin artificial ventilation.

Manual chest compression can be performed by laying the animal on its side and pushing down firmly on the chest, 15–20 times per minute. Other methods include:

- folding, then raising and pulling forward on the front legs in a pumping motion OR

An endotracheal tube and resuscitation bag are far more efficient than chest compressions for increasing and maintaining oxygenation. However, you need to be equipped with the correct size of tube and the knowledge of how to insert it!

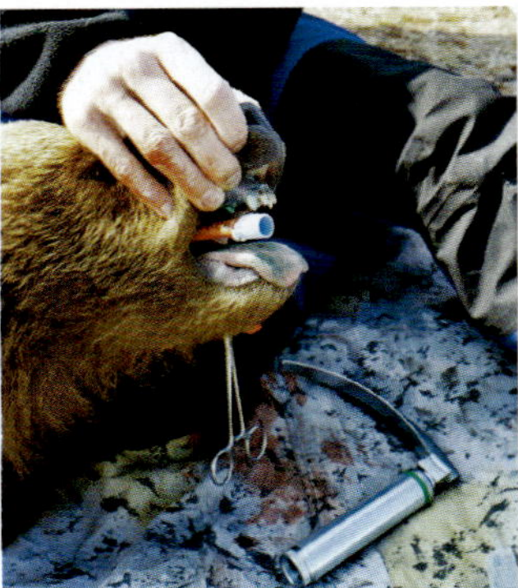

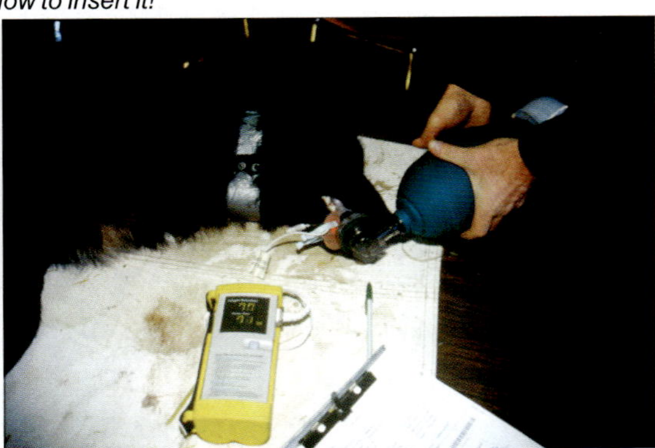

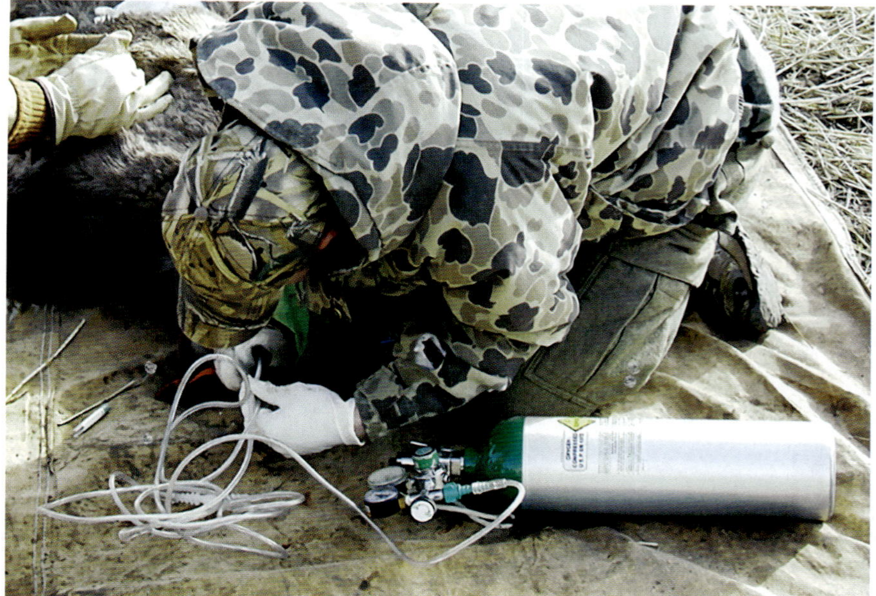

Bighorn sheep being given oxygen via portable oxygen tank and nasal cannula.

- mouth-to-mouth or mouth-to-nose resuscitation OR
- insert endotracheal tube and ventilate with air (from mouth, resuscitation bag) or from oxygen supply OR
- attempt tracheotomy if laryngeal area is hopelessly blocked.

After artificial ventilation has returned normal color to mucous membranes (gums pinkish), stop ventilation for at least one minute to see if the animal will begin breathing on its own. If no respirations are noted, resume ventilation, stopping periodically to allow the animal to breathe without your intervention.

4. *Administer oxygen*

Oxygen can be administered by passing a plastic tube of appropriate size into the nasal cavity, stopping the tip at the level of the eyes. Secure the tube with tape or gauze. Administer oxygen with a D- or E-type oxygen cylinder containing 100% oxygen and equipped with an ambulance pressure regulator. Use a flow rate of 50–100 ml/kg body weight (approximately 15 l/min for large cervids and bison and 10 l/min for deer, bighorn sheep). Adjust flow rate until cyanosis disappears and/or oxygen saturation is >90% (Cattet et al., 2005).

5. *Administer 1-2 mg/kg doxapram (Dopram®) IV.*

Give doxapram only if artificial resuscitation did not cause the animal to start breathing on its own.

6. *Try acupuncture.*

Acupunture has been used with mixed success to stimulate respiration in immo-

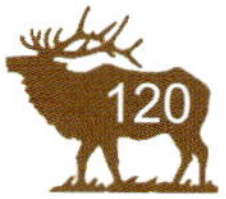

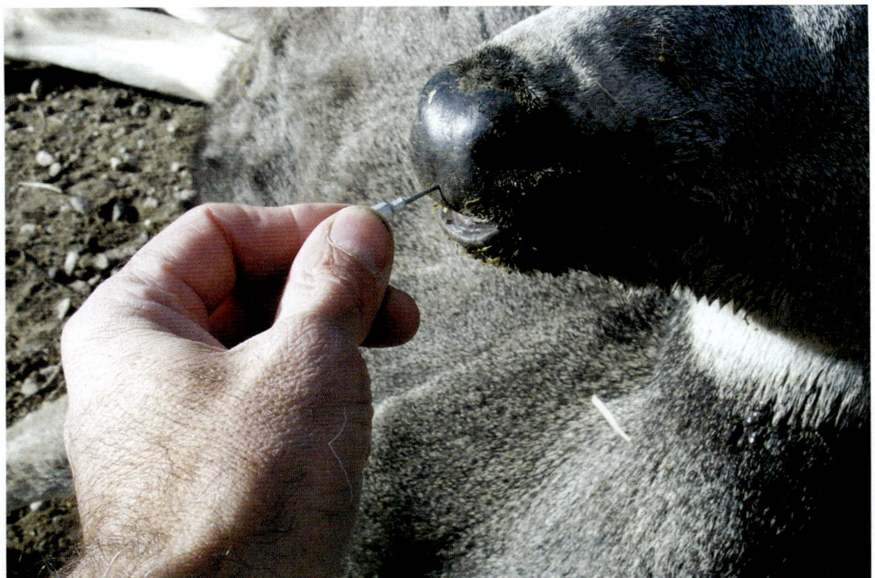

Respiration can be stimulated in ungulates by inserting a needle in the middle of the upper lip just under the nostrils. Upon insertion, the animal should take a breath; further respirations can be stimulated by moving or twirling the needle.

bilized ungulates. Insert a needle (18-20 ga) into the upper lip just between and below the nares (see picture). If just the act of inserting the needle does not cause the animal to take a breath, try twirling it or moving it in and out. If neither of these actions work, relocate the needle and try again.

7. *Administer nalorphine.*

If available, you can administer *nalorphine* IV at a rate of 5 mg nalorphine for every mg of opioid given. Nalorphine will reverse respiratory depression *without* waking the animal up completely.

8. *Administer appropriate antagonist IV.*

If artificial resuscitation or doxapram did not cause the animal to start breathing on its own, your next recourse is to antagonize the immobilizing drugs, even though it means that the animal must be released. If you cannot hit a vein within *30 seconds*, split the dose and give the antagonist in two sites in the shoulder or hip muscles:

- Etorphine: administer 2 mg diprenorphine (or 20 mg naloxone or naltrexone) for every mg of etorphine given.
- Carfentanil: administer 100 mg naltrexone or naloxone for every mg carfentanil given.
- Thiafentanil: administer 10 mg naltrexone or naloxone for every mg thiafentanil given.
- Xylazine: administer 0.125 mg/kg yohimbine; or 1 mg atipamezole for every 10 mg xylazine given.

- Medetomidine or detomidine: administer 5 mg atipamezole for every mg of medetomidine or detomidine given.

Comments:

Respiratory depression/arrest is probably the most common complication encountered in wild animal immobilization. The best advice we can give concerning respiratory arrest is not to panic. You probably have up to 5 minutes before irreversible, hypoxic brain damage occurs. This is really a very long time in which to take corrective action. Panic serves only to confuse your thinking and diffuse your efforts – both of which cost the animal time. Having an IV drip line in place could also prove invaluable in these cases.

Hyperthermia

Definition:

Body temperature increases to point where oxygen demand exceeds supply due to increased metabolism.

Causes:

- Metabolic heat generated by physical exertion
- Heat absorption from environment
  - warm ambient temperatures, direct exposure to sun
  - confinement in poorly ventilated space
- Drug-induced alteration of thermoregulatory centers
- Bacterial/viral infection

The fastest way to lower elevated body temperatures is to immerse as much of the animal as possible in water. In the winter, packing snow around the animal is preferable to wetting the animal which could lead to the opposite problem - hypothermia!

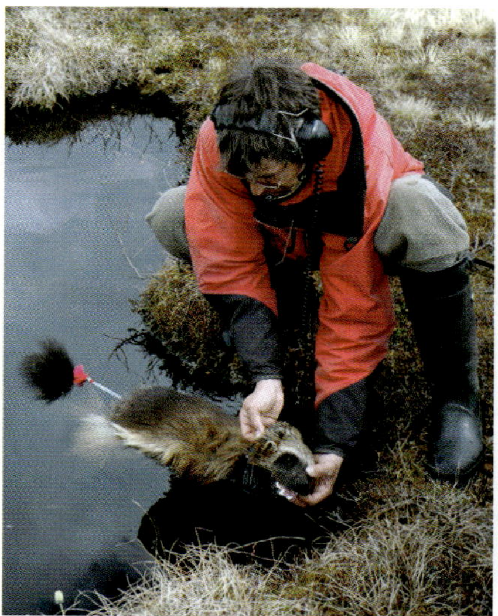

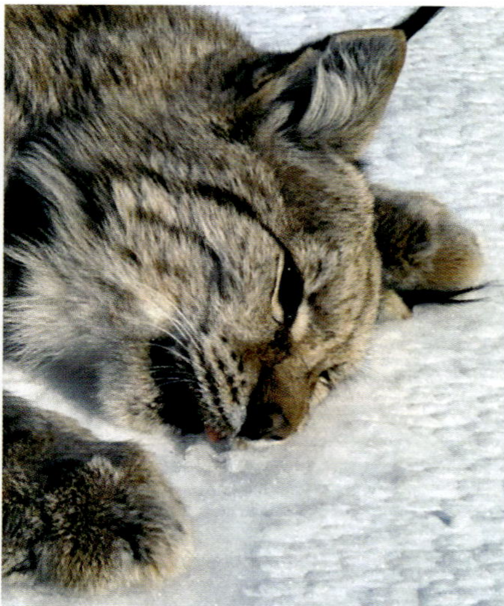

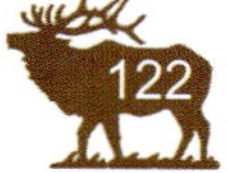

Signs:

- Elevated rectal temperature (>40.5° C/105° F)
- Extremities (ears, feet) very warm to the touch
- Rapid, shallow breathing
- Rapid heart rate, irregular pulse
- Coma, death

Treatment:

1. *Cease all further administration of immobilizing drugs.*

2. *Cool the animal.*

First move the animal out of direct sunlight, if possible. Then employ one or more of the following methods to cool the animal. Whole body immersion in water is probably the most rapid means of decreasing the temperature. Moving air ("fanning") over a wet animal will increase cooling efficiency.

- immerse animal in water (pond, stream, water tank)
- spray entire animal with water, particularly the groin and belly
- pack ice or cold water bags on groin, head
- douse with isopropyl alcohol (rapid evaporation cools quicker)
- administer cold water enema
- administer cold lactated Ringer's solution IV or IP (also see Dehydration)

3. *Administer appropriate antagonist IV.*

Immobilizing drugs not only disrupt the thermoregulatory center, but they prevent the animal from using its normal cooling mechanisms such as sweating and panting. If the above cooling steps did not lower the animal's temperature, your next recourse is to antagonize the immobilizing drugs even though it means that the animal must be released. If you cannot hit a vein within 30 seconds, split the dose and give the antagonist in two sites in the shoulder or hip muscles:

- Etorphine: administer 2 mg diprenorphine (or 20 mg naloxone or naltrexone) for every mg of etorphine given.
- Carfentanil: administer 100 mg naltrexone or naloxone for every mg carfentanil given.
- Thiafentanil: administer 10 mg naltrexone or naloxone for every mg thiafentanil given.
- Xylazine: administer 0.125 mg/kg yohimbine; or 1 mg atipamezole for every 10 mg xylazine given.
- Medetomidine or detomidine: administer 5 mg atipamezole for every mg of medetomidine or detomidine given.

Comments:

Severe hyperthermia (>41° C/106° F) is a medical emergency and you must cool the animal immediately. Obtaining a rectal temperature should be one of the first steps taken as soon as the animal can be safely handled. Monitor the temperature throughout the immobilization period.

Hypothermia/Frostbite

Definition:

Decreased body temperature to point of cellular death due to decreased metabolism, freezing of cellular water, and/or vascular damage.

Causes:

- Drug-induced
  - decreased metabolism and/or endogenous heat production
  - alteration of thermoregulatory center
- Cold ambient temperature
- Loss of insulation
  - wet, soaked coat
  - oiled fur or feathers
  - malnourished (decreased fat)
  - recumbent in one position for too long (compresses downside fur)
- Inadequate circulation
  - shock
  - foothold trap

Signs:

- Decreased rectal temperature (<35° C/95° F)
- Shivering
- Decreased heart rate
- Decreased blood pressure (pulse difficult to feel)

Prevention of hypothermia is usually preferred over having to somehow warm the animal. This bear is covered to prevent heat loss.

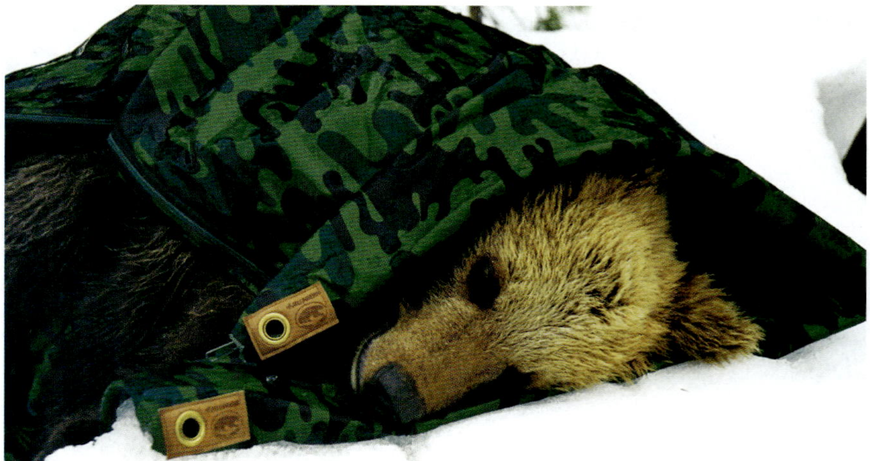

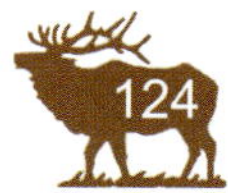

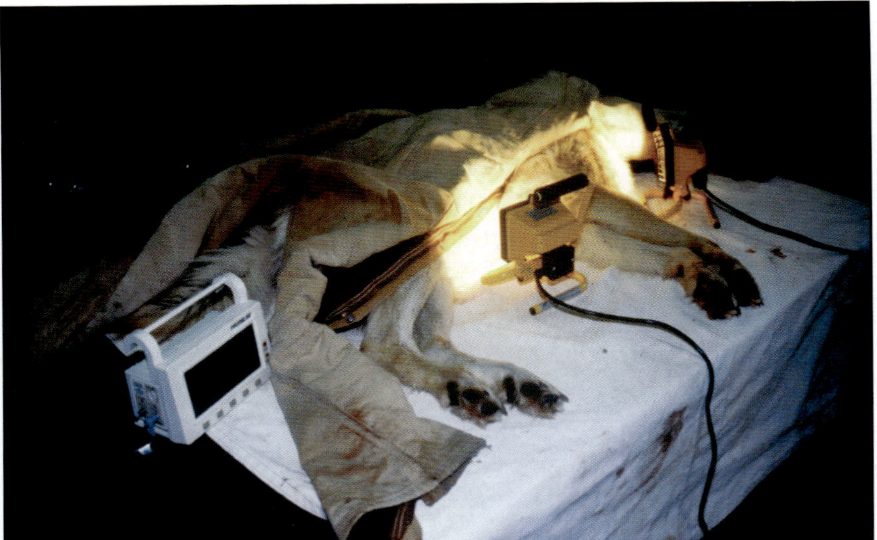

Treating hypothermia is not easy. An external source of heat needs to be applied because the animal is not generating sufficient endogenous heat. Covering the animal to retain heat is advisable. Also, the heart rate should be monitored in severe cases. Drug metabolism will be slowed so recovery will be prolonged.

- Extremities cold to touch
- Extremities firm (frostbite)

Treatment:

1. *Warm the animal.*

The only treatment for hypothermia or frostbite is warming the animal or affected part. One or more of the below methods can be employed to accomplish this. Regardless of the method(s) used, expect a slow recovery back to temperatures suitable for release of the animal (38° C/100° F).

- *containers* of warm water (do not wet the animal unless you can dry it also!)
- blankets
- foam pads (place under animal)
- hand warmers
- body heat (put small animal inside of your coat)
- electric heat pads, lights

Comments:

Antagonism of immobilizing drugs is *not* recommended for hypothermia cases. This is because recovery is invariably slow and if you release the animal with depressed temperature, it may walk away appearing normal only to succumb to hypothermia later because it was unable to produce enough endogenous heat to

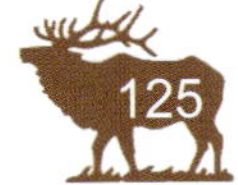

rewarm itself. Still, warming may be difficult, if not impossible, for large animals such as deer. In this case, your only recourse may be to antagonize (if possible) the drugs and release the animal. You may actually have to give boosters of immobilizing drugs to keep the animal unconscious until warmed. However, because the animal's metabolism is slowed by the hypothermia, drug effect is usually prolonged and recovery will be slow anyway. Chilling below 24° C/75° F invariably results in death. Hypothermia is not as common of a problem as is hyperthermia. Because of this, many overlook this problem in the field - much to their chagrin. Very cold weather (<-18° C/0° F) is hard on animals, people, and equipment.

Shock

Definition:

Shock is a clinical syndrome characterized by ineffective blood perfusion of tissues resulting in cellular hypoxia. Shock is often seen in animals which have undergone a stressful or strenuous capture or handling.

Causes:

- Prolonged physical exertion
- Prolonged physiological and/or psychological stress
- Severe blood loss

Signs:

- Rapid heart rate
- Low blood pressure (slow capillary refill)
- Muscle weakness
- Depressed sensorium (often masked by drugs)
- Hyperventilation

Treatment:

1. *Cease all further administration of immobilizing drugs.*

2. *Administer 30 ml/kg Lactated Ringer's solution IV.*

If shock is due to blood loss or redistribution of blood, administer lactated Ringer's solution IV rapidly by using a large-bore (16–18-gauge) needle into a large vein such as the jugular or femoral. Infusion of fluids works best with a drip set attached to the fluids bag, but you could also use a large-capacity syringe (30–60 ml) by leaving the needle in the vein, removing only the syringe to refill, and reattaching the syringe to the needle to administer the fluids. Administering fluids to large animals may be impractical due to the amount of fluid required (often several liters). Needless to say, if blood loss is due to a wound, the wound must be corrected as well.

3. *Administer 5 mg/kg dexamethasone IV.*

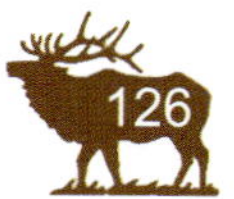

Administer slowly (app. 30 sec). Prednisolone sodium succinate at 10 mg/kg IV or methylprednisolone sodium succinate at 20 mg/kg IV can be substituted for dexamethasone.

4. *Assist ventilation if necessary.*

Comments:

Many deaths of captured animals are attributed to stress or shock but a definitive diagnosis often remains open. Like capture myopathy, there may be little that you can do to treat shock, except prevent it from happening in the first place.

Bloat

Definition:

Excess gas resulting from normal fermentation accumulating in the rumen of ungulates; the rumen enlarges compressing the diaphragm and lungs and impairing respiration.

Causes:

- Drug-induced (xylazine, opioids)
- Incorrect body position

To prevent bloat, ungulates should be kept in the sternal position. Position is less crucial in carnivores, but they can still bloat, particularly if they have recently eaten.

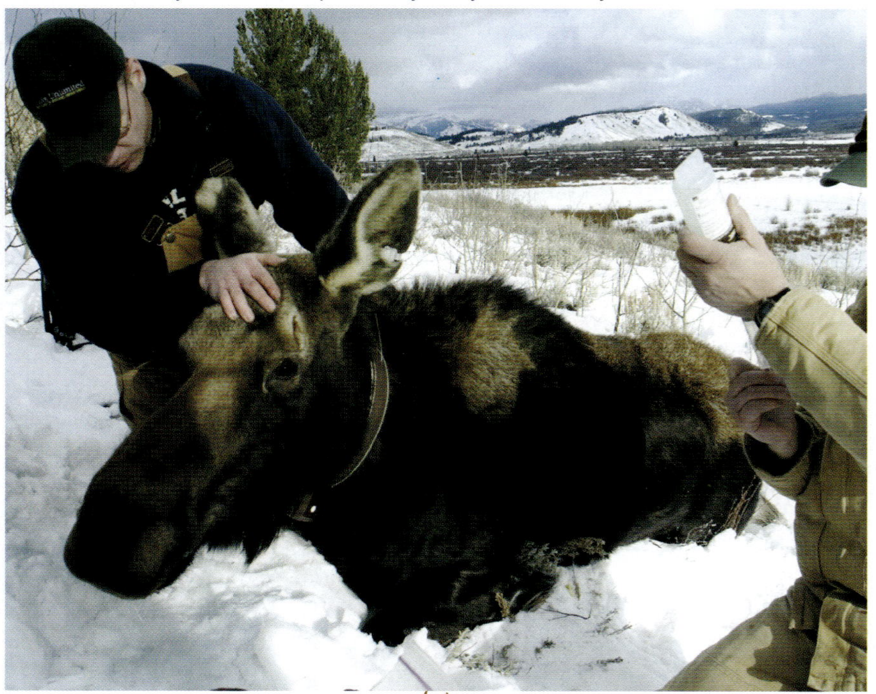

Signs:

- Increase in size of abdomen
- Labored breathing (rapid, shallow)
- Increased salivation

Treatment:

1. *Correct body position.*

If at all possible, position the animal on its sternum. Hold head up to straighten esophagus. Elephants should always be placed on their sides.

2. *Pass stomach tube.*

A fairly flexible, plastic tube (approx. 120 cm long x 1.5 cm O.D.), inserted through the esophagus into the stomach, can relieve bloat by releasing intestinal gas. Lubricate the tube with K-Y jelly and be sure that there are no sharp edges on the tube that could lacerate tissue. Be sure you are not in the trachea! If you are not sure about the placement of the tube, listen to the end of it for breathing sounds. Also, the animal will oftentimes cough if the tube is placed into the trachea.

3. *Insert large-bore needle into left side to release gas.*

If you don't have a stomach tube or can't otherwise relieve the bloat, place the animal right side down. Next, locate the highest point of the bloated rumen (which will be on the left or upper side); this essentially will be the tallest point of the animal's side if it is lying on a flat surface. Insert a 14- or 16-gauge, 1.5-inch needle straight into the rumen at this point. You should be able to hear and smell escaping rumen gas. This method is slower than a stomach tube, so continue to monitor breathing until the bloat is relieved.

4. *Administer appropriate antagonist IV.*

If the above steps did not relieve the bloat or if a respiratory crisis develops, your only recourse is to antagonize the immobilizing drugs even though it means that the animal must be released. Antagonism of the immobilizing drugs should allow the animal to eructate on its own to relieve the bloat. If you cannot hit a vein within 30 seconds, split the dose and give the antagonist in two sites in the shoulder or hip muscles:

- Etorphine: administer 2 mg diprenorphine (or 20 mg naloxone or naltrexone) for every mg of etorphine given.
- Carfentanil: administer 100 mg naltrexone or naloxone for every mg carfentanil given.
- Thiafentanil: administer 10 mg naltrexone or naloxone for every mg thiafentanil given.
- Xylazine: administer 0.125 mg/kg yohimbine; or 1 mg atipamezole for every 10 mg xylazine given.
- Medetomidine or detomidine: administer 5 mg atipamezole for every mg of medetomidine or detomidine given.

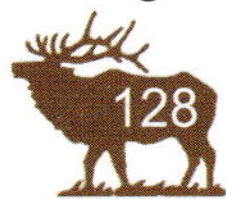

Comments:

A stomach tube should be standard equipment when immobilizing ruminants because bloat is a common sequelae to chemical capture. Often however, you will be through with the procedure and will have antagonized the capture drugs before bloat develops to the point of causing complications.

Vomiting/Aspiration

Definition:

Vomiting is the ejection of stomach contents through the esophagus and mouth; aspiration is the inspiratory sucking into the airways of foreign material, such as vomitus.

Causes:

- Drug-induced (e.g., xylazine)
- Stress, excitement
- Head positioned lower than stomach/rumen

Signs (aspiration):

- Gurgling sounds during respiration
- Choking, gasping
- Cyanosis - gums blue, gray, or "muddy"
- Presence of foreign material in larynx, trachea, nostrils
- Respiratory arrest

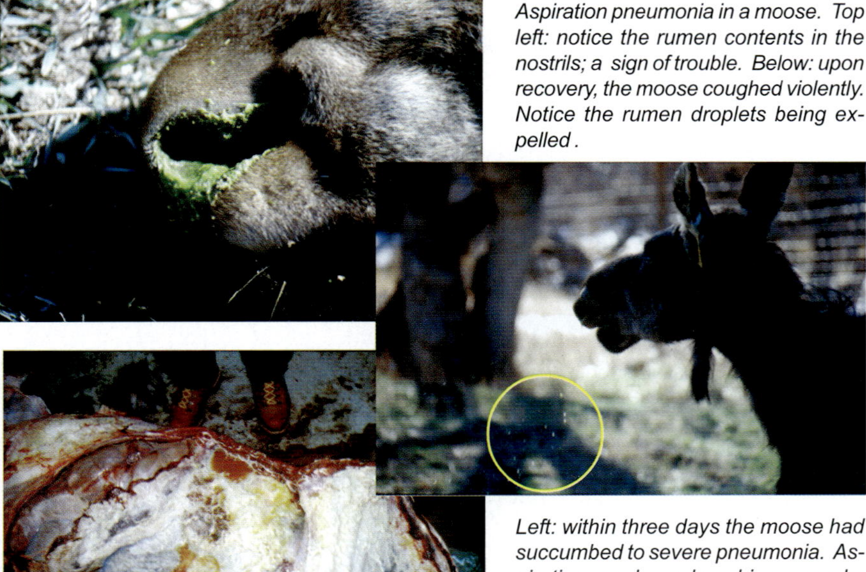

Aspiration pneumonia in a moose. Top left: notice the rumen contents in the nostrils; a sign of trouble. Below: upon recovery, the moose coughed violently. Notice the rumen droplets being expelled.

Left: within three days the moose had succumbed to severe pneumonia. Aspiration can be reduced in moose by not *adding tranquilizer to the primary anesthetic (Kreeger, 2000).*

Treatment:

1. *Cease all further administration of immobilizing drugs.*

2. *Clear airway.*

Clear vomitus, mucus, etc. as much as possible. Place the animal on its sternum with its neck down and head extended and then lift the body with head and neck remaining down, if possible, to help clear vomitus. Smaller animals can be suspended by their rear legs and shaken up and down slightly.

3. *Begin artificial ventilation, if necessary.*

If breathing has ceased, use one of the below methods to induce the animal to begin breathing on its own:

- Manual chest compression can be performed by laying the animal on its side and pushing down firmly on the chest, 15–20 times per minute OR
- folding, then raising and pulling forward on its front legs in a pumping motion OR
- mouth-to-mouth or mouth-to-nose resuscitation OR
- insert endotracheal tube and ventilate with air (from mouth, resuscitation bag) or from oxygen supply OR
- attempt tracheotomy if laryngeal area is hopelessly blocked.

4. *Administer 1-2 mg/kg doxapram (Dopram®) IV.*

Give doxapram only if artificial resuscitation did not cause the animal to start breathing on its own.

5. *Administer long-term antibiotics.*

Aspiration of vomitus can result in the development of pneumonia (see comments).

Comments:

Vomiting in and of itself may not be a problem; the aspiration of the vomitus is. Not only can the animal choke on the vomit and die, the mere aspiration of just a small amount of stomach contents can inoculate the lungs with bacteria resulting in pneumonia. The pneumonia may not develop for days - long after the animal has been released and oftentimes beyond further treatment. Thus, aspiration may result in the delayed death of the animal even though at the time of recovery it seemed perfectly healthy. Aspiration of large amounts of vomitus has a grim prognosis for the animal and euthanasia may be considered.

Capture Myopathy

Definition:

Capture myopathy (CM) is a complex condition affecting animals which usually have undergone a particularly stressful or strenuous capture or handling. It is invariably associated with severe or prolonged physical exertion, but psychologi-

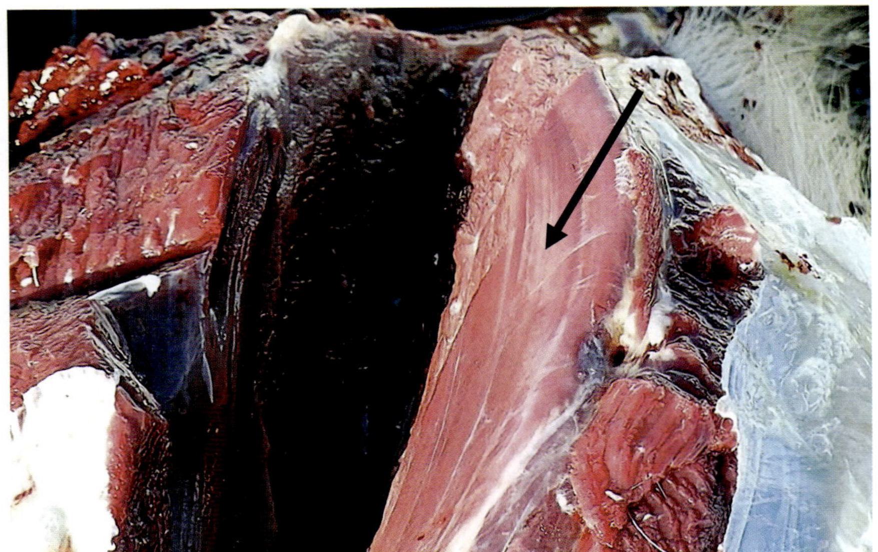

One of the few grossly observable signs of capture myopathy is pale discoloration of the large muscles (arrow) of the hindquarters. Normal musculature is to the left of the arrow.

cal stress is suspected as an important initiator of CM. The pathophysiology of CM is complex and we refer you to Spraker (1982, 1993) or Cattet et al. (2005) for excellent discussions of this topic.

Causes:

- Prolonged physical exertion
- Prolonged physiological and/or psychological stress

Signs:

- Ataxia, weakness
- Paresis or paralysis
- Myoglobinuria (dark, brownish urine)
- Death

Treatment:

1. *Administer 5 meq/kg sodium bicarbonate IV.*

Administer slowly (4–5 ml/min) to avoid cardiac arrhythmias.

2. *Administer fluids, such as Ringer's lactate.*

Comments:

Because the pathogenesis of CM is incompletely understood, treatment is difficult and often unsuccessful. There is nominal consensus that lactic acidosis (lowered blood pH) is a consistent finding in CM cases. Restoration of normal blood pH by the administration of sodium bicarbonate is thought to ameliorate much of the pathology associated with CM. Signs of CM may develop within a few hours of capture or may not appear for several days. Blood samples will show severely altered serum chemical values; necropsy of the hindquarters often reveals gross or microscopic muscle degeneration. Capture myopathy occurs predominantly in ungulates, but it has also been reported in primates, birds, marsupials, seals, raccoons, and dogs. Animals deficient in vitamin E and selenium may be more likely to develop CM. It is more frequent in animals with high metabolic rates (e.g., pronghorn) and may be higher in autumn months when the abundance and nutritional quality of forage is lower.

Seizures/Convulsions

Definition:

Transient disturbance of cerebral function characterized by a violent, involuntary contraction or series of contractions of the voluntary muscles.

Causes:

- Drug-induced (e.g., ketamine or ketamine combinations)
- Trauma
- Hypoglycemia

Signs:

- Uncontrolled muscle spasms; whole body spasms
- Rigid extension of the limbs
- Mouth gaping

Treatment:

1. Administer 10 mg diazepam (Valium®) IV slowly.

Administer the diazepam dose IV over a 10–15 second interval to prevent cardiac arrest due to a rapid IV bolus. Midazolam (Versed®) can be substituted for diazepam at the same dose. Midazolam does not have to be injected slowly. Both diazepam and midazolam can be given IM. Repeat dose if animal continues to seizure.

2. Monitor temperature.

Prolonged seizures can increase body temperature due to endogenous heat production. If temperature >41° C/105° F, refer to treatment of hyperthermia.

Comments:

Most seizures seen in chemical immobilization are due to the use of ketamine, either when used alone or in conjunction with the alpha-adrenergic or phenothiazine tranquilizers. Usually, seizures do no harm to the animal, but they disrupt handling of the animal and can lead to hyperthermia and other complications if left untreated. Seizures accompanying ketamine immobilizations are most common during induction and recovery from anesthesia.

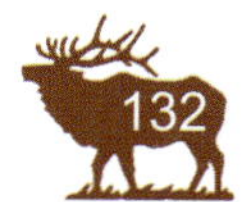

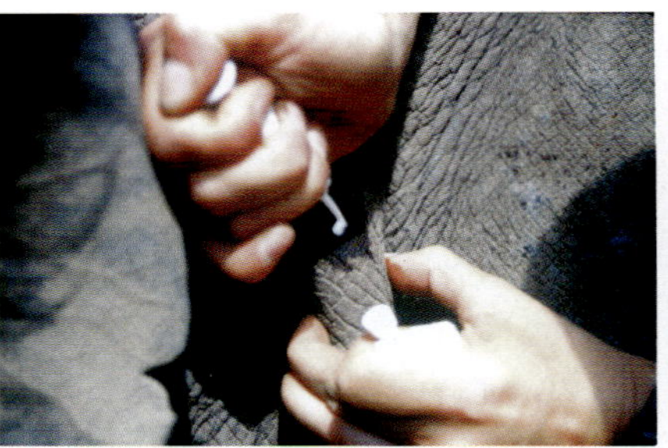

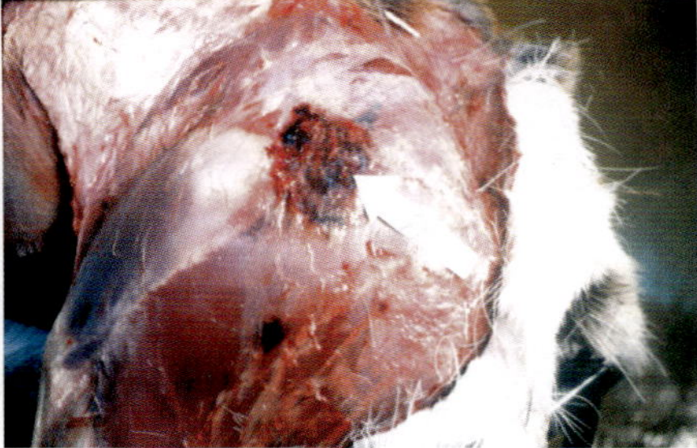

Left: treating a dart wound in a rhinoceros with a preloaded antibiotic tube intended for mastitis. Right: all darts cause injury which should be treated with long-acting antibiotics.

Wounds

Treatment:

1. *Clean the wound.*

Small, shallow lacerations can be lavaged with a povidone-iodine (Betadine®), 2% chlorhexidine (Nolvasan®) scrub solution, or sterile saline. Deeper, penetrating wounds can be flushed by diluting povidone-iodine with sterile saline to a 10% solution or 2% chlohexidine to a 0.05% (i.e., 1:40 dilution of the 2% solution) solution. If necessary, use a scalpel to cut away (debride) heavily damaged, diseased, or contaminated tissue.

2. *Suture the wound, if necessary.*

Generally, deep, penetrating wounds should *not* be sutured to allow drainage; lengthy lacerations, deep or shallow, should probably be sutured. Despite the fondness of some "old hands" to suture wounds with black thread or monofilament fishing line, there really is a rationale for using the different types of suture materials, needles, and patterns. For more information, you should consult surgery textbooks, or better, obtain first-hand experience with a veterinarian. Nonetheless, the situation is somewhat simplified under field situations. Although it is generally preferred to use *non*-absorbable sutures to close the outer skin layer and absorbable sutures for all internal layers, in the field you only need absorbable sutures for all closures since you will be releasing the animal (there is little likelihood that you could recapture the animal to remove any skin sutures!).

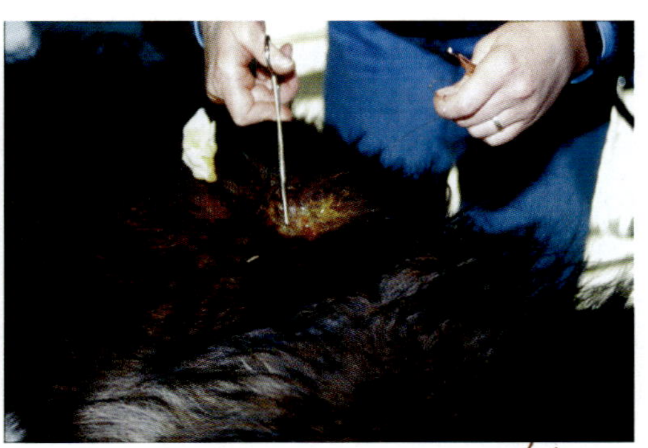

If suturing a wound is required during cold winter months, do not *shave the wound because the animal will lose tremendous amounts of heat. Rather, saturate the wound area with a mixture of iodine and sterile jelly lubricant. Then just push the sticky hair coat aside while you suture.*

If the wound is deep, suture the internal muscle layers first using a tapered needle; then suture the skin using a "cutting" needle. It can be difficult, if not impossible, to suture skin using tapered needles, so be sure that you are at least equipped with cutting needles. If suturing a long and deep laceration, leave an opening in the ventral (lower) portion of the wound to allow for drainage.

3. *Give antibiotics.*

Any animal receiving a laceration should be given antibiotics to reduce the magnitude of infection. The penicillins are the most commonly-used antibiotics since they are effective against many of the skin microbes as well as formulated in repository (long-lasting) preparations. A combination of procaine penicillin G and benzathine penicillin G provides both fast, high blood concentrations (procaine) plus prolonged therapeutic concentrations (benzathine; 5-7 days). The minimum dose should be 22,000 IU/kg (10,000 IU/lb) of the *benzathine* penicillin G in order to obtain the repository effect. That is, if a penicillin combination contains 300,000 IU/ml of both penicillin types, then there is 150,000 IU/ml of the benzathine penicillin G. A 100-kg (220 lb) animal would be given (100 kg x 22,000 IU/kg)/150,000 IU/ml = 14.6 ml of the combined antibiotic. This should be administered with a large-bore needle (18 ga) IM at *no more* than 5 ml per injection site. Inject penicillin subcutaneously (SQ) or in the large muscle masses of the proximal hind limbs (i.e., hip muscles). The penicillins need to be kept refrigerated, which is a drawback for field use.

Long-acting oxytetracycline injectable antibiotics do not require refrigeration and they are effective against a broad spectrum of bacteria. When administered IM, absorption is significantly slowed compared to other oxytetracycline formulations. Thus, a single dose may provide protective blood concentrations for up to 48 hours after administration.

Antibiotics should also be given to animals which have been darted, particularly with the powder-charged darts. The large-bore dart needles often can inoculate surface bacteria resulting in debilitating abscesses. The dose would be the same as the above dose for treating wounds. It is also helpful to have intermammary infusion tubes in your veterinary kit. These are essentially disposable syringes, pre-filled with antibiotics, and equipped with a rounded, plastic "needle" used to treat mastitis in dairy cattle. Insert the needle into the dart wound and squeeze the tube until antibiotic comes back out of the wound. The use of antibiotics in thick-skinned species such as elephant and rhino is essential.

Cardiac Arrest

Definition:

Loss of effective cardiac function resulting in cessation of circulation.

Causes:

- Drug-induced

- Hypoxia (respiratory failure)
- Acid-base imbalance
  - acidosis
  - alkalosis
- Electrolyte imbalance
  - hyperkalemia
  - hypokalemia
  - hypocalcemia
- Autonomic nervous system imbalance
  - increased sympathetic tone
  - increased parasympathetic tone
- Hypothermia

Signs:

- Weak or absent heart sounds or pulse
- Poor capillary refill (> 2 sec - see comments)
- Cyanosis - gums blue, gray, or "muddy"
- Increased respiratory rate, abnormal pattern, or apnea
- Dilated pupils
- Skin cold
- Loss of consciousness

Treatment:

1. *Cease all further administration of immobilizing drugs.*

2. *Be sure that the animal can breathe.*
   - head and neck in proper position
   - no airway obstructions
   - begin artificial respiration (see Respiratory Arrest) if apneic
   - administer doxapram (Dopram) 1–2 mg/kg IV if apneic

3. *Begin external cardiac massage.*

Place the animal on its side and apply pressure downward over the heart. Compress for a count of 1 and release for a count of 1 with 60–100 cycles/min. An assistant should palpate the femoral pulse while cardiac massage is being performed to make sure that an effective wave is being produced.

4. *Inject 0.2 mg/kg of 1:10,000 epinephrine intravenously IV or intracardially (IC) and continue massage.*

For IC injection, you may need a long needle (2–3 in) to hit the heart. Insert the needle between the 4th to 6th ribs (usually above and slightly behind the point of the elbow), pull back on the plunger to withdraw blood from the heart to confirm that you are in the heart (or at least a major vessel), and inject. Use a stethoscope to monitor the heart.

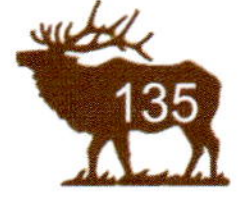

Note: many epinephrine concentrations come as 1:1,000; you should dilute each ml of this solution with 9 ml of physiological saline or lactated Ringer's solution before administering IV or IC.

5. *If no response to the above, inject 0.1 ml/kg calcium chloride solution (10% or 100 mg/ml) IV or IC.*

Calcium gluconate (10%) solution can be substituted for calcium chloride.

6. *If still no response to the above, repeat epinephrine and calcium chloride doses plus inject 10–20 mEq sodium bicarbonate IV or IC.*

Comments:

Capillary refill time (CRT) is a method to assess peripheral perfusion and, by inference, cardiac function. To evaluate CRT, locate a non-pigmented (i.e., pink) area on the gums, vulva, inner eyelid, etc. of the animal. Apply pressure to this site with your finger and the compressed area will turn pale due to blockage of blood circulation. Release finger pressure and time (by counting one-one thousand, etc.) how long it takes for the bloodless area to turn pink again as blood perfusion is restored. A CRT of <2 sec generally implies adequate blood pressure. A slower refill time indicates low blood pressure or other circulatory dysfunction.

The ideal method of cardiac dysfunction diagnosis and treatment is far more complex than presented here and in most field situations, you'll probably neither have time nor materials to follow a highly-complex treatment protocol. In the

Assessing Capillary Refill Time (CRT) in a mountain lion by applying pressure to the gum, releasing pressure, and determining how long it takes for color to return.

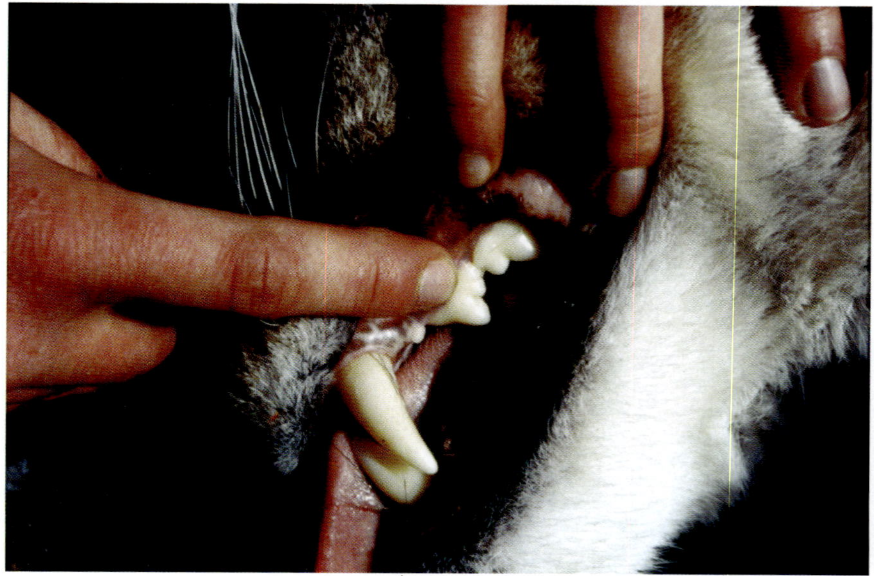

field, heart function has successfully been revived with cardiac massage and one or more epinephrine injections, but no other drugs. Those interested in a more detailed discussion of cardiac emergencies should consult an emergency treatment manual such as the *Handbook of Veterinary Procedures and Emergency Treatment* by R. B. Ford and E. Mazzaferro (8th ed., 2006, Elsevier). The occurrence of cardiac arrest in animal immobilization is fortunately rare, since odds are against saving the animal in the field.

Many cardiac problems do not arise directly from drug use but from metabolic disturbances due to extreme physical exertion and stress. The addition of drugs to a compromised physiological system often precipitates a crisis. Without an electrocardiogram or trained ear (auscultation), cardiac arrhythmias are difficult to detect or diagnose. However, many arrhythmias are probably benign in that they apparently do no long-term harm to the animal upon recovery. Again, consult the above reference if more information is desired on cardiac arrhythmias.

Dehydration

Definition:

Reduction of the body's water content

Causes:

- Decreased water intake
- Hyperthermia (increased loss of water by transpiration)
- Fever (increased loss of water by transpiration)
- Chronic vomiting
- Chronic diarrhea
- Wound drainage
- Polyuria (excessive urination)

Signs:

- Skin lacks pliability (see comments)
- Mouth, gums dry or tacky
- Weak pulse
- Depressed sensorium (may be masked by drugs)
- Signs of shock

Treatment:

1. Cease all further administration of immobilizing drugs.

Administer additional drugs to keep the animal immobilized only if necessary to initiate or maintain treatment. Often, the animal may be so depressed that additional drugs will not be necessary.

2. Determine the volume deficit (4-6-8-10 rule).

The loss of 4% of the body weight in fluid can be determined simply by a history

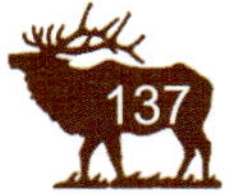

of fluid loss (e.g., held in trap or pen without water for several hours in warm weather, etc.). A 100-kg animal with a 4% loss would have a volume deficit of 4 liters (100 kg x 0.04 = 4 kg = 4 liters fluid). An animal losing about 6% of its fluid volume would have obvious fluid deficits. The mucosa of the mouth would be red and dry; the skin would be tacky and not pliable (see comments). As before, a 100-kg animal with a 6% loss would have a volume deficit of 6 liters. A loss of 8% fluid volume represents severe fluid loss. The pulse would be weak and the animal depressed. A ≥ 10% fluid loss is life threatening.

3. *Administer fluid therapy.*

Use the 4-6-8-10 rule above to calculate the amount of fluids required. Administer isotonic lactated Ringer's solution or 0.9% saline either IV, SQ, or IP.

Comments:

One of the quickest methods of diagnosing clinical dehydration in the field is to pinch the animal's skin forming a "tent." If the animal is well hydrated, the skin tent will collapse to its normal configuration almost instantly. If the tent collapses relative slowly (e.g., 1–2 sec), you can assume that the animal is dehydrated. If the tent doesn't collapse at all or very slowly (> 5 sec), assume that the animal is seriously dehydrated (≥ 8% loss).

The correct assessment of fluid loss with its concomitant electrolyte imbalance is usually beyond the capabilities of field biologists to precisely determine. Depending on the type of fluid loss, the animal's blood pH can be altered, electrolytes (e.g., sodium) lost, and the blood can be hypo- or hypertonic. Each of these conditions actually require a specific course of fluid therapy with over a dozen fluid types from which to choose. It is unlikely that you will be able to determine the osmolar deficit, special ion involvement, or acid-base status and equally unlikely that you will be lugging around several liters of the differing fluids. Thus, it seems most practical for field immobilizations to be equipped with one type of fluid (e.g., lactated Ringer's) in an amount sufficient to treat the target animal.

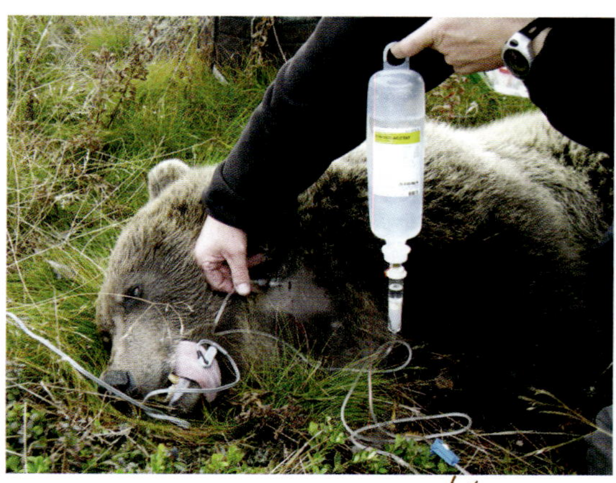

Fluids can be administered intravenously, as in the jugular vein of this bear, or subcutaneously. Fluid therapy should not be attempted without previous experience or guidance from a veterinarian or experienced technician.

Veterinary First Aid Kit Checklist

General:

16-gauge, 1-inch needles
18-gauge, 1.5-inch and 3-inch needles (for intracardiac injections)
20/21 gauge, 1-inch needles
1-, 3-, 5/6-, 10/12-, and 30/60-ml syringes
Stomach Tube
K-Y Jelly
Endotracheal Tubes - French sizes 28, 36, 44
IV Drip Set
Physiological Saline (0.9% NaCl)
Lactated Ringer's Solution
Tourniquet (for raising veins)
Thermometer (electronic or mercury)
Stethoscope
Resuscitation Bag

For Wound Management:

Povidone-iodine or 2% chlorhexidine scrub solution
Antibiotics (procaine-benzathine penicillin)
Gauze sponges, 4 cm x 4 cm
Iodine Surgical Scrubs
Needle holder or hemostats
Tissue forceps
Spools of sizes 0 and 000 chromic gut (or other absorbable suture)
Tapered (for muscle) and cutting (for skin) suture needles
Scalpel Blades
Scissors
Roll gauze
Adhesive tape
Sterile Surgical or Examination Gloves

Emergency Drugs (be sure drugs are not outdated):

Naloxone (naltrexone, nalmefene)
Diazepam or midazolam, 5 mg/ml
Epinephrine, 0.1 mg/ml (1:10,000)
Atropine Sulfate, 0.5 mg/ml
Doxapram hydrochloride, 20 mg/ml
Dexamethasone, 2 mg/ml
Calcium Chloride, 10% (100 mg/ml)
Sodium Bicarbonate, 1 mEq/m

Human Medical Treatment

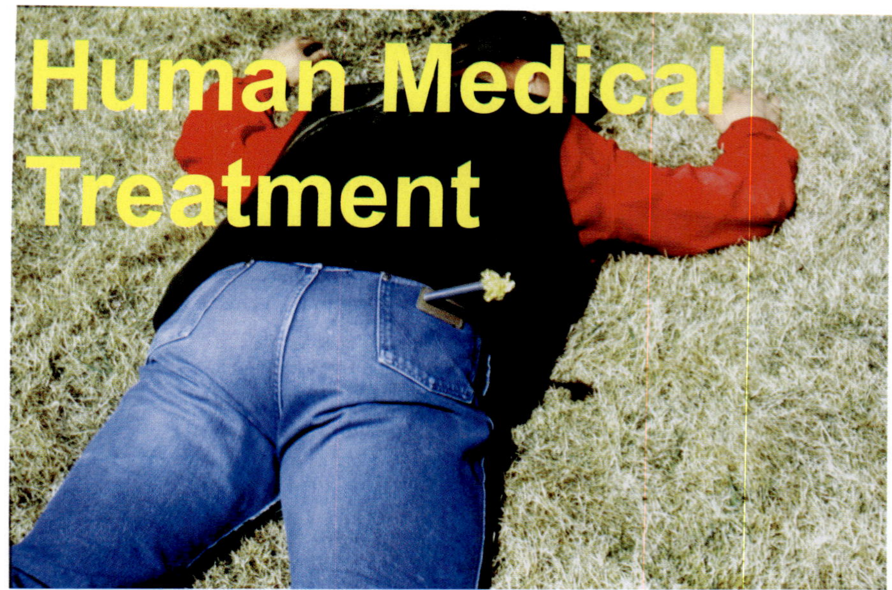

Quick Reference Guide for Human Exposure to:

Continued next page...

There are many agents used in animal anesthesia that are potentially lethal to humans. Accidental exposure can occur in many ways but, most commonly, drugs are sprayed in the eyes or mouth or injected via a syringe with an unprotected needle. Accidental injection by being hit with a dart or receiving the full dose by some other method is rare. However, there has been at least one published fatality and several accidental exposures reported (Firn, 1973; Summerhays, 1976; Allsup, 1977; Goodrich, 1977; Orr, 1977; Carruthers et al., 1979; Haigh and Haigh, 1980; Parker and Haigh, 1982; Poklis et al., 1985; Samanta et al., 1990; Petrini and Keyler, 1993). Thus, this discussion is not trivial. Following are some precautionary steps to take and rules to follow that should decrease the chances of accidental drug exposure.

Preventative Measures

Obtain competent training.

Safe drug handling and use should not be a self-taught course. Attend courses taught by experienced instructors on the use of capture drugs. Unfortunately, there are several "wannabe" individuals teaching the chemical capture of wildlife, but many of them are woefully inexperienced and misinformed. Make an effort to seek out qualified instructors.

Be trained in basic first aid and CPR techniques.

Ideally, everyone involved in the immobilization effort should have this training. Murphy's law would dictate that if only one person on the team had such training, that would be the person who needed medical help!

Always work in pairs.

This is absolutely essential when working with drugs that are potentially lethal.

Always have appropriate antagonists immediately available.

You may not have a second chance to remember the antagonist back in the truck or office. You don't need to have a syringe "preloaded" with the antagonist; just have the antagonist, syringe, and needle together and close at hand.

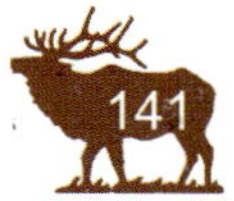

Wear protective gloves and eye protectors.

Drugs can be spilled, sprayed, dripped, dropped, slopped, and leaked in more ways than you can imagine. Don't spray drugs into the air and don't hold loaded syringes in your mouth. Also don't smoke, eat, drink, rub your eyes or mouth, or work with open sores when working with immobilizing drugs.

Carefully withdraw drugs from vials.

Do not inject excessive air into drug vials; equalize air pressure in vials with a needle before withdrawing drug. This is particularly important if you work at different altitudes with the same drug vial (vials used at low altitudes will develop high internal pressures at high altitude). Only if needed, tap the syringe to clear air bubbles. Use a small-gauge needle (e.g., 21, 22, or 25 gauge) to withdraw the drug because large-gauge needles will create holes where drug can leak.

Avoid using pressurized darts when using potent drugs.

Darts whose contents are under pressure by air, butane, or spring tension have their needles capped with a silicone plug or sleeve. When these darts are pressurized, there is a possibility that drug will leak from the sleeve or even discharge prematurely. If you must use pressurized darts, place the needle into a test tube or other device that will contain the drug should it leak.

Treat syringes and darts as if they were guns.

That is, always consider them "loaded" and watch where you point them. Don't carry loaded, unprotected syringes in your pocket; hold them in your hand with protective cap on or carry them in a protective case such as a test tube or cigar case.

Know what you are using.

Make sure the contents of bottles, tubes, and loaded syringes are marked. If you don't know what a drug is, don't use it!

If possible, notify the local emergency care center in advance.

Most physicians are ignorant of the drugs used in wildlife anesthesia and they are unfamiliar with their potency, symptoms, and antagonists. A little communication with the local hospital could save valuable time in an emergency. Either provide the staff, or have on hand, the package inserts of the drugs that you will be using; this information can help the attending physician develop an appropriate treatment. There was a case where a biologist had injected himself and was refused treatment because of the hospital staff's unfamiliarity with the drug.

Be careful with used darts, syringes, and needles.

All of these items will have residual drug remaining on them and many exposures have occurred as a result of careless handling. Store and dispose used needles and syringes with care. It may be safer not to recap the needle with the cover, rather just discard the needle into an appropriate used-needle disposal container. It is very easy to jab a finger when recapping needles – particularly when you are in a hurry or distracted. Recap used needles by placing both hands on a firm surface and carefully guide the cap into place (see picture).

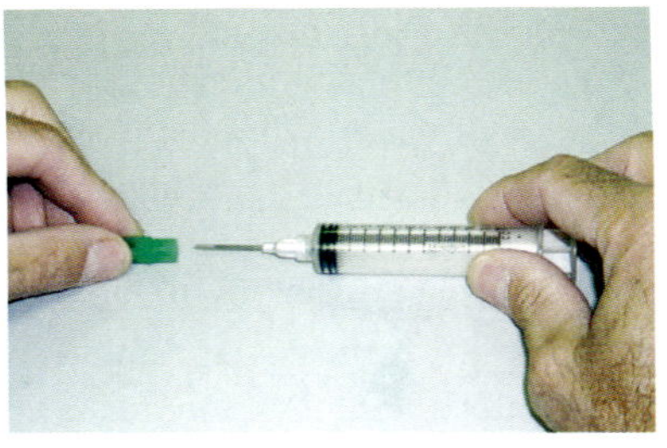

Always clean used darts with care. Cap-Chur® darts often have residual pressure remaining in them after they have been fired. With these darts, it is safer to unscrew the tailpiece first to relieve pressure. Even then, have the dart opening pointed away from you. You can also submerge the whole dart under water before disassembling. Wear gloves and goggles when cleaning darts containing potent drugs.

Rules for Accidental Exposure

The previous discussion was concerned with *preventative* measures. Below are rules to follow when there has been an actual accidental exposure. Following this section are specific treatments for the types of drugs commonly used in wildlife immobilization.

Don't panic.

Stay calm and try to determine how much drug could have been delivered. Many "exposures" are needle pricks or slight skin exposure. If there is doubt that a significant amount of drug has been absorbed, you may wish to quietly wait to determine if any signs of exposure develop. If there are no signs within 15 minutes, you can probably assume that the amount was clinically insignificant.

On the other hand, if you know that the person has received a significant drug exposure, you want to work fast, but always under control. You probably have a minimum of three minutes after complete respiratory arrest before there is irreversible brain damage. Considering the amount of time required to absorb drugs after an IM injection, you most likely have much longer than three minutes in which to get your act together. Panic can obfuscate your thinking processes which costs time. Panic by the exposed person may also cause symptoms, such as lightheadedness, fainting, hyperventilation, etc., which can be misinterpreted as a drug effect.

Tell others of the accident.

It is not the time to be embarrassed or feel stupid after you have accidentally injected yourself, particularly with any of the potentially-lethal drugs. Tell someone about the accident immediately!

Wash the site.

Irrigating the injection/exposure site (particularly mucous membranes) with large volumes of water will greatly reduce further drug absorption. An icepack applied to the site may also delay absorption.

Administer the appropriate antagonist(s).

This applies primarily to opioid exposure, but it also includes exposure to the potent alpha-adrenergic agonists such as medetomidine. The administration of opioid antagonists is probably the single most important life-saving action that you can take.

Remember your "ABCs".

A = Airway

Insure that the patient has a clear airway by placing him/her on the back and tilting the head as far back as possible. Be sure the tongue is clear of the pharynx.

B = Breathing

If respiration has ceased, you must begin artificial respiration (mouth-to-mouth) at a rate of one breath every 5 seconds.

C = Circulation

If the heart stops (no pulse, no heart sounds, color bluish), begin cardiac massage by placing the heel of your hand (with the other hand on top of the first) on the lower third of the sternum and push down every sec (i.e., 60 pushes/minute). Continue artificial respiration concurrent with cardiac massage.

Note the time.

Despite the harried circumstances surrounding accidental drug exposure, try to remember when the exposure occurred and when treatments were administered. This time could be valuable in assessing the amount of drug absorbed as well as determining an appropriate treatment regimen.

Transport the person to the nearest emergency center.

If feasible, have the person walk to the vehicle, but not at a strenuous rate. If the person requires CPR or otherwise can't be transported, send for help. If there is no one available to send, *stay with the patient!* Although the exposed person may be conscious when you leave for help, more drug will be absorbed over time and the person may lapse into a coma leading to respiratory depression and death.

The major cause of death in cases of accidental exposure is respiratory arrest, but you can artificially resuscitate a person for a long time while waiting for help to arrive. So, don't abandon an exposed person even if that person insists that he/she is all right.

Specific Emergency Treatments: Opioids

Fentanyl, Sufentanil, Carfentanil, Etorphine, Thiafentanil (A-3080)

Symptoms:

- Dizziness, incoordination, lethargy, sedation
- Nausea, vomiting
- Pinpoint pupils
- Breathing slow, shallow, or absent; bluish tinge to skin and mucous membranes;
- Cold, clammy skin; weak pulse
- Collapse, unconsciousness, and coma
- Cardiovascular collapse (secondary to hypoxia)
- Death

Treatment:

1. *Call for help.*

Appoint someone to call for help, if available. Otherwise stay with the patient until a third party arrives to help.

2. *Wash site.*

Flush mucous membranes (eyes, mouth, wound, etc.) with copious amounts of water. Use cool or room temperature water - do not use hot water. If drug was injected IM, keep the wound open and try to express blood from the site.

3. *Attempt to establish an IV line.*

Try to place a butterfly catheter in a vein and secure with adhesive tape. Use a tourniquet, if needed to raise the vein, then remove it. The veins on the back of the hand are often easier for the inexperienced to hit; otherwise try for the vein on the inside of the elbow. If you can't locate a vein within 60 seconds, administer the antagonist IM.

4. *Administer at least 10 mg naloxone, naltrexone, or nalmefene.*

Do this only if the patient is demonstrating any of the above symptoms. All these antagonists are very safe and overdosing is unlikely, regardless of the dose administered. Thus, don't waste time trying to withdraw *precisely* 10 mg. Just withdraw enough to be achieve the 10 mg minimum, but don't worry if you administer 25 mg or even 100 mg!

If the patient is asymptomatic, wait and observe the patient closely; if no symptoms develop within 15 minutes of exposure, no further treatment may be necessary. However, the patient should not be left alone for several hours even in the absence of symptoms. If there is no improvement in the patient's condition within 1 minute after giving the antagonist IV (or within 3-5 minutes for IM administra-

tion), repeat the dose. Continue to repeat this dose every 3-5 minutes until central nervous system depression is antagonized.

For IM administration, inject the antagonist into the large thigh muscles, shoulder, or other available muscle mass. Split the dose and inject into two sites. *Note:* do *not* use diprenorphine (M50-50®) as an antidote in humans due to its side effects.

5. *Place victim on side.*

Prevent vomiting and aspiration of the vomitus by keeping the individual on his/her side, if unconscious. If the person is conscious, keep him/her moving (walking), if possible.

6. *Remember your ABC's and be prepared to apply CPR.*

7. *Transfer the patient to an emergency center when feasible.*

Comments:

You should never use opioids without one of the above three antagonists available. Do not use diprenorphine (M50-50®). Naloxone, naltrexone, and nalmefene are preferred antagonists because they are "pure" antagonists, whereas diprenorphine has both antagonistic and agonistic (undesirable in case of opioid overdose) properties. There are no data on the correct dose of the above three antagonists to administer in cases of human exposure to etorphine, thiafentanil, or carfentanil. Naloxone, naltrexone, and nalmefene are all very safe drugs and humans should be able to receive amounts much higher than the dose given. If you do not see any effect after administration and the person is comatose and/or has stopped breathing, consider increasing the dose.

If you wish to have naloxone for any human exposure, be advised that naloxone is marketed worldwide in 0.4 mg/ml ampules and 1 mg/ml in some countries. To obtain the recommended 10 mg of naloxone, you would have to break open 25 glass ampules! It is doubtful that the patient will have time for this. The 1 mg/ml preparation would be preferable, even though it would still require a 10 ml injection. Although injectable naltrexone is not yet approved for human use (oral naltrexone is FDA-approved), we would not hesitate in using it in an emergency.

Cyclohexanes

Ketamine, Tiletamine

Symptoms:

- Disorientation, hallucination, excitement, abnormal behavior
- Coma
- Decreased respiratory rate

Treatment:

1. *Wash site.*

Flush mucous membranes (eyes, mouth, wound, etc.) with copious amounts of water. Use cool or room temperature water - do not use hot water. If drug was injected IM, keep the wound open and try to express blood from the site.

2. *Keep patient quiet.*

Minimize stimulation (sound, touch, light, etc.); never leave the patient unattended. Physically restrain the patient, if needed, to prevent self-inflicted injury.

3. *Give artificial resuscitation, if necessary.*

Respiratory depression may be seen only if the patient has received a large dose.

4. *Administer 10 mg of diazepam if patient has convulsions.*

You can administer 10 mg of diazepam or midazolam IV or IM. If given IV, administer *slowly* (10-15 seconds).

5. *Transport to emergency center.*

Comments:

Remember that the commonly-used cyclohexanes (ketamine, tiletamine) are congeners of phencyclidine, also known as PCP or Angel Dust. We are probably all familiar with accounts of bizarre human behavior resulting from PCP abuse and the most likely result of cyclohexane injection is such abnormal behavior.

It is unlikely that the doses of ketamine used in animal immobilization would be lethal to humans since the clinical IM dose for humans can be as high as 13 mg/kg. However, humans have died from self-administered overdoses of tiletamine-zolazepam (Cording et al., 1999; Chung et al., 2000).

Despite some common misconceptions, there is no complete antagonist for these cyclohexanes and drugs such as yohimbine, 4-aminopyridine, and atipamezole should not be given.

Neuromuscular Blocking Agents

Succinylcholine, Decamethonium

Symptoms:

- Nausea
- Progressive muscle paralysis
- Decreased respiratory rate, arrest
- Cyanosis
- Unconsciousness
- Death

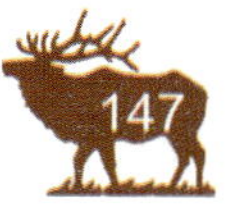

Treatment:

1. *Wash site.*

Flush mucous membranes (eyes, mouth, wound, etc.) with copious amounts of water. Use cool or room temperature water - do not use hot water. If drug was injected IM, keep the wound open and try to express blood from the site.

2. *Give artificial resuscitation.*

If the muscles of respiration become paralyzed, you will have to provide resuscitation until the drug effects wear off.

3. *Transport to emergency center.*

Comments:

Fortunately, this drug is metabolized quickly (2–5 minutes) in humans and simple maintenance of artificial resuscitation should be sufficient to allow recovery.

Gallamine, Tubocurarine

Symptoms:

- Nausea
- Progressive muscle paralysis
- Decreased respiratory rate, arrest
- Cyanosis
- Unconsciousness
- Death

Treatment:

1. *Wash site.*

Flush mucous membranes (eyes, mouth, wound, etc.) with copious amounts of water. Use cool or room temperature water - do not use hot water. If drug was injected IM, keep the wound open and try to express blood from the site.

2. *Administer antagonist.*

Do *not* give neostigmine as the antagonist *unless* you also have atropine available. The protocol for gallamine antagonism is as follows (Morkel, 1993):

a. Give 0.5 mg atropine IV *slowly* (15–30 seconds) or give IM. If given IM, wait 5 minutes before the next step.
b. Give 1 mg neostigmine IV *slowly* (15–30 seconds) or give IM.
c. Repeat steps 1 and 2 every 5 minutes until recovery, but *not to exceed* three repetitions (i.e., total atropine given is 1.5 mg and total neostigmine given is 3 mg).

3. *Give artificial resuscitation.*

If you don't have atropine and neostigmine and if the muscles of respiration become paralyzed, you will have to provide resuscitation until the drug effects wear off.

4. *Transport to emergency center.*

Comments:
Overdosing with neostigmine can be dangerous to the patient, therefore do not exceed recommended dose. Signs of neostigmine overdose include: tremors, violent stomach cramps, defecation/urination/salivation/difficult breathing, constricted pupils, very slow pulse. If you suspect neostigmine overdose, the protocol for treatment is as follows (Morkel, 1993):

- Give artificial resuscitation, if necessary.
- Give 1 mg atropine IV *slowly*
- If pulse drops below 60 bpm, give 0.5 mg additional atropine.

Continue giving increments of 0.5 mg atropine until pulse exceeds 60 bpm, but *do not exceed* 2 mg atropine total dose.

Nicotine Sulfate

Symptoms:

- Nausea, abdominal pain, vomiting, salivation, dizziness
- Headache, disturbed hearing and vision, mental confusion
- Weakness, fainting, collapse
- Difficult breathing, weak and rapid pulse, convulsions, and death due to respiratory failure

1. *Give artificial resuscitation.*

If the muscles of respiration become paralyzed, you will have to provide resuscitation until the drug effects wear off.

2. *Transport to emergency center immediately.*

Comments:
The lethal dose for humans is 60 mg of nicotine which is within the range of doses used in wildlife immobilization. There is no antidote for nicotine. If you take a lethal dose of nicotine, you will double over with agonizing cramps, vomit, defecate, and then die and there will be nothing anyone can do for you. Take home message: *never* use nicotine sulfate!

Tranquilizers/Sedatives

Xylazine, Detomidine, Medetomidine, Romifidine

Symptoms:

- Decreased respiratory and heart rate
- Decreased blood pressure
- Sedation, dizziness, nausea, slurred speech, unsteady gait
- Hypothermia

Treatment:

1. Support respiration, if necessary.

Administer artificial resuscitation if patient's respiratory rate falls below 6 breaths per minute or if lips and gums become pale or bluish.

2. Administer appropriate antagonist IV.

For any of the alpha-2 adrenoceptor tranquilizers, administer atipamezole slowly IV and monitor for antagonistic effects. An infusion rate of 5 mg atipamezole over a 5 minute period or 100 mg over a 20 minute period has been used in healthy adults. In case of medetomidine intoxication, a dose ratio of 20:1 to 50:1 for atipamezole:medetomidine is recommended (Karhuvaara et al., 1991).

For xylazine intoxication only, you can also administer 0.125 mg/kg yohimbine IV (Mackintosh, 1985). Yohimbine can be given IM, but response could take up to 20 minutes (Fyffe, 1994).

Comments:

There have been several suicide attempts with xylazine at dosages ranging from 400–2,400 mg. All of these patients survived; however, some required intensive care for up to 60 hours (Carruthers et al., 1979; Fyffe, 1994). Fatalities involving xylazine are always in association with the patient taking other drugs (Poklis et al., 1985; Fyffe, 1994). Dosages of 100–120 μg medetomidine have been well tolerated by humans (Scheinin et al., 1989). An unkown, but presumambly small, amount of detomidine caused bradycardia, hypotension, dizziness, slurred speech, and unsteadiness in one patient (Cummins, 2005).

Diazepam, Midazolam, Zolazepam (in Telazol®, Zoletil®)

Symptoms:

- Decreased respiratory rate
- Ataxia, lethargy, slurred speech
- Sleepiness, coma

Treatment:

1. Support respiration, if necessary.

Administer artificial resuscitation if patient's respiratory rate falls below 6 breaths per minute or if lips and gums become pale or bluish.

2. Administer flumazenil at 0.2 mg IV followed by 0.1 mg IV every minute until patient responds.

Flumazenil is a benzodiazepine antagonist that has been used in cases of severe benzodiazepine overdose; it has a high therapeutic index (3,000) so overdosing with this antagonist is unlikely; however, complications in humans can occur and there is some doubt as to its beneficial effect (Mathieu-Nolf, 2001)

3. Transport to emergency center.

Comments:

Death due to overdose of benzodiazepine tranquilizers is rare and highly unlikely given the doses of these drugs used in wildlife immobilization. In one case, oral ingestion of 1,500 mg diazepam caused only minor toxicity. Exposure to these agents would most likely be in conjunction with, and therefore exacerbate the effects of, primary immobilizing agents (opioids, cyclohexanes).

Promazine, Chlorpromazine, Propionylpromazine, Acetylpromazine, Haloperidol, Azaperone, Droperidol, Perphenazine

Symptoms:

- CNS stimulation (tremors, rhythmic movements, constant movement, facial grimacing, stiff neck and/or tongue)
- Tachycardia (rapid heart rate)
- Seizures
- Hyper- or hypothermia
- Ataxia, lethargy, slurred speech, akinesia (affective indifference)

Treatment:

1. *Support respiration and cardiovascular function, if necessary.*

Administer artificial resuscitation if patient's respiratory rate falls below 6 breaths per minute or if lips and gums become pale or bluish. In rare cases, ventricular fibrillation may occur requiring full CPR and immediate transport to an emergency treatment center.

2. *Administer 10 mg diazepam IV slowly (10-15 seconds) for seizures.*

This dose may be repeated every 10–15 minutes as needed to control seizures; do not exceed 30 mg total dose of diazepam.

3. *Transport to emergency center.*

Comments:

Death due to overdose of phenothiazine and butyrophenone tranquilizers is rare and highly unlikely given the doses of these drugs used in wildlife capture. Exposure to these agents would most likely be in conjunction with, and therefore exacerbate the effects of, primary immobilizing agents (opioids, cyclohexanes). In very unusual cases, a neuroleptic malignant syndrome may appear after several hours to months, most often after haloperidol overdose. This syndrome is characterized by profound hyperthermia, tachycardia, hypotension or hypertension, and fluctuating mental status progressing to coma.

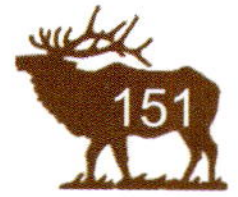

Human First Aid Kit Checklist

General:

20 or 21 ga. needles
1-ml syringes
3-ml syringes
10-ml syringes
23-ga IV Butterfly Cannulas
Adhesive Tape
IV Drip Set
Physiological Saline (0.9% NaCl)
Tourniquet (for raising vein)
Thermometer
Stethoscope
Gauze, 2-in.
Scissors
Band-aids
Topical Antibiotic
Iodine Surgical Scrubs
Forceps (tweezers)
Scalpel Blades
3-0 Absorbable Sutures with Cutting Needle
Needle holder/hemostats
Sterile Surgical or Examination Gloves

Emergency Drugs (be sure drugs are not outdated):

Naloxone (naltrexone, nalmefene)
Diazepam or midazolam, 5 mg/ml
Epinephrine, 0.1 mg/ml (1:10,000)
Atropine Sulfate, 0.5 mg/ml
Neostigmine Methylsulfate, 1 mg/ml
Methylprednisolone Sodium Succinate

Drug Dosages

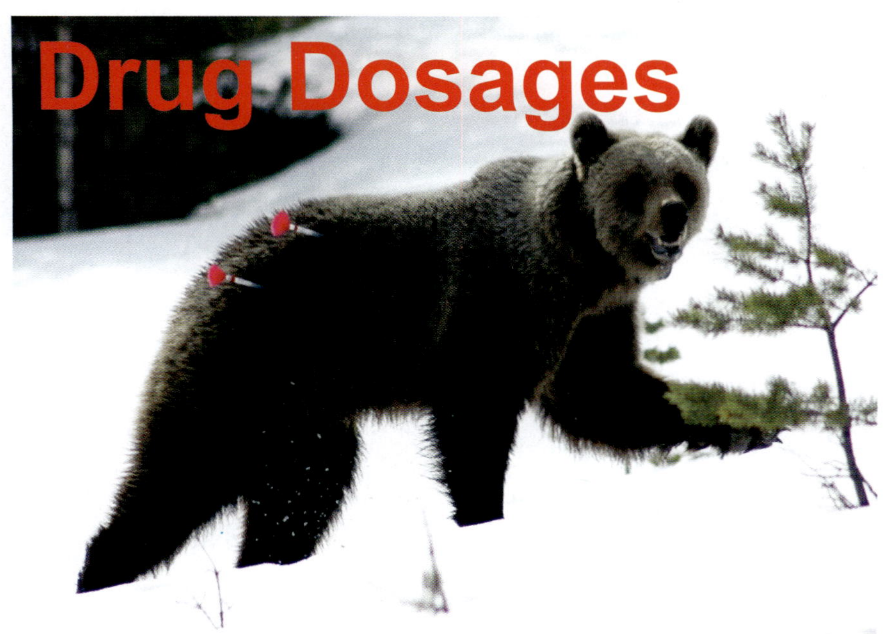

This chapter lists species by common name in alphabetical order. Scientific names are also provided should there be confusion about the common name. Scientific names were taken from *Walker's Mammals of the World* (Nowak, 1999). The information provided is intentionally designed to be brief to enable the user to quickly locate a specific animal and to simplify the decision-making process. The following information is provided for each animal, as applicable:

Weight: The average *adult* weight, or range of weights, is listed. Weights were derived either from the literature, the personal records of the author or others, or from *Walker's Mammals of the World* (Nowak, 1999). All weights are in metric units; if you need to convert pounds to kilograms, refer to the conversion chart in the back of this manual.

Recommended Drug: This is an appropriate drug and dosage for the species under most circumstances. Unless otherwise stated, it is assumed that these drugs will be administered *intramuscularly*.

Note: Be sure to read all dosages carefully. We have tried to maintain consistency by using dosages based on mg drug per kg body weight (mg/kg). Some drugs, however, are formulated as mixtures, thus dosages are given as *ml* of drug per kg body weight. Some doses are also given as *total body dose* and are based on average, adult body weights.

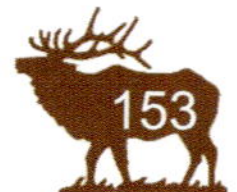

Also note the intentional inconsistency of dosages relative to style. Where dosages are fractionated (e.g., 0.125 mg/kg, 1.5 mg/kg), we have used appropriate style.

However, when dosages are in whole numbers (e.g., 5 mg/kg, 10 mg/kg), we have omitted the decimal point and the following zero (e.g., 5.0 mg/kg). The reason for this is that we did not want someone, who in haste or in poor light, to miss the decimal point and give the animal *10 times* the recommended dosage.

We have tried to use chemical names (e.g., ketamine) as opposed to trade names (e.g., Ketaset®) wherever possible. However for simplicity, we may use trade names for drugs which are a combination of two agents (e.g., Immobilon®).

Supplemental Drug: Use this drug and dose should the original dose not immobilize the animal, or if there was only partial injection.

Antagonist: If the recommended drug can be antagonized, the appropriate drugs and dosages will be listed here.

Alternative Drugs: These are drugs and dosages which also have successfully immobilized the species. Their listing as "alternative" in no way implies that they are less effective than the recommended drug. If you are more familiar with one of these alternative drugs, then by all means use it.

Comments: Additional information, particularly cautions, is provided here.

References: References applicable to the species are provided for your information and further reading. We strongly recommend obtaining and reading these references prior to immobilizing the animal. Much information is contained therein that is not presented in the *Comments* portion for each species, yet will be of use and interest to you. Some references may not contain information specifically on chemical immobilization, but they have been included for general information or historical purposes.

In general, the references that we have included in the bibliography are studies involving several animals. We intentionally omitted a large body of literature where only a single animal was immobilized for some specific purpose such as examination or surgery. Sample sizes of $n = 1$ rarely have value.

We have spent a great deal of effort to amass what we believe is the most comprehensive bibliography of chemical capture in the world. However after making that boast, we will also readily admit that we didn't find all applicable references. If you feel that we have forgotten a significant reference, please feel free to notify us and we will include it in subsequent editions.

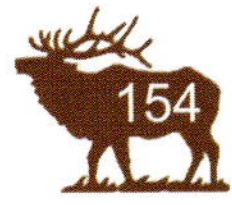

Can't Find Your Critter?

Although this chapter provides drug dosages for more than 475 species, there might not be information available for your particular animal of concern. In such cases, you could look up a closely-related species and use the provided dosages as a starting point. For example, there isn't a dosage listed for sable, *Martes zibellina*, but there is a dosage for the American pine marten, *Martes americana*. These species are similar enough that drugs and dosages for one should be safe and effective for the other.

If all else fails, you could estimate an initial dosage of ketamine and xylazine by using the below graph. To use this graph, start with the body weight (known or estimated) and draw a straight line upwards until it intersects both the ketamine and the xylazine lines. Then draw a line to both Y axes to determine the ketamine (left axis) and xylazine (right axis) dosages. Note that *all* axes are logarithmic; dosages will only be estimates due the nature of such scales. Also remember that the derived dosages will be mg of drug per kg body weight and *not* the *total* dose. The derived dosages should serve as starting dosages only; be prepared to adjust upwards or downwards based on your initial results.

Or if you prefer using ketamine and medetomidine, try an initial dosage of 3.0 mg/kg ketamine plus 0.1 mg/kg medetomidine. This dosage is based on the mean of this combination reported in 56 species.

Ketamine-xylazine doses derived from 44 mammalian species. Formulae for best-fitted curves were: ketamine (mg/kg) = 34.387BW$^{-0.369}$ and xylazine (mg/kg) = 3.454BW$^{-0.223}$. Example (dashed lines) is for a 100-kg animal. The derived dosages would be approximately 6.3 mg/kg ketamine plus 1.2 mg/kg xylazine. Note that all axes are logarithmic.

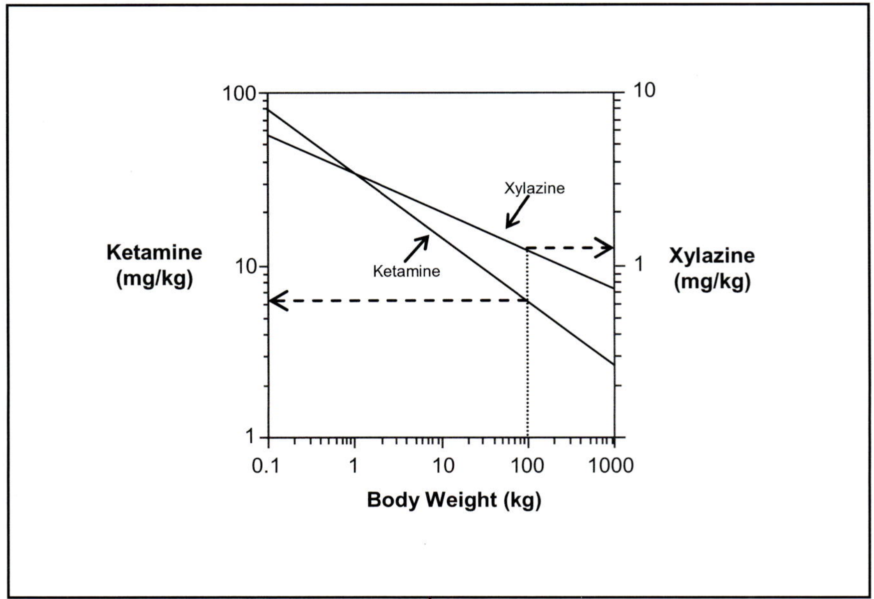

Drug Dosages by Species

AARDVARK, *Orycteropus afer*

Weight: 50–70 kg
Recommended Drug: 3 mg/kg ketamine plus 0.08 mg/kg medtomidine
Supplemental Drug: 1.5 mg/kg ketamine
Antagonist: 0.4 mg/kg atipamezole
Comments: Allow the animal to recover fully (as in a cage) before allowing it to enter its burrow; asphyxiation may occur otherwise.
References: Seal and Erickson, 1969; Seal et al., 1970; Beck, 1972; 1976; Jessup et al., 1980; IWVS, 1992; Nel et al., 2000; Vodicka, 2004

AARDWOLF, *Proteles cristatus*

Weight: 9–14 kg
Recommended Drug: 15 mg/kg ketamine plus 0.3 mg/kg acepromazine
Supplemental Drug: 8 mg/kg ketamine
Antagonist: None
Comments: Use lightweight darts with a low-impact darting system.
References: Young, 1966; Seal et al., 1970; Anderson and Richardson, 1992; IWVS, 1992; Richardson and Anderson, 1993; Kock, M., et al., 2006

ACOUCHIS (GREEN, RED), *Myoprocta spp.*

Weight: 0.6–1.3 kg
Recommended Drug: 5.5 mg/kg tiletamine-zolazepam
Supplemental Drug: 5.5 mg/kg ketamine
Antagonist: None
References: Young, 1966; Seal and Erickson, 1969; Seal et al., 1970; Gray et al., 1974; Schobert, 1987

ADDAX, *Addax nasomaculatus*

Weight: 60–125 kg
Recommended Drug: 0.025 mg/kg carfentanil
Supplemental Drug: If animal is not down in 20 minutes, repeat full dose
Antagonist: 2.5 mg/kg naltrexone
Alternative Drugs: 0.04 mg/kg etorphine plus 0.025 mg/kg detomidine; antagonize with 0.08 mg/kg diprenorphine plus 0.15 mg/kg atipamezole
• 1.5 mg/kg ketamine plus 0.07 mg/kg medetomidine; antagonize with 0.25 mg/kg atipamezole
References: Bauditz, 1972; Heck and Rivenburg, 1972; York and Huggins, 1972; Alford et al., 1974; Röken, 1975; York, 1975; Jensen, 1982; Silvestris and Heck, 1984; Densmore et al., 1987; Allen et al., 1991; Klein et al., 1994; Páras et al., 2002; Portas et al., 2003

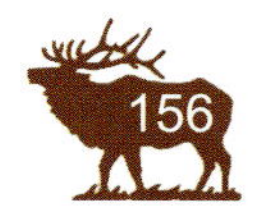

AGOUTI, *Dasyprocta spp.*

Weight: 1.3–4 kg

Recommended Drug: 10 mg/kg tiletamine-zolazepam

Supplemental Drug: 10 mg/kg ketamine

Antagonist: None

Alternative Drugs: 60 mg/kg ketamine

References: Seal and Erickson, 1969; Seal et al., 1970; Bacher et al., 1976; Genevois et al., 1984a

ALLIGATOR - SEE CROCODILIANS

ALPACA, *Lama pacos*

Weight: 55–65 kg

Recommended Drug: 1 mg/kg ketamine plus 0.05 mg/kg medetomidine

Supplemental Drug: 1 mg/kg ketamine

Antagonist: 0.25 mg/kg atipamezole

Alternative Drugs: 2 mg/kg xylazine; antagonize with 0.125 mg/kg yohimbine

• 4 mg/kg tiletamine-zolazepam

Comments: Jones (1977a) stated that the use of opioids in llama was contraindicated; assume the same for alpaca.

References: Rapley and Mehren, 1975; Dugdale, 2001

AMPHIBIANS, GENERAL

Recommended Drug: 2-10 mg/10 ml water (0.02-0.1%) tricaine methane sulfonate at pH 7.0

Antagonist: Wash amphibian repeatedly in clean, warm water (no anesthetic)

Alternative Drugs: 50 mg/kg ketamine plus 1 mg/kg diazepam

Comments: Use higher dose rates tricaine methane sulfonate for *smaller* amphibians and lower dose rates for *larger* amphibians. The longer the amphibian is immersed in the anesthetic solution, the longer the duration of effect. Always induce immobilization with the lowest effective dose possible. Adult amphibians can drown if left submerged while under general anesthesia. Eugenol (clove oil) has been found effective for leopard frogs (see Lafortune etal., 2001). Gas anesthesia works well for amphibians also. Tiletamine-zolazepamdoes not appear to be a satisfactory anesthetic for many amphibians.

References: Kaplan and Kaplan, 1961; Kaplan et al., 1962; Kaplan, 1969; Beck, 1972; Rie, 1973; Stunkard and Miller, 1974; Wass and Kaplan, 1974; Vethamany-Globus et al., 1977; Robinson and Scadding, 1983; Cooper, 1984; 1987; Sedgwick, 1986; Letcher and Amsel, 1989; Letcher, 1992; Letcher and Durante, 1995; Stetter et al., 1996; Cathers et al., 1997; Ross and Ross, 1999; Lafortune et al., 2001; Cakir and Strauch, 2005

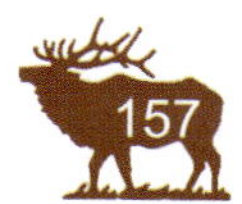

ANTEATER, GIANT, *Myrmecophaga tridactyla*

Weight: 18–39 kg
Recommended Drug: 5 mg/kg ketamine plus 3.5 mg/kg xylazine
Supplemental Drug: 5 mg/kg ketamine
Antagonist: 0.125 mg/kg yohimbine
Alternative Drugs: 11 mg/kg ketamine
References: Seal and Erickson, 1969; Seal et al., 1970; Beck, 1976; Gillepsie and Adams, 1985; Kock et al., 1989

ANTEATER, LESSER (TAMANDUA), *Tamandua tetradactyla*

Weight: 2–7 kg
Recommended Drug: 15 mg/kg tiletamine-zolazepam
Supplemental Drug: 15 mg/kg ketamine
Antagonist: None
References: Seal and Erickson, 1969; Seal et al., 1970

ANTELOPE, NORTH AMERICAN - SEE PRONGHORN

ANTELOPE, FOUR-HORNED, *Tetracerus quadricornis*

Weight: 17–21 kg
Recommended Drug: 15 mg/kg ketamine
Supplemental Drug: 8 mg/kg ketamine
Antagonist: None
References: Shashidhar, 1981

ANTELOPE, ROAN, *Hippotragus equinus*

Weight: 100–325 kg
Recommended Drug: 0.03 mg/kg thiafentanil plus 0.3 mg/kg azaperone
Supplemental Drug: 0.015 mg/kg thiafentanil
Antagonist: 0.6 mg/kg naltrexone
Alternative Drugs: 0.01 mg/kg carfentanil plus 0.1 mg/kg xylazine; antagonize with 1 mg/kg naltrexone plus 0.125 mg/kg yohimbine
• 0.025 mg/kg etorphine plus 0.3 mg/kg azaperone; antagonize with 0.05 mg /kg diprenorphine
• 0.012 mg/kg thiafentanil plus 0.005 mg/kg medetomidine plus 0.5 mg/kg ketamine; antagonize with 0.6 mg/kg naltrexone plus 0.04 mg/kg atipamezole
• 60 mg fentanyl plus 200 mg azaperone; antagonize with 0.2 mg/kg naloxone
• 3 mg/kg xylazine; antagonize with 0.125 mg/kg yohimbine (calm animals only)
Comments: Aggressive to each other when captured in groups; immediately immobilize if captured in bomas. Hyaluronidase (1,500-3,000 IU) can be added to the drug mixture to decrease induction time. If confined in bomas, the etorphine dose can be reduced. Approach downed animals

carefully; semi-immobilized animals can rake with their horns. Long-acting tranquilizer doses: zuclopenthixol (adult male, 300 mg; adult female, 225 mg; subadult, 125 mg); perphenazine (adults, 100-250 mg). The zuclopenthixol gives excellent tranquilization for three days.

References: Lanphear, 1963; Pienaar, 1968a; 1968b; 1973a; Koci, 1971b; 1972; Bauditz, 1972; Heck and Rivenburg, 1972; Jones, 1972; Hofmeyr and de Bruine, 1973; Hofmeyr, 1974; De Vos, 1975; Röken, 1975; Smuts, 1975; Haigh, 1976d; Jones, 1977; Slee and Walker, 1977; De Vos, 1978a; Hofmeyr, 1981; Silvestris and Heck, 1984; Williams and Riedesel, 1987; Kock, R. et al., 1989; IWVS, 1992; Morkel, 1992; Burroughs, 1993d; Citino et al., 2001; Kock, M., et al., 2006

AOUDAD, *Ammotragis lervia*

Weight: 40–55 (f) 100–145 (m) kg

Recommended Drug: 10 mg/kg ketamine plus 2.5 mg/kg xylazine

Supplemental Drug: 5 mg/kg ketamine

Antagonist: 0.125 mg/kg yohimbine

Alternative Drugs: 1.5 mg/kg ketamine plus 0.12 mg/kg medetomidine; antagonize with 0.6 mg/kg atipamezole

• 0.05 mg/kg carfentanil plus 0.1 mg/kg xylazine; antagonize with 5 mg/kg naltrexone plus 0.125 mg/kg yohimbine

• 3 mg etorphine plus 10 mg ketamine plus 10 mg xylazine; antagonize with 6 mg diprenorphine plus 0.15 mg/kg yohimbine

• 1.5 mg/kg xylazine; antagonize 0.2 mg/kg yohimbine (calm animals only)

• 6 mg/kg tiletamine-zolazepam

Comments: The use of xylazine without an antagonist may cause extremely prolonged recoveries (Klöppel, 1969; Gauckler and Kraus, 1970). When using ketamine-medetomidine, wait 5 minutes after recumbency before approaching animal.

References: Jarvis and Morris, 1960; Thomas, 1961; Heuschele, 1961a; Wright, 1963; Wallach et al., 1967; Wallach, 1968; 1969; Klöppel, 1969; Gauckler and Kraus, 1970; Bauditz, 1972; Heck and Rivenburg, 1972; York and Huggins, 1972; Woolf et al., 1973; Boever and Paluch, 1974; Mehren and Rapley, 1975; Rapley and Mehren, 1975; Röken, 1975; York, 1975; Wiesner, 1977; Jessup, et al., 1980; Wiesner et al., 1982; 1984; Jacobson and Kollias, 1984; Silvestris and Heck, 1984; Schobert, 1987; Williams and Riedesel, 1987; Barnett and Lewis, 1990; Jalanka and Roeken, 1990; Snyder et al., 1992; Jurczynski et al., 2006

APE, BARBARY - SEE MACAQUE, BARBARY

APE, CELEBES, *Cynopithecus niger*

Weight: 6–15 kg

Recommended Drug: 4.4 mg/kg tiletamine-zolazepam

Supplemental Drug: 4.4 mg/kg ketamine

Antagonist: None
Alternative Drugs: 25 mg/kg ketamine
References: Gray et al., 1974; Beck, 1976; Bush et al., 1977; Schobert, 1987

ARMADILLO, LONG-NOSED, *Dasypus novemcinctus*

Weight: 3–10 kg
Recommended Drug: 7.5 mg/kg ketamine plus 0.075 mg/kg medetomidine
Supplemental Drug: 5 mg/kg ketamine
Antagonist: 0.375 mg/kg atipamezole
Alternative Drugs: 8.5 mg/kg tiletamine-zolazepam
- 40 mg/kg ketamine plus 1 mg/k xylazine
- 1 mg/kg xylazine

References: Fournier-Chambrillon et al., 2000

ASS, WILD, *Equus asinus*

Weight: 200–250 kg
Recommended Drug: 3 mg etorphine plus 200 mg xylazine
Supplemental Drug: 1.5 mg etorphine
Antagonist: 2 mg diprenorphine per mg etorphine given
Alternative Drugs: 1.5 ml Large Animal Immobilon® plus 50 mg xylazine; antagonize with 7.5 mg diprenorphine
- 1 mg etorphine plus 300 mg ketamine plus 300 mg xylazine; antagonize with 2 mg diprenorphine plus 0.125 mg/kg yohimbine

References: Heuschele, 1961; Heck and Rivenburg, 1972; Röken, 1975; Jessup et al., 1980; Wiesner et al., 1982; Silvestris and Heck, 1984; Wiesner and von Hegel, 1985

BABIRUSA, *Babyrousa babysussa*

Weight: 75-100 kg
Recommended Drug: 2 mg/kg tiletamine-zolazepam plus 1.5 mg/kg xylazine
Supplemental Drug: 1.5 mg/kg ketamine
Antagonist: 0.15 mg/kg yohimbine
Alternative Drugs: 1.25 mg/kg tiletamine-zolazepam plus 0.4 mg/kg butorphanol; antagonize with 0.2 mg/kg naltrexone
Comments: Males may require lower doses than females. Flumazenil may also be given to antagonize the zolazepam. Xylazine was given as a premedication in the study of James et al., 1998; 1999. Consulting reference prior to capture is recommended.
References: James et al., 1998; 1999; Padilla, 2004

BABOON, CHACMA, *Papio ursinus*

Weight: 8–30 kg

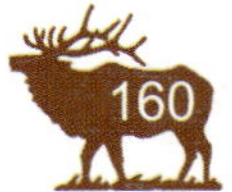

Recommended Drug: 3 mg/kg tiletamine-zolazepam
Supplemental Drug: 3 mg/kg ketamine
Antagonist: None
Alternative Drugs: 12 mg/kg ketamine
References: Kroll, 1962; Van Niekerk et al., 1963a; Van Niekerk and Pienaar, 1963a; Field et al., 1966; Steyn, 1975; Beck, 1976; Melton, 1980; Goosen et al., 1984; Van Der Merwe et al., 1987; Jessup et al., 1980; Melton and Melton, 1982; Schobert, 1987; Burroughs, 1993c

BABOON, GELADA, *Theropithecus gelada*

Weight: 13–20 kg
Recommended Drug: 2.5 mg/kg tiletamine-zolazepam
Supplemental Drug: 2.5 mg/kg ketamine
Antagonist: None
Alternative Drugs: 11 mg/kg ketamine
References: Kroll, 1962; Field et al., 1966; Gray et al., 1974; Beck, 1976; Eads, 1976; Bush et al., 1977; Schobert, 1987

BABOON, HAMADRYAS, *Papio hamadryas*

Weight: 10–18 kg
Recommended Drug: 5 mg/kg ketamine plus 0.1 mg/kg medetomidine
Supplemental Drug: 3 mg/kg ketamine
Antagonist: 0.5 mg/kg atipamezole; give 1/2 dose IV, 1/2 IM
Alternative Drugs: 12 mg/kg ketamine
- 1.3 mg/kg tiletamine-zolazepam

Comments: Ketamine-medetomidine use may not induce complete immobilization; increase amount of ketamine, if necessary.
References: Kroll, 1962; Seal and Erickson, 1969; Seal et al., 1970; Beck, 1972; 1976; Schobert, 1987; Jalanka and Roeken, 1990

BABOON, OLIVE, *Papio anubis*

Weight: 14–41 kg
Recommended Drug: 5 mg/kg ketamine plus 0.07 mg/kg medetomidine
Supplemental Drug: 3 mg/kg ketamine
Antagonist: 0.35 mg/kg atipamezole
Alternative Drugs: 4.4 mg/kg tiletamine-zolazepam
- 15 mg/kg ketamine
- 10 mg/kg ketamine plus 0.25 mg/kg diazepam

References: Kroll, 1962; Ericksen, 1968; Field et al., 1966; Bauditz, 1972; Beck, 1972; Beck and Dresner, 1972; Jessup et al., 1980; Woolfson et al., 1980; Schobert, 1987

BABOON, WESTERN, *Papio papio*

Weight: 10–30 kg
Recommended Drug: 5 mg/kg tiletamine-zolazepam

Supplemental Drug: 2.5 mg/kg ketamine
Antagonist: None
Alternative Drugs: 5 mg/kg ketamine plus 0.2 mg/kg acepromazine
Comments: Be aware of possible aggression among males during the recovery phase.
References: Heuschele, 1959; 1961a; 1961b; Kroll, 1962; Vondruska, 1965; Beck, 1976; Cohen and Bree, 1978

BABOON, YELLOW, *Papio cynocephalus*

Weight: 14–41 kg
Recommended Drug: 5 mg/kg ketamine plus 0.07 mg/kg medetomidine
Supplemental Drug: 3 mg/kg ketamine
Antagonist: 0.35 mg/kg atipamezole
Alternative Drugs: 10 mg/kg ketamine plus 0.5 mg/kg xylazine
• 4.4 mg/kg tiletamine-zolazepam
References: Beck and Dresner, 1972; Eads, 1976; White and Cummings, 1976; Schobert, 1987; Burroughs, 1993c

BADGER, EUROPEAN (OLD WORLD), *Meles meles*

Weight: 10–16 kg
Recommended Drug: 10 mg/kg tiletamine-zolazepam
Supplemental Drug: 5 mg/kg ketamine
Antagonist: None
Alternative Drugs: 20 mg/kg ketamine
• 8 mg/kg ketamine plus 0.04 mg/kg medetomidine plus 0.8 mg/kg butorphanol; antagonize with 0.2 mg/kg atipamezole
• 15 mg/kg ketamine plus 0.4 mg/kg acepromazine
• 16 mg/kg ketamine plus 6 mg/kg xylazine
Comments: Thornton et al. (2005) found that combinations of ketamine/midazolam or ketamine/medetomidine were not "convincing alternatives" to ketamine alone.
References: Seal and Erickson, 1969; Seal et al., 1970; Hunt, 1976; Mackintosh et al., 1976; Wiesner and von Hegel, 1985; Wolfensohn, 1992; Travaini et al., 1994; deLeeuw et al., 2004; Thornton et al., 2005; McLaren et al., 2005a; 2005b

BADGER, FERRET, *Melogale moschata*

Weight: 1–3 kg
Recommended Drug: 5 mg/kg tiletamine-zolazepam
Supplemental Drug: 5 mg/kg ketamine
Antagonist: None
References: Seal and Erickson, 1969; Seal et al., 1970

BADGER, HOG, *Arctonyx collaris*

Weight: 7–14 kg

Recommended Drug: 4.4 mg/kg tiletamine-zolazepam
Supplemental Drug: 2.2 mg/kg ketamine
Antagonist: None
References: Seal and Erickson, 1969; Seal et al., 1970

BADGER, HONEY, *Mellivora capensis*

Weight: 7–13 kg
Recommended Drug: 2.2 mg/kg tiletamine-zolazepam
Supplemental Drug: 2.2 mg/kg ketamine
Antagonist: None
Alternative Drugs: 6 mg/kg ketamine plus 0.5 mg/kg xylazine
Comments: Approach either darted or trapped honey badgers with care.
References: Seal and Erickson, 1969; Seal et al., 1970; Gray et al., 1974; Schobert, 1987; McKenzie and Burroughs, 1993

BADGER, *Taxidea taxus*

Weight: 4–12 kg
Recommended Drug: 4.4 mg/kg tiletamine-zolazepam
Supplemental Drug: 4.4 mg/kg ketamine
Antagonist: None
Alternative Drugs: 15 mg/kg ketamine plus 1 mg/kg xylazine
Comments: Badgers require care in drug administration because they struggle and resist handling; try to physically restrain the animal to insure accurate drug injection.
References: Seal and Erickson, 1969; Seal et al., 1970; Bailey, 1971; Fitzgerald, 1973; Boever et al., 1977; Jessup et al., 1980; Jessup, 1982b; Genevois et al., 1984b; Schobert, 1987; Seal and Kreeger, 1987; Pigozzi, 1988; Pond and O'Gara, 1994; Schwantje et al., 1998

BANDICOOT, LONG-NOSED, *Perameles gunnii*

Weight: 450–900 gm
Recommended Drug: 0.005 mg/gm tiletamine-zolazepam
Supplemental Drug: 0.005 mg/gm ketamine
Antagonist: None
References: Shima et al., 1993

BANDICOOT, SHORT-NOSED, *Isoodon macrourus*

Weight: 1–1.5 kg
Recommended Drug: 10 mg/kg tiletamine-zolazepam
Supplemental Drug: 10 mg/kg ketamine
Antagonist: None
References: Denny, 1974; Holz, 1992

BANTENG, *Bos javanicus*

Weight: 400–900 kg

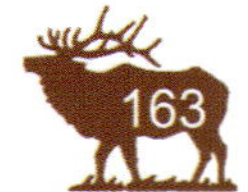

Recommended Drug: 2 ml Large Animal Immobilon® plus 50 mg xylazine
Supplemental Drug: 1 ml Large Animal Immobilon®
Antagonist: 2 mg diprenorphine per mg etorphine given plus 0.125 mg/kg yohimbine
Alternative Drugs: 1.5 mg/kg xylazine; antagonize with 0.125 mg/kg yohimbine
• 4 mg/kg tiletamine-zolazepam plus 0.2 mg/kg detomidine; antagonize with 0.2 mg/kg atipamezole
Comments: Expect prolonged recoveries when using tiletamine-zolazepam, even when the detomidine is antagonized (see Bradsha et al., 2005)
References: Göltenboth and Klös, 1970; Bauditz, 1972; Wiesner et al., 1982; Bradshaw et al., 2005

BARASINGHA, *Cervus duvauceli*

Weight: 172–181 kg
Recommended Drug: 2.1 mg carfentanil
Supplemental Drug: If animal is not down in 20 min, repeat full dose
Antagonist: 1 mg/kg naltrexone
Alternative Drugs: 0.015 mg/kg etorphine plus 0.5 mg/kg xylazine; antagonize with 0.03 mg/kg diprenorphine plus 0.125 mg/kg yohimbine
• 1 mg etorphine plus 100 mg ketamine plus 100 mg xylazine; antagonize with 2 mg diprenorphine plus 0.125 mg/kg yohimbine
Comments: Prone to sudden leg kicks when immobilized with carfentanil.
References: Jarvis and Morris, 1960; Thomas, 1961; Heck and Rivenburg, 1972; Jones, 1972; 1984; Woolf et al., 1973; Rapley and Mehren, 1975; Wiesner, 1975; 1977; Jensen, 1982; Wiesner et al., 1982; Silvestris and Heck, 1984; Wiesner and von Hegel, 1985; Seal and Bush, 1987; Allen et al., 1991

BATS, GENERAL

Recommended Drug: 10 mg/kg ketamine plus 2 mg/kg xylazine
Supplemental Drug: 5 mg/kg ketamine
Antagonist: None reported
Alternative Drugs: 10 mg/kg ketamine plus 1 mg/kg acepromazine
• 5 mg/kg ketamine plus 0.05 mg/kg medetomidine
• Isoflurane
References: Beck, 1976; Rauch and Beatty, 1977; Bassett, 1987; Wilson, 1988; Heard et al., 1996; 2006; Heard and Huft, 1998; Jonsson et al., 2004; Wimsatt et al., 2005

BEAR, ASIATIC BLACK, *Ursus thibetanus*

Weight: 65–90 (f), 110–150 (m) kg
Recommended Drug: 4.4 mg/kg tiletamine-zolazepam
Supplemental Drug: 2.2 mg/kg ketamine

Antagonist: None
References: Jarvis and Morris, 1960; Heuschele, 1961a; Kuntze, 1967; Seal and Erickson, 1969; Seal et al., 1970; Schobert, 1987

BEAR, BLACK, *Ursus americanus*

Weight: 92–140 (f), 115–270 (m) kg
Recommended Drug: 7 mg/kg tiletamine-zolazepam
Supplemental Drug: 3.5 mg/kg ketamine
Antagonist: None
Alternative Drugs: 4.4 mg/kg ketamine plus 2 mg/kg xylazine; antagonize with 0.15 mg/kg yohimbine
• 1.5 mg/kg ketamine plus 0.04 mg/kg medetomidine; antagonize with 0.2 mg/kg atipamezole
• 2 mg/kg tiletamine-zolazepam plus 0.05 mg/kg medetomidine; antagonize with 0.25 mg/kg atipamezole
• 0.02 mg/kg etorphine; antagonize with 0.04 mg/kg diprenorphine
Comments: Anesthetic induction with tiletamine-zolazepam may take up to 20 min and recoveries may be prolonged (2-4 hours). However, combining tiletamine-zolazepam with medetomidine will reduce both induction and recovery times (if atipamezole is given). Bears may arouse spontaneously when using medetomidine with either ketamine or tiletamine-zolazepam. Thus, monitor closely for signs of recovery. Respiratory depression may occur with etorphine.
References: Martyn, 1955; Erickson, 1957; Black et al., 1959; Meyer, 1959; Youatt and Erickson, 1959; Jarvis and Morris, 1960; Heuschele, 1961a; Clifford et al., 1962; Kroll, 1962; Clarke et al., 1963; Dyson, 1965; Kuntze, 1967; Pearson et al., 1968; Wallach et al., 1967; Wallach, 1968; 1969; Seal and Erickson, 1969; Rogers, 1970; Seal et al., 1970; Bauditz, 1972; Miller et al., 1973; Alford et al., 1974; Beeman et al., 1974; Miller and Will, 1974; Haigh, 1976d; Hugie et al., 1976; Miller and Will, 1976; Rogers et al., 1976; Hugie et al., 1977; Addison and Kolenosky, 1979; Barnes and Rogers, 1980; Bush et al., 1980a; Jessup, 1982b; Stewart et al., 1980; Carpenter and Lance, 1983; Lynch et al., 1982; Cook, 1984; Genevois et al., 1984b; Clutton, 1987; Garshelis et al., 1987; Schobert, 1987; Seal and Kreeger, 1987; Hellgren and Vaughn, 1989; Barnett and Lewis, 1990; Gibeau and Paquet, 1991; McLaughlin, 1993; Pond and O'Gara, 1994; Ramsay et al., 1995; White et al., 1996; Caulkett and Cattet, 1997; Black and Whiteside, 2005

BEAR, BROWN (GRIZZLY), *Ursus arctos*

Weight: 100–325 kg
Recommended Drug: 2.5 mg/kg tiletamine-zolazepam plus 0.05 mg/kg medetomidine
Supplemental Drug: 2 mg/kg ketamine plus 0.025 mg/kg medetomidine
Antagonist: 0.25 mg/kg atipamezole

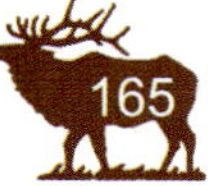

Alternative Drugs: 8 mg/kg tiletamine-zolazepam

• 3 mg/kg tiletamine-zolazepam plus 2 mg/kg xylazine; antagonize with 0.2 mg/kg atipamezole

Comments: Bears may arouse spontaneously when using tiletamine-zolazepam/medetomidine, although this was not seen in almost 600 immobilizations of European brown bears (Arnemo, pers. comm.). Thus, monitor closely for signs of recovery. Avoid loud or sharp noises; try to prevent vocalization of cubs when mother is immobilized. Recovery from high dosages of tiletamine-zolazepam may take several hours. Dosages of tiletamine-zolazepam-medetomidine were based on spring and early summer captures. Body weights can vary widely depending on geographical location. Opioids cannot be recommended (but they have been used) because of the risk of respiratory depression and hyperthermia.

References: Louw, 1957; Craighead et al., 1960; Jarvis and Morris, 1960; Heuschele, 1961a; Troyer et al., 1961; Larsen, 1963; Kuntze, 1967; Ericksen, 1968; Pearson et al., 1968; Wallach, 1968; 1969; Seal and Erickson, 1969; Seal et al., 1970; Hebert et al., 1970; Bauditz, 1972; Halloran and Pearson, 1972; Pearson and Halloran, 1972; Alford et al., 1974; Gray et al., 1974; Boever et al., 1977; Perry, 1977; Bush et al., 1980a; Hebert et al., 1980; Gatesman and Wiesner, 1982; Lynch et al., 1982; Wiesner et al., 1982; 1984; Carpenter and Lance, 1983; Genevois et al., 1984b; Duchamps, 1985; Wiesner and von Hegel, 1985; Hugues et al., 1986; Röken, 1987; Schobert, 1987; Seal, 1987; Seal and Kreeger, 1987; Carr, 1989; Taylor et al., 1989; Barnett and Lewis, 1990; Jalanka and Roeken, 1990; Tsubota and Yamamoto, 1991; Pond and O'Gara, 1994; Mortenson and Bechert, 1996; 2002; Mama et al., 2000; Arnemo et al., 2001a; 2001b; Cattet et al., 2003b; 2003c; Arnemo, 2006; Caulkett and Arnemo, 2007

BEAR, POLAR, *Ursus maritimus*

Weight: 150–300 (f), 300–800 (m) kg

Recommended Drug: 8 mg/kg tiletamine-zolazepam

Supplemental Drug: 2 mg/kg ketamine

Antagonist: None

Alternative Drugs: 2.2 mg/kg tiletamine-zolazepam plus 0.06 mg/kg medetomidine; antagonize with 0.24 mg/kg atipamezole

• 3 mg/kg tiletamine-zolazepam plus 2 mg/kg xylazine; antagonize with 0.2 mg/kg yohimbine (partial antagonism only)

• 4 mg/kg ketamine plus 0.15 mg/kg medetomidine; antagonize with 0.6 mg/kg atipamezole

• 0.035 mg/kg etorphine; antagonize with 0.07 mg/kg diprenorphine

• 7 mg/kg ketamine plus 7 mg/kg xylazine (use 3 mg/kg ketamine plus 3 mg/kg xylazine for cubs of the year)

Comments: Polar bears are subject to hyperthermia and require monitoring. Renarcotization with carfentanil is possible (Scheinsburg and Haigh, 1982), thus it is recommended to give an additional dose of the antagonist SC or IM

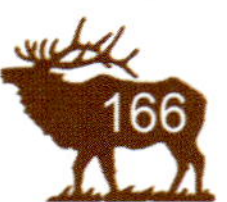

to prolong absorption. Severe respiratory depression is also possible with carfentanil use. Spontaneous recovery may occur when using medetomidine combinations (more likely with ketamine-medatomidine than tiletamine-zolazepam-medetomidine); avoid loud or sharp noises; try to prevent vocalization of cubs when mother is immobilized. Use long needles (i.e., >4 cm) to avoid injection into subcutaneous fat. Although safe and efficacious, tiletamine-zolazepam alone can result in prolonged recovery times (>2 hr). If quicker recoveries are required, use the tiletamine-zolazepam-medetomidine combination with atipamezole antagonism (Cattet et al., 1999).

References: Heck, 1965; Larsen, 1966; Flyger et al., 1967; Kuntze, 1967; Larsen, 1967; 1971; Lentfer, 1968; Seal and Erickson, 1969; Seal et al., 1970; Treimo, 1970; Kistchinski and Uspenski, 1970; Treimo, 1971; Bauditz, 1972; Robinson and Sedgwick, 1973; Alford et al., 1974; Beck, 1976; Eriksen, 1976; Kuntze, 1976; Boever et al., 1977; Patenaude, 1979; Lee et al., 1981; Gatesman and Wiesner, 1982; Scheinsburg et al., 1982; Taylor et al., 1982; Wiesner et al., 1982; Haigh et al., 1983; 1984; 1985; Ramsay et al., 1985; Stirling et al., 1985; 1989; Wiesner and von Hegel, 1985; Ramsay and Stirling, 1986; Schobert, 1987; Seal and Kreeger, 1987; Barnett and Lewis, 1990; Jalanka and Roeken, 1990; Torgerson, 1990; Williams et al., 1990a; Caulkett et al., 1996c; 1998b; 1999; Cattet et al., 1997; 1998; 1999a; 1999b; 2003a; Semple et al., 2000; Black and Whiteside, 2005

BEAR, SLOTH, *Melurus ursinus*

Weight: 55–145 kg
Recommended Drug: 6 mg/kg tiletamine-zolazepam
Supplemental Drug: 2 mg/kg ketamine
Antagonist: None
Alternative Drugs: 7.5 mg/kg ketamine plus 2 mg/kg xylazine; antagonize with 0.125 mg/kg yohimbine
References: Jarvis and Morris, 1960; Heuschele, 1961a; Kuntze, 1967; Seal and Erickson, 1969; Seal et al., 1970; Nair, 1977; Bush et al., 1980a; Page, 1986; Schobert, 1987; Black and Whiteside, 2005

BEAR, SPECTACLED, *Tremarctos ornatus*

Weight: 60–140 kg
Recommended Drug: 6 mg/kg tiletamine-zolazepam
Supplemental Drug: 2 mg/kg ketamine
Antagonist: None
References: Jarvis and Morris, 1960; Pistey and Wright, 1961; Graham-Jones, 1964; Kuntze, 1967; Wallach, 1968; 1969; Seal and Erickson, 1969; Seal et al., 1970; Bauditz, 1972; Boever et al., 1977; Nair, 1977; Bush et al., 1980a; Genevois et al., 1984b; Schobert, 1987; Black and Whiteside, 2005

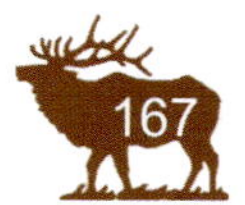

BEAR, SUN, *Ursus malayanus*

Weight: 50–73 kg

Recommended Drug: 3 mg/kg ketamine plus 0.07 mg/kg medetomidine

Supplemental Drug: 2 mg/kg ketamine

Antagonist: 0.35 mg/kg atipamezole; give 1/2 dose IV, 1/2 IM

Alternative Drugs: 2 mg/kg tiletamine-zolazepam plus 0.05 mg/kg medetomidine; antagonize with 0.25 mg/kg atipamezole

References: Jarvis and Morris, 1960; Kroll, 1962; Seal and Erickson, 1969; Seal et al., 1970; Pistey and Wright, 1961; Kuntze, 1967; Beck, 1976; Boever et al., 1977; Bush et al., 1980a; Schobert, 1987; Barnett and Lewis, 1990; Onuma, 2003

BEAVER, *Castor canadensis*

Weight: 12–25 kg

Recommended Drug: 10 mg/kg ketamine plus 1 mg/kg xylazine

Supplemental Drug: 5 mg/kg ketamine

Antagonist: None reported

Alternative Drugs: Isoflurane (see Breck and Gaynor, 2003)

- 5 mg/kg tiletamine-zolazepam
- 11 mg/kg ketamine plus 0.22 mg/kg acepromazine

References: Allen, 1965; Seal and Erickson, 1969; Seal et al., 1970; Beck, 1972; 1976; Lancia et al., 1978; Jessup et al., 1980; Hoilien and Oates, 1982; Jessup, 1982b; Wright, 1983; Seal and Kreeger, 1987; Eisele et al., 1997; Breck and Gaynor, 2003

BEAVER, EUROPEAN, *Castor fiber*

Weight: 18–25 kg

Recommended Drug: 5 mg/kg ketamine plus 0.05 mg/kg medetomidine plus 0.1 mg/kg butorphanol plus 0.25 mg/kg midazolam

Antagonist: 0.25 mg/kg atipamezole

Comments: This combination has been used for surgical implantation of radio transmitters (Ranheim et al., 2004). Anesthetized beavers may develop severe hypoxemia (SpO <80%) and supplemental oxygen should be considered.

References: Ranheim et al., 2004

BETTONG, BRUSH-TAILED, *Bettongia penicillata*

Weight: 1.1–1.6 kg

Recommended Drug: 10 mg/kg tiletamine-zolazepam

Supplemental Drug: 10 mg/kg ketamine

Antagonist: None

References: Holz, 1992

BINTURONG, *Arctictus binturong*

Weight: 16–28 kg

Recommended Drug: 2 mg/kg tiletamine-zolazepam
Supplemental Drug: 2 mg/kg ketamine
Antagonist: None
Alternative Drugs: 2 mg/kg ketamine plus 0.04 mg/kg medetomidine plus 0.2 mg/kg butorphanol
References: Seal and Erickson, 1969; Seal et al., 1970; Gray et al., 1974; Schobert, 1987; Moresco, 2002; Moresco and Larsen, 2003

BIRDS, GENERAL NONPASSERINE

Weight: < 30 gm
Recommended Drug: 0.035 mg/gm ketamine
Supplemental Drug: 0.02 mg/gm ketamine
Alternative Drugs: 0.02 mg/gm ketamine plus 0.004 mg/gm xylazine

Weight: 30–100 gm
Recommended Drug: 0.025 mg/gm ketamine
Supplemental Drug: 0.015 mg/gm ketamine
Alternative Drugs: 0.015 mg/gm ketamine plus 0.003 mg/gm xylazine

Weight: 100–200 gm
Recommended Drug: 0.02 mg/gm ketamine
Supplemental Drug: 0.01 mg/gm ketamine
Alternative Drugs: 0.01 mg/gm ketamine plus 0.002 mg/gm xylazine

Weight: 200–800 gm
Recommended Drug: 0.015 mg/gm ketamine
Supplemental Drug: 0.008 mg/gm ketamine
Alternative Drugs: 0.01 mg/gm ketamine plus 0.002 mg/gm xylazine

Weight: 0.8–5 kg
Recommended Drug: 10 mg/kg ketamine
Supplemental Drug: 5 mg/kg ketamine
Alternative Drugs: 5 mg/kg ketamine plus 1 mg/kg xylazine

Weight: 5–100 kg
Recommended Drug: 2.5 mg/kg ketamine plus 0.5 mg/kg xylazine
Supplemental Drug: 1.25 mg/kg ketamine
Antagonist: None reported
References: Borg, 1955; Marsboom et al., 1964; Smith, 1967; Williams and Phillips, 1972; 1973; Cooper and Frank, 1973; Webster and Hollard, 1973; Stunkard and Miller, 1974; Boever and Wright, 1975; Jones, 1977b; Amand, 1980; Smith et al., 1980; Neal et al., 1981; Hartsfield, 1982; Samour et al., 1984; Allen and Oosterhuis, 1986; Freeman, 1986; Linn, 1986; Sedgwick, 1986; Taylor, 1987; Degernes et al., 1988; Stouffer and Caccamise, 1991; Hochleithner, 1993; Cooke, 1995; Bailey et al., 1999;

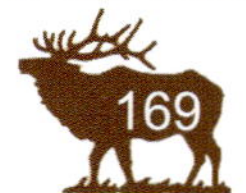

Belant et al., 1999; Quandt and Greenacre, 1999; Hayes et al., 2003; Mulcahy et al., 2003; Machin, 2004

BIRDS, GENERAL PASSERINE

Weight: < 30 gm
Recommended Drug: 0.06 mg/gm ketamine
Supplemental Drug: 0.003 mg/gm ketamine
Alternative Drugs: 0.03 mg/gm ketamine plus 0.006 mg/gm xylazine

Weight: 30–100 gm
Recommended Drug: 0.045 mg/gm ketamine
Supplemental Drug: 0.025 mg/gm ketamine
Alternative Drugs: 0.025 mg/gm ketamine plus 0.005 mg/gm xylazine

Weight: 100–200 gm
Recommended Drug: 0.035 mg/gm ketamine
Supplemental Drug: 0.02 mg/gm ketamine
Alternative Drugs: 0.02 mg/gm ketamine plus 0.004 mg/gm xylazine

Weight: 200–500 gm
Recommended Drug: 0.03 mg/gm ketamine
Supplemental Drug: 0.015 mg/gm ketamine
Alternative Drugs: 0.015 mg/gm ketamine plus 0.003 mg/gm xylazine

Weight: 0.5–1 kg
Recommended Drug: 10 mg/kg ketamine plus 2 mg/kg xylazine
Supplemental Drug: 5 mg/kg ketamine
Antagonist: None reported
References: Schafer et al., 1967; Smith, 1967; Peek, 1972; Schafer and Cunningham, 1972; Williams and Phillips, 1972; Stunkard and Miller, 1974; Boever and Wright, 1975; Jones, 1977b; Amand, 1980; Krechetov, 1980; Hartsfield, 1982; Mueller, 1982; Cooper, 1984; Samour et al., 1984; Allen and Oosterhuis, 1986; Linn, 1986; Sedgwick, 1986; Taylor, 1987; Degernes et al., 1988; Cyr and Brunet, 1992; Avery, 1993b; Hochleithner, 1993; Day and Roge, 1996; Belant et al., 1999

BIRDS, GENERAL PET

Weight: < 100 gm
Recommended Drug: 0.2 mg/gm ketamine
Supplemental Drug: 0.1 mg/gm ketamine

Weight: 100–500 gm
Recommended Drug: 0.1 mg/gm ketamine
Supplemental Drug: 0.05 mg/gm ketamine
Weight: 0.5–3 kg

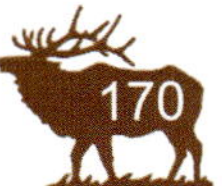

Recommended Drug: 80 mg/kg ketamine
Supplemental Drug: 40 mg/kg ketamine

Weight: > 3 kg
Recommended Drug: 50 mg/kg ketamine
Supplemental Drug: 25 mg/kg ketamine
References: Kittle, 1971; Stunkard and Miller, 1974; Boever and Wright, 1975; Beck, 1976; Boever, 1979; Amand, 1980; Hartsfield. 1982; Cooper, 1984; Samour et al., 1984; Garver and Jackson, 1985; Linn, 1986; Schobert, 1987; Taylor, 1987; Heaton and Brauth, 1992; Felkai, 1993; Hochleithner, 1993; Curro, 1998; Quandt and Greenacre, 1999; Sandmeier, 2000

BISON, AMERICAN, *Bison bison*

Weight: 350–1,000 kg
Recommended Drug: 0.005 mg/kg carfentanil plus 0.07 mg/kg xylazine
Supplemental Drug: 0.005 mg/kg carfentanil
Antagonist: 0.5 mg/kg naltrexone plus 0.125 mg/kg yohimbine
Alternative Drugs: 0.01 mg/kg etorphine plus 0.05 mg/kg xylazine; antagonize with 0.02 mg/kg diprenorphine plus 0.125 mg/kg yohimbine
• 1.2 mg/kg tiletamine-zolazepam plus 0.06 mg/kg medetomidine; antagonize with 0.18 mg/kg atipamezole
• 3 mg/kg tiletamine-zolazepam plus 1.5 mg/kg xylazine; antagonize with 3 mg/kg tolazoline (calm animals only)
Comments: The tiletamine-zolazepam dosages were based on captive wood bison (Caulkett et al., 1998; 2000).
References: Jarvis and Morris, 1960; Wallach et al., 1967; Wallach, 1968; 1969; Gauckler and Kraus, 1970; Jones, 1971; Thomas, 1961; Sedgwick and Acosta, 1969; Bauditz, 1972; Heck and Rivenburg, 1972; Jones, 1972; Gray et al., 1974; Hertzog, 1975; Rapley and Mehren, 1975; Haigh, 1976d; Haugen et al., 1976; Wiesner, 1977; Jessup et al., 1980; Thorne, 1982; Wiesner et al., 1982; Carpenter and Lance, 1983; Silvestris and Heck, 1984; Wiesner and von Hegel, 1985; Hugues et al., 1986; Sedgwick, 1986; Kock and Berger, 1987; Schobert, 1987; Williams and Riedesel, 1987; Berger and Kock, 1988; Renecker et al., 1992; Pond and O'Gara, 1994; Haigh and Gates, 1995; Caulkett et al., 1998a; 2000a; Shury, 1998; Páras et al., 2002; Shury and Caulkett, 2006

BISON, EUROPEAN, *Bison bonasus*

Weight: 350–1,000 kg
Recommended Drug: 1.5 mg carfentanil plus 35 mg xylazine
Supplemental Drug: If animal is not down in 20 min, repeat full dose
Antagonist: 100 mg naltrexone per mg carfentanil given plus 0.125 mg/kg yohimbine
Alternative Drugs: 0.01 mg/kg etorphine plus 0.5 mg/kg xylazine; antagonize with 0.02 mg/kg diprenorphine plus 0.125 mg/kg yohimbine

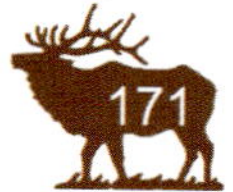

• 1.8 ml Large Animal Immobilon® plus 50 mg xylazine; antagonize with 2 mg diprenorphine per mg etorphine given plus 0.125 mg/kg yohimbine
• 2.5 mg/kg ketamine plus 0.08 mg/kg medetomidine; antagonize with 0.4 mg/kg atipamezole
References: Jaczewski and Swierzynski, 1955; Piwowarczyk, 1967; Zaniewski, 1967; Gauckler and Kraus, 1970; Göltenboth and Klös, 1970; Jones, 1971; Bauditz, 1972; Heck and Rivenburg, 1972; Kania et al., 1973; 1985; Kania and Teuchman, 1975; Rapley and Mehren, 1975; Wentges, 1975; Wiesner, 1975; 1977; Krasinski et al., 1982; Wiesner et al., 1982; Duchamps, 1985; Wiesner and von Hegel, 1985; Sedgwick, 1986; Strauss, 1987; Kock et al., 1989; Jalanka and Roeken, 1990

BLACKBUCK, *Antilope cervicapra*

Weight: 32–43 kg
Recommended Drug: 6 mg/kg tiletamine-zolazepam
Supplemental Drug: 3 mg/kg ketamine
Antagonist: None
Alternative Drugs: 1.5 mg carfentanil; antagonize with 1 mg/kg naltrexone
• 2 mg/kg ketamine plus 0.25 mg/kg medetomidine; antagonize with 1 mg/kg atipamezole
• 4 mg/kg xylazine; antagonize with 0.2 mg/kg yohimbine (calm animals)
• 0.3 ml Large Animal Immobilon® plus 10 mg xylazine; antagonize with 2 mg diprenorphine per mg etorphine given plus 0.125 mg/kg yohimbine
• 3 mg etorphine; antagonize with 6 mg diprenorphine
References: Larsen, 1963; Wright, 1963; Wallach et al., 1967; Wallach, 1968; 1969; Gauckler and Kraus, 1970; Bauditz, 1972; Heck and Rivenburg, 1972; York and Huggins, 1972; Rapley and Mehren, 1975; Wiesner, 1977; Jones, 1978; Jessup et al., 1980; Wiesner et al., 1982; Silvestris and Heck, 1984; Wiesner and von Hegel, 1985; Allen, 1986b; Hugues et al., 1986; Strauss, 1987; Williams and Riedesel, 1987; Arora, 1988; Jalanka and Roeken, 1990; Allen et al., 1991; Páras et al., 2002

BLESBOK, *Damaliscus dorcas*

Weight: 60–75 kg
Recommended Drug: 0.05 mg/kg etorphine plus 0.15 mg/kg xylazine
Supplemental Drug: If animal is not down in 20 minutes, repeat full dose
Antagonist: 2 mg diprenorphine per mg etorphine given plus 0.125 mg/kg yohimbine
Alternative Drugs: 0.01 mg/kg carfentanil plus 0.1 mg/kg xylazine; antagonize with 1 mg/kg naltrexone plus 0.125 mg/kg yohimbine
• 1.25 mg etorphine plus 15 mg ketamine plus 15 mg xylazine; antagonize with 2.5 mg diprenorphine plus 0.125 mg/kg yohimbine
• 0.6 ml Large Animal Immobilon® plus 10 mg xylazine; antagonize with 2 mg diprenorphine per mg etorphine given plus 0.125 mg/kg yohimbine
• 15 mg fentanyl plus 50 mg azaperone

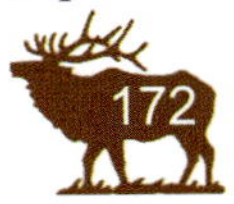

• 8 mg/kg tiletamine-zolazepam

Comments: High impact darting systems should not be used. Long-acting tranquilizer doses: haloperidol (adult male, 15 mg; adult female, 10 mg, subadult, 7.5 mg; neonate, 5 mg); zuclopenthixol, 1 mg/kg; perphenazine (adults, 50-80 mg).

References: Van Niekerk et al., 1963a; Pienaar, 1969b; 1973a; Barkhuizen, 1972; Bauditz, 1972; Heck and Rivenburg, 1972; Harthoorn and Van der Walt, 1974; De Vos, 1975; Röken, 1975; York, 1975; Haigh, 1976d; Hofmeyr, 1981; Wiesner et al., 1982; Silvestris and Heck, 1984; Wiesner and von Hegel, 1985; Schobert, 1987; Williams and Riedesel, 1987; Ganhao et al., 1988; Allen et al., 1991; IWVS, 1992; Snyder et al., 1992; Burroughs, 1993d; Kock, M., et al., 2006

BOBCAT, *Felis rufus*

Weight: 4.1–15.3 kg

Recommended Drug: 10 mg/kg tiletamine-zolazepam

Supplemental Drug: 5 mg/kg ketamine

Antagonist: None

Alternative Drugs: 10 mg/kg ketamine plus 1.5 mg/kg xylazine

• 20 mg/kg ketamine plus 0.1 mg/kg acepromazine

References: Kroll, 1962; Seal and Erickson, 1969; Seal et al., 1970; Bailey, 1971; Beck, 1976; Boever et al., 1977; Jessup et al., 1980; Hoilien and Oates, 1982; Jessup, 1982b; Fuller et al., 1985; Kocan et al., 1985; Schobert, 1987; Seal and Kreeger, 1987; Pond and O'Gara, 1994; Beltrán and Tewes, 1995

BONGO, *Tragelaphus eurycerus*

Weight: 150–200 kg

Recommended Drug: 1.4 mg carfentanil plus 80 mg ketamine plus 20 mg xylazine (adults)

Supplemental Drug: If animal is not down in 20 minutes, repeat full dose

Antagonist: 140 mg naltrexone plus 1.5 mg/kg yohimbine

Alternative Drugs: 2 mg carfentanil (males); 1.5 mg carfentanil (females)

• 0.023 mg/kg etorphine; antagonize with 0.05 mg/kg

References: Röken, 1975; Gray, 1974; Haigh, 1976b; 1976d; Slee and Walker, 1977; Allen et al, 1991; Miller-Edge and Amsel, 1994; Schumacher et al., 1997; Mikota et al., 1999

BONTEBOK - SEE BLESBOK

BUFFALO, AFRICAN, *Syncerus caffer*

Weight: 600–900 kg

Recommended Drug: 0.005 mg/kg carfentanil plus 0.05 mg/kg xylazine

Supplemental Drug: If animal is not down in 20 minutes, repeat full dose

Antagonist: 0.5 mg/kg naltrexone plus 0.05 mg/kg yohimbine

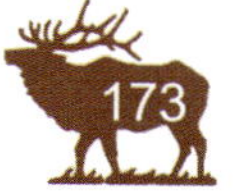

Alternative Drugs: 0.02 mg/kg thiafentanil plus 0.1 mg/kg azaperone; antagonize with 0.2 mg/kg naltrexone

- 0.0125 mg/kg etorphine plus 0.1 mg/kg xylazine; antagonize with 0.025 mg/kg diprenorphine plus 0.05 mg/kg yohimbine
- 0.015 mg/kg etorphine plus 0.15 mg/kg azaperone; antagonize with 0.03 mg/kg diprenorphine
- 5 mg/kg tiletamine-zolazepam
- 60 mg fentanyl plus 300 mg azaperone

Comments: Maintain in sternal recumbency. Change body position of large bulls every 10 minutes to maintain blood flow. Xylazine can induce regurgitation and possible aspiration pneumonia. The addition of hyaluronidase to the drug mixture is beneficial. If ambient temperature is >28.5 C, be prepared to cool the animal with water. Etorphine dose can be reduced to 0.006 mg/kg for captive buffalo. Long-acting tranquilizer doses: zuclopenthixol, 1 mg/kg (not to exceed 600 mg total); perphenazine (adult male, 400 mg; adult female, 200 mg; subadult, 100 mg; calf, 50 mg). Zuclopenthixol gave adequate tranquilization for three days.

References: Buechner et al., 1960c; 1960d; Harthoorn and Lock, 1961; Talbot and Talbot, 1962; Van Niekerk et al., 1963a; Van Niekerk and Pienaar, 1963a; Condy, 1964; Graham-Jones, 1964; Pienaar et al., 1966a; Pienaar, 1968a; 1969a; 1969b; Jones, 1971; 1972; Bauditz, 1972; Harthoorn, 1972a; 1973a; 1973b; 1974; Heck and Rivenburg, 1972; Woodford et al., 1972; York and Huggins, 1972; Young and Whyte, 1973; Eltringham, 1974; Gray et al., 1974; Manton and Jones, 1974; De Vos, 1975; 1985; Rapley and Mehren, 1975; Röken, 1975; Smuts, 1975; York, 1975; Drager et al., 1976; Haigh, 1976d; Hattingh et al., 1984; Silvestris and Heck, 1984; Schobert, 1987; Kock, R., et al., 1989; Allen et al., 1991; Janssen et al., 1991; IWVS, 1992; Bengis, 1993; Kock, 2001; Kock, M., et al., 2006

BURRO - SEE ASS, WILD

BUSH BABY - SEE GALAGO

BUSHBUCK, *Tragelaphus scriptus*

Weight: 24–42 (f), 30–77 (m) kg

Recommended Drug: 1.5 mg etorphine plus 50 mg azaperone, total dose

Supplemental Drug: 1 mg etorphine

Antagonist: 2 mg diprenorphine per mg etorphine given

Alternative Drugs: 2 mg thiafentanil; antagonize with 150 mg naltrexone

- 15 mg fentanyl plus 80 mg azaperone
- 12 mg/kg tiletamine-zolazepam

Comments: If captured by net first, immobilization can be achieved by administering 0.5 mg etorphine IV. Avoid high-impact darting systems.

References: Ebedes, 1962; Bauditz, 1972; Pienaar, 1973a; Röken, 1975; Smuts, 1975; Haigh, 1976d; Schobert, 1987; IWVS, 1992; Burroughs,

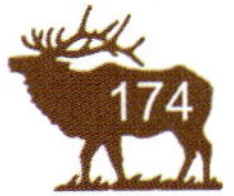

1993d; Kock et al., 2006

BUSH PIG, AFRICAN, *Potamochoerus porcus*

Weight: 46–130 kg
Recommended Drug: 2 mg/kg tiletamine-zolazepam
Supplemental Drug: 1 mg/kg tiletamine-zolazepam
Antagonist: None
Comments: Do not use etorphine in bush pigs.
References: Van Rensburg, 1993; Kock, M., et al., 2006

CAIMAN - SEE CROCODILIANS, GENERAL

CAMEL, BACTRIAN, *Camelus bactrianus*

Weight: 300–690 kg
Recommended Drug: 2 mg/kg ketamine plus 2 mg/kg xylazine
Supplemental Drug: 1 mg/kg ketamine
Antagonist: 0.125 mg/kg yohimbine
Alternative Drugs: 1.5 mg/kg xylazine
Comments: Although opioids have been used on the Camelidae (Schels and Nowrouzian, 1977; Wiesner et al., 1982), some feel that their use is contraindicated (Jones, 1977a).
References: Gates, 1970; Bauditz, 1972; Jones, 1972; Heck and Rivenburg, 1972; Rapley and Mehren, 1975; Custer et al., 1977; Held and Paddleford, 1982; Wiesner et al., 1982; Higgins and Kock, 1984; Wiesner and von Hegel, 1985; Allen, 1986b; Kock et al., 1989; Jalanka and Roeken, 1990

CAMEL, DROMEDARY, *Camelus dromedarius*

Weight: 300–690 kg
Recommended Drug: 2 mg/kg ketamine plus 2 mg/kg xylazine
Supplemental Drug: 1 mg/kg ketamine
Antagonist: 0.125 mg/kg yohimbine
Alternative Drugs: 1 mg/kg ketamine plus 0.05 mg/kg medetomidine; antagonize with 0.15 mg/kg atipamezole
Comments: Although opioids have been used on the Camelidae (Schels and Nowrouzian, 1977; Wiesner et al., 1982), some feel that their use is contraindicated (Jones, 1977a).
References: Metcalfe, et al., 1968; Bhargava et al., 1969; Hime and Jones, 1970; Bauditz, 1972; Dennig, 1972; Gates, 1972; Heck and Rivenburg, 1972; Khamis et al., 1973; Alford et al., 1974; Rosborough et al., 1974; Hertzog, 1975; Mehren and Rapley, 1975; Rapley and Mehren, 1975; Röken, 1975; Schels and Nowrouzian, 1977; Peshin et al., 1980; 1992; Wiesner et al., 1982; Higgins and Kock, 1984; Jacobson and Kollias, 1984; Wiesner and von Hegel, 1985; White, 1986; Dioloi, 1992; Peshin et al., 1992; Singh et al., 1994; Bonath, 1995; deMaar et al., 1998; Al Busadah, 2001; El Maghraby and Al Qudah, 2005

CAPYBARA, *Hydrochoerus hydrochaeris*

Weight: 27–79 kg
Recommended Drug: 5 mg/kg tiletamine-zolazepam
Supplemental Drug: 2.5 mg/kg ketamine
Antagonist: None
Alternative Drugs: 15 mg/kg ketamine plus 0.1 mg/kg acepromazine
References: Seal and Erickson, 1969; Seal et al., 1970; Szabuniewicz et al., 1978; Stoskopf, 1979; Wiesner and von Hegel, 1985

CARACAL, *Felis caracal*

Weight: 13–19 kg
Recommended Drug: 6.6 mg/kg tiletamine-zolazepam
Supplemental Drug: 6.6 mg/kg ketamine
Antagonist: None
Alternative Drugs: 10 mg/kg ketamine plus 1 mg/kg xylazine
References: Seal et al., 1970; Ebedes, 1973b; Genevois et al., 1984b; Gray et al., 1974; Schobert, 1987; McKenzie and Burroughs, 1993; Kock, M., et al., 2006

CARIBOU, *Rangifer tarandus*

Weight: 80–318 kg
Recommended Drug: 2.5 mg/kg ketamine plus 0.25 mg/kg medetomidine
Supplemental Drug: 1.5 mg/kg ketamine
Antagonist: 1.25 mg/kg atipamezole
Alternative Drugs: 0.06 mg/kg etorphine plus 0.3 mg/kg xylazine, antagonize with 0.12 mg/kg diprenorphine plus 0.125 mg/kg yohimbine

- 6 mg/kg ketamine plus 1.2 mg/kg xylazine; antagonize with 0.125 mg/kg yohimbine
- 5 mg/kg tiletamine-zolazepam
- 5 mg/kg xylazine; antagonize with 0.06 mg/kg idazoxan or 0.2 mg/kg yohimbine (calm animals only)

Comments: Concentrated xylazine (300 mg/ml) worked better in darts than did the standard 100 mg/ml solution (Doherty and Tweedie, 1989).
References: Bergerud et al., 1964; Wallach et al., 1967; Wallach, 1968; 1969; Gauckler and Kraus, 1970; Des Meules et al., 1971; Bauditz, 1972; Heck and Rivenburg, 1972; Jones, 1972; 1978; Laisher, 1972; Gray et al., 1974; Hertzog, 1975; Rapley and Mehren, 1975; Haigh, 1976d; 1978c; Wiesner, 1977; Jarofke, 1980; Fuller and Keith, 1981; Fong, 1982; Patenaude, 1982a; Thorne, 1982; Wiesner et al., 1982; Carpenter and Lance, 1983; Valkenburg et al., 1983; Jones, 1984; Röken, 1987; Schobert, 1987; Williams and Riedesel, 1987; Doherty and Tweedie, 1989; Kock et al., 1989; Jalanka, 1989d; Barnett and Lewis, 1990; Jalanka and Roeken, 1990; Tyler et al., 1990; Caulkett et al., 1996a; Ranheim et al., 1997; Arnemo and Ranheim, 1999; Soveri et al., 1999; Ranheim, 1999; Valkenburg et al., 1999; Ryeng et al., 2001a; 2001b; 2002; Caulkett and Arnemo, 2007

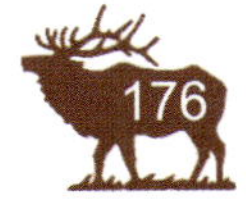

CASSOWARY, DOUBLE-WATTLED, *Casuarius casuarius*

Weight: 40–85 kg
Recommended Drug: 10 mg etorphine plus 200 mg ketamine
Supplemental Drug: 2 mg etorphine plus 100 mg ketamine
Antagonist: 20 mg diprenorphine
Alternative Drugs: 0.5 mg/kg medetomidine; antagonize with 2.5 mg/kg atipamezole (provides heavy sedation, not anesthesia)
References: Beck, 1976; Ensley, 1984; Stoskopf et al., 1982; Westcott and Reid, 2002

CAT, BLACK-FOOTED, *Felis nigripes*

Weight: 1.5–2.75 kg
Recommended Drug: 5 mg/kg tiletamine-zolazepam
Supplemental Drug: 2.5 mg/kg ketamine
Antagonist: None
Alternative Drugs: 25 mg/kg ketamine plus 1 mg/kg xylazine
References: Seal et al., 1970; Kock, M., et al., 2006

CAT, FISHING, *Felis viverrina*

Weight: 7.7–14 kg
Recommended Drug: 4.4 mg/kg tiletamine-zolazepam
Supplemental Drug: 4.4 mg/kg ketamine
Antagonist: None
Alternative Drugs: 22 mg/kg ketamine
References: Seal and Erickson, 1969; Seal et al., 1970; Dolensek, 1971; Beck, 1972; 1976; Gray et al., 1974; Jessup et al., 1980; Genevois et al., 1984b; Schobert, 1987

CAT, FLAT-HEADED, *Felis planiceps*

Weight: 1.6–2.1 kg
Recommended Drug: 8 mg/kg ketamine
Supplemental Drug: 4 mg/kg ketamine
Antagonist: None
References: Beck, 1972; 1976; Jessup et al., 1980

CAT, GEOFFREY, *Felis geoffroyi*

Weight: 3–7 kg
Recommended Drug: 4 mg/kg tiletamine-zolazepam
Supplemental Drug: 4 mg/kg ketamine
Antagonist: None
References: Seal et al., 1970; Gray et al., 1974; Schobert, 1987

CAT, ASIAN GOLDEN, *Felis temmincki*

Weight: 12–15 kg
Recommended Drug: 4 mg/kg ketamine plus 0.1 mg/kg medetomidine

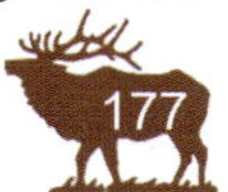

Supplemental Drug: 2 mg/kg ketamine
Antagonist: 0.5 mg/kg atipamezole; give 1/2 dose IV, 1/2 IM
Alternative Drugs: 4.4 mg/kg tiletamine-zolazepam
References: Seal and Erickson, 1969; Seal et al., 1970; Gray et al., 1974; Boever et al., 1977; Schobert, 1987; Jalanka and Roeken, 1990; Grassman et al., 2004

CAT, JUNGLE, *Felis chaus*

Weight: 4–16 kg
Recommended Drug: 5 mg/kg tiletamine-zolazepam
Supplemental Drug: 5 mg/kg ketamine
Antagonist: None
Alternative Drugs: 2.5 mg/kg ketamine plus 0.1 mg/kg medetomidine; antagonize with 0.5 mg/kg atipamezole
References: Graham-Jones, 1964; Seal and Erickson, 1969; Seal et al., 1970; Gray et al., 1974; Boever et al., 1977; Genevois et al., 1984b; Schobert, 1987; Barnett and Lewis, 1990

CAT, LEOPARD, *Felis bengalensis*

Weight: 2–5 kg
Recommended Drug: 25 mg/kg ketamine plus 2 mg/kg xylazine
Supplemental Drug: 12 mg/kg ketamine
Antagonist: None
References: Grassman et al., 2004

CAT, MARBLED, *Felis marmorata*

Weight: 1.4–5 kg
Recommended Drug: 12 mg/kg tiletamine-zolazepam
Supplemental Drug: 12 mg/kg ketamine
Antagonist: None
Alternative Drugs: 25 mg/kg ketamine plus 2 mg/kg xylazine
References: Seal and Erickson, 1969; Seal et al., 1970; Gray et al., 1974; Hime, 1974; Beck, 1976; Boever et al., 1977; Genevois et al., 1984b; Schobert, 1987; Grassman et al., 2004

CAT, PAMPAS, *Felis manul*

Weight: 3–7 kg
Recommended Drug: 5 mg/kg tiletamine-zolazepam
Supplemental Drug: 5 mg/kg ketamine
Antagonist: None
References: Gray et al., 1974; Genevois et al., 1984b; Schobert, 1987

CAT, SPOTTED, *Felis tigrina*

Weight: 1.75–2.75 kg
Recommended Drug: 8 mg/kg ketamine

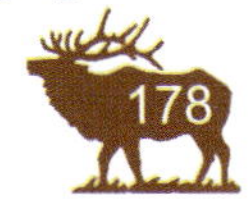

Supplemental Drug: 4 mg/kg ketamine
Antagonist: None
References: Seal and Erickson, 1969; Seal et al., 1970

CAT, WILD, *Felis sylvestris*

Weight: 3–8 kg
Recommended Drug: 5 mg/kg tiletamine-zolazepam
Supplemental Drug: 5 mg/kg ketamine
Antagonist: None
Alternative Drugs: 25 mg/kg ketamine plus 1 mg/kg xylazine
References: Seal et al., 1970; Gray et al., 1974; Wiesner, 1977; Genevois et al., 1984b; Schobert, 1987; Kock, M., et al., 2006

CATTLE, FERAL, *Bos taurus*

Weight: 500–1,000 kg
Recommended Drug: 0.004 mg/kg carfentanil plus 0.07 mg/kg xylazine
Supplemental Drug: 0.004 mg/kg carfentanil
Antagonist: 0.4 mg/kg naltrexone plus 0.125 mg/kg yohimbine or 2 mg/kg tolazoline
Alternative Drugs: 0.08 mg/kg medetomidine; antagonize with 0.24 mg/kg atipamezole
• 0.5 mg/kg xylazine; antagonize with 2 mg/kg tolazoline (or 0.05 mg/kg atipamezole)
Comments: Resedation may occur with the xylazine or medetomidine dosages and administration of additional atipamezole SC should be considered.
References: Arnemo and Søli, 1993; 1995b

CAVY, PATAGONIAN, *Dolichatis patagonum*

Weight: 9–16 kg
Recommended Drug: 10 mg/kg tiletamine-zolazepam
Supplemental Drug: 5 mg/kg ketamine
Antagonist: None
Alternative Drugs: 10 mg/kg ketamine plus 12 mg/kg xylazine
References: Gray et al., 1974; Kock et al., 1989

CHAMOIS, *Rupricapra rupricapra*

Weight: 24–50 kg
Recommended Drug: 2 mg/kg ketamine plus 0.1 mg/kg medetomidine
Supplemental Drug: 1 mg/kg ketamine
Antagonist: 0.5 mg/kg atipamezole; give 1/2 dose IV, 1/2 IM
Alternative Drugs: 0.013 mg/kg carfentanil plus 0.08 mg/kg xylazine; antagonize with 1.3 mg/kg naltrexone plus 0.125 mg/kg yohimbine
• 0.8 ml Large Animal Immobilon®; antagonize with 2 mg diprenorphine per mg etorphine given

• 0.05 mg/kg fentanyl plus 0.5 mg/kg xylazine; antagonize with 0.2 mg/kg naloxone plus 0.125 mg/kg yohimbine

References: Boch et al., 1961; Bauditz, 1972; Wiesner, 1977; Clarke and Henderson, 1979; Jensen, 1982; Wiesner et al., 1982; Duchamps, 1985; Jalanka and Roeken, 1990; Moran et al., 1994; Walzer et al., 1996

CHEETAH, *Acinonyx jubatu*

Weight: 35–72 kg

Recommended Drug: 2.5 mg/kg ketamine plus 0.07 mg/kg medetomidine

Supplemental Drug: 1.5 mg/kg ketamine

Antagonist: 0.3 mg/kg atipamezole

Alternative Drugs: 1.5 mg/kg v plus 0.03 mg/kg medetomidine; antagonize with 0.15 mg/kg atipamezole

• 10 mg/kg ketamine plus 1 mg/kg xylazine

• 4 mg/kg tiletamine-zolazepam

Comments: Partial antagonism of tiletamine-zolazepam may be achieved with 0.03 mg/kg flumazenil or 0.1 mg/kg sarmazenil (see Walzer and Huber, 2002). In a few cases, cheetah have stopped breathing 60-90 minutes after given tiletamine-zolazepam and they do not respond to doxapram (Kock, M., et al., 2006). Perphenazine enanthate (3 mg/kg) has been used as a long-acting tranquilizer in captive cheetah (Huber et al., 2001)

References: Young, 1966; Ericksen, 1968; Pienaar et al., 1969; Seal and Erickson, 1969; Ebedes, 1970; 1973b; Seal et al., 1970; Dolensek, 1971; Bauditz, 1972; Beck, 1972; 1976; York and Huggins, 1972; Holmes and Ngethe, 1973; Smuts et al., 1973; York, 1973; Alford et al., 1974; Gray et al., 1974; Hime, 1974; Wentges, 1975; Boever et al., 1977; Nair, 1977; Smeller and Bush, 1977; Wiesner, 1977; Jessup et al., 1980; Button et al., 1981; Genevois et al., 1984b; Wiesner and von Hegel, 1985; Schobert, 1987; Kock, R., et al., 1989; Barnett and Lewis, 1990; IWVS, 1992; Klein and Stover, 1993; McKenzie and Burroughs, 1993; Deem et al., 1998; Rogers, 1998; Walzer and Huber, 1999; 2002; Huber et al., 1999; 2001; Lewandowski et al., 2002; Lafortune et al., 2005; Kock, M., et al., 2006

CHIMPANZEE, *Pan troglodytes*

Weight: 35–70 kg

Recommended Drug: 5 mg/kg ketamine plus 0.05 mg/kg medetomidine

Supplemental Drug: 3 mg/kg ketamine

Antagonist: 0.2 mg/kg atipamezole; give 1/2 dose IV, 1/2 IM

Alternative Drugs: 10 mg/kg ketamine plus 1 mg/kg xylazine

• 2.5 mg/kg tiletamine-zolazepam plus 0.04 mg/kg medetomidine; antagonize with 0.2 mg/kg atipamezole

• 15 mg/kg ketamine

Comments: Good induction and relaxation with ketamine/medetomidine.

References: Heuschele, 1959; Wallach et al., 1960; Marsboom et al., 1962; 1963; Larsen, 1963; Coetzee, 1964; Ericksen, 1968; Wallach et al., 1967;

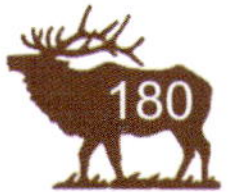

Wallach, 1968; 1969; Seal et al., 1970; Bauditz, 1972; Beck, 1972; Beck and Dresner, 1972; Gray et al., 1974; Bush et al., 1977; Vercruysse and Mortelmans, 1978; Jessup et al., 1980; April et al., 1982; Hugues et al., 1986; Robinson and Lambert, 1986; Göltenboth and Klös, 1987; Hess et al., 1987; Röken, 1987; Schobert, 1987; Kock, R. et al., 1989; Jalanka and Roeken, 1990; Lewis, 1993; Kearns et al., 1996; 1998; 1999; 2000; Horne et al., 1997; 1998; Adams et al., 2003; Hunter et al., 2004; Kock, M. et al., 2006

CHINCHILLA, *Chinchilla spp.*

Weight: 0.5–0.8 kg
Recommended Drug: 35 mg/kg tiletamine-zolazepam
Supplemental Drug: 20 mg/kg ketamine
Antagonist: None
Alternative Drugs: 40 mg/kg ketamine plus 0.5 mg/kg acepromazine
References: Gray et al., 1974; Schulz and Fowler, 1974; Morgan et al., 1981; Genevois et al., 1984a; Schobert, 1987

CHITAL - SEE DEER, AXIS

CHOUSINGHA - SEE FOUR-HORNED ANTELOPE

CIVET, AFRICAN PALM, *Nandinia binotata*

Weight: 1.7–2.1 kg
Recommended Drug: 8.8 mg/kg tiletamine-zolazepam
Supplemental Drug: 8.8 mg/kg ketamine
Antagonist: None
References: Seal et al., 1970; Gray et al., 1974; Beck, 1976; Genevois et al., 1984b; Schobert, 1987

CIVET, AFRICAN, *Civettictis civetta*

Weight: 7–20 kg
Recommended Drug: 4.4 mg/kg tiletamine-zolazepam
Supplemental Drug: 4.4 mg/kg ketamine
Antagonist: None
Alternative Drugs: 10 mg/kg ketamine plus 0.5 mg/kg xylazine
Comments: Darting of free-ranging civets is not recommended because they can easily become lost before the drug takes effect (McKenzie and Burroughs, 1993).
References: Seal and Erickson, 1969; Seal et al., 1970; McKenzie and Burroughs, 1993

CIVET, BANDED PALM, *Hemigalus derbyanus*

Weight: 1.75–3.0 kg
Recommended Drug: 6.6 mg/kg tiletamine-zolazepam

Supplemental Drug: 6.6 mg/kg ketamine
Antagonist: None
References: Seal and Erickson, 1969; Gray et al., 1974; Schobert, 1987

CIVET, BROWN PALM, *Paradoxurus jerdoni*

Weight: 1.2–3.5 kg
Recommended Drug: 15 mg/kg ketamine plus 1.5 mg/kg xylazine
Supplemental Drug: One-half of original dose
Antagonist: None reported
References: Mudappa and Chellam, 2001

CIVET, LESSER ORIENTAL, *Viverricula indica*

Weight: 2–4 kg
Recommended Drug: 4.4 mg/kg tiletamine-zolazepam
Supplemental Drug: 4.4 mg/kg ketamine
Antagonist: None
References: Seal and Erickson, 1969; Seal et al., 1970; Gray et al., 1974; Genevois et al., 1984b; Schobert, 1987

CIVET, MALAGASY, *Fossa fossa*

Weight: 1.5–2 kg
Recommended Drug: 6 mg/kg tiletamine-zolazepam
Supplemental Drug: 6 mg/kg ketamine
Antagonist: None
References: Seal et al., 1970; Gray et al., 1974; Schobert, 1987

CIVET, MASKED PALM, *Paguma larvata*

Weight: 3.6–5 kg
Recommended Drug: 4 mg/kg tiletamine-zolazepam
Supplemental Drug: 4 mg/kg ketamine
Antagonist: None
References: Seal and Erickson, 1969; Seal et al., 1970; Gray et al., 1974; Schobert, 1987

CIVET, ORIENTAL, *Viverra zibetha*

Weight: 5–11 kg
Recommended Drug: 4.4 mg/kg tiletamine-zolazepam
Supplemental Drug: 4.4 mg/kg ketamine
Antagonist: None
References: Seal and Erickson, 1969; Seal et al., 1970

CIVET, PALM, *Paradoxurus hermaphroditus*

Weight: 1.5–4.5 kg
Recommended Drug: 5 mg/kg tiletamine-zolazepam
Supplemental Drug: 5 mg/kg ketamine

Antagonist: None
References: Kroll, 1962; Seal and Erickson, 1969; Seal et al., 1970; Gray et al., 1974; Genevois et al., 1984b; Schobert, 1987

COATIMUNDI, *Nasua spp.*

Weight: 3–6 kg
Recommended Drug: 20 mg/kg ketamine plus 1 mg/kg xylazine
Supplemental Drug: 10 mg/kg ketamine
Antagonist: None reported
Alternative Drugs: 15 mg/kg ketamine plus 0.1 mg/kg acepromazine
Comments: Keep separate from other coatis for 24 hours after immobilization, if possible.
References: Graham-Jones, 1964; Dyson, 1965; Seal and Erickson, 1969; Seal et al., 1970; Beck, 1976; Jessup et al., 1980; Seal and Kreeger, 1987; Georoff et al., 2004

COUGAR - SEE LION, MOUNTAIN

COYOTE, *Canis latrans*

Weight: 7–18 kg
Recommended Drug: 10 mg/kg tiletamine-zolazepam
Supplemental Drug: 5 mg/kg ketamine
Alternative Drugs: 10 mg/kg ketamine plus 0.1 mg/kg acepromazine
• 4 mg/kg ketamine plus 2 mg/kg xylazine, antagonize with 0.15 mg/kg yohimbine
Comments: If using xylazine, wait at least 45 min after last ketamine injection before administering yohimbine.
References: Kroll, 1962; Balser, 1965; Seal and Erickson, 1969; Seal et al., 1970; Bailey, 1971; Gray et al., 1974; Ramsden et al., 1976; Baer et al., 1978; Mulder, 1978a; Cornely, 1979; Hallett et al., 1979; Jessup et al., 1980; Hoilien and Oates, 1982; Jessup, 1982b; Genevois et al., 1984b; Kreeger and Seal, 1986b; Schobert, 1987; Seal and Kreeger, 1987; Servin et al., 1990; Servin and Huxley, 1992; Pond and O'Gara, 1994

COYPU - SEE NUTRIA

CROCODILIANS, GENERAL

Recommended Drug: 15 mg/kg ketamine plus 1 mg/kg xylazine
Supplemental Drug: 8 mg/kg ketamine
Antagonist: None
Alternative Drugs: 15 mg/kg tiletamine-zolazepam
• 7.5 mg/kg ketamine plus 0.13 mg/kg medetomidine; antagonize with 0.7 mg/kg atipamezole (see Comments)
Comments: Expect prolonged induction times (20-30 min) when using either cyclohexane drug combination. Paralytic agents such as succinylcho-

line, gallamine, or atracurium may be more effective in crocodiles than other drugs. See Kock, M., et al., 2006 for precise gallamine and neostigmine doses. Decrease the dose of gallamine as size of crocodile increases (see Blake, 1993; Kock, M., et al., 2006). Pole syringes are safe and effective means of drug delivery, although darts also can be used. Sites of injection are hind legs, the side of the tail just behind the hind legs, or the large jaw muscles. Gallamine should be used with caution in American alligators. The ketamine-medetomidine dosages were developed for adult American alligators; juvenile alligators require higher dosages (10 mg/kg ketamine plus 0.22 mg/kg medetomidine; antagonize with 1.2 mg/kg atipamezole [see Heaton-Jones et al., 2002]).

References: Brisbin, 1966; Wallach and Hoessle, 1970; Calderwood, 1971; Klide and Klein, 1971; Loveridge and Blake, 1972; 1987; Woodford, 1972; Stunkard and Miller, 1974; Beck, 1976; Haigh, 1976d; Jones, 1977b; Terpin et al., 1978; Loveridge, 1979; Messel et al., 1980; Morgan-Davies, 1980; Lee, 1981; Jacobson, 1984; Spiegel et al., 1984a; 1984b; Idowu and Akinrinmade, 1985; Whitaker and Andrews, 1989; Bonath et al., 1990; Clyde et al., 1990; 1994; Bennett, 1991; Bonath et al., 1991; Johnson, 1991; Flamand et al., 1992; Haager and Reynolds, 1992; Blake, 1993; Page, 1993; Lloyd et al., 1994; Fleming, 1996; Heaton-Jones, 1996; Smith et al., 1998; Lloyd, 1999; Heaton-Jones et al., 2002; Kock, M., et al., 2006

CRUSTACEANS (CRABS, LOBSTER, CRAYFISH)

Recommended Drug: 25 mg/kg procaine

Comments: Administer by injection with 27-gauge needle through a coxoarthrodial membrane of a walking leg (not a swimming appendage) into a lateral sinus.

References: Sedgwick, 1986

CUSCUS, *Phalanger spp.*

Weight: 1–5 kg

Recommended Drug: 10 mg/kg ketamine

Supplemental Drug: 5 mg/kg ketamine

Antagonist: None

References: Salas and Stephens, 2004

DEER, AXIS, *Axis axis*

Weight: 40–110 kg

Recommended Drug: 3.5 mg/kg ketamine plus 0.1 mg/kg medetomidine

Supplemental Drug: 2 mg/kg ketamine

Antagonist: 0.5 mg/kg atipamezole

Alternative Drugs: 4 mg/kg ketamine plus 4 mg/kg xylazine; antagonize with 0.125 mg/kg yohimbine

• 0.004 mg/kg carfentanil plus 0.125 mg/kg xylazine; antagonize with 0.4 mg/kg naltrexone plus 0.125 mg/kg yohimbine

• 2.6 mg/kg tiletamine-zolazepam
• 1.7 ml Large Animal Immobilon® plus 30 mg xylazine; antagonize with 2 mg diprenorphine per mg etorphine given plus 0.125 mg/kg yohimbine
• 3 mg fentanyl plus 24 mg azaperone plus 30 mg xylazine (i.e., Fentaz® plus xylazine); antagonize with 10 mg naloxone per mg fentanyl given plus 2 mg/kg tolazoline
• 3 mg/kg xylazine (calm animals only); antagonize with 0.2 mg/kg yohimbine
References: Jarvis and Morris, 1960; Thomas, 1961; Heuschele, 1961a; Kroll, 1962; Bauditz, 1972; Jones, 1972; Gray et al., 1974; Sutherland and Hodgkin, 1974; Rapley and Mehren, 1975; Nair, 1977; Presidente et al., 1978c; Keep, 1979; Jessup et al., 1980; Singh and Singh, 1982; Arora et al., 1983; Jones, 1984; Wiesner et al., 1982; 1984; Kock and Pearce, 1985; Wiesner and von Hegel, 1985; Karesh et al., 1986; Röken, 1987; Schobert, 1987; Seal and Bush, 1987; Arora, 1988; Franzmann and Lance, 1988; Van Mourik et al., 1988; Jalanka and Roeken, 1990; Arnemo et al., 1993c; Haigh et al., 1993; Páras et al., 2002; Smith, K. et al., 2005; 2006

DEER, BLACK-TAILED - SEE DEER, MULE

DEER, BROCKET, *Mazama rufina*

Weight: 8–25 kg
Recommended Drug: 1 mg etorphine plus 5 mg ketamine plus 5 mg xylazine
Supplemental Drug: 15 mg ketamine IV, if possible
Antagonist: 2 mg diprenorphine plus 0.125 mg/kg yohimbine
References: Snyder et al., 1992

DEER, BROW-ANTLERED, *Cervus eldi*

Weight: 75–150 kg
Recommended Drug: 3 mg/kg ketamine plus 0.1 mg/kg medetomidine
Supplemental Drug: 1.5 mg/kg ketamine
Antagonist: 0.4 mg/kg atipamezole
Alternative Drugs: 3 mg/kg tiletamine-zolazepam plus 0.3 mg/kg xylazine; antagonize with 0.125 mg/kg yohimbine
• 6 mg/kg tiletamine-zolazepam
• 0.06 mg/kg etorphine plus 0.25 mg/kg acepromazine; antagonize with 0.12 mg/kg diprenorphine
References: Bush et al., 1992; Klein et al., 1996

DEER, CHINESE WATER, *Hydropotes inermis*

Weight: 11–30 kg
Recommended Drug: 0.06 mg/kg etorphine plus 0.25 mg/kg acepromazine Supplemental Drug: If not down in 20 min, repeat full dose
Antagonist: 2 mg diprenorphine per mg etorphine given

Alternative Drugs: 7 mg/kg ketamine plus 7 mg/kg xylazine
References: Rapley and Mehren, 1975; Jones, 1978; 1984; Seal and Bush, 1987; Hastings et al., 1989; Kock et al., 1989

DEER, ELD'S - SEE DEER, BROW-ANTLERED

DEER, FALLOW, *Dama dama*

Weight: 40–100 kg
Recommended Drug: 1 mg/kg tiletamine-zolazepam plus 0.1 mg/kg medetomidine
Supplemental Drug: 1.5 mg/kg ketamine
Antagonist: 0.5 mg/kg atipamezole; give 1/2 dose IV, 1/2 IM
Alternative Drugs: 2.5 mg/kg ketamine plus 0.1 mg/kg medetomidine; antagonize with 0.5 mg/kg atipamezole

- 5 mg/kg tiletamine-zolazepam plus 1 mg/kg xylazine
- 5 mg/kg ketamine plus 5 mg/kg xylazine; antagonize with 0.125 mg/kg yohimbine
- 0.013 mg/kg carfentanil plus 0.125 mg/kg xylazine; antagonize with 1.3 mg/kg naltrexone plus 0.125 mg/kg yohimbine
- 0.02 mg/kg etorphine plus 0.3 mg/kg xylazine; antagonize with 0.04 mg/kg diprenorphine plus 0.125 mg/kg yohimbine

Comments: No entirely satisfactory combination of drugs has been found for the immobilization of fallow deer; be prepared for less-than-satisfactory immobilizations. The use of acepromazine is contraindicated in fallow deer because of hyperthermia and respiratory depression. Xylazine alone gives unpredictable results.
References: Pistey and Wright, 1959; Jarvis and Morris, 1960; Heuschele, 1961a; 1961b; Thomas, 1961; Wallach et al., 1967; Wallach, 1968; 1969; Eriksen, 1970; Gauckler and Kraus, 1970; Göltenboth and Klös, 1970; Honich, 1970; Klide and Klein, 1971; Mulling and Henning, 1971; Bauditz, 1972; Fessel, 1972; Jones, 1972; 1978; Heck and Rivenburg, 1972; Chapman, 1973; Kilde and Klein, 1973; York and Huggins, 1972; Scanlon, 1973; Woolf et al., 1973; Alford et al., 1974; Gray et al., 1974; Harrington, 1974; Done et al., 1975; Hertzog, 1975; Rapley and Mehren, 1975; Geiger, 1976; Haigh, 1976d; 1977; Wiesner, 1977; Presidente et al., 1978b; Keep, 1979; Pertz and Sundberg, 1978; Jarofke, 1980; Jessup, et al., 1980; Schulz and Dingeldein, 1980; Wiesner et al., 1982; 1984; Jones, 1984; Silvestris and Heck, 1984; Duchamps, 1985; Kock and Pearce, 1985; Pearce et al., 1985; Wiesner and von Hegel, 1985; Hugues et al., 1986; Röken, 1987; Schobert, 1987; Seal and Bush, 1987; Williams and Riedesel, 1987; Sancken and Fischer, 1988; Van Mourik et al., 1988; Kock et al., 1989; Barnett and Lewis, 1990; Jalanka and Roeken, 1990; Stewart and English, 1990; Allen et al., 1991; Tung et al., 1993; Fernandez-Moran and Peinado, 1996; Galka et al., 1999; Fernandez-Moran et al., 2000; Páras et al., 2002; Haefele et al., 2005

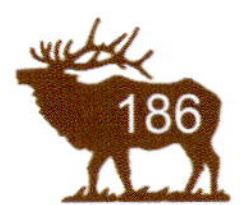

DEER, HIMALAYAN MUSK, *Moschus chrysogasters*

Weight: 7–17 kg
Recommended Drug: 4.5 mg/kg ketamine plus 1.5 mg/kg xylazine
Supplemental Drug: 2.5 mg/kg ketamine
Antagonist: 0.125 mg/kg yohimbine
References: Green, 1986; Kattel and Alldredge, 1991

DEER, HOG, *Axis porcinus*

Weight: 27–110 kg
Recommended Drug: 0.45 mg carfentanil
Supplemental Drug: If animal is not down in 20 min, repeat full dose
Antagonist: 1 mg/kg naltrexone
Alternative Drugs: 1.5 mg/kg ketamine plus 0.05 mg/kg medetomidine; antagonize with 0.25 mg/kg atipamezole
• 4 mg/kg xylazine; antagonize with 0.2 mg/kg yohimbine (calm deer only)
References: Göltenboth and Klös, 1970; Bauditz, 1972; Heck and Rivenburg, 1972; Presidente et al., 1978b; Keep, 1979; Jarofke, 1980; Singh and Singh, 1982; Jones, 1984; Dhungel, 1985 Allen et al., 1991; Arnemo et al., 2005a

DEER, MULE, *Odocoileus hemionus*

Weight: 75–135 kg
Recommended Drug: 3 mg/kg ketamine plus 0.1 mg/kg medetomidine
Supplemental Drug: 2 mg/kg ketamine
Antagonist: 0.5 mg/kg atipamezole
Alternative Drugs: 4.4 mg/kg tiletamine-zolazepam plus 2.2 mg/kg xylazine; antagonize with 0.125 mg/kg yohimbine (or 2 mg/kg tolazoline)
• 7 mg/kg ketamine plus 0.7 mg/kg xylazine; antagonize with 0.125 mg/kg yohimbine (or 2 mg/kg tolazoline)
• 0.03 mg/kg carfentanil plus 0.7 mg/kg xylazine; antagonize with 3 mg/kg naltrexone plus 0.125 mg/kg yohimbine
• 0.15 mg/kg thiafentanil plus 1 mg/kg xylazine; antagonize with 2 mg/kg naltrexone plus 2 mg/kg tolazoline
• 3 mg etorphine plus 30 mg xylazine; antagonize with 6 mg diprenorphine plus 0.125 mg/kg yohimbine
• 3 mg/kg xylazine, antagonize with 0.2 mg/kg yohimbine or 2 mg/kg tolazoline (calm deer only)
Comments: Deer immobilized with etorphine may run long distances and/or have an extended period (10+ min) of hyperactivity before recumbency. This hyperactivity can result in hyperthermia. All opioid agents can result in respiratory depression. When using ketamine-xylazine or tiletamine-zolazepam-xylazine for highly excited deer, the xylazine dose can be increased up to the dose of ketamine or tiletamine-zolazepam given (i.e., 7 mg/kg or 4.4 mg/kg, respectively). An effective standard dose for most adult mule deer is 1.5 ml of 200 mg/ml ketamine (i.e., 300 mg ketamine) plus 0.5

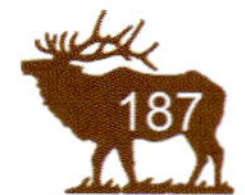

ml of 20 mg/ml medetomidine (i.e., 10 mg medetomidine). This will fit nicely in a 2 ml dart. Antagonize the medetomidine with 0.5 mg/kg atipamezole.

References: Heuschele, 1959; 1961a; 1961b; Jarvis and Morris, 1960; Anderson, 1961; Boyd, 1962; Cowan et al., 1962; Kroll, 1962; Merriam, 1962; Nordan et al., 1962; Pearson et al., 1963; Denney, 1965; Dyson, 1965; Siglin, 1965; Wolff et al., 1965; Kitchen, 1966; Miller, 1968; Day, 1969; Heck and Rivenburg, 1972; Dean et al., 1973; Gray et al., 1974; Rapley and Mehren, 1975; Haigh, 1976d; Richter, 1977; Wiesner, 1977; Trindle and Lewis, 1978; Jarofke, 1980; Lange, 1982; Jessup et al., 1980; 1982a; 1983; 1984; 1985a; Thorne, 1982; Carpenter and Lance, 1983; Jacobsen, 1983; Gullett, 1984; Krausman et al., 1984; Seidel and Strauss, 1984; Renecker and Olsen, 1985; Krausman et al., 1986; Schobert, 1987; Seal and Bush, 1987; Williams and Riedesel, 1987; Franzmann and Lance, 1988; Greene, 1988; DelGiudice et al., 1989; Smits et al., 1989; Caulkett et al., 1995; 1996b; 2000b; Wolfe et al., 2004

DEER, PAMPAS, *Ozotoceros bezoarticus*

Weight: 25–40 kg

Recommended Drug: 0.3 ml Large Animal Immobilon®

Supplemental Drug: If not down in 20 min, repeat full dose

Antagonist: 2 mg diprenorphine per mg etorphine given

References: Wiesner et al., 1982

DEER, PÉRE DAVID'S, *Elaphurus davidianus*

Weight: 159–214 kg

Recommended Drug: 1 mg/kg ketamine plus 0.03 mg/kg medetomidine

Supplemental Drug: 0.5 mg/kg ketamine

Antagonist: 0.15 mg/kg atipamezole; give 1/2 dose IV, 1/2 IM

Alternative Drugs: 3 mg/kg tiletamine-zolazepam plus 0.2 mg/kg xylazine; antagonize with 0.125 mg/kg yohimbine

- 5 mg/kg tiletamine-zolazepam
- 0.03 mg/kg etorphine plus 0.2 mg/kg xylazine; antagonize with 0.06 mg/kg diprenorphine plus 0.125 mg/kg yohimbine
- 1 mg/kg xylazine; antagonize with 0.2 mg/kg yohimbine (calm deer only)

References: Heck and Rivenburg, 1972; Jones, 1972; 1978; Rapley and Mehren, 1975; Smeller et al., 1976; Wiesner, 1977; Jarofke, 1980; Bush, 1982; Jacobson and Kollias, 1984; Jensen, 1982; Wiesner et al., 1982; Jacobson and Kollias, 1984; Jones, 1984; Kock and Pearce, 1985; Seal and Bush, 1987; Kock et al., 1989; Jalanka and Roeken, 1990; Bush et al., 1992; Lu et al., 1992

DEER, RED, *Cervus elaphus hippelaphus*

Weight: 60–180 kg

Recommended Drug: 2.2 mg/kg ketamine plus 0.11 mg/kg medetomidine

Supplemental Drug: 1.1 mg/kg ketamine
Antagonist: 0.5 mg/kg atipamezole
Alternative Drugs: 2.4 mg/kg tiletamine-zolazepam plus 2.4 mg/kg xylazine; antagonize with 0.125 mg/kg yohimbine
• 4 mg/kg ketamine plus 4 mg/kg xylazine; antagonize with 0.125 mg/kg yohimbine
• 0.004 mg/kg carfentanil plus 0.15 mg/kg xylazine; antagonize with 0.4 mg/kg naltrexone plus 0.125 mg/kg yohimbine
• 0.035 mg/kg etorphine plus 0.14 mg/kg acepromazine (Large Animal Immobilon®); antagonize with 0.7 mg/kg diprenorphine
• 0.21 mg/kg fentanyl plus 1.7 mg/kg azaperone
• 3 mg/kg xylazine, antagonize with 0.125 mg/kg yohimbine (calm deer only)
• 0.08 mg/kg medetomidine, antagonize with 0.3 mg/kg atipamezole (calm or captive deer only)
References: Schloeth et al., 1960; Boch et al., 1961; Thomas, 1961; Jewell et al., 1965; Jewell and Lowe, 1965; Taylor and Magnussen, 1965; Eriksen, 1968b; Eriksen, 1970; Gauckler and Kraus, 1970; Honich, 1970; Mulling and Henning, 1971; Bauditz, 1972; Fessel. 1972; Heck and Rivenburg, 1972; Jones, 1972; 1978; Woolf et al., 1973; Fletcher, 1974; 1986; McAllum, 1977; Wiesner, 1977; Presidente et al., 1978b; Keep, 1979; Jarofke, 1980; Van Reenen, 1982; Wiesner et al., 1982; 1984; Dickson et al., 1983; Simpson et al., 1983; Jones, 1984; MacKintosh and Van Reenen, 1984a; 1984b; Duchamps, 1985; Kock and Pearce, 1985; McKelvey and Simpson, 1985; Wiesner and von Hegel, 1985; Sedgwick, 1986; Röken, 1987; Seal and Bush, 1987; Cross et al., 1988; Koubek and Mrlik, 1988; Van Mourik et al., 1988; Kock et al., 1989; Jalanka and Roeken, 1990; Diverio et al., 1993; 1996; Haigh and Hudson, 1993; Zomborszky et al., 1993; Arnemo et al., 1994b; Wolkers et al., 1994; Wiesner, 1998; Janovsky et al., 2000; Walsh and Wilson, 2002; Johnson et al., 2005; Woodbury et al., 2005

DEER, ROE, *Capreolus capreolus*

Weight: 15–50 kg
Recommended Drug: 5 mg/kg ketamine plus 3 mg/kg xylazine
Supplemental Drug: 2.5 mg/kg ketamine
Antagonist: 0.15 mg/kg yohimbine
Alternative Drugs: 1.5 mg/kg ketamine plus 0.05 mg/kg medetomidine; antagonize with 0.25 mg/kg atipamezole
• 0.06 mg carfentanil; antagonize with 6 mg/kg naltrexone
• 0.3 ml Large Animal Immobilon® plus 5 mg xylazine; antagonize with 2 mg diprenorphine per mg etorphine given plus 0.125 mg/kg yohimbine
• 0.002 mg/kg etorphine plus 0.2 mg/kg xylazine; antagonize with 2 mg diprenorphine per mg etorphine given plus 0.125 mg/kg yohimbine
• 3 mg/kg xylazine; antagonize with 0.2 mg/kg yohimbine (calm deer only)
References: Gauckler and Kraus, 1970; Marma, 1970; Mulling and

Henning, 1971; Blazhis et al., 1972; Fessel, 1972; Heck and Rivenburg, 1972; Rapley and Mehren, 1975; Schultze, 1976; Wiesner, 1977; Keep, 1979; Jarofke, 1980; Wiesner et al., 1982; Jones, 1984; Seidel and Strauss, 1984; Duchamps, 1985; Röken, 1987; Seal and Bush, 1987; Jalanka and Roeken, 1990; Allen et al., 1991; Montané et al., 2003

DEER, RUSA - SEE SAMBAR, SUNDA

DEER, SIKA, *Cervus nippon*

Weight: 40–80 kg

Recommended Drug: 4 mg/kg ketamine plus 0.06 mg/kg medetomidine

Supplemental Drug: 2 mg/kg ketamine

Antagonist: 0.3 mg/kg atipamezole

Alternative Drugs: 2.5 mg/kg ketamine plus 3 mg/kg xylazine; antagonize with 0.125 mg/kg yohimbine

- 5 mg/kg tiletamine-zolazepam
- 0.01 mg/kg carfentanil; antagonize with 1 mg/kg naltrexone
- 0.05 mg/kg etorphine plus 0.2 mg/kg acepromazine; antagonize with 0.1 mg/kg diprenorphine
- 4 mg/kg xylazine; antagonize with 0.2 mg/kg yohimbine (calm deer only)

References: Jarvis and Morris, 1960; Heuschele, 1961a; Thomas, 1961; Seal and Erickson, 1969; Eriksen, 1970; Gauckler and Kraus, 1970; Göltenboth and Klös, 1970; Seal et al., 1970; Bauditz, 1972; Heck and Rivenburg, 1972; Jones, 1972; 1978; 1984; York and Huggins, 1972; Woolf et al., 1973; Gray et al., 1974; Rapley and Mehren, 1975; Haigh, 1976d; Wiesner, 1977; Paponov, 1978; Keep, 1979; Jarofke, 1980; Arora et al., 1983; Jacobson and Kollias, 1984; Silvestris and Heck, 1984; Kock and Pearce, 1985; Wiesner and von Hegel, 1985; Zabarain, 1985; Allen, 1986b; Schobert, 1987; Seal and Bush, 1987; Strauss, 1987; Barnett and Lewis, 1990; Allen et al., 1991; Tung et al., 1993; Tsuruga et al., 1999; Páras et al., 2002; Suzuki et al., 2001

DEER, SWAMP - SEE BARASINGHA

DEER, TIMOR - SEE SAMBAR, SUNDA

DEER, WHITE-TAILED, *Odocoileus virginianus*

Weight: 60–150 kg

Recommended Drug: 4.4 mg/kg tiletamine-zolazepam plus 2.2 mg/kg xylazine

Supplemental Drug: 2.2 mg/kg ketamine

Antagonist: 0.125 mg/kg yohimbine or 2 mg/kg tolazoline

Alternative Drugs: 7.5 mg/kg ketamine plus 1.5 mg/kg xylazine, antagonize with 0.125 mg/kg yohimbine (or 2 mg/kg tolazoline)

- 2 mg/kg ketamine plus 0.07 mg/kg medetomidine; antagonize with 0.35

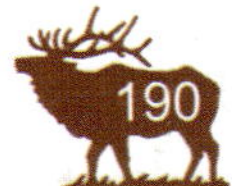

mg/kg atipamezole

- 0.1 mg/kg thiafentanil plus 1 mg/kg xylazine; antagonize with 2 mg/kg naltrexone plus 0.125 mg/kg yohimbine (or 2 mg/kg tolazoline)
- 0.03 mg/kg carfentanil plus 0.3 mg/kg xylazine; antagonize with 3 mg/kg naltrexone plus 0.15 mg/kg yohimbine
- 6 mg etorphine; antagonize with 12 mg diprenorphine
- 3 mg/kg xylazine, antagonize with 0.2 mg/kg yohimbine or 2 mg/kg tolazoline (calm deer only)

Comments: When using xylazine alone, young deer (< 1 yr) may require higher doses (i.e., 6 mg/kg; Bubenick, 1982). Immobilization with xylazine alone is unreliable, particularly when the animal is excited or has been chased. When using ketamine-xylazine or tiletamine-zolazepam-xylazine for highly excited deer, the xylazine dose can be increased up to the dose of ketamine or tiletamine-zolazepam given (i.e., 7.5 mg/kg or 4.4 mg/kg, respectively). Deer immobilized with etorphine may run long distances and/or have an extended period (10+ min) of hyperactivity before recumbency. This hyperactivity can result in hyperthermia. All opioid agents can result in respiratory depression. Long-acting tranquilizers (0.3 mg/kg azaperone plus 1 mg/kg zuclopenthixol) has been effective for translocating deer (see Read and McCorkell, 2002).

References: Severinghaus, 1950; Hall et al., 1953; Jenkins et al., 1955; Crockford et al., 1957a; 1957b; Feurt et al., 1958; Jarvis and Morris, 1960; Montgomery, 1961; Cowan et al., 1962; Nordan et al., 1962; Green, 1963; Murry and Dennett, 1963; Murray, 1964; 1965; Thomas and Marburger, 1964; Behrend, 1965; Dyson, 1965; Kitchen, 1966; Fletch et al., 1967; Hawkins et al., 1967; 1968; Montgomery and Hawkins, 1967; Thomas et al., 1967; Day, 1969b; Liscinsky et al., 1969; Seal and Erickson, 1969; Short, 1969; Allen, 1970; Göltenboth and Klös, 1970; Seal et al., 1970; 1972; Woolf, 1970; 1974; Bauditz, 1972; Beck, 1972; Heck and Rivenburg, 1972; York and Huggins, 1972; Dean et al., 1973; Presidente et al., 1973; 1978a; 1978b; Presnell et al., 1973; Woolf et al., 1973; Gray et al., 1974; Scanlon and Mirarchi, 1974; Wesson et al., 1974; 1976; 1979a; 1979b; Hertzog, 1975; Rapley and Mehren, 1975; Roughton, 1975; Haigh, 1976d; Jacobsen et al., 1976; Scanlon et al., 1977; Wiesner, 1977; Jones, 1978; 1984; Presidente and Draisma, 1978; Gibson et al., 1979; 1980a; 1980b; 1982; Hawkins et al., 1979; Jarofke, 1980; Kocan et al., 1980; 1981; Mautz et al., 1980; Kopf et al., 1981a; 1981b; Bubenik, 1982; Jensen, 1982; Nielsen, 1982; Thorne, 1982; Carpenter and Lance, 1983; Jensen, et al., 1983; Samuelson, 1983; Chao et al., 1984; Hsu and Shulaw, 1984; Mech et al., 1984; 1985; Silvestris and Heck, 1984; Scanlon and Brunjak, 1984; Warren et al., 1984; Renecker and Olsen, 1985; Scanlon and Vaughan, 1985; Zabarain, 1985; Van Der Eems and Brown, 1986; Kreeger et al., 1986a; 1986b; 1987b; DelGiudice et al., 1986; 2001; 2005; Schobert, 1987; 1988; Seal and Bush, 1987; Strauss, 1987; Williams and Riedesel, 1987; Dew, 1988; Diehl, 1988; Green, 1988; Bubenik and Brown, 1989; Smits and Haigh, 1989; Barnett and Lewis, 1990;

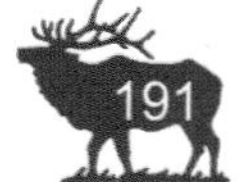

Jalanka and Roeken, 1990; Schultz et al., 1991; Pond and O'Gara, 1994; Wallingford et al., 1996; Kilpatrick et al., 1996; 1997; Schwartz et al., 1997; Ballard et al., 1998; Kilpatrick and Spohr, 1999; Murray et al., 2000; Haulton et al., 2001; Páras et al., 2002; Read and McCorkell, 2002; Miller et al., 2003; 2004; Posner et al., 2005; Millspaugh et al., 2005; Storms et al., 2004; 2005; 2006

DEGU, *Octodon degus*

Weight: 170–300 gm
Recommended Drug: 40 mg/kg ketamine plus 1 mg/kg diazepam
Supplemental Drug: 20 mg/kg ketamine only
Antagonist: None
References: Stoskopf, 1979

DEVIL, TASMANIAN, *Sarcophilus harrisii*

Weight: 4.1–11.8 kg
Recommended Drug: 5.5 mg/kg tiletamine-zolazepam
Supplemental Drug: 5 mg/kg ketamine
Antagonist: None
Alternative Drugs: 4.5 mg/kg ketamine plus 0.6 mg/kg xylazine
References: Denny, 1974; Gray et al., 1974; Smeller et al., 1977; Schobert, 1987; Bush et al., 1990; Pemberton and Gales, 1991; Holz, 1992

DHOLE, *Cuon alpinus*

Weight: 15–24 kg
Recommended Drug: 10 mg/kg tiletamine-zolazepam
Supplemental Drug: 10 mg/kg ketamine
Alternative Drugs: 5 mg/kg ketamine plus 0.04 mg/kg medetomidine; antagonize with 0.2 mg/kg atipamezole
• 20 mg/kg ketamine plus 0.2 mg/kg acepromazine
References: Böer et al., 2002

DIK-DIK, *Madoqua kirki*

Weight: 3–7 kg
Recommended Drug: 3 mg fentanyl plus 5 mg azaperone
Supplemental Drug: 1.5 mg fentanyl
Antagonist: 0.2 mg/kg naloxone
Alternative Drugs: 6 mg/kg tiletamine-zolazepam
• 0.2 mg/kg fentanyl plus 0.4 mg/kg xylazine
• 0.01 mg/kg etorphine plus 0.4 mg/kg xylazine; antagonize with 0.02 mg/kg diprenorphine plus 0.125 mg/kg yohimbine
Comments: Monitor for respiratory depression when using opioids.
References: Hofmeyr, 1981; IWVS, 1992; Burroughs, 1993d; Kock et al., 2006

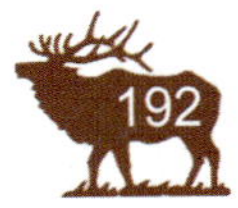

DINGO, *Canis dingo*

Weight: 12–15 kg

Recommended Drug: 5 mg/kg ketamine plus 2 mg/kg xylazine, antagonize with 0.15 mg/kg yohimbine

Supplemental Drug: 2.5 mg/kg ketamine

Alternative Drugs: 10 mg/kg tiletamine-zolazepam

- 10 mg/kg ketamine plus 0.1 mg/kg acepromazine
- 0.04 mg/kg etorphine plus 1 mg/kg promazine, antagonize with 0.08 mg/kg diprenorphine

Comments: If using xylazine, wait at least 45 min after last ketamine injection before administering yohimbine.

References: Heuschele, 1961a; 1961b; Wentges, 1975; Wiesner, 1975; Green, 1976; Hess and Knakal, 1985

DOG, BUSH, *Speothos venaticus*

Weight: 5–7 kg

Recommended Drug: 10 mg/kg tiletamine-zolazepam

Supplemental Drug: 10 mg/kg ketamine

Alternative Drugs: 20 mg/kg ketamine plus 0.2 mg/kg acepromazine

References: Seal and Erickson, 1969; Seal et al., 1970

DOG, AFRICAN HUNTING, *Lycaon pictus*

Weight: 17–36 kg

Recommended Drug: 5 mg/kg ketamine plus 0.05 mg/kg medetomidine

Supplemental Drug: 2.5 mg/kg ketamine

Antagonist: 0.15 mg/kg atipamezole

- 0.1 mg/kg fentanyl plus 1 mg/kg xylazine; antagonize with 0.04 mg/kg naloxone and 0.125 mg/kg yohimbine
- 3 mg/kg tiletamine-zolazepam
- 2 mg/kg ketamine plus 2 mg xylazine; antagonize with 0.2 mg/kg yohimbine

Comments: Monitor anesthetized animals for hyperthermia. The fentanyl/xylazine dose is highly recommended by Van Heerden (1993) for immobilizing free-ranging adult animals. Vocalization may occur with fentanyl immobilization

References: Kroll, 1962; Seal and Erickson, 1969; Seal et al., 1970; Gray et al., 1974; Ebedes and Grobler, 1979; Van Heerden and de Vos, 1981; Genevois et al., 1984b; Schobert, 1987; Kock et al., 1989; Van Heerden et al., 1991a; 1991b; Raath et al., 1993; 1995; Vahala, 1993; Van Heerden, 1993; Osofsky et al., 1995; 1996; Devilliers et al., 1997; Woodroffe, 2001; Fleming et al., 2006; Kock, M., et al., 2006; Ward et al., 2006

DOG, FERAL DOMESTIC, *Canis lupus familiaris*

Weight: 5–50 kg

Recommended Drug: 10 mg/kg ketamine plus 1 mg/kg xylazine

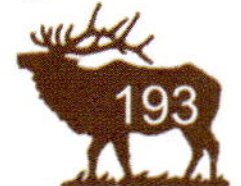

Supplemental Drug: 5 mg/kg ketamine only
Antagonist: 0.125 mg/kg yohimbine
Alternative Drugs: 10 mg/kg tiletamine-zolazepam
References: Ortega and Otter, 1967; McWade, 1982

DOG, RACCOON, *Nyctereutes procyonoides*

Weight: 5–8.5 kg
Recommended Drug: 5 mg/kg ketamine plus 0.1 mg/kg medetomidine
Supplemental Drug: 2.5 mg/kg ketamine
Antagonist: 1 mg/kg atipamezole
Alternative Drugs: 6.6 mg/kg tiletamine-zolazepam
• 20 mg/kg ketamine plus 2 mg/kg promazine
Comments: Monitor body temperature for hypo/hyperthermia during periods of extreme ambient temperatures.
References: Seal and Erickson, 1969; Seal et al., 1970; Gray et al., 1974; Schobert, 1987; Arnemo et al., 1993a

DOG, SMALL-EARED, *Atelocynus microtis*

Weight: 9–10 kg
Recommended Drug: 10 mg/kg tiletamine-zolazepam
Supplemental Drug: 10 mg/kg ketamine
Alternative Drugs: 20 mg/kg ketamine plus 2 mg/kg promazine
References: Seal et al., 1970

DOLPHIN, BOTTLENOSED, *Tursiops truncatus*

Weight: 150–200 kg
Recommended Drug: 0.23 mg/kg meperidine
Alternative Drugs: 5.5 mg/kg propofol, IV
References: Ridgway and McCormick, 1967; Ridgway et al., 1975; Meshcherskii et al., 1978; Joseph and Cornell, 1988; Linnehan and MacMillan, 1991; Reynolds, 1992; Haulena and Heath, 2001

DOUROUCOULIS, *Aotus spp.*

Weight: 0.6–1 kg
Recommended Drug: 9 mg/kg ketamine
Supplemental Drug: 4.5 mg/kg ketamine
Antagonist: None
References: Bush et al., 1977

DRAGON, KOMODO, *Varanus komodoensis*

Weight: 11–55 kg
Recommended Drug: 5.5 mg/kg tiletamine-zolazepam
Supplemental Drug: 2.5 mg/kg ketamine
Antagonist: None
Alternative Drugs: 12 mg/kg ketamine plus 0.5 mg/kg midazolam

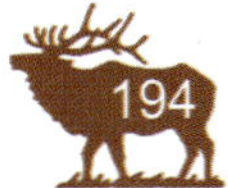

References: Spelman et al., 1996

DUCK, MALLARD, *Anas platyrhynchos*

Weight: 1–1.3 kg
Recommended Drug: 50 mg/kg tiletamine-zolazepam
Supplemental Drug: 25 mg/kg ketamine
Antagonist: None
Alternative Drugs: 40 mg/kg alpha-choralose given orally
Comments: Oral administration of immobilizing drugs is generally an ineffective method of capturing birds, but may be employed when no other alternatives exist. Be prepared for extreme variability of effects, ranging from little or no sedation to relatively high mortality.
References: Crider et al., 1968; Crider and McDaniel, 1968; Cline and Greenwood, 1972; Krapu, 1976; Gordon, 1977; Camburn and Stead, 1978; Hofman and Weaver, 1980; Schobert, 1987; Rotella and Ratti, 1990; Machin and Caulkett, 1996; 1998a; 1998b

DUCK, MUSCOVY, *Cairina moschata*

Weight: 1.1–4 kg
Recommended Drug: 15 mg/kg tiletamine-zolazepam
Supplemental Drug: 15 mg/kg ketamine
Antagonist: None
Comments: Muscovy ducks may be sensitive to tiletamine-zolazepam dose. Insure that body weight is accurate.
References: Crider et al., 1968; Schobert, 1987

DUCK, WOOD, *Aix sponsa*

Weight: 0.9–1.1 kg
Recommended Drug: 10 mg/kg propofol IV
Antagonist: None
Comments: Alternatively, ducks can be anesthetized with methoxyflurane.
References: Hepp and Manlove, 2001

DUIKER, BLACK, *Cephalophorus niger*

Weight: 20–40 kg
Recommended Drug: 0.026 mg/kg carfentanil
Supplemental Drug: If animal is not down in 20 minutes, repeat full dose
Antagonist: 2.6 mg/kg naltrexone
Alternative Drugs: 0.02 mg/kg etorphine plus 1 mg/kg xylazine
Comments: Monitor for respiratory depression when using opioids.
References: Haigh, 1976d; Frahm, 1999

DUIKER, BLUE, *Cephalophorus monticola*

Weight: 3.5–9 kg
Recommended Drug: 2.2 mg/kg ketamine plus 0.2 mg/kg medetomidine

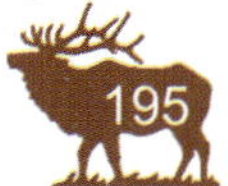

Supplemental Drug: 1.1 mg/kg ketamine
Antagonist: 1 mg/kg atipamezole
Alternative Drugs: 3 mg fentanyl plus 5 mg azaperone; antagonize with 0.2 mg/kg naloxone
- 6 mg/kg tiletamine-zolazepam
- 0.2 mg/kg fentanyl plus 0.4 mg/kg xylazine
- 0.03 mg/kg etorphine plus 0.4 mg/kg xylazine; antagonize with 0.06 mg/kg diprenorphine plus 0.125 mg/kg yohimbine

Comments: Monitor for respiratory depression when using opioids.
References: IWVS, 1992; Burroughs, 1993d; Bailey et al., 1995; Frahm, 1999; Kock, M., et al., 2006

DUIKER, COMMON (GRAY), *Silivicapra grimmia*

Weight: 12–25 kg
Recommended Drug: 2.2 mg/kg ketamine plus 0.2 mg/kg medetomidine
Supplemental Drug: 2.0 mg/kg ketamine
Antagonist: 1 mg/kg atipamezole
Alternative Drugs: 1 mg etorphine plus 2 mg xylazine; antagonize with 2 mg diprenorphine plus 0.125 mg/kg yohimbine
- 13 mg/kg ketamine plus16 mg/kg xylazine
- 10 mg/kg tiletamine-zolazepam

Comments: Monitor for respiratory depression when using opioids. Long-acting tranquilizer doses: haloperidol (adult male, 15 mg; adult female, 10 mg); zuclopenthixol, 1 mg/kg; perphenazine (adults, 20-40 mg).
References: Wilson, 1967; Haigh, 1976d; Hofmeyr, 1981; Schobert, 1987; IWVS, 1992; Burroughs, 1993d; Nicholls et al., 1996; Frahm, 1999; Kock, 2001; Kock, M., et al., 2006

DUIKER, JENTINK'S, *Cephalophorus jentinki*

Weight: 20–40 kg
Recommended Drug: 0.026 mg/kg carfentanil
Supplemental Drug: If animal is not down in 20 minutes, repeat full dose
Antagonist: 2.6 mg/kg naltrexone
Comments: Monitor for respiratory depression when using opioids.
References: Haigh, 1976d

DUIKER, MAXWELL'S, *Cephalophorus maxwelli*

Weight: 10–15 kg
Recommended Drug: 0.026 mg/kg carfentanil
Supplemental Drug: If animal is not down in 20 minutes, repeat full dose
Antagonist: 2.6 mg/kg naltrexone
Alternative Drugs: 10 mg/kg tiletamine-zolazepam
- 0.02 mg/kg etorphine plus 1 mg/kg xylazine; antagonize with 0.04 mg/kg diprenorphine plus 0.125 mg/kg yohimbine

Comments: Monitor for respiratory depression when using opioids.

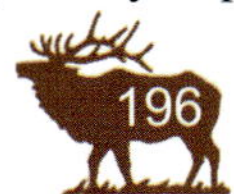

References: Bauditz, 1972; Haigh, 1976d; Schobert, 1987; Frahm, 1999

DUIKER, RED, *Cephalophorus natalensis*

Weight: 20–40 kg
Recommended Drug: 5 mg fentanyl plus 5 mg azaperone
Supplemental Drug: 2.5 mg fentanyl
Antagonist: 0.2 mg/kg naloxone
Alternative Drugs: 6 mg/kg tiletamine-zolazepam
• 0.2 mg/kg fentanyl plus 0.4 mg/kg xylazine
• 0.01 mg/kg etorphine plus 0.4 mg/kg xylazine; antagonize with 0.02 mg/kg diprenorphine plus 0.125 mg/kg yohimbine
References: IWVS, 1992; Burroughs, 1993d; Frahm, 1999; Kock et el., 2006

DUIKER, RED-FLANKED, *Cephalophorus rufilatus*

Weight: 20–40 kg
Recommended Drug: 0.026 mg/kg carfentanil
Supplemental Drug: If animal is not down in 20 minutes, repeat full dose
Antagonist: 2.6 mg/kg naltrexone
Alternative Drugs: 0.02 mg/kg etorphine plus 1 mg/kg xylazine; antagonize with 0.04 mg diprenorphine plus 0.125 mg/kg yohimbine
Comments: Monitor for respiratory depression when using opioids.
References: Young and Whyte, 1973; Haigh, 1976d

DUIKER, YELLOW-BACK, *Cephalophorus sylvicultor*

Weight: 45–80 kg
Recommended Drug: 0.026 mg/kg carfentanil
Supplemental Drug: If animal is not down in 20 minutes, repeat full dose
Antagonist: 2.6 mg/kg naltrexone
Alternative Drugs: 0.02 mg/kg etorphine plus 1 mg/kg xylazine; antagonize with 0.04 mg/kg diprenorphine plus 0.125 mg/kg yohimbine
Comments: Monitor for respiratory depression when using opioids.
References: Haigh, 1976d

DUIKER, ZEBRA, *Cephalophorus zebra*

Weight: 20–40 kg
Recommended Drug: 0.026 mg/kg carfentanil
Supplemental Drug: If animal is not down in 20 minutes, repeat full dose
Antagonist: 2.6 mg/kg naltrexone
Alternative Drugs: 0.02 mg/kg etorphine plus 1 mg/kg xylazine; antagonize with 0.04 mg/kg diprenorphine plus 0.125 mg/kg yohimbine
Comments: Monitor for respiratory depression when using opioids.
References: Haigh, 1976d; Frahm, 1999

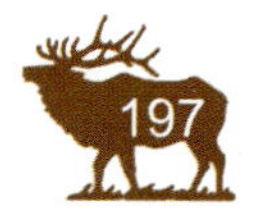

EAGLE, BALD, *Haliaetus leucocephalus*

Weight: 3–4 kg
Recommended Drug: 15 mg/kg tiletamine-zolazepam
Supplemental Drug: 15 mg/kg ketamine
Antagonist: None
References: Schobert, 1987; Aguilar et al., 1996

EAGLE, GOLDEN, *Aguila chrysaetos*

Weight: 3.5–5 kg
Recommended Drug: 44 mg/kg ketamine
Supplemental Drug: 22 mg/kg ketamine
Antagonist: None
Alternative Drugs: Sevoflurane, 7% or isoflurane, 4%
References: Haupert and Lindeen, 1974; Frank and Cooper, 1974; Beck, 1976, Clutton, 1986; Joyner et al., 2006

ECHIDNA, *Tachyglossus aculeatus*

Weight: 2.5–6 kg
Recommended Drug: 5 mg/kg tiletamine-zolazepam
Supplemental Drug: 5 mg/kg ketamine
Antagonist: None
References: Denny, 1974; Shima et al., 1993

ELAND, *Taurotragus oryx*

Weight: 400–700 kg
Recommended Drug: 0.008 mg/kg carfentanil plus 0.2 mg/kg xylazine
Supplemental Drug: If animal is not down in 20 min, repeat full dose
Antagonist: 0.8 mg/kg naltrexone plus 0.1 mg/kg yohimbine
Alternative Drugs: 0.02 mg/kg etorphine plus 0.4 mg/kg xylazine; antagonize with 0.04 mg/kg diprenorphine plus 0.125 mg/kg yohimbine

- 0.03 mg/kg thiafentanil plus 0.15 mg/kg xylazine; antagonize with 1 mg/kg naltrexone plus 0.1 mg/kg yohimbine
- 4 mg/kg ketamine plus 0.8 mg/kg xylazine; antagonize with 0.125 mg/kg yohimbine
- 11.5 mg/kg tiletamine-zolazepam

Comments: Prone to excessive running during induction with opioids, particularly if underdosed; monitor for hyperthermia. Opioids may increase probability of regurgitation. Do not use opioids without xylazine or similar neuroleptic. The addition of hyaluronidase (1,500-3,000 IU) is recommended (Kock et al., 2006). Azaperone (200 mg) may be substituted for xylazine when using opioids. Semi-immobilized animals can be aggressive towards humans. Yohimbine must be given to antagonize xylazine, if given. Long-acting tranquilizer doses: haloperidol (adults, 20 mg; subadult, 10 mg); zuclopenthixol, 1 mg/kg; perphenazine (adults, 100 mg; subadults, 50 mg).
References: Pistey and Wright, 1959; Jarvis and Morris, 1960; Thomas,

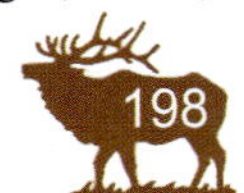

1961; Larsen, 1963; Van Niekerk et al., 1963a; Wright, 1963; Bigalke, 1965; Hirst et al., 1965; Pienaar et al., 1966a; Wallach et al., 1967; Keep and Keep, 1968; Wallach, 1968; 1969; Pienaar, 1968a; 1969b; 1973a; Gauckler and Kraus, 1970; Harthoorn, 1971; Bauditz, 1972; Heck and Rivenburg, 1972; Jones, 1972; York and Huggins, 1972; Abbott, 1973; Smuts, 1973; Woolf et al., 1973; Young and Whyte, 1973; Drevemo and Karstad, 1974; Manton and Jones, 1974; De Vos, 1975; Hertzog, 1975; Röken, 1975; York, 1975; Grootenhuis et al., 1976; Haigh, 1976d; Jones, 1977; Slee and Walker, 1977; Hofmeyr, 1981; Jensen, 1982; Janssen and Oosterhuis, 1984; Silvestris and Heck, 1984; Sedgwick, 1986; Schobert, 1987; Williams and Riedesel, 1987; Ganhao et al., 1988; Allen et al., 1991; Janssen et al., 1991; IWVS, 1992; Burroughs, 1993d; Kock, 2001; Pye et al., 2001; Páras et al., 2002; Cole et al., 2005; 2006; Kock, M., et al., 2006

ELEPHANT, AFRICAN, *Loxodonta africana*

Weight: 2,000–4,000 (f), 4,000–6,000 (m) kg
Recommended Drug: 0.0021 mg/kg carfentanil
Supplemental Drug: 0.0005 mg/kg carfentanil
Antagonist: 0.08 mg/kg naltrexone or nalmefene
Alternative Drugs: 0.003 mg/kg etorphine; antagonize with 0.009 mg/kg diprenorphine plus 0.03 mg/kg naltrexone
- 0.003 mg/kg thiafentanil; antagonize with 0.06 mg/kg naltrexone
- 1.14 mg/kg ketamine plus 0.14 mg/kg xylazine; antagonize with 0.13 mg/kg yohimbine

Comments: Hyaluronidase may be added (1,000-4,500 IU) to hasten induction. Tranquilizers need not be added to opioids because they may prolong recovery. However, azaperone (50 mg in an adult bull) should probably be given IV after the animal has become immobilized to decrease the high mean arterial blood pressure apparently caused by opioids which can result in lung edema and capillary bleeding (see Raath, 1993). Dart needles should be ≥ 60 mm in length and 3 mm in diameter. Avoid shoulder shots which may strike the ear or the dart may be reached and pulled out by the trunk. Place immobilized elephant in lateral recumbency; do not allow animal to remain in sternal recumbency. Insure that breathing through the trunk is unimpaired. Body temperature ranges from 37–39.9° C (96.3–99.5° F), but may decline during immobilization to 35° C (95° F). Agitated or aggressive animals may require higher doses of recommended drug. Be sure to flush all dart wounds with antimicrobial solution to prevent abcesses. The mother of a calf to be immobilized must also be immobilized because she will not leave it.

References: Harthoorn, 1960; 1963d; 1965a; 1972a; 1973a; 1973b; 1974; 1976; Harthoorn et al., 1961; Harthoorn and Luck, 1962; Pienaar, 1963; 1967b; 1969a; 1969b; Harthoorn and Bligh, 1965; Somers, 1965; Pienaar et al., 1966a; 1966b; Ericksen, 1968; Pienaar, 1968a; Wallach, 1968; 1969; Wallach and Anderson, 1968; Lietsch, 1969; Woodford et al., 1972; Young,

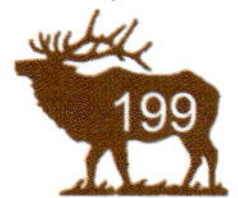

1972; Alford et al., 1974; Elder and Rogers, 1974; Eltringham, 1974; Gray et al., 1974; De Vos, 1975; 1985a; Ebedes, 1975b; Röken, 1975; Smuts, 1975; Haigh, 1976d; Silberman, 1977; Haigh et al., 1979; Fowler, 1981b; Wiesner et al., 1982; Tamas and Geiser, 1983; Dunlop et al., 1984; Hattingh et al., 1984; Jacobson and Kollias, 1984; Bengis et al., 1985; Jacobson et al., 1985; 1986; 1987; 1988; Trembath, 1985; Wiesner and von Hegel, 1985; Allen, 1986a; 1986b; Heard et al., 1986; 1988; Göltenboth and Klös, 1987; Schobert, 1987; Kock, R. et al., 1989; 1993; Welsch et al., 1989; Janssen et al., 1991; IWVS, 1992; Raath, 1993; Still, 1993; Hattingh et al., 1994a; 1994b; Osofsky, 1995; 1997; Schumacher et al., 1996; Still et al., 1996; Raath, 1999; Horne et al., 2001; Ramsay, 2000; Neiffer et al., 2005; Kock, M., et al., 2006

ELEPHANT, ASIAN, *Elaphus maximus*

Weight: 2,300–3,700 kg (f), 3,700–4,500 (m) kg
Recommended Drug: 0.003 mg/kg etorphine
Supplemental Drug: 2 mg etorphine, as needed to maintain immobilization
Antagonist: 2 mg diprenorphine per mg etorphine given
Alternative Drugs: 1 ml Large Animal Immobilon® per 1,000 kg BW; antagonize with equal volume of diprenorphine
Comments: Xylazine (0.1 mg/kg) or medetomidine (0.005 mg/kg) are capable of producing profound sedation (see Bongso, 1979; Schmidt, 1975; 1983; Sarma et al., 2002; 2004). Hyaluronidase may be added (4,500 IU) to hasten induction. Immobilized elephants suffer fewer respiratory problems when in lateral, as opposed to sternal, recumbency. Body temperature ranges from 37–39.9½ C (96.3–99.5½ F), but may decline during immobilization to 35½ C (95½ F).
References: Kodituwakku et al., 1961; Larsen, 1963; Wallach, 1969; Gray and Nettashinghe, 1970; Jainudeen, 1970; Jainudeen et al., 1971; Fowler, 1973; 1981b; Fowler and Hart, 1973; Alford et al., 1974; Schmidt, 1975a; 1975b; 1985; Jainudeen and Khan, 1977; Bongso et al., 1978; Bongso 1979; 1980; Muraleedharan et al., 1979; Jarofke, 1981a; 1981b; Byron et al., 1985; Lateur and Stolk, 1986; Sale, et al., 1986; Göltenboth and Klös, 1987; Kock et al., 1993; Johnsingh et al., 1993; Silva and Kuruwita, 1993; Page, 1994; Schmitt et al., 1996; Fowler et al., 1999; Fowler et al., 2000; Dangolla et al., 2004; Sarma et al., 2002; 2004

ELK, NORTH AMERICAN, *Cervus elaphus*

Weight: 230–318 kg
Recommended Drug: 0.01 mg/kg carfentanil plus 0.1 mg/kg xylazine
Supplemental Drug: 0.005 mg/kg carfentanil
Antagonist: 1 mg/kg naltrexone plus 0.125 mg/kg yohimbine
Alternative Drugs: 0.04 mg/kg thiafentanil; antagonize with 1 mg/kg naltrexone
• 2 mg/kg ketamine plus 0.07 mg/kg medetomidine; antagonize with 0.35

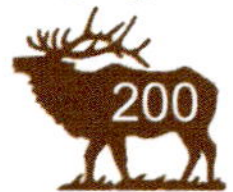

mg/kg atipamezole

- 3 mg/kg tiletamine-zolazepam plus 0.4 mg/kg xylazine; antagonize with 0.125 mg/kg yohimbine
- 4 mg/kg ketamine plus 2 mg/kg xylazine; antagonize with 0.125 mg/kg yohimbine
- 6 mg etorphine plus 50 mg xylazine; antagonize with 12 mg diprenorphine plus 0.125 mg/kg yohimbine
- 2 mg/kg xylazine, antagonize with 0.125 mg/kg yohimbine (calm or captive elk only)

Comments: Monitor elk carefully for overheating or bloat. Underdosing with etorphine can cause hyperexcitability; use a minimum of 0.02 mg/kg etorphine. For highly excited elk, the carfentanil dose can be increased to 0.013 mg/kg; the xylazine dose remains the same (i.e., 0.1 mg/kg). Long-acting tranquilizers have been used successfully to reduce stress in wild-caught elk (Read et al., 2000a; 2000b). Once immobilized, the addition of a small amount of *naloxone* (2 mg naloxone per mg carfentanil given) may improve oxygenation (Moresco et al., 2001); however, monitor the animal closely for spontaneous recovery. Walter et al. (2005) used tiletamine-zolazepam plus xylazine in transmitter darts.

References: Post, 1959; Heuschele, 1961a; Thomas, 1961; Flook et al., 1962; Larsen, 1963; Harper, 1964; 1965; Denney, 1965; 1966; Day, 1969; Seal and Erickson, 1969; Sedgwick and Acosta, 1969; Gauckler and Kraus, 1970; Seal et al., 1970; Woolf and Swart, 1970; Guinness et al., 1971; Bauditz, 1972; Heck and Rivenburg, 1972; Thurmon et al., 1972; York and Huggins, 1972; Woolf et al., 1973; Gray et al., 1974; Woolf, 1974; Coggins, 1975; Hertzog, 1975; Pedersen and Pedersen, 1975; Pedersen and Thomas, 1975; Rapley and Mehren, 1975; Wentges, 1975; Wiesner, 1975; 1977; Farnsworth and Stowe, 1976; Haigh, 1976d; 1990b; 1991; 1993; Varland, 1976; Magonigle et al., 1977; Keep, 1979; Jarofke, 1980; Jessup et al., 1980; 1985b; Amstrup et al., 1982; Hebert et al., 1982; Thorne, 1982; Wiesner et al., 1982; 1984; Carpenter and Lance, 1983; Jones, 1984; Meulman et al., 1984; Silvestris and Heck, 1984; Stanley et al., 1984; 1988; 1989; Bailey et al., 1985; Olsen and Renecker, 1985; Rolfe and Haigh, 1985; Renecker and Olsen, 1986; Sedgwick, 1986; Haigh, 1987; Schobert, 1987; Williams and Riedesel, 1987; Franzmann and Lance, 1988; McCorquodale et al., 1988; Greene, 1988; Golightly and Hofstra, 1989; Jalanka and Roeken, 1990; Starke, 1991; Renecker et al., 1992; Haigh and Hudson, 1993; McJames et al., 1993; Smith et al., 1993; Pond and O'Gara, 1994; Millspaugh et al., 1995; Miller et al., 1996; Moresco et al., 2000; 2001; Read et al., 2000a; 2000b; 2001; Cattet et al., 2004; Walter et al., 2005; Paterson et al., 2006

ELK, ROOSEVELT, *Cervus elaphus roosevelti*

Weight: 265–284 (f), 318–499 (m) kg
Recommended Drug: 10 mg etorphine plus 20 mg acepromazine
Supplemental Drug: 5 mg etorphine

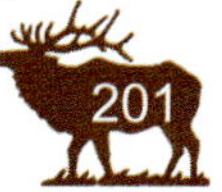

Antagonist: 2 mg diprenorphine per mg etorphine given
Alternative Drugs: 4 ml Large Animal Immobilon®
Comments: Roosevelt elk appear to require a higher dose of etorphine compared to North American elk (Hebert et al., 1982).
References: Harper, 1965; Thorne, 1982; Hebert et al., 1982; Carpenter and Lance, 1983

ELK, TULE, *Cervus elaphus nannodes*

Weight: 150–182 kg
Recommended Drug: 0.02 mg/kg carfentanil plus 0.24 mg/kg xylazine
Supplemental Drug: If animal is not down in 20 min, repeat full dose
Antagonist: 2 mg/kg naltrexone plus 0.125 mg/kg yohimbine
Alternative Drugs: 4 mg etorphine plus 20 mg acepromazine, antagonize with 8 mg diprenorphine
References: Alford et al., 1974; Hebert et al., 1982; Thorne, 1982; Carpenter and Lance, 1983; Greene, 1988

EMU, *Dromiceius novachollandie*

Weight: 40–55 kg
Recommended Drug: 22 mg/kg tiletamine-zolazepam
Supplemental Drug: 11 mg/kg ketamine
Antagonist: None
Alternative Drugs: 10 mg/kg ketamine plus 0.5 mg/kg xylazine
Comments: Xylazine use should be avoided in very sick birds. Also see Ostrich for additional comments
References: Beck, 1972; 1976; Schobert, 1987; Matthews, 1993; Jensen et al., 1994

ERMINE, *Mustela erminea*

Weight: 50–365 gm
Recommended Drug: 0.005 mg/gm ketamine plus 0.0001 mg/gm medetomidine
Supplemental Drug: 0.0025 mg/gm ketamine
Antagonist: 0.0005 mg/gm atipamezole; give 1/2 dose IV, 1/2 IM
Alternative Drugs: 0.03 mg/gm ketamine
References: Seal and Erickson, 1969; Seal et al., 1970; Genevois et al., 1984b; Seal and Kreeger, 1987; Jalanka and Roeken, 1990; Belant, 1992

ESEL - SEE ASS, WILD

FALCON, PEREGRINE, *Falco peregrinus*

Weight: 0.6–1.1 kg
Recommended Drug: 30 mg/kg ketamine plus 1.2 mg/kg diazepam, IV
Supplemental Drug: 5 mg/kg ketamine, IV
Antagonist: None

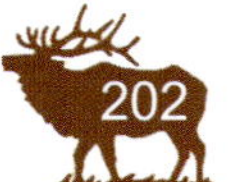

Alternative Drugs: 20 mg/kg ketamine
References: Borzio, 1973; Beck, 1976; Redig and Duke, 1976

FALCON, PRAIRIE, *Falco mexicanus*

Weight: 0.6–1.1 kg
Recommended Drug: 30 mg/kg ketamine plus 1.2 mg/kg diazepam, IV
Supplemental Drug: 5 mg/kg ketamine, IV
Antagonist: None
Alternative Drugs: 20 mg/kg ketamine
References: Borzio, 1973; Beck, 1976; Redig and Duke, 1976

FANALOKA - SEE FOSSA

FERRET, BLACK-FOOTED, *Mustela nigripes*

Weight: 0.7–1.5 kg
Recommended Drug: 3 mg/kg ketamine plus 0.075 mg/kg medetomidine
Supplemental Drug: 1.5 mg/kg ketamine
Antagonist: 0.45 mg/kg atipamezole
Alternative Drugs: 35 mg/kg ketamine plus 0.2 mg/kg diazepam
References: Thorne et al., 1985; Seal and Kreeger, 1987; Gaynor et al., 1997; Kreeger et al., 1998

FERRET, *Mustela putorius*

Weight: 0.6–1.2 kg
Recommended Drug: 25 mg/kg ketamine plus 2 mg/kg xylazine
Supplemental Drug: 12 mg/kg ketamine
Antagonist: None reported
Alternative Drugs: 25 mg/kg ketamine plus 1.1 mg/kg acepromazine

- 15 mg/kg tiletamine-zolazepam
- 5 mg/kg ketamine plus 0.1 mg/kg medetomidine

References: Seal et al., 1970; Beck, 1972; 1976; Boever et al., 1977; Carpenter and Hillman, 1978; Garver and Jackson, 1985; Moreland and Glaser, 1985; Schobert, 1987; Payton and Pick, 1989; Jalanka and Roeken, 1990; Marini et al., 1994; Gaynor et al., 1997; Fournier-Chambrillon et al., 2003

FISH, GENERAL

Recommended Drug: Tricaine methane sulfonate, 3–10 mg/100 ml water (0.003–0.01%)
Antagonist: Place fish in clean water (no anesthetic)
Comments: Use higher dose rates for *smaller* fish and lower dose rates for *larger* fish. The longer the fish is immersed in the anesthetic solution, the longer the duration of effect.
Comments: Propofol may be considered for larger fish (see Miller, S. M. et al., 2005)

References: McFarland and Klontz, 1969; Wedemeyer, 1970; Houston et al., 1971; Jolly et al., 1972; Stunkard and Miller, 1974; Sylvester, 1975; Smit et al., 1979; Smit and Hattingh, 1979; Genevois et al., 1983a; Cooper, 1984; Sedgwick, 1986; Harvey et al., 1988; Akhari and Dehghani, 1993; Brown, 1993; Malmstrom et al., 1993; Williams et al., 1993; Harms and Bakal, 1994; Sylvia et al., 1994; Redman et al., 1998; Sladky et al., 1999a; 2001; Harms, 1999; Ross and Ross, 1999; Chittick et al., 2000a; Fleming et al., 2003; Hansen et al., 2003; Iversen et al., 2003; Pirhonen and Schreck, 2003; Small, 2003; Bressler and Ron, 2004; Davis and Griffin, 2004; Williams et al., 2004; Miller et al., 2005; Roubach et al., 2005; Velisek et al., 2005

FISHER, *Martes pennanti*

Weight: 2.6–5.5 kg

Recommended Drug: 4 mg/kg ketamine plus 0.08 mg/kg medetomidine

Supplemental Drug: 2 mg/kg ketamine

Antagonist: 0.4 mg/kg atipamezole

Alternative Drugs: 11 mg/kg tiletamine-zolazepam

- 20 mg/kg ketamine

Comments: Lower doses of ketamine-medetomidine (e.g., 10 mg/kg ketamine plus 0.2 mg/kg medetomidine) may be effective in females.

References: Seal and Erickson, 1969; Seal et al., 1970; Jessup et al., 1980; Jessup, 1982b; Seal and Kreeger, 1987; Belant, 1991; Schwantje et al., 1998; Mitcheltree et al., 1999; Dzialak et al., 2001; 2002; Dzialak and Serfass, 2003

FOX, ARCTIC, *Alopex lagopus*

Weight: 2.5–9 kg

Recommended Drug: 2.5 mg/kg ketamine plus 0.05 mg/kg medetomidine

Supplemental Drug: 2.5 mg/kg ketamine

Antagonist: 0.25 mg/kg atipamezole; give 1/2 dose IV, 1/2 IM

Alternative Drugs: 20 mg/kg ketamine plus 0.2 mg/kg acepromazine

- 10 mg/kg tiletamine-zolazepam

Comments: Lower doses of tiletamine-zolazepam (e.g., 5 mg/kg) may be effective on calm animals.

References: Heuschele, 1959; Seal and Erickson, 1969; Seal et al., 1970; Jalanka, 1987; Röken, 1987; Seal and Kreeger, 1987; Barnett and Lewis, 1990; Jalanka and Roeken, 1990; Aguirre et al., 1998; 2000; Fuglei et al., 2002; Samelius et al., 2003

FOX, BAT-EARED, *Otocyon megalotis*

Weight: 3–5.3 kg

Recommended Drug: 5 mg/kg tiletamine-zolazepam

Supplemental Drug: 5 mg/kg ketamine

Alternative Drugs: 8 mg/kg ketamine and 0.5 mg/kg xylazine

- 20 mg/kg ketamine plus 0.2 mg/kg acepromazine

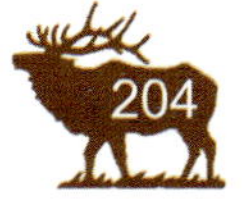

References: Seal and Erickson, 1969; Seal et al., 1970; McKenzie and Burroughs, 1993

FOX, CAPE, *Vulpes chama*

Weight: 4 kg
Recommended Drug: 5 mg/kg tiletamine-zolazepam
Supplemental Drug: 5 mg/kg ketamine
Alternative Drugs: 8 mg/kg ketamine and 0.5 mg/kg xylazine
• 20 mg/kg ketamine plus 0.2 mg/kg acepromazine
Comments: Use lightweight darts at low power settings.
References: McKenzie and Burroughs, 1993

FOX, CRAB-EATING, *Cerdocyon thous*

Weight: 6–7 kg
Recommended Drug: 10 mg/kg tiletamine-zolazepam
Supplemental Drug: 10 mg/kg ketamine
Alternative Drugs: 20 mg/kg ketamine plus 0.2 mg/kg acepromazine
References: Seal and Erickson, 1969; Seal et al., 1970

FOX, FENNEC, *Fennecus zerda*

Weight: 1–1.5 kg
Recommended Drug: 10 mg/kg tiletamine-zolazepam
Supplemental Drug: 10 mg/kg ketamine
Alternative Drugs: 20 mg/kg ketamine plus 0.2 mg/kg acepromazine
References: Seal and Erickson, 1969; Seal et al., 1970; Boever et al., 1977; Schobert, 1987

FOX, FLYING - SEE BATS, GENERAL

FOX, GRAY, *Urocyon cinereoargenteus*

Weight: 2.5–7 kg
Recommended Drug: 8.8 mg/kg tiletamine-zolazepam
Supplemental Drug: 8.8 mg/kg ketamine
Alternative Drugs: 20 mg/kg ketamine plus 0.2 mg/kg acepromazine
References: Kroll, 1962; Murry and Dennett, 1963; Seal and Erickson, 1969; Seal et al., 1970; Gray et al., 1974; Brooks and Morris, 1979; Jessup et al., 1980; Jessup, 1982b; Hoilien and Oates, 1982; Schobert, 1987; Seal and Kreeger, 1987; Servin and Huxley, 1992

FOX, KIT, *Vulpes macrotis*

Weight: 3 kg
Recommended Drug: 10 mg/kg tiletamine-zolazepam
upplemental Drug: 10 mg/kg ketamine
Alternative Drugs: 20 mg/kg ketamine plus 0.2 mg/kg acepromazine
References: Seal and Erickson, 1969; Seal et al., 1970; Jessup et al., 1980;

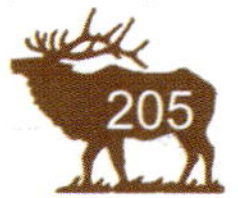

Jessup, 1982b; Seal and Kreeger, 1987

FOX, RED, *Vulpes vulpes*

Weight: 4.1–4.5 (f), 4.5–5.4 (m) kg
Recommended Drug: 10 mg/kg tiletamine-zolazepam
Supplemental Drug: 10 mg/kg ketamine
Alternative Drugs: 20 mg/kg ketamine plus 0.2 mg/kg acepromazine
• 20 mg/kg ketamine plus 1 mg/kg xylazine, antagonize with 0.15 mg/kg yohimbine
• 25 mg/kg ketamine plus 1 mg/kg midazolam
Comments: If using xylazine, wait at least 45 min after last ketamine injection before administering yohimbine.
References: Seal and Erickson, 1969; Göltenboth and Klös, 1970; Seal et al., 1970; Gray et al., 1974; Ramsden et al., 1976; Boever et al., 1977; Brooks and Morris, 1979; Jessup et al., 1980; Jessup, 1982b; Hoilien and Oates, 1982; Genevois et al., 1984b; Wiesner and von Hegel, 1985; Schobert, 1987; Seal and Kreeger, 1987; Kreeger et al., 1989b; 1990a; 1990b; 1990c; Travaini et al., 1992; Travaini and Delibes, 1994

FOX, SOUTH AMERICAN, *Pseudalopex culpaeus*

Weight: 8–13 kg
Recommended Drug: 10 mg/kg tiletamine-zolazepam
Supplemental Drug: 5 mg/kg ketamine
Alternative Drugs: 20 mg/kg ketamine plus 0.2 mg/kg acepromazine
References: Seal and Erickson, 1969; Seal et al., 1970

FOX, SWIFT, *Vulpes velox*

Weight: 1.8–3 kg
Recommended Drug: 10 mg/kg ketamine plus 1 mg/kg xylazine
Supplemental Drug: 5 mg/kg ketamine
Antagonist: 0.125 mg/kg yohimbine
Alternative Drugs: 20 mg/kg ketamine plus 0.2 mg/kg acepromazine
• 10 mg/kg tiletamine-zolazepam
References: Seal and Erickson, 1969; Seal et al., 1970; Jessup et al., 1980; Jessup, 1982b; Seal and Kreeger, 1987; Telesco and Sovada, 2002

FROGS - SEE AMPHIBIANS, GENERAL

GALAGO, *Galago senegalensis*

Weight: 120–300 gm
Recommended Drug: 0.005 mg/gm tiletamine-zolazepam
Supplemental Drug: 0.005 mg/gm ketamine
Antagonist: None
Alternative Drugs: 0.015 mg/gm ketamine

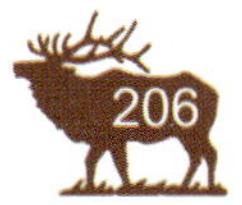

References: Seal et al., 1970; Beck, 1972; 1976; Gray et al., 1974; Schobert, 1987

GALAGO, THICK-TAILED, *Otolemur crassicaudatus*

Weight: 0.6–2 kg
Recommended Drug: 8 mg/kg tiletamine-zolazepam
Supplemental Drug: 8 mg/kg ketamine
Antagonist: None
Comments: Also known as greater bush baby.
References: Kroll, 1962; Seal and Erickson, 1969; Seal et al., 1970; Gray et al., 1974; Burroughs, 1993c

GAUR, *Bos gaurus*

Weight: 650–1,000 kg
Recommended Drug: 0.0075 mg/kg carfentanil plus 0.1 mg/kg xylazine
Supplemental Drug: 0.0075 mg/kg carfentanil
Antagonist: 0.75 mg/kg naltrexone 0.1 mg/kg yohimbine
Alternative Drugs: 2.5 ml Large Animal Immobilon® plus 100 mg xylazine; antagonize with 2 mg diprenorphine per mg etorphine given plus 0.125 mg/kg yohimbine

- 1 mg/kg xylazine; antagonize with 0.125 mg/kg yohimbine (calm animals only)

References: Bauditz, 1972; Rapley and Mehren, 1975; Wiesner, 1975; Wiesner et al., 1982; Conroy, 1986; Williams and Riedesel, 1987; Armstrong, 1981; Allen et al., 1991; Wilson, et al. 1993

GAZELLE, DAMA, *Gazella dama*

Weight: 20–60 kg
Recommended Drug: 0.035 mg/kg carfentanil
Supplemental Drug: If animal is not down in 20 minutes, repeat full dose
Antagonist: 3.5 mg/kg naltrexone
Alternative Drugs: 0.4 ml Large Animal Immobilon® plus 2 mg xylazine; antagonize with 2 mg diprenorphine per mg etorphine given plus 0.125 mg/kg yohimbine

- 2.4 mg etorphine; antagonize with 5.8 mg diprenorphine
- 4 mg/kg xylazine; antagonize with 0.125 mg/kg yohimbine (calm animals only)

Comments: Prone to excessive running during induction with carfentanil; monitor for hyperthermia. A lower carfentanil dosage (0.018 mg/kg) may be suitable for captive animals.
References: Bauditz, 1972; Heck and Rivenburg, 1972; Röken, 1975; Jensen, 1982; Wiesner et al., 1982; Silvestris and Heck, 1984; Wiesner and von Hegel, 1985; Wallace and Bush, 1987; Jacobson and Lukas, 1988; Allen et al., 1991; Schumacher et al., 1995; Schumacher et al., 1997a

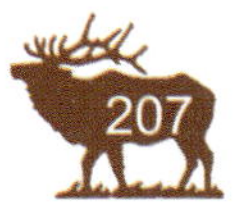

GAZELLE, DORCAS, *Gazella dorcas*

Weight: 20–60 kg

Recommended Drug: 0.035 mg/kg carfentanil

Supplemental Drug: If animal is not down in 20 minutes, repeat full dose

Antagonist: 3.5 mg/kg naltrexone

Alternative Drugs: 0.1 ml Large Animal Immobilon® plus 2.5 mg xylazine; antagonize with 2 mg diprenorphine per mg etorphine given plus 0.125 mg/kg yohimbine

- 10 mg/kg tiletamine-zolazepam
- 0.5 mg/kg fentanyl plus 1.56 mg/kg azaperone

Comments: Prone to excessive running during induction with carfentanil; monitor for hyperthermia.

References: Gray et al., 1974; Wiesner et al., 1982; Wiesner and von Hegel, 1985; Schobert, 1987; Greth et al., 1993

GAZELLE, GRANT'S, *Gazella granti*

Weight: 20–60 kg

Recommended Drug: 0.035 mg/kg carfentanil

Supplemental Drug: If animal is not down in 20 minutes, repeat full dose

Antagonist: 3.5 mg/kg naltrexone

Alternative Drugs: 10 mg/kg tiletamine-zolazepam

Comments: Prone to excessive running during induction with carfentanil; monitor for hyperthermia.

References: Talbot and Lamprey, 1961; Talbot and Talbot, 1962; Gray et al., 1974; Jensen, 1982; Schobert, 1987

GAZELLE, MOUNTAIN, *Gazella gazella*

Weight: 20 kg

Recommended Drug: 0.035 mg/kg carfentanil

Supplemental Drug: If animal is not down in 20 minutes, repeat full dose

Antagonist: 3.5 mg/kg naltrexone

Alternative Drugs: 10 mg/kg ketamine plus 12 mg/kg xylazine

- 2.5 mg etorphine; antagonize with 5 mg diprenorphine
- 0.5 mg/kg fentanyl plus 1.56 mg/kg azaperone

Comments: Prone to excessive running during induction with carfentanil; monitor for hyperthermia.

References: Baharav and Tadmor, 1981; Wiesner et al., 1982; Furley, 1986; Greth et al., 1993; Rietjkerk and Delima, 1994; Rietjkerk et al., 1994; Foster, 1999

GAZELLE, PERSIAN, *Gazella subgutturosa*

Weight: 20–60 kg

Recommended Drug: 0.035 mg/kg carfentanil

Supplemental Drug: If animal is not down in 20 minutes, repeat full dose

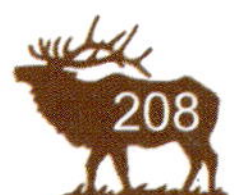

Antagonist: 3.5 mg/kg naltrexone
Alternative Drugs: 10 mg/kg tiletamine-zolazepam plus 1 mg/kg xylazine
• 0.5 mg/kg fentanyl plus 1.56 mg/kg azaperone
• 6 mg/kg ketamine plus 6 mg/kg xylazine
Comments: Prone to excessive running during induction with carfentanil; monitor for hyperthermia.
References: York and Huggins, 1972; Gray et al., 1974; Rapley and Mehren, 1975; Schobert, 1987; Allen et al., 1991; Greth et al., 1993; Foster, 1999; Yaralioglu-Gurgoze et al., 2005

GAZELLE, SLENDER-HORNED, *Gazella leptoceros*

Weight: 20–60 kg
Recommended Drug: 0.035 mg/kg carfentanil
Supplemental Drug: If animal is not down in 20 minutes, repeat full dose
Antagonist: 3.5 mg/kg naltrexone
Alternative Drugs: 10 mg/kg tiletamine-zolazepam
Comments: Prone to excessive running during induction with carfentanil; monitor for hyperthermia.
References: Gray et al., 1974; Schobert, 1987; Allen et al., 1991

GAZELLE, SOEMMERINGS, *Gazella soemmerringi*

Weight: 20–60 kg
Recommended Drug: 0.035 mg/kg carfentanil
Supplemental Drug: If animal is not down in 20 minutes, repeat full dose
Antagonist: 3.5 mg/kg naltrexone
• 0.5 mg/kg fentanyl plus 1.56 mg/kg azaperone
Comments: Prone to excessive running during induction with carfentanil; monitor for hyperthermia.
References: Schobert, 1987; Greth et al., 1993

GAZELLE, THOMSON'S, *Gazella thomsonii*

Weight: 20–27 kg
Recommended Drug: 1.2 mg carfentanil (males); 1 mg carfentanil (females)
Supplemental Drug: If animal is not down in 20 minutes, repeat full dose
Antagonist: 120 mg naltrexone (both sexes)
Alternative Drugs: 1.5 mg etorphine plus 10 mg ketamine plus 10 mg xylazine; antagonize with 3 mg diprenorphine plus 0.125 mg/kg yohimbine
• 8.8 mg/kg tiletamine-zolazepam
• 0.5 mg/kg fentanyl plus 1.56 mg/kg azaperone
• 3.6 mg/kg ketamine plus 4.6 mg/kg xylazine; antagonize with 0.125 mg/kg yohimbine
Comments: Prone to excessive running during induction with carfentanil; monitor for hyperthermia.
References: Kroll, 1962; Talbot and Talbot, 1962; Bauditz, 1972; Jones,

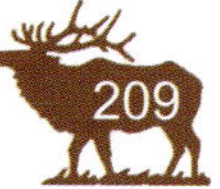

1972; 1978; Gray et al., 1974; Haigh, 1976d; Schobert, 1987; Kock et al., 1989; Allen et al., 1991; Snyder et al., 1992; Greth et al., 1993; Chittick et al., 2002a

GEMSBOK, *Oryx gazella*

Weight: 150–240 kg

Recommended Drug: 0.01 mg/kg carfentanil plus 0.1 mg/kg xylazine

Supplemental Drug: If animal is not down in 20 minutes, repeat full dose

Antagonist: 1 mg/kg naltrexone plus 0.125 mg/kg yohimbine

Alternative Drugs: 0.04 mg/kg thiafentanil plus 0.04 mg/kg medetomidine plus 1 mg/kg ketamine; antagonize with 1.2 mg/kg mg naltrexone plus 0.16 mg/kg atipamezole

• 0.03 mg/kg etorphine plus 0.25 mg/kg xylazine; antagonize with 0.06 mg/kg diprenorphine plus 0.125 mg/kg yohimbine

• 3.5 mg etorphine plus 50 mg ketamine plus 50 mg xylazine; antagonize with 7 mg diprenorphine plus 0.125 mg/kg yohimbine

• 2 mg/kg tiletamine-zolazepam plus 0.2 mg/kg xylazine; antagonize with 0.125 mg/kg yohimbine

Comments: Gemsbok are profoundly sensitive to xylazine; antagonism is essential. Azaperone (100 mg) or detomidine (10 mg) may be substituted for xylazine. Hyaluronidase (1,500-3,000 IU) may be added to dart to increase drug absorption. Semi-immobilized animals may show aggression towards humans; when immobilized restrain horns at all times. Once down, 100 mg ketamine IV may improve immobilization. Long-acting tranquilizer doses: haloperidol (adults, not to exceed 20 mg); zuclopenthixol, 1 mg/kg; perphenazine (adults, 100-200 mg).

References: Heuschele, 1961a; Ebedes, 1962; 1966b; 1967; 1969; 1975a; Talbot and Talbot, 1962; Lanphear, 1963; Pienaar, 1968a; 1969b; 1973a; Bauditz, 1972; Heck and Rivenburg, 1972; Jones, 1972; York and Huggins, 1972; Lyon and Dinning, 1973; Smuts, 1973; Young and Whyte, 1973; Gray et al., 1974; De Vos, 1975; Hertzog, 1975; Rapley and Mehren, 1975; Röken, 1975; Haigh, 1976d; De Vos 1978; Jessup et al., 1980; Hofmeyr, 1981; Jensen, 1982; Wiesner et al., 1982; Silvestris and Heck, 1984; Wiesner and von Hegel, 1985; Sedgwick, 1986; Schobert, 1987; Kock, R., et al., 1989; Allen et al., 1991; Berry, 1992; IWVS, 1992; Snyder et al., 1992; Majonica and Bonath, 1993; Burroughs, 1993d; Grobler et al., 2001; Kock, M., et al., 2006

GENET, *Genetta spp.*

Weight: 1–3 kg

Recommended Drug: 5 mg/kg tiletamine-zolazepam

Supplemental Drug: 5 mg/kg ketamine

Antagonist: None

Alternative Drugs: 30 mg/kg ketamine plus 0.3 mg/kg acepromazine

• 30 mg/kg ketamine plus 0.5 mg/kg xylazine

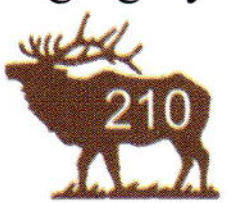

References: Seal and Erickson, 1969; Seal et al., 1970; Gray et al., 1974; Genevois et al., 1984b; Schobert, 1987; Maddock, 1989; Fuller et al., 1990; McKenzie and Burroughs, 1993; Palomares, 1993; Kock, M., et al., 2006

GERBILS, GENERAL

Weight: 30–200 gm

Recommended Drug: 0.044 mg/gm ketamine plus 0.006 mg/gm xylazine

Supplemental Drug: 0.022 mg/gm ketamine

Antagonist: None reported

Alternative Drugs: 0.05 mg/gm ketamine plus 0.002 mg/gm xylazine

- 0.05 mg/gm ketamine plus 0.005 mg/gm diazepam
- 0.075 mg/gm ketamine plus 0.003 mg/gm acepromazine
- 0.005 mg/gm tiletamine-zolazepam

References: Beck, 1976; Lightfoote and Molinari, 1978; Flecknell et al., 1983; Genevois et al., 1984a; Garver and Jackson, 1985

GIBBON, SIAMANG, *Hylobates syndactylus*

Weight: 8–13 kg

Recommended Drug: 4.4 mg/kg tiletamine-zolazepam

Supplemental Drug: 4.4 mg/kg ketamine

Antagonist: None

References: Kroll, 1962; Gray et al., 1974; Bush et al., 1977; Schobert, 1987

GIBBON, WHITE-CHEEKED (CRESTED), *Hylobates concolor*

Weight: 4–8 kg

Recommended Drug: 3.3 mg/kg tiletamine-zolazepam

Supplemental Drug: 3.3 mg/kg ketamine

Antagonist: None

Alternative Drugs: 16 mg/kg ketamine

References: Gray et al., 1974; Bush et al., 1977; Schobert, 1987

GIBBON, WHITE-HANDED (LAR), *Hylobates lar*

Weight: 4–8 kg

Recommended Drug: 3 mg/kg ketamine plus 0.07 mg/kg medetomidine

Supplemental Drug: 1.5 mg/kg ketamine

Antagonist: 0.35 mg/kg atipamezole; give 1/2 dose IV, 1/2 IM

Alternative Drugs: 4.4 mg/kg tiletamine-zolazepam

- 12 mg/kg ketamine

References: Kroll, 1962; Seal and Erickson, 1969; Seal et al., 1970; Beck, 1972; 1976; Beck and Dresner, 1972; Jessup et al., 1980; Schobert, 1987; Jalanka and Roeken, 1990; Mortenson, 1994

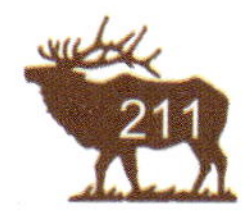

GIRAFFE, *Giraffa camelopardalis*

Weight: 550–1,800 kg

Recommended Drug: 20 mg thiafentanil

Supplemental Drug: 5 mg thiafentanil

Antagonist: 150 mg naltrexone

Alternative Drugs: 8 mg carfentanil plus 100 mg xylazine plus 10 mg atropine; antagonize with 800 mg naltrexone plus 0.05 mg/kg yohimbine

• 11 mg etorphine (bull), 9 mg etorphine (cow), 6 mg etorphine (young); antagonize with 22 mg (bull), 18 mg (cow), 12 mg (young) diprenorphine; or 100 mg naltrexone for every mg etorphine given

• 8 mg/kg tiletamine-zolazepam

Comments: Immobilization mortality can be as high as 35% in giraffes. The current capture philosophy for giraffes is to dose high and *quickly antagonize* (i.e., within 15-20 min) after physical restraint has been achieved. If possible, a physical restraining device should be used in preference to, or in conjunction with, chemical immobilization. Do not attempt immobilization without expert consultation and thorough familiarity with the literature (e.g., Morkel, 1993b; Kock et al., 2006) and always work with someone with experience. Blood pressure must be maintained in order to perfuse the brain. Opioids cause profound respiratory depression. Capture must *not* be attempted if ambient temperature is >25½ C (77½ F). Hyaluronidase (2,000 IU) can be added to the drug mixture to increase absorption. Ketamine-medetomidine combinations have been used on captive giraffe (see Lamberski et al., 2004). Long-acting tranquilizer doses: haloperidol (adult male, 30 mg; adult female, 20 mg); zuclopenthixol, 1 mg/kg; perphenazine (adult male, 100 mg; subadults, 150 mg).

References: Goetz, 1955; Buechner et al., 1960a; 1960c; Harthoorn, 1960; 1963a; 1965a; 1973a; 1973b; Harthoorn and Lock, 1961; Talbot and Lamprey, 1961; Talbot and Talbot, 1962; Larsen, 1963; Van Niekerk et al., 1963a; Van Niekerk and Pienaar, 1963a; 1969a; Pienaar and Fairall, 1963; Wright, 1963; Graham-Jones, 1964; Harthoorn and Bligh, 1965; Hirst et al., 1965; Hirst, 1966; Pienaar et al., 1966a; Wallach et al., 1967; Wallach, 1968; 1969; Williamson and Wallach, 1968; 1969; Sedgwick and Acosta, 1969; York and Kidder, 1971; Harthoorn, 1972a; Jones, 1972; Langman, 1973; Alford et al., 1974; De Vos, 1975; Hertzog, 1975; Mehren and Rapley, 1975; Rapley and Mehren, 1975; Röken, 1975; York, 1975; Bush, 1976; Bush et al., 1976; 1980; 2001; Haigh, 1976d; Wiesner et al., 1982; Citino et al., 1984; Meltzer et al., 1985; Savage, 1985; Hugues et al., 1986; Sedgwick, 1986; Bush and De Vos, 1987; Calle and Bornmann, 1988; Wiesner and von Hegel, 1989; Geiser et al., 1992; Morkel, 1992b; IWVS, 1992; Morkel, 1993b; Kato and Seino, 1996; Fischer et al., 1997; Vogelnest and Ralph, 1997; Lamberski et al., 2004; Citino et al., 2006; Kock, M., et al., 2006

GLIDER, SUGAR, *Petaruus breviceps*

Weight: 90–130 gm

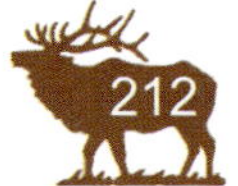

Recommended Drug: 0.011 mg/gm tiletamine-zolazepam
Supplemental Drug: 0.01 mg/gm ketamine
Antagonist: None
Comments: Caution: Holz (1992) reported 100% mortality ($n = 3$) in squirrel gliders (*Petaurus norfolcensis*) given 10 mg/kg tiletamine-zolazepam
References: Bush et al., 1990; Holz, 1992

GNU - SEE WILDEBEEST

GOAT, FERAL, *Capra hircus*

Weight: 20–80 kg
Recommended Drug: 2 mg/kg ketamine plus 0.05 mg/kg medetomidine
Supplemental Drug: If not down in 15 minutes, repeat full dose
Antagonist: 0.25 mg/kg atipamezole
Alternative Drugs: 20 mg/kg ketamine
- 15 mg/kg tiletamine-zolazepam
- 0.04 mg/kg carfentanil; antagonize with 4 mg/kg naltrexone
- 0.028 mg/kg etorphine; antagonize with 0.056 mg/kg diprenorphine

References: Jarvis and Morris, 1960; Gauckler and Kraus, 1970; Rudge and Joblin, 1976; Jessup et al., 1980; Merilan, 1986; Schobert, 1987; Sleeman and Ramsay, 1995; Sleeman et al., 1997a; Mutlow et al., 2004

GOAT, MOUNTAIN, *Oreamnos americanus*

Weight: 46–140 kg
Recommended Drug: 0.035 mg/kg carfentanil
Supplemental Drug: If not down in 20 minutes, repeat full dose
Antagonist: 3.5 mg/kg naltrexone
Alternative Drugs: 4 mg etorphine plus 30 mg xylazine antagonize with 8 mg diprenorphine plus 0.15 mg/kg yohimbine
- 1.5 mg/kg ketamine plus 0.07 mg/kg medetomidine; antagonize with 0.35 mg/kg atipamezole; give 1/2 dose IV, 1/2 IM
- 5 mg/kg xylazine (trapped animals only; see Haviernick et al., 1998)

References: Hebert and Cowan, 1971; McKean and Magonigle, 1978; Jessup et al., 1980; Thorne, 1982; Carpenter and Lance, 1983; Côté et al., 1998; Haviernick et al., 1998; Jessup, 1999

GOOSE, CANADA, *Branta canadensis*

Weight: 3.3–3.8 kg
Recommended Drug: 20 mg/kg tiletamine-zolazepam
Supplemental Drug: 20 mg/kg ketamine
Antagonist: None
Alternative Drugs: Gas anesthesia
References: Crider and McDaniel, 1966; 1967; 1968; Crider et al., 1968; Krapu, 1976; Belant and Seamans, 1997

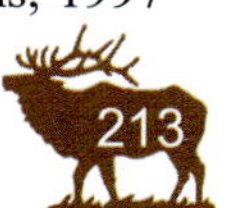

GOOSE, EGYPTIAN, *Alopechen aegyptiacus*

Weight: 1.2–1.5 kg
Recommended Drug: 22 mg/kg tiletamine-zolazepam
Supplemental Drug: 22 mg/kg ketamine
Antagonist: None
References: Schobert, 1987

GOOSE, LESSER MAGELLAN, *Chlorphaga picta*

Weight: 2.7–3.2 kg
Recommended Drug: 8.8 mg/kg tiletamine-zolazepam
Supplemental Drug: 8.8 mg/kg ketamine
Antagonist: None
References: Schobert, 1987

GOOSE, WHITE-FRONTED, *Anserini albiforns frontalis*

Weight: 1.3–2.3 kg
Recommended Drug: 2.7 mg/kg tiletamine-zolazepam
Supplemental Drug: 2.7 mg/kg ketamine
Antagonist: None
References: Schobert, 1987

GORILLA, *Gorilla gorilla*

Weight: 70–140 (f), 135–275 (m) kg
Recommended Drug: 5 mg/kg ketamine plus 0.05 mg/kg medetomidine
Supplemental Drug: 2.5 mg/kg ketamine
Antagonist: 0.25 mg/kg atipamezole; give 1/2 dose IV, 1/2 IM
Alternative Drugs: 2.2 mg/kg tiletamine-zolazepam
• 10 mg/kg ketamine
Comments: Oral ketamine and detomidine have been used with partial success in captive gorillas (Miller et al., 2000).
References: Jarvis and Morris, 1960; Marsboom et al., 1962; 1963; Seal et al., 1970a; 1970b; Beck, 1972; Bush et al., 1971; 1977; Beck and Dresner, 1972; Gray et al., 1974; Vercruysse and Mortelmans, 1978; Jessup et al., 1980; Ludders et al., 1982; Cook and Clarke, 1984; 1985; Hess and Knakal, 1985; Robinson and Lambert, 1986; Schobert, 1987; Jalanka and Roeken, 1990; Horne et al., 1997; Sleeman et al., 1998; 2000; Vogelnest, 1998; Miller et al., 2000; Raphael et al., 2001; Hunter et al., 2004

GOSHAWK, *Accipiter gentilis*

Weight: 0.9–1.5 kg
Recommended Drug: 20 mg/kg ketamine
Supplemental Drug: 10 mg/kg ketamine
Antagonist: None
References: Borzio, 1973; Beck, 1976; Lumeij, 1986

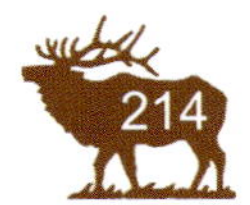

GRIVET, *Cercopithecus aethiops*

Weight: 5–9 kg
Recommended Drug: 8.8 mg/kg tiletamine-zolazepam
Supplemental Drug: 4.4 mg/kg ketamine
Antagonist: None
Alternative Drugs: 12 mg/kg ketamine
References: Beck, 1976; Schobert, 1987

GRYSBOK, *Raphicerus melanotis*

Weight: 7–16 kg
Recommended Drug: 5 mg fentanyl plus 10 mg azaperone
Supplemental Drug: 2.5 mg/kg fentanyl
Antagonist: 0.2 mg/kg naloxone
Alternative Drugs: 8 mg/kg tiletamine-zolazepam
Comments: Monitor for respiratory depression when using opioids.
References: Burroughs, 1993d

GRYSBOK, SHARPE'S, *Raphicerus sharpei*

Weight: 7–16 kg
Recommended Drug: 5 mg fentanyl plus 10 mg azaperone
Supplemental Drug: 2.5 mg/kg fentanyl
Antagonist: 0.2 mg/kg naloxone
Alternative Drugs: 8 mg/kg tiletamine-zolazepam
Comments: Monitor for respiratory depression when using opioids.
References: Burroughs, 1993d; Kock et el., 2006

GUANACO, *Lama guanicoe*

Weight: 100–120 kg
Recommended Drug: 2 mg/kg ketamine plus 0.1 mg/kg medetomidine
Supplemental Drug: 1 mg/kg ketamine
Antagonist: 0.5 mg/kg atipamezole; give 1/2 dose IV, 1/2 IM
Alternative Drugs: 6 mg/kg tiletamine-zolazepam
• 3.25 mg/kg xylazine; antagonize with 0.125 mg/kg yohimbine
Comments: Jones (1977a) stated that the use of opioids in llama was contraindicated; assume the same for guanaco.
References: Larsen, 1963; Bauditz, 1972; Beck, 1972; Jones, 1972; Hertzog, 1975; Haigh, 1976d; Rapley and Mehren, 1975; De Lamo and Garrido, 1983; Wiesner and von Hegel, 1985; Kock et al., 1989; Jalanka and Roeken, 1990; Sarno et al., 1996; Karesh et al., 1998

GUENONS - SEE MONKEY (GUENON)

GUINEA PIG, *Cavia spp.*

Weight: 0.5–1.5 kg
Recommended Drug: 40 mg/kg ketamine plus 5 mg/kg xylazine

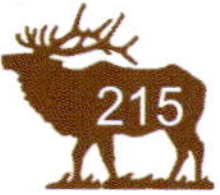

Supplemental Drug: 20 mg/kg ketamine
Antagonist: None
Alternative Drugs: 40 mg/kg ketamine plus 2 mg/kg acepromazine
• 50 mg/kg tiletamine-zolazepam
References: Love, 1970; Rubright and Thayer, 1970; Weisbroth and Fudens, 1972; Stunkard and Miller, 1974; Hughes et al., 1975; Mulder et al., 1979; Gilroy and Varga, 1980; Genevois et al., 1984a; Garver and Jackson, 1985; Henke et al., 1996

GUINEAFOWL, *Numida meleagris*

Weight: 3–5 kg
Recommended Drug: 25 mg/kg ketamine plus 1 mg/kg xylazine
Supplemental Drug: 12.5 mg/kg ketamine
Antagonist: 0.15 mg/kg yohimbine
References: Teare, 1987

GYRFALCON, *Falco rusticolus*

Weight: 1.4–1.6 kg
Recommended Drug: 20 mg/kg ketamine plus 1.2 mg/kg diazepam, IV
Supplemental Drug: 5 mg/kg ketamine, IV
Antagonist: None
Alternative Drugs: 20 mg/kg ketamine
References: Borzio, 1973; Beck, 1976; Redig and Duke, 1976

HAMSTERS, GENERAL

Weight: 112–908 gm
Recommended Drug: 0.044 mg/gm ketamine plus 0.006 mg/gm xylazine
Supplemental Drug: 0.022 mg/gm ketamine
Antagonist: None reported
Alternative Drugs: 0.01 mg/gm tiletamine-zolazepam
References: Hughes et al., 1975; Mulder et al., 1979; Genevois et al., 1984a; Garver and Jackson, 1985; Forsyth et al., 1992

HARTEBEEST, *Alcelaphus buselaphus*

Weight: 140–170 kg
Recommended Drug: 6 mg etorphine plus 10 mg xylazine (bull); 5 mg etorphine plus 10 mg xylazine (cow)
Supplemental Drug: 2 mg etorphine
Antagonist: 2 mg diprenorphine per mg etorphine given plus 0.15 mg/kg yohimbine
Alternative Drugs: 5 mg thiafentanil; antagonize with 1 mg/kg naltrexone
• 0.01 mg/kg carfentanil plus 0.1 mg/kg xylazine; antagonize with 1 mg/kg naltrexone plus 0.15 mg/kg yohimbine
Comments: Difficult to immobilize, often struggle against recumbency and

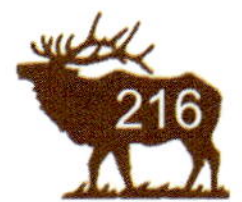

continue to run. Azaperone (70 mg) may be substituted for xylazine. Long-acting tranquilizer doses: haloperidol (adult male, 30 mg; adult female, 20 mg; subadult, 10 mg); zuclopenthixol (adults, 100 mg); perphenazine (adults, 100 mg).

References: Buechner et al., 1960a; 1960c; Lanphear, 1963; Bigalke, 1965; Pienaar et al., 1966a; Pienaar, 1969b; 1973a; Harthoorn, 1971; Bartmann, 1972; Bauditz, 1972; Heck and Rivenburg, 1972; Kok, 1973; Hirst et al., 1965; De Vos, 1975; Röken, 1975; Grootenhuis et al., 1976; Haigh, 1976d; Slee and Walker, 1977; Hofmeyr, 1981; Kupper et al., 1981; Jensen, 1982; Ganhao et al., 1988; Berry, 1992; IWVS, 1992; Burroughs, 1993d; Kock, M., et al., 2006

HARTEBEEST, LICHTENSTEIN'S, *Sigmoceros lichtensteinii*

Weight: 135–245 kg

Recommended Drug: 0.02 mg/kg thiafentanil plus 0.008 mg/kg medetomidine plus 1 mg/kg ketamine

Supplemental Drug: repeat full dose if not down in 15 minuntes

Antagonist: 0.6 mg/kg naltrexone plus 0.035 mg/kg atipamezole

Alternative Drugs: 5 mg etorphine plus 80 mg azaperone; antagonize with 1 mg/kg naltrexone

References: Citino et al., 2002; Kock, M., et al., 2006

HAWK, BROAD-WINGED, *Buteo platypterus*

Weight: 0.3–0.5 kg

Recommended Drug: 45 mg/kg ketamine plus 1.25 mg/kg diazepam, IV

Supplemental Drug: 5 mg/kg ketamine, IV

Antagonist: None

lternative Drugs: 20 mg/kg ketamine plus 2 mg/kg acepromazine

References: Mattingly, 1972; Redig and Duke, 1976; Freed and Baker, 1980; 1989; Jessup et al., 1980

HAWK, RED-SHOULDERED, *Buteo lineatus*

Weight: 0.5–1.3 kg

Recommended Drug: 20 mg/kg ketamine plus 2 mg/kg acepromazine

Supplemental Drug: 10 mg/kg ketamine

Antagonist: None

Alternative Drugs: 15 mg/kg tiletamine-zolazepam

References: Jessup et al., 1980

HAWK, RED-TAILED, *Buteo jamaicensis*

Weight: 0.6–1.4 kg

Recommended Drug: 4.4 mg/kg ketamine plus 2.2 mg/kg xylazine

Supplemental Drug: 2.2 mg/kg ketamine

Antagonist: 0.1 mg/kg yohimbine

Alternative Drugs: 35 mg/kg ketamine plus 1.5 mg/kg diazepam, IV

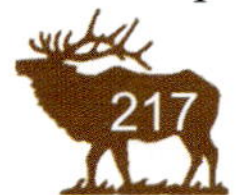

• 10 mg/kg ketamine plus 2 mg/kg xylazine
• 20 mg/kg ketamine plus 2 mg/kg acepromazine
Comments: Tiletamine-zolazepam in these hawks caused copious salivation and less than satisfactory immobilization (Kreeger et al., 1993).
References: Kittle, 1972; Mattingly, 1972; Borzio, 1973; Frank and Cooper, 1974; Haupert and Lindeen, 1974; Cooper and Redig, 1975; Beck, 1976; Redig and Duke, 1976; Kollias and McLeish, 1978; Freed and Baker, 1980; 1989; Jessup et al., 1980; Degernes et al., 1988; Fitzgerald, 1993; Kreeger et al., 1993; Hawkins et al., 2003

HAWK, ROUGH-LEGGED, *Buteo lagopus*

Weight: 700 gm
Recommended Drug: 0.03 mg/gm ketamine plus 0.0012 mg/gm diazepam IV
Supplemental Drug: 0.005 mg/gm ketamine IV
Antagonist: None
Alternative Drugs: 0.02 mg/gm ketamine plus 0.002 mg/gm acepromazine
References: Redig and Duke, 1976

HAWKS, GENERAL

Recommended Drug: 30 mg/kg ketamine plus 1.5 mg/kg diazepam, IV
Supplemental Drug: 5 mg/kg ketamine, IV
Antagonist: None
Alternative Drugs: 20 mg/kg ketamine plus 2 mg/kg acepromazine
• 15 mg/kg tiletamine-zolazepam
Comments: Tiletamine-zolazepam in some hawks may cause copious salivation and less than satisfactory immobilization. Oral tiletamine-zolazepam in baits might be effective in hawks (see Janovsky et al., 2002)
References: Redig and Duke, 1976; Jessup et al., 1980; Amand, 1982a; Janovsky et al., 2002

HEDGEHOG, *Erinaceus europaeus*

Weight: 0.4–1.1 kg
Recommended Drug: 2 mg/kg ketamine plus 0.2 mg/kg medetomidine plus 0.1 mg/kg fentanyl
Supplemental Drug: 1 mg/kg ketamine
Antagonist: 1 mg/kg atipamezole plus 0.16 mg/kg naloxone
Alternative Drugs: 5 mg/kg ketamine plus 0.2 mg/kg medetomidine; antagonize with 1 mg/kg atipamezole
• 5 mg/kg tiletamine-zolazepam
Comments: Expect prolonged recoveries with tiletamine-zolazepam
References: Seal and Erickson, 1969; Seal et al., 1970; Schobert, 1987; Jalanka and Roeken, 1990; Arnemo and SØli, 1995a

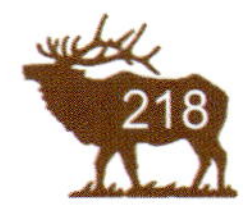

HERON, GREEN, *Butorides virescens*

Weight: 100 gm
Recommended Drug: 0.075 mg/gm tiletamine-zolazepam
Supplemental Drug: 0.075 mg/kg ketamine
Antagonist: None
References: Kittle, 1972; Schobert, 1987

HIPPOPOTAMUS, *Hippopotamus amphibius*

Weight: 1,000–2,000 kg
Recommended Drug: 2 mg etorphine plus 200 mg azaperone plus 250 mg succinylcholine (adult)
Supplemental Drug: 1 mg etorphine
Antagonist: 200 mg naltrexone
Alternative Drugs: 0.7 ml Large Animal Immobilon® plus 8 mg xylazine; antagonize with 85 mg naloxone
• 5 mg etorphine plus 200 mg azaperone (on land, away from water)
Comments: Hippos are very difficult to chemically immobilize; physical capture (boma) is preferred. Mortalities can be as high as 35%. Induction times can be prolonged (30–60 min) if drug is not administered intramuscularly. Inject in the neck just caudal to ear. Estimate drug doses carefully; etorphine is not tolerated well by hippos, respiratory arrest can occur even at low doses - minimize immobilization time if at all possible (preferably less than 30 min.). Administer doxapram (400 mg) or nalorphine (100 mg) for severe respiratory depression (Kock, M., et al., 2006). Etorphine and acepromazine mixtures and fentanyl and azaperone mixtures have caused side effects such as sweating, salivation, and muscular hypertonicity. Use long darts (6–9 cm). Hippos are very sensitive to diazepam; good sedation can be obtained using 10 mg increments.
References: Buechner et al., 1960c; 1960d; Harthoorn, 1960; 1963d; 1965a; 1972a; 1973a; 1973b; Harthoorn and Lock, 1961; Buck et al., 1963; Van Niekerk et al., 1963a; 1963b; Van Niekerk and Pienaar, 1963a; Pienaar et al., 1966a; Pienaar, 1967a; 1969a; 1969b; Jones, 1972; York and Huggins, 1972; York, 1973b; Alford et al., 1974; Haigh, 1976d; Reed, 1978; Stoskopf and Bishop, 1978; Wiesner et al., 1982; Jarofke and Klos, 1983; Pearce et al., 1985; Wiesner and von Hegel, 1985; Sedgwick, 1986; IWVS, 1992; Ramsay et al., 1998; Loomis and Ramsay, 1999; Kock, 2001; Kock, M., et al., 2006

HIPPOPOTAMUS, PYGMY, *Choeropsis liberiensis*

Weight: 160–270 kg
Recommended Drug: 2.5 mg etorphine plus 125 mg xylazine
Supplemental Drug: 1.5 mg etorphine
Antagonist: 5 mg diprenorphine plus 0.125 mg/kg yohimbine
Alternative Drugs: 0.25 ml Large Animal Immobilon®; antagonize with 2 mg diprenorphine per mg etorphine given
Comments: See comments on Hippopotamus above.

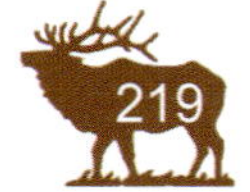

References: Jones, 1972; Wiesner et al., 1982; Pearce et al., 1985; Weston et al., 1996

HOG, EUROPEAN WILD, *Sus scrofa*

Weight: 100–350 kg
Recommended Drug: 5 mg/kg ketamine plus 0.2 mg/kg medetomidine
Supplemental Drug: 2 mg/kg ketamine
Antagonist: 0.5 mg/kg atipamezole
Alternative Drugs: 5 mg/kg tiletamine-zolazepam plus 0.1 mg/kg medetomidine; antagonize with 0.5 mg/kg atipamezole

- 3 mg/kg tiletamine-zolazepam plus 0.05 mg/kg medetomidine plus 0.2 mg/kg; antagonize with 0.25 mg/kg atipamezole
- 4.4 mg/kg tiletamine-zolazepam plus 2.2 mg/kg xylazine; antagonize with 0.15 mg/kg yohimbine
- 0.4 mg/kg butorphanol plus 0.125 mg/kg detomidine plus 0.4 mg/kg midazolam; antagonize with 5 mg/kg naltrexone plus 0.3 mg/kg yohimbine
- 10 mg/kg ketamine plus 0.5 mg/kg xylazine
- 0.022 mg/kg etorphine plus 0.11 mg/kg acepromazine; antagonize with 0.044 mg/kg diprenorphine

Comments: Hogs can overheat readily, particulary when using etorphine or xylazine. The tiletamine-zolazepam-medetomidine dosages were used only on juveniles (Enqvist et al., 2000).
References: Zurowski and Sakowicz, 1965; Austin and Peoples, 1967; Henry and Matschke, 1968; 1972; Matschke and Henry, 1969a; 1969b; Seal et al., 1970; Vertessen, 1970; Jones, 1972; Alford et al., 1974; Wood et al., 1977; Jessup et al., 1980; Baber and Coblentz, 1982; Wiesner et al., 1982; Wiesner and von Hegel, 1985; Macek, 1987; Strauss, 1987; Bonath et al., 1992; Siemon et al., 1992; Wolkers et al., 1994; Walzer, 1995; Gabor et al., 1997; Sweitzer et al., 1997; Calle and Morris, 1999; Enqvist et al., 2000; Arnemo, 2004a

HORSE, FERAL, *Equus caballus*

Weight: 250–530 kg
Recommended Drug: 0.02 mg/kg carfentanil plus 0.6 mg/kg xylazine
Supplemental Drug: If animal is not down in 20 min, repeat full dose
Antagonist: 2 mg/kg naltrexone
Alternative Drugs: 5.5 mg etorphine plus 1,300 mg xylazine plus 7.5 mg atropine; antagonize with 11 mg diprenorphine plus 0.1 mg/kg yohimbine
Comments: Yohimbine must be administered to horses receiving xylazine.
References: Alford et al., 1974; Jones, 1978; Borchard, 1980; Jessup et al., 1980; 1985b; Berger et al., 1983; Seal et al., 1985a; Plotka et al., 1987; Matthews and Meyers, 1993; Shaw et al., 1995; Linklater et al., 1998

HORSE, PRZEWALSKI, *Equus caballus*

Weight: 275–455 kg

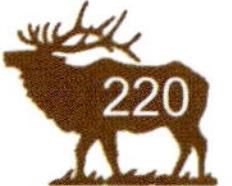

Recommended Drug: 2 mg/kg ketamine plus 0.08 mg/kg medetomidine
Supplemental Drug: 1 mg/kg ketamine
Antagonist: 0.4 mg/kg atipamezole; give 1/2 dose IV, 1/2 IM
Alternative Drugs: 0.02 mg/kg carfentanil; antagonize with 2 mg/kg naltrexone
• 0.02 mg/kg etorphine plus 0.2 mg/kg xylazine plus 0.08 mg/kg acepromazine; antagonize with 0.04 mg/kg diprenorphine plus 0.125 mg/kg yohimbine
Comments: These horses are difficult animals to immobilize. No ideal drug combination has yet been determined. Be prepared for ataxia and especially hyperthermia. Have cooling water available. Muscle relaxation is notoriously poor, even when midazolam/diazepam is employed. Split opioid antagonists equally IV and IM to reduce renarcotization.
References: Larsen, 1963; Bauditz, 1972; Heck and Rivenburg, 1972; Alford et al., 1974; Jones, 1976; 1978; Oosterhuis, 1979; Wright, 1981; Wiesner et al., 1982; Janssen and Oosterhuis, 1984; Kock and Pearce, 1985; Wiesner and von Hegel, 1985; Kuttner and Wiesner, 1987; Jalanka and Roeken, 1990; Allen, 1990a; 1992a; Morris, 1992; Wiesner, 1993; Matthews et al., 1995

HUTIA, HISPANOLIA, *Plagiodontia aedium*

Weight: 1–1.3 kg
Recommended Drug: 6.6 mg/kg tiletamine-zolazepam
Supplemental Drug: 6.6 mg/kg ketamine
Antagonist: None
References: Schobert, 1987

HYENA, BROWN, *Hyaena brunnea*

Weight: 37–47.5 kg
Recommended Drug: 5 mg/kg tiletamine-zolazepam
Supplemental Drug: 2 mg/kg ketamine
Antagonist: None
Alternative Drugs: 10 mg/kg ketamine plus 1 mg/kg xylazine; antagonize with 0.11 mg/kg yohimbine
Comments: The long coat of the brown hyena may lead to overestimation of weight and interfere with accurate dart placement.
References: Seal and Erickson, 1969; Seal et al., 1970; Ebedes, 1973b; Wiesner, 1977; Wiesner and von Hegel, 1985; McKenzie and Burroughs, 1993; Kock, M., et al., 2006

HYENA, SPOTTED, *Crocuta crocuta*

Weight: 40–86 kg
Recommended Drug: 5 mg/kg tiletamine-zolazepam
Supplemental Drug: 2 mg/kg ketamine
Antagonist: None

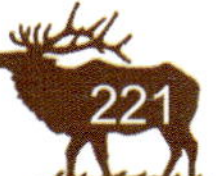

Alternative Drugs: 10 mg/kg ketamine plus 1 mg/kg xylazine; antagonize with 0.11 mg/kg yohimbine
• 0.05 mg/kg etorphine plus 0.6 mg/kg xylazine; antagonize with 0.1 mg/kg diprenorphine plus 0.15 mg/kg yohimbine
Comments: Respiratory depression can occur with etorphine and xylazine
References: Heuschele, 1961a; Kroll, 1962; Talbot and Talbot, 1962; Ericksen, 1968; Seal and Erickson, 1969; Pienaar et al., 1969; Seal et al., 1970; Ebedes, 1973b; Smuts, 1973b; Young and Whyte, 1973; Gray et al., 1974; Beck, 1976; Whately, 1979; Genevois et al., 1984b; Schobert, 1987; Van Jaarsveld, 1988; Stander and Gasawy, 1991; IWVS, 1992; Van Jaarsveld and Skinner, 1992; McKenzie and Burroughs, 1993; Kock, M., et al., 2006

HYENA, STRIPED, *Hyaena hyaena*

Weight: 25–55 kg
Recommended Drug: 5 mg/kg tiletamine-zolazepam
Supplemental Drug: 2 mg/kg ketamine
Antagonist: None
Alternative Drugs: 10 mg/kg ketamine plus 1 mg/kg xylazine; antagonize with 0.11 mg/kg yohimbine
References: Larsen, 1963; Seal and Erickson, 1969; Göltenboth and Klös, 1970; Seal et al., 1970; Bauditz, 1972; Nair, 1977; Genevois et al., 1984b

IBEX, ALPINE, *Capra ibex*

Weight: 35–150 kg
Recommended Drug: 0.04 mg/kg carfentanil plus 0.15 mg/kg xylazine
Supplemental Drug: If animal is not down in 20 minutes, repeat full dose
Antagonist: 4 mg/kg naltrexone plus 0.125 mg/kg yohimbine
Alternative Drugs: 1.5 mg/kg ketamine plus 0.11 mg/kg medetomidine; antagonize with 0.5 mg/kg atipamezole
• 2 mg etorphine plus 20 mg ketamine plus 20 mg xylazine; antagonize with 4 mg diprenorphine plus 0.15 mg/kg yohimbine
• 0.8 ml Large Animal Immobilon® plus 10 mg xylazine; antagonize with 2 mg diprenorphine per mg etorphine given plus 0.125 mg/kg yohimbine
• 0.05 mg/kg fentanyl plus 0.5 mg/kg xylazine; antagonize with 0.2 mg/kg naloxone plus 0.125 mg/kg yohimbine
Comments: Monitor for hyperthermia and respiratory depression.
References: Boch et al., 1961; Gauckler and Kraus, 1970; Bauditz, 1972; Heck and Rivenburg, 1972; Mehren and Rapley, 1975; Rapley and Mehren, 1975; Wentges, 1975; Jensen, 1982; Wiesner et al., 1982; 1984; Duchamps, 1985; De Meneghi et al., 1987; Barnett and Lewis, 1990; Jalanka and Roeken, 1990; Allen et al., 1991; Snyder et al., 1992; Escos and alados, 1993; Peinado et al., 1993

IGUANA, *Iguana iguana*

Weight: 0.5–1.5 kg

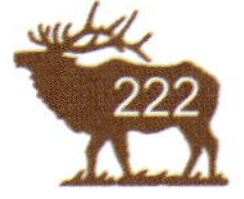

Recommended Drug: 10 mg/kg tiletamine-zolazepam
Supplemental Drug: 10 mg/kg ketamine
Antagonist: None
Alternative Drugs: 35 mg/kg ketamine
• 2 mg/kg butorphanol (induction); maintain on sevoflurane or isoflurane (see Mosley et al., 2004 or HernandezDivers et al., 2005)
• 10 mg/kg propofol (intraosseous)
References: Cooper, 1971; Beck, 1972; 1976; Gray et al., 1974; Jessup et al., 1980; Schobert, 1987; Smith et al., 1997; Bennett et al., 1998a; 1998b; Vienet, 2001; Hernandez-Divers et al., 2003; 2005; Mosley, 2003a; 2003b; 2004; vonDegerfeld, 2004; Barter et al., 2006

IMPALA, *Aepyceros melampus*

Weight: 40–60 kg
Recommended Drug: 0.04 mg/kg thiafentanil
Supplemental Drug: 0.02 mg/kg carfentanil
Antagonist: 0.8 mg/kg naltrexone
Alternative Drugs: 0.006 mg/kg carfentanil plus 0.15 mg/kg xylazine; antagonize with 0.6 mg/kg naltrexone plus 0.125 mg/kg yohimbine
• 1.5 mg etorphine plus 20 mg azaperone; antagonize with 3 mg diprenorphine
• 5 mg/kg tiletamine-zolazepam
• 8 mg/kg ketamine plus 0.04 mg/kg medetomidine; antagonize with 0.12 mg/kg atipamezole
Comments: Monitor for respiratory depression when opioids are used. Impala are small, so accurate dart placement is critical to avoid injury. Impala often move into brush after being struck, making location difficult. Long-acting tranquilizer doses: haloperidol (adult male, 20 mg; adult female, 15 mg, subadult, 10 mg; neonate, 5 mg); zuclopenthixol, 1 mg/kg; perphenazine, 2-5 mg/kg; pipothiazine, 2 mg/kg.
References: Talbot and Lamprey, 1961; Kroll, 1962; Van Niekerk et al., 1963a; 1963b; Van Niekerk and Pienaar, 1963a; Pienaar and Fairall, 1963; Graham-Jones, 1964; Harthoorn and Bligh, 1965; Hirst et al., 1965; Pienaar et al., 1966a; Ables, 1969; Pienaar, 1968a; 1969b; 1973a; Bauditz, 1972; Heck and Rivenburg, 1972; Jones, 1972; 1978; York and Huggins, 1972; Hofmeyr and de Bruine, 1973; Smuts, 1973a; Smuts et al., 1973; Young and Whyte, 1973; Drevemo and Harstad, 1974; De Vos, 1975; Röken, 1975; York, 1975; Grootenhuis et al., 1976; Haigh, 1976d; Murray et al., 1971; Hofmeyr, 1981; Wiesner et al., 1982; 1984; 1985; Wiesner and von Hegel, 1985; Schobert, 1987; Williams and Riedesel, 1987; Cheney and Hattingh, 1988; Hattingh et al., 1988; Gandini et al., 1989; Knox, et al., 1989, 1990, 1991; Raath and Knox, 1989; Allen et al., 1991; Janssen et al., 1991; IWVS, 1992; Janssen et al., 1993; Burroughs, 1993d; Vahala, 1994; Phillips et al., 1998; Páras et al., 2002; Bush et al., 2004b; Kock, M., et al., 2006

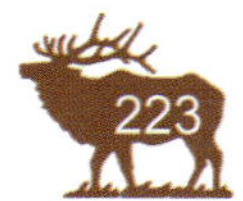

JACKAL, BLACK-BACKED, *Canis mesomelas*

Weight: 7–13.5 kg
Recommended Drug: 8 mg/kg tiletamine-zolazepam
Supplemental Drug: 8 mg/kg ketamine
Alternative Drugs: 20 mg/kg ketamine plus 0.2 mg/kg acepromazine
References: Young, 1966; Rowe-Rowe and Green, 1980; IWVS, 1992; McKenzie and Burroughs, 1993; Kaunda, 2001

JACKAL, GOLDEN, *Canis aureus*

Weight: 7–15 kg
Recommended Drug: 10 mg/kg tiletamine-zolazepam
Supplemental Drug: 10 mg/kg ketamine
Alternative Drugs: 20 mg/kg ketamine plus 0.2 mg/kg acepromazine
• 8 mg/kg ketamine plus 0.5 mg/kg xylazine
References: Seal and Erickson, 1969; Seal et al., 1970; Genevois et al., 1984b

JACKAL, SIDE STRIPED, *Canis adustus*

Weight: 6.5–14 kg
Recommended Drug: 8 mg/kg tiletamine-zolazepam
Supplemental Drug: 8 mg/kg ketamine
Alternative Drugs: 20 mg/kg ketamine plus 0.2 mg/kg acepromazine
• 8 mg/kg ketamine plus 0.5 mg/kg xylazine
References: IWVS, 1992; McKenzie and Burroughs, 1993

JACKAL, SIMIEN, *Canis simensis*

Weight: 10–18 kg
Recommended Drug: 4 mg/kg tiletamine-zolazepam
Supplemental Drug: 4 mg/kg ketamine
Alternative Drugs: 20 mg/kg ketamine plus 0.2 mg/kg acepromazine
References: Boever et al., 1977; Sillero-Zubiri, 1996

JAGUAR, *Panthera onca*

Weight: 64–114 kg
Recommended Drug: 5 mg/kg tiletamine-zolazepam
Supplemental Drug: 2 mg/kg ketamine
Antagonist: None
Alternative Drugs: 2.5 mg/kg ketamine plus 0.07 mg/kg medetomidine
• 4 mg/kg ketamine plus 2 mg/kg xylazine
References: Larsen, 1963; Seal and Erickson, 1969; Seal et al., 1970; Bauditz, 1972; Gray et al., 1974; Hime, 1974; Beck, 1976; Boever et al., 1977; Wiesner, 1977; Genevois et al., 1984b; Arora et al., 1983; Wiesner and von Hegel, 1985; Gonzales and McDonnel, 1986; Göltenboth and Klös, 1987; Schobert, 1987; Seal and Kreeger, 1987; Kock et al., 1989; Barnett and Lewis, 1990; Jalanka and Roeken, 1990

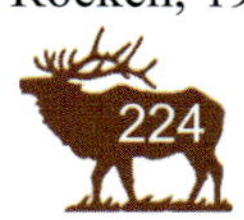

JAGUARUNDI, *Felis yagouaroundi*

Weight: 4.5–9 kg
Recommended Drug: 6.6 mg/kg tiletamine-zolazepam
Supplemental Drug: 3.3 mg/kg ketamine
Antagonist: None
Alternative Drugs: 15 mg/kg ketamine plus 1 mg/kg xylazine
References: Dyson, 1965; Seal and Erickson, 1969; Seal et al., 1970; Genevois et al., 1984b; Gray et al., 1974; Schobert, 1987; Seal and Kreeger, 1987

JAVELINA - SEE PECCARY

KANGAROO, BENNETT'S TREE, *Dendrolagus bennettianus*

Weight: 6.7–10 kg
Recommended Drug: 5 mg/kg tiletamine-zolazepam
Supplemental Drug: 2.5 mg/kg ketamine
Antagonist: None
References: Shima et al., 1993

KANGAROO, EASTERN GREY, *Macropus giganteus*

Weight: 30–55 kg
Recommended Drug: 4 mg/kg ketamine plus 0.04 mg/kg medetomidine
Supplemental Drug: 2 mg/kg ketamine
Antagonist: 0.2 mg/kg atipamezole
Alternative Drugs: 9 mg/kg ketamine
• 6 mg/kg tiletamine-zolazepam
Comments: Give atipamezole >30 min after the last ketamine dose when using ketamine-medetomidine.
References: Larsen, 1963; Wellington, 1972; Denny, 1974; Finnie, 1976; Bush et al., 1990; Shima et al., 1993; Pye and Booth, 1998

KANGAROO, RED, *Macropus rufus*

Weight: 20–40 kg
Recommended Drug: 7 mg/kg tiletamine-zolazepam
Supplemental Drug: 3.5 mg/kg ketamine
Antagonist: None
Alternative Drugs: 8 mg/kg ketamine plus 8 mg/kg xylazine
Comments: Immobilon® has been shown to be unsatisfactory..
References: Heuschele, 1961; Larsen, 1963; Seal and Erickson, 1969; Seal et al., 1970; Denny, 1973; 1974; Wilson, 1974; 1976; Beck, 1976; Finnie, 1976; 1986; Wilson, 1976; Boever et al., 1977; Smeller et al., 1977; Wiesner, 1977; Wiesner and von Hegel, 1985; Schobert, 1987; Bush et al., 1990; Shima et al., 1993

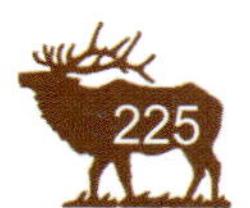

KANGAROO, TREE, *Dendrolagus matschiei*

Weight: 6.7–10 kg
Recommended Drug: 5 mg/kg tiletamine-zolazepam
Supplemental Drug: 2.5 mg/kg ketamine
Antagonist: None
Alternative Drugs: 5 mg/kg ketamine
Comments: Sometimes referred to as Goodfellows' tree kangaroo
References: Smeller et al., 1977; Schobert, 1987; Bush et al., 1990; Shima et al., 1993

KANGAROO, WESTERN GREY, *Macropus fuliginosus*

Weight: 30–50 kg
Recommended Drug: 5 mg/kg tiletamine-zolazepam
Supplemental Drug: 2.5 mg/kg ketamine
Antagonist: None
References: Watson and Way, 1973; Denny, 1974; Finnie, 1976; Arnold et al., 1986; Bush et al., 1990

KESTREL, AMERICAN, *Falco sparverius*

Weight: 0.1–0.12 kg
Recommended Drug: 5 mg/kg ketamine plus 2.2 mg/kg diazepam, IV
Supplemental Drug: 5 mg/kg ketamine, IV
Antagonist: None
References: Redig and Duke, 1976; Camburn and Stead, 1978; Freed and Baker, 1989

KINKAJOU, *Potus flavus*

Weight: 1.4–4.6 kg
Recommended Drug: 5.5 mg/kg ketamine plus 0.1 mg/kg medetomidine
Supplemental Drug: 3 mg/kg ketamine
Antagonist: 0.5 mg/kg atipamezole
Alternative Drugs: 10 mg/kg tiletamine-zolazepam
• 25 mg/kg ketamine
References: Seal and Erickson, 1969; Seal et al., 1970; Beck, 1976; Gray et al., 1974; Genevois et al., 1984b; Hugues et al., 1986; Schobert, 1987; Fournier et al., 1998

KLIPSPRINGER, *Oreotragus oreotragus*

Weight: 8–14 kg
Recommended Drug: 0.1 mg/kg thiafentanil plus 1 mg/kg azaperone
Supplemental Drug: 0.05 mg/kg thiafentanil
Antagonist: 2 mg/kg naltrexone
Alternative Drugs: 0.6 mg/kg fentanyl plus 2.5 mg/kg azaperone; antagonize with 0.2 mg/kg naltrexone
• 0.01 mg/kg etorphine plus 0.4 mg/kg xylazine; antagonize with 0.02 mg/

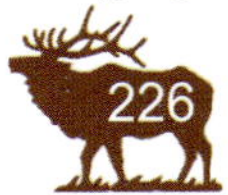

kg diprenorphine plus 0.15 mg/kg yohimbine
• 2.1 mg/kg ketamine plus 0.16 mg/kg medetomidine; antagonize with 0.8 mg/kg atipamezole
Comments: Monitor for respiratory depression when using opioids. Fentanyl is superior to etorphine. Klipspringer are sensitive to capture myopathy. Long-acting tranquilizer doses: haloperidol (adults, 5 mg).
References: IWVS, 1992; Kock, 2001; Kock, M., et al., 2006

KOALA, *Phascolarctos cinereus*

Weight: 8.2–10.4 kg
Recommended Drug: 7 mg/kg tiletamine-zolazepam
Supplemental Drug: 3.5 mg/kg ketamine
Antagonist: None
Alternative Drugs: 16 mg/kg ketamine plus 0.6 mg/kg xylazine
References: Robinson, 1981; Wildt et al., 1988; Bush et al., 1990; Holz, 1992; Shima et al., 1993

KOB, UGANDA, *Kobus kob*

Weight: 100–300 kg
Recommended Drug: 0.06 mg/kg thiafentanil plus 0.5 mg/kg azaperone
Supplemental Drug: If animal is not down in 15 minutes, repeat full dose
Antagonist: 1 mg/kg naltrexone
Alternative Drugs: 2.1 mg carfentanil (males); 1.5 mg carfentanil (females); plus 5 mg xylazine (both sexes); antagonize with 1 mg/kg naltrexone plus 0.125 mg/kg yohimbine
• 5 mg/kg tiletamine-zolazepam
• 1 mg etorphine plus 80 mg xylazine; antagonize with 2 mg diprenorphine plus 0.125 mg/kg yohimbine
• 1 ml Large Animal Immobilon®; antagonize with 2 mg diprenorphine per mg etorphine given
• 1 mg/kg xylazine; antagonize with 0.125 mg/kg yohimbine
References: Buechner et al., 1960a; 1960b; 1960c; 1960d; Harthoorn, 1960; Talbot and Lamprey, 1961; Bauditz, 1972; Röken, 1975; Küpper et al., 1981; Hugues et al., 1986; Wanzie, 1986; Okaeme et al., 1988; Allen et al., 1991; Caulkett et al., 2006

KUDU, *Tragelaphus strepsiceros*

Weight: 160–250 kg
Recommended Drug: 0.01 mg/kg carfentanil plus 0.1 mg/kg xylazine
Supplemental Drug: If animal is not down in 20 minutes, repeat full dose
Antagonist: 1 mg/kg naltrexone plus 0.125 mg/kg yohimbine
Alternative Drugs: 0.04 mg/kg thiafentanil plus 0.05 mg/kg detomidine; antagonize with 0.8 mg/kg naltrexone plus 0.2 mg/kg atipamezole
• 10 mg etorphine plus 70 mg xylazine; antagonize with 20 mg diprenorphine plus 0.125 mg/kg yohimbine

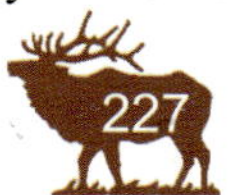

• 2.5 mg carfentanil plus 40 mg ketamine plus 40 mg xylazine; antagonize with 1 mg/kg naltrexone plus 0.125 mg/kg yohimbine
• 1.4 ml Large Animal Immobilon® plus 5 mg xylazine; antagonize with 2 mg diprenorphine per mg etorphine given plus 0.125 mg/kg yohimbine
• 3 mg etorphine plus 150 mg ketamine plus 150 mg xylazine; antagonize with 6 mg diprenorphine plus 0.125 mg/kg yohimbine
• 6 mg/kg tiletamine-zolazepam
Comments: Prone to excessive running during induction with opioids; monitor for hyperthermia. When darting from helicopter, consider increasing the dose by 20% (Kock et al., 2006). A muscle relaxant (xylazine, etc.) is essential to prevent capture myopathy. Hyaluronidase (1,500-3,000 IU) may be added to the drug mixture to hasten induction. Long-acting tranquilizer doses: haloperidol (adults, 20 mg; subadult, 10 mg); zuclopenthixol, 1 mg/kg; perphenazine (adult male, 200 mg; adult female, 100 mg; subadult, 50 mg).
References: Heuschele, 1959; Lanphear, 1963; Bigalke, 1965; Harthoorn and Bligh, 1965; Pienaar et al., 1966a; Pienaar, 1969b; 1973a; Wallach et al., 1967; Hime and Jones, 1970; Bauditz, 1972; Heck and Rivenburg, 1972; Jones, 1972; 1978; York and Huggins, 1972; Smuts, 1973; 1975; Young and Whyte, 1973; De Vos, 1975; Röken, 1975; Wiesner, 1975; York, 1975; Haigh, 1976d; Hofmeyr, 1981; Wiesner et al., 1982; Silvestris and Heck, 1984; Hess and Knakal, 1985; Schobert, 1987; Kock, R., et al., 1989; Allen et al., 1991; Janssen et al., 1991; IWVS, 1992; Snyder et al., 1992; Burroughs, 1993d; Kock, M., et al., 2006

KULAN, *Equus hemionus*

Weight: 180–250 kg
Recommended Drug: 1.7 ml Large Animal Immobilon® plus 30 mg xylazine
Supplemental Drug: 1 ml Large Animal Immobilon®
Antagonist: 2 mg diprenorphine per mg etorphine given plus 0.125 mg/kg yohimbine
Alternative Drugs: 1.5 mg etorphine plus 50 mg xylazine; antagonize with 3 mg diprenorphine plus 0.125 mg/kg yohimbine
• 3 mg etorphine antagonize with 6 mg diprenorphine
References: Lanphear, 1963; Göltenboth and Klös, 1970; Bauditz, 1972; Heck and Rivenburg, 1972; Hertzog, 1975; Jones, 1976; Oosterhuis, 1979; Wiesner et al., 1982; Kock and Pearce, 1985; Allen, 1990a

LANGUR, HANUMAN (INDIAN), *Semnopithecus entellus*

Weight: 10–23.6 kg
Recommended Drug: 3.3 mg/kg tiletamine-zolazepam
Supplemental Drug: 3.3 mg/kg ketamine
Antagonist: None
Alternative Drugs: 5 mg/kg ketamine

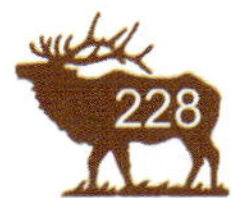

References: Beck, 1972; Beck and Dresner, 1972; Gray et al., 1974; Singh and Singh, 1982; Schobert, 1987

LECHWE, *Kobus leche*

Weight: 80–125 kg
Recommended Drug: 0.018 mg/kg carfentanil
Supplemental Drug: If animal is not down in 20 minutes, repeat full dose
Antagonist: 2 mg/kg naltrexone plus 0.125 mg/kg yohimbine
Alternative Drugs: 0.08 mg/kg thiafentanil; antagonize with 0.4 mg/kg naltrexone

- 1.5 mg etorphine plus 30 mg ketamine plus 30 mg xylazine; antagonize with 3 mg diprenorphine plus 0.15 mg/kg yohimbine
- 4 mg etorphine plus 10 mg xylazine; antagonize with 8 mg diprenorphine plus 0.15 mg/kg yohimbine

Comments: Prone to excessive running during induction; monitor for hyperthermia. Also prone to sudden rear leg kicking when immobilized.
References: Kock et al., 1989; Allen et al., 1991; Snyder et al., 1992; Burroughs, 1993d; Kock, M., et al., 2006

LECHWE, NILE, *Kobus megaceros*

Weight: 50–125 kg
Recommended Drug: 2.1 mg carfentanil (males); 1.5 mg carfentanil (females)
Supplemental Drug: If animal is not down in 20 minutes, repeat full dose
Antagonist: 1 mg/kg naltrexone
Comments: Prone to excessive running during induction; monitor for hyperthermia. Also prone to sudden rear leg kicking when immobilized.
References: Allen et al., 1991; Clippinger et al., 1998

LEMMING, *Lemmus lemmus*

Weight: 40–112 gm
Recommended Drug: 0.003 mg/gm medetomidine
Supplemental Drug: 0.0015 mg/gm medetomidine
Antagonist: 0.015 mg/gm atipamezole
References: Love, 1970; Genevois et al., 1984a; Jalanka and Roeken, 1990

LEMUR, BLACK, *Eulemur macaco*

Weight: 2–3 kg
Recommended Drug: 6.6 mg/kg tiletamine-zolazepam
Supplemental Drug: 6.6 mg/kg ketamine
Antagonist: None
Alternative Drugs: 12 mg/kg ketamine
References: Beck, 1972; Eads, 1976; Hugues et al., 1986; Schobert, 1987

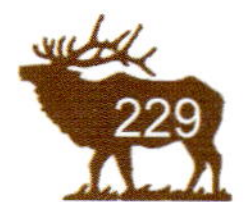

LEMUR, RING-TAILED, *Lemur catta*

Weight: 2.3–3.5 kg
Recommended Drug: 4.4 mg/kg tiletamine-zolazepam
Supplemental Drug: 4.4 mg/kg ketamine
Antagonist: None
Alternative Drugs: 10 mg/kg ketamine plus 1 mg/kg xylazine; antagonize with 1 mg/kg tolazoline
• 0.04 mg/kg medetomidine plus 0.4 mg/kg butorphanol plus 0.3 mg/kg midazolam; antagonize with 0.2 mg/kg atipamezole plus 0.02 mg/kg naloxone plus 0.02 mg/kg IV flumazenil (captive lemurs only; see Williams et al., 2003)
• 12 mg/kg ketamine
References: Seal and Erickson, 1969; Seal et al., 1970; Beck and Dresner, 1972; Gray et al., 1974; Beck, 1976; Schobert, 1987; Strauss, 1987; Williams et al., 2003

LEMUR, RUFFED, *Varecia variegata*

Weight: 3.2–4.5 kg
Recommended Drug: 5 mg/kg tiletamine-zolazepam
Supplemental Drug: 5 mg/kg ketamine
Antagonist: None
Alternative Drugs: 12 mg/kg ketamine
References: Beck, 1976

LEOPARD, CLOUDED, *Panthera nebulaosa*

Weight: 10–20 kg
Recommended Drug: 10 mg/kg tiletamine-zolazepam
Supplemental Drug: 5 mg/kg ketamine
Antagonist: None
Alternative Drugs: 20 mg/kg ketamine plus 2 mg/kg xylazine
References: Seal and Erickson, 1969; Seal et al., 1970; Bauditz, 1972; Beck, 1972; 1976; Hime, 1974; Boever et al., 1977; Nair, 1977; Jessup et al., 1980; Schobert, 1987; Grassman et al., 2004

LEOPARD, *Panthera pardus*

Weight: 50–80 kg
Recommended Drug: 3 mg/kg ketamine plus 0.07 mg/kg medetomidine
Supplemental Drug: 2 mg/kg ketamine
Antagonist: 0.35 mg/kg atipamezole; give 1/2 dose IV, 1/2 IM
Alternative Drugs: 6.6 mg/kg tiletamine-zolazepam
• 10 mg/kg ketamine plus 1 mg/kg xylazine
Comments: Leopards tend to fight rather than flee; always use caution when approaching. Trapping before darting should be considered (see Kock et al., 2006). Long-acting tranquilizer doses: zuclopenthixol (adult male, 70 mg; adult female, 50 mg).

References: Kroll, 1962; Young, 1966; Ericksen, 1968; Bennett and Tillotson, 1969; Pienaar et al., 1969; Seal and Erickson, 1969; Ebedes, 1970; 1973b; Göltenboth and Klös, 1970; Seal et al., 1970; Mathews, 1971; Bauditz, 1972; Beck, 1972; 1976; Holmes and Ngethe, 1973; Smuts et al., 1973; Foster, 1974; Gray et al., 1974; Hime, 1974; Seidensticker et al., 1974; Wentges, 1975; Wiesner, 1975; Bertram and King, 1976; Boever et al., 1977; King et al., 1977; Kuntze, 1977; Nair, 1977; Wiesner, 1977; Jessup et al., 1980; Genevois et al., 1984b; Pathak et al., 1985; Singh and Singh, 1985; Wiesner and von Hegel, 1985; Hugues et al., 1986; Göltenboth and Klös, 1987; Schobert, 1987; Barnett and Lewis, 1990; Jalanka and Roeken, 1990; IWVS, 1992; Rogers, 1992; McKenzie and Burroughs, 1993; Sabapara, 1995; Singh et al., 1995; Kock, M., et al., 2006

LEOPARD, SNOW, *Panthera uncia*

Weight: 25–75 kg
Recommended Drug: 3 mg/kg ketamine plus 0.08 mg/kg medetomidine
Supplemental Drug: 2 mg/kg ketamine
Antagonist: 0.4 mg/kg atipamezole; give 1/2 dose IV, 1/2 IM
Alternative Drugs: 4 mg/kg tiletamine-zolazepam
• 10 mg/kg ketamine plus 2.2 mg/kg xylazine
References: Seal and Erickson, 1969; Seal et al., 1970; Dolensek, 1971; Beck, 1972; 1976; Wentges, 1975; Boever et al., 1977; Jessup et al., 1980; Fanton et al., 1984; Wiesner and von Hegel, 1985; Jalanka, 1987; 1989b; 1989c; Röken, 1987; Schobert, 1987; Barnett and Lewis, 1990; Jackson et al., 1990; Jalanka and Roeken, 1990

LINSANG, BANDED, *Prionodon linsang*

Weight: 0.6–0.8 kg
Recommended Drug: 4.4 mg/kg tiletamine-zolazepam
Supplemental Drug: 4.4 mg/kg ketamine
Antagonist: None
References: Seal and Erickson, 1969; Seal et al., 1970; Gray et al., 1974; Genevois et al., 1984b; Schobert, 1987

LION, *Panthera leo*

Weight: 100–250 kg
Recommended Drug: 2.5 mg/kg ketamine plus 0.07 mg/kg medetomidine
Supplemental Drug: 1.5 mg/kg ketamine
Antagonist: 0.35 mg/kg atipamezole; give 1/2 dose IV, 1/2 IM
Alternative Drugs: 2 mg/kg tiletamine-zolazepam plus 0.07 mg/kg medetomidine; antagonize with 0.35 mg/kg atipamezole
• 5 mg/kg tiletamine-zolazepam
• 7.5 mg/kg ketamine plus 3.5 mg/kg xylazine; antagonize with 0.125 mg/kg yohimbine
Comments: Maintain vigilance for other members of the pride when

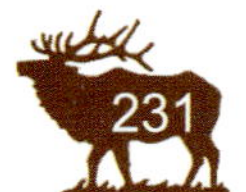

working with an immobilized lion. When using medetomidine, constantly monitor depth of anesthesia as time goes on; animals can wake up suddenly when stimulated. Long-acting tranquilizer doses: zuclopenthixol, 1 mg/kg.
References: Heuschele, 1959; 1961a; Pistey and Wright, 1959; Clifford et al., 1960; 1962; Jarvis and Morris, 1960; Thomas, 1961; Harthoorn and Campbell, 1962; Campbell and Harthoorn, 1963; Larsen, 1963; Graham-Jones, 1964; Young, 1966; Wallach et al., 1967; Ericksen, 1968; Wallach, 1968; 1969; Bennett and Tillotson, 1969; Pienaar et al., 1969; Seal and Erickson, 1969; Krahwinkel, 1970; Seal et al., 1970; Ebedes, 1970; 1973b; Gass, 1970; Göltenboth and Klös, 1970; Krahwinkel, 1970; Bennet et al., 1971; Harthoorn et al., 1971; Bauditz, 1972; Beck, 1972; 1976; York and Huggins, 1972; Holmes and Ngethe, 1973; Smuts et al., 1973; York, 1973; Young and Whyte, 1973; Alford et al., 1974; Eltringham, 1974; Gray et al., 1974; Hime, 1974; Wentges, 1975; Bertram, 1976; Bertram and King, 1976; Boever et al., 1977; King et al., 1977; Kuntze, 1977; Nair, 1977; Wiesner, 1977; Bush et al., 1978; Jessup et al., 1980; Arora et al., 1983; Genevois et al., 1984b; Herbst et al., 1985; Wiesner and von Hegel, 1985; Hugues et al., 1986; Gonzales and McDonnel, 1986; Van Wyk and Berry, 1986; Röken, 1987; Schobert, 1987; Kock et al., 1989; Barnett and Lewis, 1990; Jalanka and Roeken, 1990; Joubert and Stander, 1990; Stander and Morkel, 1991; IWVS, 1992; Chandrasekara Pillai, 1992; Quandt, 1992; Rogers, 1992; McKenzie and Burroughs, 1993; Tomizawa et al., 1997; Ofri et al., 1998; Bengis and Keet, 2000; Stegmann et al., 2000; Epstein et al., 2002; Fahlman et al., 2005a; Jacquier et al., 2006; Kock, M., et al., 2006

LION, MOUNTAIN, *Felis concolor*

Weight: 30–75 kg
Recommended Drug: 2 mg/kg ketamine plus 0.075 mg/kg medetomidine
Supplemental Drug: 1 mg/kg ketamine
Antagonist: 0.3 mg/kg atipamezole
Alternative Drugs: 5 mg/kg tiletamine-zolazepam plus 1 mg/kg xylazine; antagonize with 0.125 mg/kg yohimbine
• 10 mg/kg ketamine plus 2 mg/kg xylazine; antagonize with 0.125 mg/kg yohimbine
References: Heuschele, 1959; Graham-Jones, 1964; Hornocker et al., 1965; Young, 1966; Seal and Erickson, 1969; Göltenboth and Klös, 1970; Seal et al., 1970; Bauditz, 1972; Hornocker and Wiles, 1972; Gray et al., 1974; Hime, 1974; Beck, 1976; Boever et al., 1977; Kuntze, 1977; Wiesner, 1977; Jessup et al., 1980; Jessup, 1982b; Genevois et al., 1984b; Wiesner and von Hegel, 1985; Gonzales and McDonnel, 1986; Logan et al., 1986; Logan et al., 1987; Schobert, 1987; Seal and Kreeger, 1987; Pond and O'Gara, 1994; Davis et al., 1996; Taylor et al., 1998; Schumacher et al., 1999; Wolfe and Miller, 2005

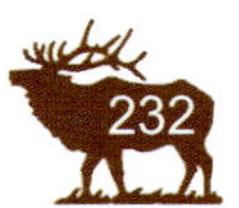

LIZARDS/SKINKS, GENERAL

Recommended Drug: 50 mg/kg ketamine
Supplemental Drug: 25 mg/kg ketamine
Antagonist: None
Alternative Drugs: 30 mg/kg tiletamine-zolazepam
References: Brazenor and Kaye, 1953; Cooper, 1974; Beck, 1976; Wang et al., 1977; Throckmorton, 1981; Amand, 1982b; Garver and Jackson, 1985; Ogunranti, 1987; Arena et al., 1988; Johnson, 1991; Page, 1993; Spelman et al., 1996

LLAMA, *Lama glama*

Weight: 130–155 kg
Recommended Drug: 2 mg/kg ketamine plus 0.07 mg/kg medetomidine
Supplemental Drug: 1 mg/kg ketamine
Antagonist: 0.35 mg/kg atipamezole
Alternative Drugs: 2 mg/kg xylazine; antagonize with 0.125 mg/kg yohimbine
• 4 mg/kg tiletamine-zolazepam
Comments: The dosage for captive, calm llamas can be reduced to 1 mg/kg ketamine plus 0.05 mg/kg medetomidine; antagonize with 0.25 mg/kg atipamezole. The use of opioids in llama is contraindicated (Jones, 1977a).
References: Jarvis and Morris, 1960; Kroll, 1962; Seal and Erickson, 1969; Seal et al., 1970; Gauckler and Kraus, 1970; Bauditz, 1972; Heck and Rivenburg, 1972; Beck, 1972; 1976; York and Huggins, 1972; Rapley and Mehren, 1975; Jones, 1977a; Slee and Walker, 1977; Jessup et al., 1980; Wiesner et al., 1982; Silvestris and Heck, 1984; Wiesner and von Hegel, 1985; Gavier et al., 1986; Hugues et al., 1986; Riebold et al., 1986; Jalanka and Roeken, 1990: Duke et al., 1997; Waldridge et al., 1997; Páras et al., 2002; Arnemo, 2005

LORIS, SLOW, *Nycticebus coucang*

Weight: 0.4–2 kg
Recommended Drug: 11 mg/kg ketamine
Supplemental Drug: 5 mg/kg ketamine
Antagonist: None
References: Seal and Erickson, 1969; Seal et al., 1970; Schulz and Silverman, 1973; Beck, 1976

LYNX, EUROPEAN, *Felis lynx*

Weight: 8–38 kg
Recommended Drug: 5 mg/kg ketamine plus 0.2 mg/kg medetomidine
Supplemental Drug: 2.5 mg/kg ketamine
Antagonist: 1 mg/kg atipamezole
Alternative Drugs: 5 mg/kg tiletamine-zolazepam
• 10 mg/kg ketamine plus 1.5 mg/kg xylazine

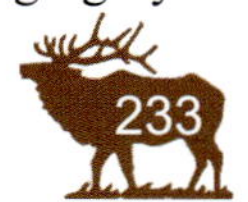

Comments: The ketamine-medetomidine dose can be reduced by 50% for captive lynx. Arnemo et al. (1999) used 5 mg/kg ketamine plus 0.08 mg/kg medetomidine on lynx kittens (4-5 weeks old).
References: Heuschele, 1961; Wiesner, 1977; Oen, 1980; Wiesner and von Hegel, 1985; Jalanka and Roeken, 1990; Arnemo et al., 1999; Schöne et al., 2002; Ryser et al., 2005; Arnemo, 2006

LYNX, IBERIAN, *Felis pardina*

Weight: 10–12 kg
Recommended Drug: 4 mg/kg ketamine plus 4 mg/kg xylazine
Supplemental Drug: 2 mg/kg ketamine
Antagonist: 0.125 mg/kg yohimbine
Alternative Drugs: 5 mg/kg tiletamine-zolazepam
• 10 mg/kg ketamine plus 1.5 mg/kg xylazine
References: Ferreras et al., 1994

LYNX, *Lynx canadensis*

Weight: 5.1–17.2 kg
Recommended Drug: 5 mg/kg tiletamine-zolazepam
Supplemental Drug: 2 mg/kg ketamine
Antagonist: None
Alternative Drugs: 10 mg/kg ketamine plus 2 mg/kg xylazine
References: Heuschele, 1961b; Seal and Erickson, 1969; Seal et al., 1970; Berrie, 1972; Jessup, 1982b; Duchamps, 1985; Seal and Kreeger, 1987; Poole et al., 1993; Pond and O'Gara, 1994

MACAQUE, BARBARY, *Macaca sylvanus*

Weight: 6–15 kg
Recommended Drug: 5 mg/kg ketamine plus 0.07 mg/kg medetomidine
Supplemental Drug: 3 mg/kg ketamine
Antagonist: 0.35 mg/kg atipamezole
Alternative Drugs: 4.4 mg/kg tiletamine-zolazepam
• 15 mg/kg ketamine
References: Bauditz, 1972; Gray et al., 1974; Bush et al., 1977; Schobert, 1987

MACAQUE, BONNET, *Macaca radiata*

Weight: 5–15 kg
Recommended Drug: 6 mg/kg ketamine plus 0.09 mg/kg medetomidine
Supplemental Drug: 3 mg/kg ketamine
Antagonist: 0.45 mg/kg atipamezole
Alternative Drugs: 5 mg/kg tiletamine-zolazepam
• 25 mg/kg ketamine
References: Beck, 1972; Gray et al., 1974; Beck and Dresner, 1972; Jessup et al., 1980; Schobert, 1987

MACAQUE, CRAB-EATING (CYNOMOLGUS), *Macaca fascicularis*

Weight: 5–15 kg
Recommended Drug: 8 mg/kg ketamine plus 0.1 mg/kg medetomidine
Supplemental Drug: 3 mg/kg ketamine
Antagonist: 0.5 mg/kg atipamezole
Alternative Drugs: 5 mg/kg tiletamine-zolazepam
• 20 mg/kg ketamine
References: Graham-Jones, 1964; Beck, 1972; 1976; Beck and Dresner, 1972; Gray et al., 1974; Eads, 1976; Vercruysse and Mortelmans, 1978; Jessup et al., 1980; Castro et al., 1981; Schobert, 1987; Kim et al., 2005

MACAQUE, JAPANESE, *Macaca fuscata*

Weight: 5–15 kg
Recommended Drug: 5 mg/kg ketamine plus 0.1 mg/kg medetomidine
Supplemental Drug: 3 mg/kg ketamine
Antagonist: 0.5 mg/kg atipamezole
Alternative Drugs: 5 mg/kg tiletamine-zolazepam
• 22 mg/kg ketamine
References: Seal et al., 1970; Beck, 1972; 1976; Jessup et al., 1980; Miyabe et al., 2001

MACAQUE, LION-TAIL, *Macaca silenus*

Weight: 5–15 kg
Recommended Drug: 4.4 mg/kg tiletamine-zolazepam
Supplemental Drug: 4.4 mg/kg ketamine
Antagonist: None
Alternative Drugs: 22 mg/kg ketamine
References: Gray et al., 1974; Beck, 1976; Eads, 1976; Bush et al., 1977; Jessup et al., 1980; Singh and Singh, 1982; Schobert, 1987; Smith, J. et al., 2005

MACAQUE, PIG-TAIL, *Macaca nemestrina*

Weight: 5–15 kg
Recommended Drug: 6 mg/kg ketamine plus 0.09 mg/kg medetomidine
Supplemental Drug: 3 mg/kg ketamine
Antagonist: 0.45 mg/kg atipamezole
Alternative Drugs: 4.4 mg/kg tiletamine-zolazepam
• 22 mg/kg ketamine
References: Heuschele, 1961a; 1961b; Larsen, 1963; Field et al., 1966; Seal et al., 1970; Bauditz, 1972; Beck, 1972; Beck and Dresner, 1972; Crittal and Smith, 1972; Gray et al., 1974; Eads, 1976; Bush et al., 1977; Jessup et al, 1980; Schobert, 1987

MACAQUE, RHESUS, *Macaca mulatta*

Weight: 9–12 kg

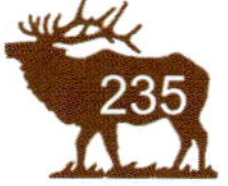

Recommended Drug: 6 mg/kg ketamine plus 0.09 mg/kg medetomidine
Supplemental Drug: 3 mg/kg ketamine
Antagonist: 0.45 mg/kg atipamezole
Alternative Drugs: 2.5 mg/kg ketamine plus 2 mg/kg xylazine
- 6.6 mg/kg tiletamine-zolazepam
- 22 mg/kg ketamine

References: Marsboom et al., 1963; Ericksen, 1968; Seal and Erickson, 1969; Seal et al., 1970; Bauditz, 1972; Beck, 1972; Beck and Dresner, 1972; Alford et al., 1974; Gray et al., 1974; Eads, 1976; Ferin et al., 1976; Channing et al., 1977; Banknieder et al., 1978; Cohen and Bree, 1978; Naccarato and Hunter, 1979; Jessup et al., 1980; Puri et al., 1981; Porter, 1982a; 1982b; Fuller et al., 1984; Hess and Knakal, 1985; Hess et al., 1987; Schobert, 1987; Pulley et al., 2004

MACAQUE, STUMP-TAILED, *Macaca arctoides*

Weight: 5–15 kg
Recommended Drug: 5 mg/kg tiletamine-zolazepam
Supplemental Drug: 5 mg/kg ketamine
Antagonist: None
Alternative Drugs: 22 mg/kg ketamine
References: Beck, 1972; 1976; Beck and Dresner, 1972; Gray et al., 1974; Eads, 1976; Jessup et al., 1980; Schobert, 1987

MACAQUE, TOQUE, *Macaca sinica*

Weight: 2.5–6.1 kg
Recommended Drug: 2.6 mg/kg tiletamine-zolazepam
Supplemental Drug: 2.6 mg/kg ketamine
Antagonist: None
References: Gray et al., 1974; Schobert, 1987

MANATEE, *Trichechus manatus*

Weight: 400–600 kg
Recommended Drug: 0.08 mg/kg diazepam for intubation preceding isoflurane anesthesia
Antagonist: None
References: Walsh and Bossart, 1999

MANDRILL, *Mandrillus sphinx*

Weight: 20–54 kg
Recommended Drug: 2.2 mg/kg tiletamine-zolazepam
Supplemental Drug: 2.2 mg/kg ketamine
Antagonist: None
Alternative Drugs: 15 mg/kg ketamine
References: Seal and Erickson, 1969; Seal et al., 1970; Beck, 1976; Schobert, 1987

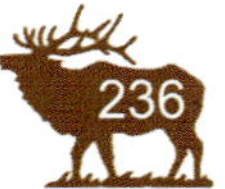

MANGABEY, BLACK, *Lophocebus aterrimus*

Weight: 4–11 kg
Recommended Drug: 7 mg/kg ketamine plus 0.1 mg/kg medetomidine
Supplemental Drug: 3 mg/kg ketamine
Antagonist: 0.5 mg/kg atipamezole

MANGABEY, GRAY-CHEEKED, *Cercocebus albigena*

Weight: 5–20 kg
Recommended Drug: 3 mg/kg tiletamine-zolazepam
Supplemental Drug: 3 mg/kg ketamine
Antagonist: None
References: Schobert, 1987

MANGABEY, SOOTY, *Cercocebus torquatis*

Weight: 5–20 kg
Recommended Drug: 4.4 mg/kg tiletamine-zolazepam
Supplemental Drug: 4.4 mg/kg ketamine
Antagonist: None
Alternative Drugs: 12.5 mg/kg ketamine
References: Marsboom et al., 1963; Seal and Erickson, 1969; Seal et al., 1970; Field et al., 1966; Beck, 1972; Beck and Dresner, 1972; Gray et al., 1974; Schobert, 1987

MARA - SEE CAVY

MARGAY, *Felis tiedii*

Weight: 2.6–3.4 kg
Recommended Drug: 8.8 mg/kg tiletamine-zolazepam
Supplemental Drug: 8.8 mg/kg ketamine
Antagonist: None
Alternative Drugs: 15 mg/kg ketamine plus 1 mg/kg xylazine
References: Seal and Erickson, 1969; Seal et al., 1970; Hime, 1974; Beck, 1976; Seal and Kreeger, 1987

MARKHOR, *Capra falconeri*

Weight: 80–100 kg
Recommended Drug: 2 mg/kg ketamine plus 0.08 mg/kg medetomidine
Supplemental Drug: 1 mg/kg ketamine only
Antagonist: 0.4 mg/kg atipamezole; give 1/2 dose IV, 1/2 IM
Alternative Drugs: 0.022 mg/kg carfentanil; antagonize with 2 mg/kg naltrexone

- 2 mg etorphine plus 20 mg ketamine plus 20 mg xylazine; antagonize with 4 mg diprenorphine plus 0.15 mg/kg yohimbine
- 0.7 ml Large Animal Immobilon® plus 10 mg xylazine; antagonize with 2 mg diprenorphine per mg etorphine given plus 0.15 mg/kg yohimbine

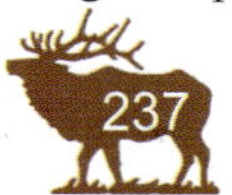

Comments: Rapid, smooth induction (< 5 min) and antagonism (< 10 min) with ketamine/medetomidine.
References: Wiesner, 1975; 1977; Jensen, 1982; Wiesner et al., 1982; 1984; Jalanka, 1987; 1988; 1989a; Barnett and Lewis, 1990; Jalanka and Roeken, 1990; Allen et al., 1991; Snyder et al., 1992

MARMOSET, COTTON TOP - SEE TAMARIN, COTTON HEADED

MARMOSET, GOLDEN - SEE TAMARIN, GOLDEN LION

MARMOSET, SHORT-TUSKED, *Callithrix jacchus*

Weight: 230–453 gm
Recommended Drug: 0.0022 mg/gm tiletamine-zolazepam
Supplemental Drug: 0.0022 mg/gm ketamine
Antagonist: None
Alternative Drugs: 0.005 mg/gm ketamine plus 0.0001 mg/gm medetomidine
References: Gray et al., 1974; Jalanka and Roeken, 1990

MARMOT, ALPINE, *Marmota marmota*

Weight: 1–4 kg
Recommended Drug: 20 mg/kg tiletamine-zolazepam plus 10 mg/kg xylazine
Supplemental Drug: 10 mg/kg tiletamine-zolazepam plus 5 mg/kg xylazine (or isoflurane)
Antagonist: 2 mg/kg tolazoline
Alternative Drugs: 80 mg/kg ketamine plus 20 mg/kg xylazine; antagonize with 2 mg/kg tolazoline
• 70 mg/kg ketamine plus 0.5 mg/kg medetomidine; antagonize with 2 mg/kg atipamezole
Comments: Dosages listed are for late summer or autumn use; dosages may be decreased earlier in the year or for minor procedures (see Beiglböck and Zenker, 2003). Hypothermia was observed for all drug combinations.
References: Beiglböck and Zenker, 2003

MARMOT, HOARY, *Marmota caligata*

Weight: 3–7.5 kg
Recommended Drug: 0.3 ml/kg Innovar-Vet®
Antagonist: 0.2 mg/kg naloxone
References: Noyes and Siekierski, 1975

MARMOT, YELLOW-BELLIED, *Marmota flaviventris*

Weight: 2–5 kg
Recommended Drug: 50 mg/kg ketamine

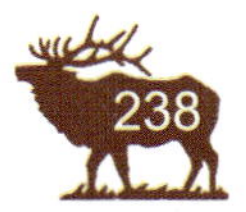

Supplemental Drug: 25 mg/kg ketamine
Antagonist: None
References: Frase and Van Vuren, 1989

MARTEN, PINE, *Martes americanas*

Weight: 0.5–1.5 kg
Recommended Drug: 10 mg/kg ketamine plus 0.2 mg/kg medetomidine
Supplemental Drug: 5 mg/kg ketamine
Antagonist: 1 mg/kg atipamezole
Alternative Drugs: 18 mg/kg ketamine plus 1.6 mg/kg xylazine
• 3 mg/kg tiletamine-zolazepam plus 2 mg/kg xylazine
Comments: A gas-anesthesia machine designed for field use has been successfully used on marten (Herman et al., 1982). Avoid overheating.
References: Jonkel and Weckworth, 1963; Birnbaum et al., 1969; Seal and Erickson, 1969; Seal et al., 1970; Mech, 1974; Wilson, 1976; More, 1977; Jessup et al., 1980; Herman et al., 1982; Jessup, 1982b; Wiesner and von Hegel, 1985; Seal and Kreeger, 1987; Jalanka and Roeken, 1990; Belant, 1992; 2005; Arnemo et al., 1994c; Flynn and Schumacher, 1994; Bull et al., 1996

MINK, *Mustela vison*

Weight: 0.8–1.1 kg
Recommended Drug: 15 mg/kg tiletamine-zolazepam
Supplemental Drug: 15 mg/kg ketamine
Antagonist: None
Alternative Drugs: 5 mg/kg ketamine plus 0.1 mg/kg medetomidine
• 40 mg/kg ketamine plus 1 mg/kg xylazine
References: Fuhrman and Stuhr, 1941; Sandelien, 1966; Graham et al., 1967; Seal and Erickson, 1969; Seal et al., 1970; Beck, 1972; 1976; Gray et al., 1974; Ramsden et al., 1976; Boever et al., 1977; Jessup et al., 1980; Jepsen et al., 1981; Hoilien and Oates, 1982; Jessup, 1982b; Wright, 1983; Genevois et al., 1984b; Schobert, 1987; Seal and Kreeger, 1987; Jalanka and Roeken, 1990; Arnemo and Søli, 1992; Lariviere et al., 2000; 2001

MINK, EUROPEAN, *Mustela lutreola*

Weight: 0.4–1.0 kg
Recommended Drug: 10 mg/kg ketamine plus 0.2 mg/kg medetomidine
Supplemental Drug: 5 mg/kg ketamine
Antagonist: 1 mg/kg atipamezole
Comments: Monitor for hypothermia
References: Fournier-Chambrillon et al., 2003

MONGOOSE, AFRICAN WATER, *Atilax paludinosus*

Weight: 2.5–4.1 kg
Recommended Drug: 5.5 mg/kg tiletamine-zolazepam

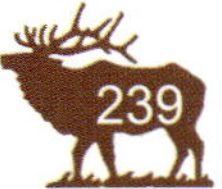

Supplemental Drug: 5.5 mg/kg ketamine
Antagonist: None
Alternative Drugs: 45 mg/kg ketamine
References: Seal et al., 1970; Gray et al., 1974; Genevois et al., 1984b; Schobert, 1987; Maddock, 1989

MONGOOSE, BLACK-LEGGED, *Bdeogale spp.*

Weight: 0.9–3 kg
Recommended Drug: 4.4 mg/kg tiletamine-zolazepam
Supplemental Drug: 4.4 mg/kg ketamine
Antagonist: None
References: Seal et al., 1970; Gray et al., 1974; Schobert, 1987

MONGOOSE, *Herpestes spp.*

Weight: 0.4–4 kg
Recommended Drug: 5 mg/kg tiletamine-zolazepam
Supplemental Drug: 5 mg/kg ketamine
Antagonist: None
Alternative Drugs: 30 mg/kg ketamine plus 0.75 mg/kg acepromazine
- 6 mg/kg ketamine plus 6 mg/kg xylazine
- 45 mg/kg ketamine

References: Seal and Erickson, 1969; Seal et al., 1970; Beltrán et al., 1985; Maddock, 1989; Palomares and Delibes, 1992; McKenzie and Burroughs, 1993

MONGOOSE, MALAGASY RING-TAILED, *Galidia elegans*

Weight: 0.7–0.9 kg
Recommended Drug: 5 mg/kg tiletamine-zolazepam
Supplemental Drug: 5 mg/kg ketamine
Antagonist: None
References: Seal et al., 1970; Gray et al., 1974; Genevois et al., 1984b

MONKEY, AFRICAN GREEN - SEE MONKEY (GUENON), GREEN

MONKEY, ALLEN'S, *Allenopithecus nigroviridis*

Weight: 3.5–6 kg
Recommended Drug: 2.2 mg/kg tiletamine-zolazepam
Supplemental Drug: 2.2 mg/kg ketamine
Antagonist: None
References: Gray et al., 1974; Schobert, 1987

MONKEY (GUENON), BLACK-CHEEKED, *Cercopithecus ascanius*

Weight: 1.8–6.4 kg
Recommended Drug: 18 mg/kg ketamine plus 1.8 mg/kg xylazine
Supplemental Drug: 9 mg/kg ketamine

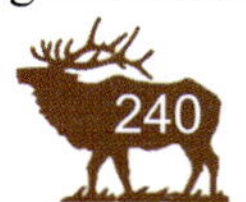

Antagonist: None reported
References: Jones and Bush, 1988

MONKEY (GUENON), BLUE, *Cercopithecus mitis*

Weight: 6–12 kg
Recommended Drug: 9 mg/kg ketamine plus 0.1 mg/kg medetomidine
Supplemental Drug: 3 mg/kg ketamine
Antagonist: 0.5 mg/kg atipamezole

MONKEY, CAPUCHIN, *Cebus spp.*

Weight: 1.1–3.3 kg
Recommended Drug: 10 mg/kg ketamine plus 0.1 mg/kg medetomidine
Supplemental Drug: 3 mg/kg ketamine
Antagonist: 0.5 mg/kg atipamezole
Alternative Drugs: 10 mg/kg tiletamine-zolazepam
• 25 mg/kg ketamine
References: Seal and Erickson, 1969; Seal et al., 1970; Beck, 1972; Beck and Dresner, 1972; Gray et al., 1974; Eads, 1976; Jessup et al., 1980; Schobert, 1987

MONKEY, COLOBUS, *Colobus spp.*

Weight: 5.4–14.5 kg
Recommended Drug: 4.4 mg/kg tiletamine-zolazepam
Supplemental Drug: 4.4 mg/kg ketamine
Antagonist: None
Alternative Drugs: 10 mg/kg ketamine
References: Kroll, 1962; Gray et al., 1974; Bush et al., 1977; Schobert, 1987; Carpenter, 1998

MONKEY (GUENON), DEBRAZZA'S, *Cercopithecus neglectus*

Weight: 4.5–7.8 kg
Recommended Drug: 4.75 mg/kg tiletamine-zolazepam
Supplemental Drug: 4.75 mg/kg ketamine
Antagonist: None
References: Schobert, 1987

MONKEY (GUENON), DIANA, *Cercopithecus diana*

Weight: 3–6 kg
Recommended Drug: 5 mg/kg tiletamine-zolazepam
Supplemental Drug: 5 mg/kg ketamine
Antagonist: None
References: Eads, 1976; Schobert, 1987

MONKEY (GUENON), GREEN, *Chlorocebus sabaeus*

Weight: 3–7 kg

Recommended Drug: 8 mg/kg ketamine plus 0.1 mg/kg medetomidine
Supplemental Drug: 3 mg/kg ketamine
Antagonist: 0.5 mg/kg atipamezole
Alternative Drugs: 5 mg/kg tiletamine-zolazepam
• 15 mg/kg ketamine
References: Seal et al., 1970; Beck, 1972; Gray et al., 1974; Eads, 1976; Bush et al., 1977; Jessup et al., 1980; Schobert, 1987

MONKEY (GUENON), GRIVET, *Cercopithecus aethiops*

Weight: 5–9 kg
Recommended Drug: 7 mg/kg tiletamine-zolazepam
Supplemental Drug: 4 mg/kg ketamine
Antagonist: None
Alternative Drugs: 27 mg/kg ketamine
References: Seal and Erickson, 1969; Beck and Dresner, 1972

MONKEY, HOWLER, *Alouatta spp.*

Weight: 4–10 kg
Recommended Drug: 4 mg/kg ketamine plus 0.15 mg/kg medetomidine
Supplemental Drug: 2 mg/kg ketamine
Antagonist: 0.75 mg/kg atipamezole
Alternative Drugs: 30 mg/kg tiletamine-zolazepam
References: Bush et al., 1977; Schobert, 1987; Glander et al., 1991; Agoramoorthy and Rudran, 1994; Vie and Thoisy, 1996; Vie et al., 1998; Larsen et al., 1999

MONKEY (GUENON), LESSER WHITE-NOSED, *Cercopithecus petaurista*

Weight: 4–8 kg
Recommended Drug: 5 mg/kg ketamine plus 0.08 mg/kg medetomidine
Supplemental Drug: 3 mg/kg ketamine
Antagonist: 0.4 mg/kg atipamezole
Alternative Drugs: 2 mg/kg tiletamine-zolazepam
References: Schobert, 1987

MONKEY (GUENON), MONA, *Cercopithecus mona*

Weight: 3–6 kg
Recommended Drug: 5 mg/kg tiletamine-zolazepam
Supplemental Drug: 5 mg/kg ketamine
Antagonist: None
References: Gray et al., 1974; Schobert, 1987

MONKEY, NIGHT (DOUROUCOULIS), *Aotus trivirgatus*

Weight: 0.6–1 kg
Recommended Drug: 22 mg/kg ketamine

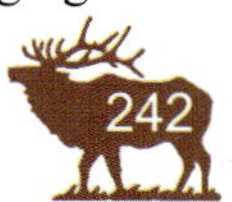

Supplemental Drug: 11 mg/kg ketamine
Antagonist: None
References: Beck, 1972; Beck and Dresner, 1972; Jessup et al., 1980

MONKEY, PATAS, *Erythrocebus patus*

Weight: 4–13 kg
Recommended Drug: 5 mg/kg tiletamine-zolazepam
Supplemental Drug: 5 mg/kg ketamine
Antagonist: None
Alternative Drugs: 10 mg/kg ketamine
References: Seal and Erickson, 1969; Seal et al., 1970; Beck, 1972; 1976; Beck and Dresner, 1972; Gray et al., 1974; Eads, 1976; Bush et al., 1977; Jessup et al., 1980; Schobert, 1987; Kalema-Zikusoka et al., 2003

MONKEY, PROBOSCIS, *Nasalis larvatus*

Weight: 7–11 (f), 16–22.5 (m) kg
Recommended Drug: 22 mg/kg ketamine
Supplemental Drug: 11 mg/kg ketamine
Antagonist: None
References: Heuschele, 1961; Beck, 1976

MONKEY, SPIDER, *Ateles spp.*

Weight: 4–6 kg
Recommended Drug: 5 mg/kg tiletamine-zolazepam
Supplemental Drug: 5 mg/kg ketamine
Antagonist: None
Alternative Drugs: 30 mg/kg ketamine
References: Jarvis and Morris, 1960; Thomas, 1961; Kroll, 1962; Wallach et al., 1967; Wallach, 1968; 1969; Seal et al., 1970; Bauditz, 1972; Beck, 1976; Gray et al., 1974; Eads, 1976; Bush et al., 1977; Schobert, 1987; Karesh et al., 1998; Karesh et al., 1998a

MONKEY, SQUIRREL, *Saimiri spp.*

Weight: 0.7–1.1 kg
Recommended Drug: 10 mg/kg tiletamine-zolazepam
Supplemental Drug: 10 mg/kg ketamine
Antagonist: None
Alternative Drugs: 25 mg/kg ketamine
References: Marsboom et al., 1963; Wallach, 1968; 1969; Seal and Erickson, 1969; Seal et al., 1970; Beck, 1972; Beck and Dresner, 1972; Gray et al., 1974; Eads, 1976; Jessup et al., 1980; Schobert, 1987

MONKEY (GUENON), SYKES, *Cercopithecus albogularis*

Weight: 3–6 kg
Recommended Drug: 3 mg/kg tiletamine-zolazepam

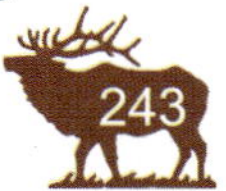

Supplemental Drug: 3 mg/kg ketamine
Antagonist: None
Alternative Drugs: 25 mg/kg ketamine
References: Gray et al., 1974; Beck, 1976; Schobert, 1987

MONKEY, TOQUE - SEE MACAQUE, TOQUE

MONKEY (GUENON), WHITE-NOSED, *Cercopithecus nictitans*

Weight: 2–8 kg
Recommended Drug: 4.4 mg/kg tiletamine-zolazepam
Supplemental Drug: 4.4 mg/kg ketamine
Antagonist: None
References: Schobert, 1987

MONKEY, WOOLY, *Lagothrix spp.*

Weight: 5.5–10.8 kg
Recommended Drug: 7 mg/kg tiletamine-zolazepam
Supplemental Drug: 7 mg/kg ketamine
Antagonist: None
Alternative Drugs: 20 mg/kg ketamine
References: Wallach et al., 1967; Wallach, 1968; 1969; Beck, 1972; 1976; Gray et al., 1974; Jessup et al., 1980; Schobert, 1987

MOOSE, *Alces alces*

Weight: 300–500 kg
Recommended Drug: 0.01 mg/kg carfentanil
Supplemental Drug: If animal is not down in 15 min, repeat full dose
Antagonist: 1 mg/kg naltrexone
Alternative Drugs: 10 mg thiafentanil total dose (yearlings and adults); antagonize with 1 mg/kg naltrexone

- 7.5 mg etorphine (adults) total dose; antagonize with 12 mg diprenorphine
- 1.5 mg/kg ketamine plus 0.1 mg/kg medetomidine; antagonize with 0.3 mg/kg atipamezole
- 4 mg/kg ketamine plus 1 mg/kg xylazine; antagonize with 0.25 mg/kg tolazoline

Comments: The addition of xylazine to carfentanil decreases muscle rigidity caused by using carfentanil alone, but xylazine increases the probability of aspiration pneumonia (Kreeger, 2000). Problems were also observed by Arnemo (unpubl. data) when using etorphine-xylazine and, thus, the addition of xylazine to opioids is not recommended unless there are overriding considerations. Increased mortality and complications have been observed when *underdosing* with etorphine. Renarcotization is possible with either opioid anesthetic; give equal doses of the antagonists both IV and IM.
References: Pimlott and Carberry, 1958; Rausch and Ritcey, 1961; Bergerud et al., 1964; Nielson and Shaw, 1967; Houston, 1969; 1970;

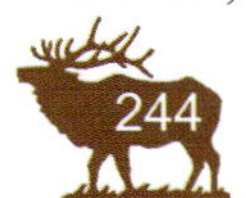

Bauditz, 1972; Alford et al., 1974; Franzmann and Arneson, 1974; Gray et al., 1974; Roussel and Pichette, 1974; Franzmann et al., 1975; 1982; 1984; 1987; Roussel and Patenaude, 1975; Rapley and Mehren, 1975; Wiesner, 1975; 1977; Haigh, 1976d; Haigh et al., 1977; Gasaway et al., 1978; Joyal et al., 1978; Haigh, 1979; Smith and Franzmann, 1979; Jarofke, 1980; Jones, 1978; 1984; Jessup et al., 1980; Ballard and Tobey, 1981; Lynch and Hanson, 1981; Franzmann, 1982; Thorne, 1982; Schwab et al., 1984; Wiesner et al., 1984; Kock and Pearce, 1985; Röken, 1985; Seal et al., 1985b; Sedgwick, 1986; Schmitt and Dalton, 1987; Sandegren et al., 1987; Schobert, 1987; Seal and Bush, 1987; Williams and Riedesel, 1987; Franzmann and Lance, 1988; Schmitt and Aho, 1988; Doherty and Tweedie, 1989; Stanley et al., 1989; Jalanka and Roeken, 1990; Schwartz et al., 1991; Arnemo et al., 1994a; 2003; 2004; Garner and Addison, 1994a; 1994b; McJames et al., 1994; Pond and O'Gara, 1994; Schwartz et al., 1997; Delvaux et al., 1999; Kreeger, 2000; Roffe et al., 2001

MOUFLON, *Ovis musimon*

Weight: 20–32 kg
Recommended Drug: 2.5 mg/kg ketamine plus 0.125 mg/kg medetomidine
Supplemental Drug: 1.5 mg/kg ketamine
Antagonist: 0.6 mg/kg atipamezole
Alternative Drugs: 0.01 mg/kg carfentanil plus 0.25 mg/kg xylazine; antagonize with 1 mg/kg naltrexone plus 0.125 mg/kg yohimbine
• 7 mg/kg tiletamine-zolazepam
• 0.7 ml Large Animal Immobilon® plus 20 mg xylazine; antagonize with 2 mg diprenorphine per mg etorphine given plus 0.125 mg/kg yohimbine
• 2 mg etorphine; antagonize with 2 mg diprenorphine per mg etorphine given
• 0.05 mg/kg fentanyl plus 0.5 mg/kg xylazine; antagonize with 0.2 mg/kg naloxone plus 0.125 mg/kg yohimbine
References: Honich, 1970; Bauditz, 1972; Heck and Rivenburg, 1972; York and Huggins, 1972; Boever and Paluch, 1974; Gray et al., 1974; York, 1975; Wiesner, 1977; Jessup, et al., 1980; Wiesner et al., 1982; 1984; Duchamps, 1985; Hugues et al., 1986; Macek, 1987; Röken, 1987; Schobert, 1987; Barnett and Lewis, 1990; Jalanka and Roeken, 1990; Allen et al., 1991

MOUSE, BRUSH-TAILED MARSUPIAL, *Phascogale tapoatafa*

Weight: 110–135 gm
Recommended Drug: 0.01 mg/gm tiletamine-zolazepam
Supplemental Drug: 0.01 mg/gm ketamine
Antagonist: None
References: Holz, 1992

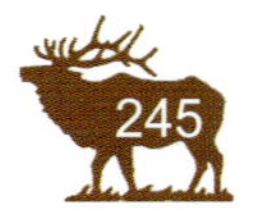

MOUSE, GENERAL

Weight: 5–110 gm

Recommended Drug: 0.044 mg/gm ketamine plus 0.006 mg/gm xylazine

Supplemental Drug: 0.022 mg/gm ketamine

Antagonist: None reported

Alternative Drugs: Ether or methoxyflurane gas anesthesia

• 0.05 mg/gm ketamine plus 0.001 mg/gm medetomidine

Comments: Mice can be effectively anesthetized using a jar and cotton swabs soaked in ether or methoxyflurane; monitor closely and remove as soon as the animal becomes unconscious.

References: Weisbroth and Fudens, 1972; Stunkard and Miller, 1974; Hughes et al., 1975; Mulder, 1978b; Baumgardner and Dewsbury, 1979; Genevois et al., 1984a; Garver and Jackson, 1985; Hahn et al., 2005

MUNTJAC, *Muntiacus muntjak*

Weight: 14–28 kg

Recommended Drug: 3.3 mg/kg ketamine plus 3.3 mg/kg xylazine

Supplemental Drug: 2 mg/kg ketamine

Antagonist: 0.125 mg/kg yohimbine

Alternative Drugs: 0.007 mg/kg carfentanil plus 0.05 mg/kg xylazine; antagonize with 0.7 mg/kg naltexone plus 0.125 mg/kg yohimbine

• 0.1 ml Large Animal Immobilon® plus 3 mg xylazine; antagonize with 2 mg diprenorphine per mg etorphine given

References: Heck and Rivenburg, 1972; Cooper et al., 1984; Seidel and Strauss, 1984; Jensen, 1982; Wiesner et al., 1982; 1984; Arora et al., 1983; Wiesner and von Hegel, 1985; Göltenboth and Klös, 1987; Seal and Bush, 1987

MUNTJAC, REEVES, *Muntiacus reevesi*

Weight: 14–28 kg

Recommended Drug: 3.3 mg/kg ketamine plus 3.3 mg/kg xylazine

Supplemental Drug: 2 mg/kg ketamine

Antagonist: 0.125 mg/kg yohimbine

Alternative Drugs: 8 mg/kg tiletamine-zolazepam

• 0.06 mg/kg etorphine plus 0.025 mg/kg acepromazine; antagonize with 2 mg diprenorphine per mg etorphine given

References: Heck and Rivenburg, 1972; Jones, 1972; 1984; Beck, 1976; Seidel and Strauss, 1984; Cooper et al., 1986; Seal and Bush, 1987; Kock et al., 1989; Bush et al., 1992

MUSKOX, *Ovibos moschatus*

Weight: 200–410 kg

Recommended Drug: 0.0125 mg/kg etorphine plus 0.1 mg/kg xylazine

Supplemental Drug: If not down in 20 min, repeat full dose

Antagonist: 2 mg diprenorphine per mg etorphine givenplus 0.125 mg/kg

yohimbine
Alternative Drugs: 1.5 mg/kg xylazine; antagonize with 0.125 mg/kg yohimbine
Comments: Muskoxen easily overheat in warm weather. It is best to capture them on cool days or during the coolest part of the day. During the rutting season, bulls may require less xylazine (0.5 mg/kg) if you choose to use xylazine alone.
References: Jones, 1971a; 1971b; Bauditz, 1972; Heck and Rivenburg, 1972; Jonkel et al., 1975; Seidel, 1979; Patenaude, 1982b; Wiesner et al., 1982; Reynolds and Garner, 1983; Clausen et al., 1984; Dieterich, 1984; White et al., 1985; Jingfors and Gunn, 1989; Kock et al., 1989; Clausen, 1994

MUSKRAT, *Ondatra zibethicus*

Weight: 0.7–1.8 kg
Recommended Drug: 50 mg/kg ketamine plus 5 mg/kg xylazine
Supplemental Drug: 25 mg/kg ketamine plus 2.5 mg/kg xylazine
Antagonist: 0.125 mg/kg yohimbine
Alternative Drugs: Gas anesthesia such as methoxyflurane or isoflurane
References: Hoilien and Oates, 1982; Seal and Kreeger, 1987; Blanchette, 1989; Lacki et al., 1989; Belant, 1995; 1996; Sleeman et al., 1997b

NILGAI, *Boselaphus tragocamelus*

Weight: 170–240 kg
Recommended Drug: 3.9 mg carfentanil (males); 3 mg carfentanil (females)
Supplemental Drug: If animal is not down in 20 min, repeat full dose
Antagonist: 100 mg naltrexone or naloxone per mg carfentanil given
Alternative Drugs: 6 mg etorphine; antagonize with antagonize with 2 mg diprenorphine per mg etorphine given
• 1.8 ml Large Animal Immobilon® plus 10 mg xylazine antagonize with 2 mg diprenorphine per mg etorphine given plus 0.125 mg/kg yohimbine
• 3 mg/kg xylazine; antagonize with 0.2 mg/kg yohimbine (calm animals only)
Comments: Prone to excessive running during induction with opioids; monitor for hyperthermia.
References: Jarvis and Morris, 1960; Heuschele, 1961a; Wright, 1963; Gauckler and Kraus, 1970; Bauditz, 1972; Heck and Rivenburg, 1972; York and Huggins, 1972; Hertzog, 1975; Mehren and Rapley, 1975; Rapley and Mehren, 1975; York, 1975; Jessup et al., 1980; Singh and Singh, 1982; Wiesner et al., 1982; Silvestris and Heck, 1984; Althouse et al., 1987; Arora, 1988; Kock et al., 1989; Allen et al., 1991; Páras et al., 2002

NUTRIA, *Myocastor coypus*

Weight: 5–10 kg

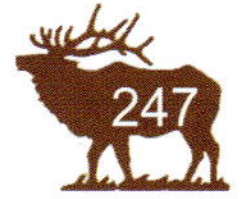

Recommended Drug: 5 mg/kg tiletamine-zolazepam
Supplemental Drug: 5 mg/kg ketamine
Antagonist: None
Alternative Drugs: 4 mg/kg ketamine plus 0.5 mg/kg xylazine
• 5 mg/kg ketamine plus 0.1 mg/kg medetomidine
References: Murry and Dennett, 1963; Van Foreest, 1980; Seal and Kreeger, 1987; Jalanka and Roeken, 1990; Bó et al., 1994

NYALA, *Tragelaphus angasi*

Weight: 60–110 kg
Recommended Drug: 0.1 mg/kg thiafentanil plus 0.2 mg/kg xylazine
Supplemental Drug: 0.05 mg/kg thiafentanil
Antagonist: 2 mg/kg naltrexone plus 0.125 mg/kg yohimbine
Alternative Drugs: 0.08 mg/kg etorphine plus 0.2 mg/kg xylazine; antagonize with 2 mg diprenorphine per mg etorphine given plus 0.125 mg/kg yohimbine
• 1 mg etorphine plus 60 mg ketamine plus 60 mg xylazine; antagonize with 2 mg diprenorphine per mg etorphine given plus 0.15 mg/kg yohimbine
• 0.7 ml Large Animal Immobilon® plus 5 mg xylazine; antagonize with 2 mg diprenorphine per mg etorphine given plus 0.15 mg/kg yohimbine
• 11 mg/kg tiletamine-zolazepam
• 0.045 mg/kg thiafentanil plus 0.07 mg/kg medetomidine plus 200 mg (total) ketamine; antagonize with 1 mg/kg naltrexone plus 5 mg/kg atipamezole
Comments: Nyala are prone to capture myopathy. Use careful dart placement to avoid trauma in small- to medium-sized animals. Hyaluronidase (1,500-3,000 IU) may be added to hasten induction. Long-acting tranquilizer doses: haloperidol (adult male, 15 mg; adult female, 10 mg); zuclopenthixol, 1 mg/kg; perphenazine (adults, 100-150 mg). The use of zuclopenthixol significantly reduces mortalities.
References: Bauditz, 1972; Heck and Rivenburg, 1972; Pienaar, 1973a; Gray et al., 1974; Rapley and Mehren, 1975; Röken, 1975; York, 1975; Haigh, 1976d; Wiesner et al., 1982; Silvestris and Heck, 1984; Schobert, 1987; Kock, R., et al., 1989; Flamand and Rogers, 1992; IWVS, 1992; Burroughs, 1993d; Cooper et al., 2005; Kock, M., et al., 2006

OCEOLOT, *Felis pardalis*

Weight: 11.3–15.8 kg
Recommended Drug: 5 mg/kg tiletamine-zolazepam
Supplemental Drug: 5 mg/kg ketamine
Antagonist: None
Alternative Drugs: 15 mg/kg ketamine plus 1 mg/kg xylazine
References: Larsen, 1963; Seal and Erickson, 1969; Seal et al., 1970; Hime, 1974; Wiesner and von Hegel, 1985; Seal and Kreeger, 1987; Crawshaw and Quigley, 1989; Beltrán and Tewes, 1995; Shindle and Tewes,

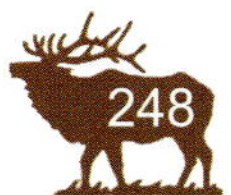

2000; Selmi et al., 2004a

OKAPI, *Okapia johnstoni*

Weight: 200–350 kg

Recommended Drug: 2 mg/kg ketamine plus 0.075 mg/kg medetomidine

Supplemental Drug: 2 mg/kg ketamine

Antagonist: 0.4 mg/kg atipamezole

Alternative Drugs: 0.005 mg/kg carfentanil plus 0.08 mg/kg xylazine; antagonize with 0.5 mg/kg naltrexone plus 0.125 mg/kg yohimbine

Comments: Okapi can be difficult to immobilize; complications secondary to anesthesia are the most significant single cause of death.

References: Mortelmans, 1978; Raphael, 1999

OLINGO, *Bassaricyon gabbii*

Weight: 0.9–1.5 kg

Recommended Drug: 5 mg/kg tiletamine-zolazepam

Supplemental Drug: 5 mg/kg ketamine

Antagonist: None

References: Seal and Erickson, 1969; Seal et al., 1970

ONAGER - SEE KULAN

OPOSSUM, NORTH AMERICAN, *Didelphis virginianus*

Weight: 2–5.5 kg

Recommended Drug: 10 mg/kg ketamine plus 2 mg/kg xylazine

Supplemental Drug: 5 mg/kg ketamine

Antagonist: None reported

Alternative Drugs: 15 mg/kg tiletamine-zolazepam

• 20 mg/kg ketamine

References: Mosby and Cantner, 1956; Seal and Erickson, 1969; Seal et al., 1970; Feldman and Self, 1971; Beck, 1972; 1976; Haupert and Lindeen, 1974; Hughes et al., 1975; Smeller et al., 1977; Hoilien and Oates, 1982; Scott and Kolata, 1982; Wright, 1983; Seal and Kreeger, 1987; Stoskopf et al., 1999

ORANGUTAN, *Pongo pygmaeus*

Weight: 30–50 (f), 50–70 (m) kg

Recommended Drug: 3.5 mg/kg tiletamine-zolazepam

Supplemental Drug: 3.5 mg/kg ketamine

Antagonist: None

Alternative Drugs: 6.5 mg/kg ketamine plus 0.8 mg/kg xylazine

References: Kroll, 1962; Wallach et al., 1967; Seal et al., 1970; Beck, 1972; Beck and Dresner, 1972; Gray et al., 1974; Bush et al., 1977; Vercruysse and Mortelmans, 1978; Jessup et al., 1980; Robinson and Lambert, 1986; Göltenboth and Klös, 1987; Schobert, 1987; Kock et al.,

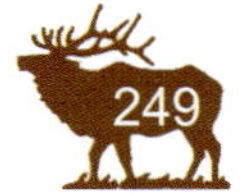

1989; Andau et al., 1994; Hunter et al., 2004

ORIBI, *Ourebia ourebi*

Weight: 8–15 kg
Recommended Drug: 0.1 mg/kg etorphine plus 2 mg/kg azaperone
Supplemental Drug: 0.05 mg/kg etorphine
Antagonist: 2 mg diprenorphine per mg etorphine given
Alternative Drugs: 0.8 mg/kg fentanyl plus 2 mg/kg azaperone
• 6 mg/kg tiletamine-zolazepam
Comments: Monitor for respiratory depression when using opioids.
References: Van Niekerk et al., 1963a; Pienaar and Van Niekerk, 1963; Viljoen, 1981; IWVS, 1992; Burroughs, 1993d; Kock et al., 2006

ORYX, ARABIAN, *Oryx leucoryx*

Weight: 80–120 kg
Recommended Drug: 3 mg carfentanil plus 5 mg xylazine
Supplemental Drug: If animal is not down in 15 minutes, repeat full dose
Antagonist: 3 mg/kg naltexone plus 0.125 mg/kg yohimbine
Alternative Drugs: 2 mg/kg tiletamine-zolazepam plus 0.2 mg/kg xylazine; antagonize with 0.125 mg/kg yohimbine
• 0.03 mg/kg etorphine plus 0.3 mg/kg xylazine; antagonize with 0.06 mg/kg diprenorphine plus 0.125 mg/kg yohimbine
• 0.05 mg/kg etorphine plus 0.05 mg/kg medetomidine; antagonize with 0.1 mg/kg diprenorphine plus 0.025 mg/kg atipamezole
• 0.5 mg/kg xylazine; antagonize with 0.09 mg/kg atipamezole or 0.125 mg/kg yohimbine (calm animals only)
• 0.06 mg/kg medetomidine; antagonize with 0.25 mg/kg atipamezole (calm animals only)
References: Graham-Jones, 1964; Machado et al., 1983; Kock et al., 1989; Allen et al., 1991; Bush et al., 1992; Greth et al., 1993; Ancrenaz, 1994; Ancrenaz et al., 1995; 1996; Flamand, 1999

ORYX, SCIMITAR-HORNED, *Oryx dammah*

Weight: 100–210 kg
Recommended Drug: 3 mg carfentanil plus 10 mg xylazine (males); 2.5 mg carfentanil (females)
Supplemental Drug: If animal is not down in 15 minutes, repeat full dose
Antagonist: 3 mg/kg naltrexone plus 0.125 mg/kg yohimbine
Alternative Drugs: 0.04 mg/kg etorphine plus 0.05 mg/kg xylazine; antagonize with 0.08 mg/kg diprenorphine plus 0.125 mg/kg yohimbine
• 9.4 mg/kg tiletamine-zolazepam
• 3 mg/kg xylazine; antagonize with 0.125 mg/kg yohimbine (calm animals only)
References: Bauditz, 1972; Heck and Rivenburg, 1972; Rapley and Mehren, 1975; Röken, 1975; Silvestris and Heck, 1984; Kock et al., 1989;

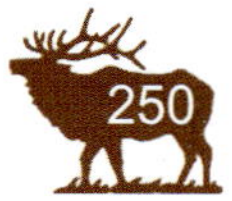

Allen et al., 1991; Majonica and Bonath, 1993; Páras et al., 2002

OSTRICH, *Struthio camelus*

Weight: 100–150 kg

Recommended Drug: 3 mg carfentanil plus 150 mg xylazine

Supplemental Drug: 1.5 mg carfentanil

Antagonist: 300 mg naltrexone plus 20 mg yohimbine

Alternative Drugs: 3.6 mg etorphine plus 25 mg acepromazine plus 200 mg xylazine; antagonize with 7.6 mg diprenorphine plus 0.125 mg/kg yohimbine

- 10 mg/kg ketamine plus 0.5 mg/kg xylazine; antagonize with 0.125 mg/kg yohimbine
- 10 mg/kg tiletamine-zolazepam

Comments: Ostriches have thin skin; use low-impact darts. They are also highly susceptible to complications and capture myopathy if pursued or handled roughly. Avoid capture at temperatures > 28½ C (82.4½ F). Upon induction and recovery, ostriches may thrash with their head and neck, resulting in injury; underdosing tends to exacerbate this head thrashing. Attempt to immobilize and restrain the bird as quickly as possible. Do not approach birds until fully recumbent because this may stimulate them to rise and prolong induction. Ostriches have a thick (50 mm) layer of fat under the skin in the abdominal region which can slow down drug absorption if injected in this site. The primary targets are the muscle masses of the legs and back. Tiletamine-zolazepam or ketamine may result in prolonged and/or rough recoveries; diazepam (1 mg/kg) may be given IV as soon as the animal attempts to rise to smooth recovery. If diprenorphine is used to antagonize opioid anesthesia, monitor for 24 hours for renarcotization. Xylazine should be avoided in very sick birds.

References: Harthoorn, 1971; Blackshaw and Wakeman, 1972; York and Huggins, 1972; Robinson and Fairfield, 1974; Beck, 1976; Stoskopf et al., 1982; Gandini et al., 1986; Schobert, 1987; Samour et al., 1990; Van Heerden and Keffen, 1991; Cornick and Jensen, 1992; IWVS, 1992; Raath et al., 1992; Keffen, 1993; Matthews, 1993; Jensen et al., 1994; Ostrowski and Ancrenaz, 1995; Burroughs, 1996; Lin and Ko, 1997; Lin et al., 1997; Langan et al., 2000; Stegman, 2000; Kock, M., et al., 2006

OTTER, AMERICAN RIVER, *Lontra canadensis*

Weight: 7–9 kg

Recommended Drug: 2.5 mg/kg ketamine plus 0.025 mg/kg medetomidine

Supplemental Drug: 2 mg/kg ketamine

Antagonist: 0.1 mg/kg atipamezole

Alternative Drugs: 4 mg/kg tiletamine-zolazepam

- 10 mg/kg ketamine plus 0.25 mg/kg midazolam
- 7.5 mg/kg ketamine plus 1.5 mg/kg xylazine

References: Seal and Erickson, 1969; Seal et al., 1970; Gray et al., 1974;

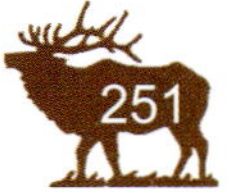

Boever et al., 1977; Kane, 1979; Jessup et al., 1980; Jenkins and Gorman, 1981; Jessup, 1982b; Elmore et al., 1985; Genevois et al., 1984b; Hoover, 1984; 1985; Hoover et al., 1984; Woolf et al., 1984; Elmore et al., 1985; Hoover and Jones, 1986; Erickson and McCullough, 1987; Göltenboth and Klös, 1987; Schobert, 1987; Spelman et al., 1993a; 1993b; 1994; 1997a; 1997b; Spelman, 1999; Muller et al., 2005

OTTER, ASIAN SMALL-CLAWED, *Aonyx cinerea*

Weight: 1–5 kg
Recommended Drug: 5 mg/kg ketamine plus 0.12 mg/kg medetomidine
Supplemental Drug: 2.5 mg/kg ketamine
Antagonist: 0.6 mg/kg atipamezole
Alternative Drugs: 5.5 mg/kg tiletamine-zolazepam
• 10 mg/kg ketamine
References: Seal and Erickson, 1969; Seal et al., 1970; Beck, 1976; Kane, 1979; Lindsay and Lloyd, 1991; Spelman, 1999

OTTER, CLAWLESS, *Aonyx capensis*

Weight: 13–34 kg
Recommended Drug: 5 mg/kg tiletamine-zolazepam
Supplemental Drug: 2.5 mg/kg ketamine
Antagonist: None
Alternative Drugs: 8 mg/kg ketamine plus 1 mg/kg xylazine
References: McKenzie and Burroughs, 1993

OTTER, EUROPEAN, *Lutra lutra*

Weight: 3–14 kg
Recommended Drug: 5 mg/kg ketamine plus 0.05 mg/kg medetomidine
Supplemental Drug: 2.5 mg/kg ketamine
Antagonist: 0.25 mg/kg atipamezole
Alternative Drugs: 20 mg/kg ketamine plus 2 mg/kg xylazine
• 15 mg/kg ketamine plus 0.5 mg/kg diazepam
References: Holmes, 1974; Jenkins and Gorman, 1981; Reuther, 1983; Reuther and Brandes, 1984; Wiesner and von Hegel, 1985; Kuiken, 1988; Arnemo, 1989; 1990; Spelman, 1999; Fernandez-Moran et al., 2001; 2002; 2004

OTTER, SEA, *Enhydra lutris*

Weight: 15–32 (f), 22–45 (m) kg
Recommended Drug: 0.3 mg/kg fentanyl plus 0.1 mg/kg diazepam
Supplemental Drug: 0.15 mg/kg fentanyl
Antagonist: 0.6 mg/kg naltrexone
Alternative Drugs: 0.2 mg/kg fentanyl plus 1 mg/kg xylazine, antagonize with 0.2 mg/kg naloxone and 0.15 mg/kg yohimbine
• 0.3 mg/kg fentanyl plus 0.25 mg/kg azaperone

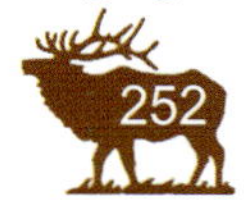

• 3 mg/kg tiletamine-zolazepam

Comments: Avoid overheating by monitoring rectal temperature.

References: Stullken and Kirkpatrick, 1955; Williams, 1978; 1990; Williams and Kocher, 1978; Jessup et al., 1980; Williams et al., 1981; 1990a; 1990b; 1992; Jessup, 1982b; Joseph et al., 1987; Schobert, 1987; Seal and Kreeger, 1987; Sawyer and Williams, 1996; Spelman, 1999; Haulena and Heath, 2001; Monson et al., 2002

OTTER, SPOTTED-NECKED, *Lutra maculicollis*

Weight: 3–14 kg

Recommended Drug: 5 mg/kg tiletamine-zolazepam

Supplemental Drug: 5 mg/kg ketamine

Antagonist: None

Alternative Drugs: 8 mg/kg ketamine plus 1 mg/kg xylazine

References: McKenzie and Burroughs, 1993

OWL, BARN, *Tyto alba*

Weight: 600–800 gm

Recommended Drug: 0.03 mg/gm tiletamine-zolazepam

Supplemental Drug: 0.03 mg/gm ketamine

Antagonist: None

References: Camburn and Stead, 1978; Schobert, 1987; Mama et al., 1996

OWL, BARRED, *Strix varia*

Weight: 500–900 gm

Recommended Drug: 0.01 mg/gm ketamine plus 0.001 mg/gm diazepam, IV

Supplemental Drug: 0.005 mg/gm ketamine, IV

Antagonist: None

Alternative Drugs: 0.02 mg/gm ketamine plus 0.002 mg/gm acepromazine

References: Mattingly, 1972; Redig and Duke, 1976; Jessup et al., 1980; Freed and Baker, 1989

OWL, GREAT HORNED, *Bubo virgianus*

Weight: 1.1–1.4 kg

Recommended Drug: 10 mg/kg tiletamine-zolazepam

Supplemental Drug: 10 mg/kg ketamine

Antagonist: None

Alternative Drugs: 25 mg/kg ketamine plus 1.2 mg/kg diazepam, IV

• 20 mg/kg ketamine plus 2 mg/kg acepromazine

References: Mattingly, 1972; Borzio, 1973; Frank and Cooper, 1974; Redig and Duke, 1976; Jessup et al., 1980; Redig et al., 1984; Freed and Baker, 1989; Kreeger et al., 1993; Hawkins et al., 2003

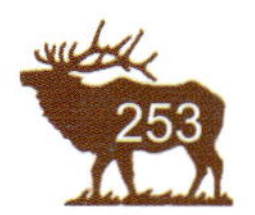

OWL, SCREECH, *Otus asio*

Weight: 150–300 gm
Recommended Drug: 0.01 mg/gm tiletamine-zolazepam
Supplemental Drug: 0.01 mg/gm ketamine
Antagonist: None
Alternative Drugs: 0.02 mg/gm ketamine plus 0.002 mg/gm acepromazine
References: Kittle, 1972; Mattingly, 1972; Borzio, 1973; Beck, 1976; Jessup et al., 1980; Kreeger et al., 1993

OWL, SNOWY, *Nyctea scandiaca*

Weight: 1.8–2.1 kg
Recommended Drug: 18 mg/kg ketamine plus 1.2 mg/kg diazepam, IV
Supplemental Drug: 5 mg/kg ketamine, IV
Antagonist: None
References: Redig and Duke, 1976

OWLS, GENERAL

Recommended Drug: 20 mg/kg ketamine plus 2 mg/kg acepromazine
Supplemental Drug: 10 mg/kg ketamine
Antagonist: None
References: Borzio, 1973; Camburn and Stead, 1978; Amand, 1982a

PACA, *Agouti paca*

Weight: 6–10 kg
Recommended Drug: 25 mg/kg ketamine plus 0.125 mg/kg acepromazine
Supplemental Drug: 15 mg/kg ketamine
Antagonist: None
References: Pachaly and Werner, 1998

PACARANA, *Dinomys branickii*

Weight: 10–15 kg
Recommended Drug: 4.4 mg/kg tiletamine-zolazepam
Supplemental Drug: 4.4 mg/kg ketamine
References: Schobert, 1987

PADEMELON, RED-LEGGED, *Thylogale stigmatica*

Weight: 2–12 kg
Recommended Drug: 6 mg/kg tiletamine-zolazepam
Supplemental Drug: 6 mg/kg ketamine
Antagonist: None
References: Shima et al., 1993

PANDA, GIANT, *Ailuropoda melanoleuca*

Weight: 75–160 kg
Recommended Drug: 5 mg/kg ketamine plus 0.4 mg/kg xylazine

Supplemental Drug: 2.5 mg/kg ketamine
Antagonist: None reported
Alternative Drugs: 6.6 mg/kg tiletamine-zolazepam
References: Graham-Jones, 1964; Schaller et al., 1985; Fan et al., 1987; Schobert, 1987; Yu and Yu, 1987; Qiu, 1990; Zhu and Wang, 1992; Mainka and He, 1993

PANDA, LESSER, *Ailurus fulgens*

Weight: 3–6 kg
Recommended Drug: 5 mg/kg tiletamine-zolazepam
Supplemental Drug: 5 mg/kg ketamine
Antagonist: None
Alternative Drugs: 4 mg/kg ketamine plus 0.1 mg/kg medetomidine; antagonize with 0.5 mg/kg atipamezole
• 10 mg/kg ketamine plus 2 mg/kg xylazine
References: Seal et al., 1970; Custer et al., 1978; Schobert, 1987; Jalanka and Roeken, 1990; Chakraborty, 1993

PANGOLIN, *Manis tetradactyla*

Weight: 2–2.5 kg
Recommended Drug: 22 mg/kg ketamine
Supplemental Drug: 11 mg/kg ketamine
Antagonist: None
References: Seal and Erickson, 1969; Seal et al., 1970; Robinson, 1983; IWVS, 1992

PARROTS, GENERAL

Recommended Drug: 10 mg/kg ketamine plus 1 mg/kg diazepam
Supplemental Drug: 5 mg/kg ketamine
Antagonist: None
Alternative Drugs: 10 mg/kg tiletamine-zolazepam
References: Beck, 1976; Amand, 1982a; Schobert, 1987

PECCARY, CHACOAN, *Catagonus wagneri*

Weight: 29.5–40 kg
Recommended Drug: 2.2 mg/kg tiletamine-zolazepam
Supplemental Drug: 2.2 mg/kg ketamine
Antagonist: None
References: Allen, 1992b; Sutherland-Smith et al., 2004

PECCARY, COLLARED, *Tayassu tajacu*

Weight: 14–30 kg
Recommended Drug: 4.4 mg/kg tiletamine-zolazepam plus 2.2 mg/kg xylazine
Supplemental Drug: If not down in 15 minutes, repeat full dose

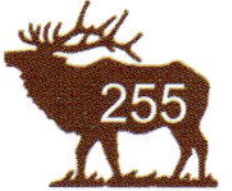

Antagonist: 0.15 mg/kg yohimbine
Alternative Drugs: 8 mg/kg ketamine plus 10 mg/kg xylazine
References: Kroll, 1962; Dyson, 1965; Jewell et al., 1965; Day, 1969; Seal et al., 1970; Jones, 1972; Gray et al., 1974; Gallagher et al., 1985; Hellgren et al., 1985; Schobert, 1987; Kock et al., 1989; Gabor et al., 1997; Páras et al., 2002; Selmi et al., 2003

PECCARY, WHITE-LIPPED, *Tayassu pecari*

Weight: 20–50 kg
Recommended Drug: 1.5 mg/kg tiletamine-zolazepam plus 0.14 mg/kg butorphanol
Supplemental Drug: If not down in 15 minutes, repeat full dose
Antagonist: None reported
References: Selmi et al., 2003

PENGUIN, KING, *Aptenodytes patagonicus*

Weight: 12–14 kg
Recommended Drug: 5 mg/kg tiletamine-zolazepam
Supplemental Drug: 5 mg/kg ketamine
Antagonist: None
References: Thil and Groscolas, 2002

PIG, WILD - SEE HOG, EUROPEAN WILD

POLECAT - SEE FERRET

PORCUPINE, CAPE, *Hystrix africaeustralis*

Weight: 12–18 kg
Recommended Drug: 5 mg/kg ketamine plus 0.05 mg/kg medetomidine
Supplemental Drug: 2.5 mg/kg ketamine
Antagonist: 0.2 mg/kg atipamezole
Alternative Drugs: 5 mg/kg ketamine plus 1.5 mg/kg xylazine
• 0.16 mg/kg fentanyl plus 0.66 mg/kg xylazine; antagonize with 0.2 mg/kg naloxone plus 0.2 mg/kg yohimbine
References: Van Aarde, 1985

PORCUPINE, CRESTED, *Hystrix cristata*

Weight: 9–15 kg
Recommended Drug: 10 mg/kg ketamine plus 2 mg/kg xylazine
Supplemental Drug: 5 mg/kg ketamine only
Antagonist: None reported
Alternative Drugs: 7.25 mg/kg tiletamine-zolazepam
Comments: Porcupines require high doses for complete immobilization. The recommended dose may only heavily sedate the animal and additional ketamine may be required for surgery or other manipulations.

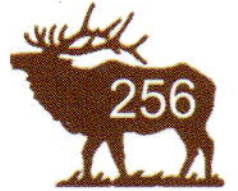

References: Beck, 1976; Stoskopf, 1979; Pigozzi, 1987; Massolo et al., 2003

PORCUPINE, INDIA CRESTED, *Hystrix indica*

Weight: 10–30 kg
Recommended Drug: 15 mg/kg ketamine plus 1 mg/kg xylazine
Supplemental Drug: 10 mg/kg ketamine
Antagonist: None reported
References: Bose et al., 1982; Alkon, 1984

PORCUPINE, NORTH AMERICAN, *Erethizon dorsatum*

Weight: 3.5–11 kg
Recommended Drug: 5 mg/kg ketamine plus 2 mg/kg xylazine
Supplemental Drug: 5 mg/kg ketamine
Antagonist: 0.15 mg/kg yohimbine
Alternative Drugs: 10 mg/kg tiletamine-zolazepam
Comments: The tail muscles are the optimal injection site for porcupines (see Morin and Berteaux. 2003)
References: Seal and Erickson, 1969; Seal et al., 1970; Hale et al., 1994; Griesemer et al., 1999; Morin and Berteaux. 2003

POSSUM, BRUSH-TAIL, *Trichosurus vulpecula*

Weight: 1.3–5 kg
Recommended Drug: 10 mg/kg tiletamine-zolazepam
Supplemental Drug: 5 mg/kg ketamine
Antagonist: None
Alternative Drugs: 50 mg/kg ketamine
References: Denny, 1974; Smeller et al., 1977; Shima et al., 1993; Viggers and Lindenmayer, 1995

POSSUM, MOUNTAIN PYGMY, *Burramys parvus*

Weight: 30–60 gm
Recommended Drug: 0.007 mg/gm tiletamine-zolazepam
Supplemental Drug: 0.003 mg/gm ketamine
Antagonist: None
References: Holz, 1992

POSSUM, RINGTAIL, *Pseudocheirus peregrinus*

Weight: 0.7–1 kg
Recommended Drug: 7.5 mg/kg tiletamine-zolazepam
Supplemental Drug: 7.5 mg/kg ketamine
Antagonist: None
Alternative Drugs: 10 mg/kg ketamine
References: Bush et al., 1990; Holz, 1992; Salas and Stephens, 2004

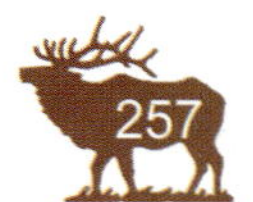

POTOROO, *Potorous spp.*

Weight: 0.5–2.2 kg
Recommended Drug: 9.5 mg/kg tiletamine-zolazepam
Supplemental Drug: 5 mg/kg ketamine
Antagonist: None
References: Bush et al., 1990

POTOROO, LONG-NOSED, *Potorous tridactylus*

Weight: 0.7–1.3 kg
Recommended Drug: 15 mg/kg tiletamine-zolazepam
Supplemental Drug: 15 mg/kg ketamine
Antagonist: None
Alternative Drugs: 25 mg/kg ketamine plus 0.2 mg/kg acepromazine
References: Alford et al., 1974; Finnie, 1976; Smeller et al., 1977; Ludders and Ojerio, 1980; Schobert, 1987

PRAIRIE DOG, BLACK-TAILED, *Cynomys ludovicianus*

Weight: 0.7–1.5 kg
Recommended Drug: 30 mg/kg ketamine plus 0.5 mg/kg diazepam
Supplemental Drug: 15 mg/kg ketamine only
Antagonist: None
Alternative Drugs: 20 mg/kg tiletamine-zolazepam
References: Roslyn et al., 1979; Stoskopf, 1979

PRONGHORN, *Antilocapra americana*

Weight: 40–50 kg
Recommended Drug: 0.05 mg/kg carfentanil plus 1 mg/kg xylazine
Supplemental Drug: If animal is not down in 20 min, repeat full dose
Antagonist: 5 mg/kg naltrexone plus 0.125 mg/kg yohimbine
Alternative Drugs: 0.1 mg/kg thiafentanil; antagonize with 2 mg/kg naltrexone

- 0.1 mg/kg etorphine plus 1 mg/kg xylazine, antagonize with 0.2 mg/kg diprenorphine plus 0.125 mg/kg yohimbine
- 5 mg/kg ketamine plus 0.3 mg/kg medetomidine; antagonize with 1.5 mg/kg atipamezole

Comments: In our experience, thiafentanil (A-3080) has been the most satisfactory drug for pronghorn, followed by carfentanil-xylazine. However, thiafentanil is not yet readily available. To reduce renarcotization with carfentanil, give a double dose of the antagonists, one IV and the other IM. Even after antagonism, expect the animal to undergo a period (up to 30 min) of excitement (rapid pacing, tongue hanging out, etc.). Do *not* give xylazine to a pronghorn if you are not going to use an antagonist - prolonged hyperexcitability may ensue. We have also used the ketamine-medetomidine combination with some success on captive (not excited) pronghorn. In general, combinations like ketamine-xylazine and tiletamine-zolazepam-xylazine give

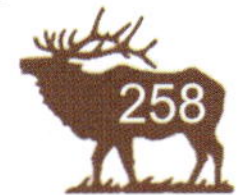

unpredicatable results; the animal becomes recumbent only to stumble away when you try to approach it. Pronghorn are extraordinarily difficult to immobilize; be prepared for less than satisfactory results.
References: Jarvis and Morris, 1960; Thomas, 1961; Dyson, 1965; Beale and Smith, 1967; Gray et al., 1974; Chalmers and Barrett, 1977; Copeland et al., 1978; Seal and Hoskinson, 1978; Amstrup and Segerstrom, 1981; Autenrieth et al., 1981; Pusateri et al., 1982; Thorne, 1982; Carpenter and Lance, 1983; O'Gara, 1987; Schobert, 1987; Williams and Riedesel, 1987; Pond and O'Gara, 1994; Kreeger et al., 1999; 2001

PUDU, *Pudu puda*

Weight: 6–13 kg
Recommended Drug: 2.5 mg/kg ketamine plus 0.07 mg/kg medetomidine plus 0.3 mg/kg butorphanol
Supplemental Drug: 2.5 mg/kg ketamine
Antagonist: 0.35 mg/kg atipamezole plus 0.1 mg/kg naltrexone
Comments: Dosage based on ten captive pudu.
References: Fabry et al., 2001

PUKU, *Kobus vardoni*

Weight: 50–90 kg
Recommended Drug: 25 mg fentanyl plus 150 mg azaperone
Supplemental Drug: If animal is not down in 20 minutes, repeat full dose
Antagonist: 0.2 mg/kg naltrexone or naloxone
References: Hanks and Dowsett, 1969; Haigh, 1976d

PUMA - SEE LION, MOUNTAIN

QUOKKA, *Setonix brachyurus*

Weight: 2–5 kg
Recommended Drug: 8 mg/kg ketamine plus 8 mg/kg xylazine
Supplemental Drug: 4 mg/kg ketamine only
Antagonist: None reported
References: Richardson and Cullen, 1984

RABBIT, COTTONTAIL, *Sylvilagus floridanus*

Weight: 0.8–1.5 kg
Recommended Drug: 44 mg/kg ketamine plus 5 mg/kg xylazine
Supplemental Drug: 22 mg/kg ketamine
Antagonist: None
Alternative Drugs: 44 mg/kg ketamine plus 5 mg/kg acepromazine
• 44 mg/kg ketamine plus 10 mg/kg diazepam
References: Wesson et al., 1977; Garver and Jackson, 1985

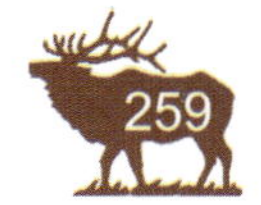

RABBIT, *Oryctolagus cuniculus*

Weight: 1.3–2.2 kg
Recommended Drug: 30 mg/kg ketamine plus 6 mg/kg xylazine
Supplemental Drug: 15 mg/kg ketamine
Antagonist: 0.22 mg/kg yohimbine
Alternative Drugs: 44 mg/kg ketamine plus 5 mg/kg acepromazine

- 44 mg/kg ketamine plus 10 mg/kg diazepam
- 22 mg/kg tiletamine-zolazepam

References: Weisbroth and Fudens, 1972; Stunkard and Miller, 1974; Hughes et al., 1975; Kisloff, 1975; White and Holmes, 1976; Garver and Jackson, 1985; Wiesner and von Hegel, 1985; Schobert, 1987; Hellebrekers et al., 1997; Keller et al., 1988; Flecknell et al., 1996; 1999

RACCOON, *Procyon lotor*

Weight: 2–12 kg
Recommended Drug: 20 mg/kg ketamine plus 4 mg/kg xylazine
Supplemental Drug: 10 mg/kg ketamine
Antagonist: 0.15 mg/kg yohimbine
Alternative Drugs: 20 mg/kg ketamine plus 0.1 mg/kg acepromazine

- 3 mg/kg tiletamine-zolazepam plus 2 mg/kg xylazine

References: Murry and Dennett, 1963; Mech, 1965; Seal and Erickson, 1969; Seal et al., 1970; Bigler and Hoff, 1974; Gray et al., 1974; Haupert and Lindeen, 1974; Gregg and Olson, 1975; Hughes et al., 1975; Speckmann, 1975; Beck, 1976; Ramsden et al., 1976; Boever et al., 1977; Jessup et al., 1980; Hoilien and Oates, 1982; Jessup, 1982b; Wright, 1983; Genevois et al., 1984b; Wiesner and von Hegel, 1985; Clutton and Duggan, 1986; Schobert, 1987; Seal and Kreeger, 1987; Deresienki and Rupprecht, 1989; Servin and Huxley, 1992; Taulman and Williamson, 1993; Norment et al., 1994; Pond and O'Gara, 1994; Belant, 1995a; 2004; Gehrt et al., 2001

RAPTORS, GENERAL

Recommended Drug: 5 mg/kg ketamine plus 0.5 mg/kg xylazine IV
Supplemental Drug: 2.5 mg/kg ketamine IV
Antagonist: None
Alternative Drugs: 30 mg/kg ketamine plus 1 mg/kg diazepam IM
References: Haigh, 1980

RAT, NORWAY, *Rattus norvegicus*

Weight: 200–400 gm
Recommended Drug: 0.025 mg/gm tiletamine-zolazepam
Supplemental Drug: 0.025 mg/gm ketamine
Antagonist: None
Alternative Drugs: 0.044 mg/gm ketamine
References: Weisbroth and Fudens, 1972; Hughes et al., 1975; Genevois et al., 1984a; Schobert, 1987

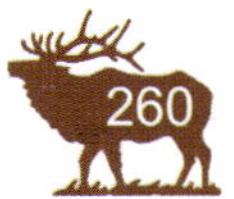

RAT, BUSHY-TAILED WOOD, *Neotoma cinerea*

Weight: 115–350 gm
Recommended Drug: 0.075 mg/gm ketamine
Supplemental Drug: 0.035 mg/gm ketamine
Antagonist: None
References: Frase and Van Vuren, 1989

RATEL - SEE BADGER, HONEY

RATITES, GENERAL

Recommended Drug: 40 mg/kg ketamine plus 1 mg/kg diazepam
Supplemental Drug: 20 mg/kg ketamine
Antagonist: None
References: Amand, 1982a

RATS, GENERAL

Weight: 0.2–1 kg
Recommended Drug: 50 mg/kg ketamine
Supplemental Drug: 25 mg/kg ketamine
Antagonist: None
Alternative Drugs: 50 mg/kg ketamine plus 1 mg/kg medetomidine
References: Stunkard and Miller, 1974; Mulder and Johnson, 1978; Garver and Jackson, 1985; Hahn et al., 2005

REEDBUCK, *Redunca arundinum*

Weight: 50–75 kg
Recommended Drug: 0.04 mg/kg thiafentanil plus 1 mg/kg azaperone
Supplemental Drug: If not down in 15 minutes, repeat full dose
Antagonist: 0.8 mg/kg naltrexone
Alternative Drugs: 3 mg etorphine plus 5 mg xylazine; antagonize with 6 mg diprenorphine plus 0.15 mg/kg yohimbine
• 1 mg/kg ketamine plus 0.1 mg/kg medetomidine; antagonize with 0.25 mg/kg atipamezole
• 12 mg fentanyl plus 75 mg azaperone
References: Pienaar, 1968a; 1973; Jones, 1972; Röken, 1975; Haigh, 1976d; Hofmeyr, 1981; Flamand and Rogers, 1992; IWVS, 1992; Burroughs, 1993d; Kock, 2001; Kock, M., et al., 2006

REEDBUCK, MOUNTAIN, *Redunca fulvorufula*

Weight: 25–35 kg
Recommended Drug: 2 mg etorphine plus 40 mg azaperone
Supplemental Drug: 1 mg etorphine
Antagonist: 2 mg diprenorphine per mg etorphine given
Alternative Drugs: 0.04 mg/kg thiafentanil plus 1 mg/kg azaperone; antagonize with 0.8 mg/kg naltrexone

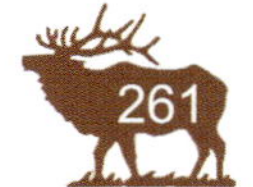

Comments: Long-acting tranquilizer doses: haloperidol (adult male, 20 mg; adult female, 15 mg; subadult, 10 mg; neonate, 5 mg); zuclopenthixol, 1 mg/kg; perphenazine (adults, 30 mg).
References: Burroughs, 1993d; Kock, M., et al., 2006

REINDEER - SEE CARIBOU

REPTILES, GENERAL

Weight: <50 gm
Recommended Drug: 0.1 mg/gm ketamine
Supplemental Drug: 0.05 mg/gm ketamine
Alternative Drugs: 0.04 mg/gm ketamine plus 0.008 mg/gm xylazine

Weight: 50 gm–1 kg
Recommended Drug: 0.05 mg/gm ketamine
Supplemental Drug: 0.025 mg/gm ketamine
Alternative Drugs: 0.025 mg/gm ketamine plus 0.005 mg/gm xylazine

Weight: 1–20 kg
Recommended Drug: 25 mg/kg ketamine
Supplemental Drug: 12 mg/kg ketamine
Alternative Drugs: 10 mg/kg ketamine plus 2 mg/kg xylazine

Weight: 20–50 kg
Recommended Drug: 12 mg/kg ketamine
Supplemental Drug: 6 mg/kg ketamine
Alternative Drugs: 7.5 mg/kg ketamine plus 1.5 mg/kg xylazine

Weight: 50–100 kg
Recommended Drug: 8 mg/kg ketamine
Supplemental Drug: 4 mg/kg ketamine
Alternative Drugs: 5 mg/kg ketamine plus 1 mg/kg xylazine
Comments: Reptiles should be acclimated to their preferred ambient temperature (30–35 ½C/86–95½ F) prior to immobilization. Complete behavioral recovery from anesthesia can take *days*. Never assume an anesthetized, venomous reptile is incapable of biting – take appropriate precautions when handling such animals. Alphaxalone/alphadolone has been shown effective in many reptiles (see Lawrence, 1988). Gas anesthesia may be preferable over injectables for many reptiles.
References: Hinsch and Gandal, 1969; Kaplan, 1969; Beck, 1976; Ahmad et al., 1977; Jones, 1977b; Boever, 1979; Sedgwick, 1980b; Jackson et al., 1981; Boever and Caputo, 1982; Genevois et al., 1983a; Lawrence, 1983; Cooper, 1984; 1987; Harper, 1984; Sedgwick, 1986; Adest et al., 1988; Arena et al., 1988; Bennett, 1991; 1993a; 1994; 1998; Bienzle and Boyd, 1991; Frye, 1991; Boyer, 1992; Pietrak, 1992; Avery, 1993a; Hochleithner,

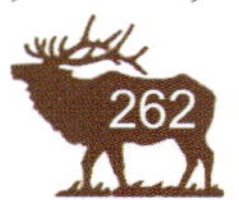

1993; Schildger et al., 1993; Holz and Holz, 1994; Schumacher, 1999; Heard, 2001; Maas and Brunson, 2002; Bertelsen et al., 2004; 2005

RHEA, *Rhea americana*

Weight: 15–25 kg
Recommended Drug: 22 mg/kg tiletamine-zolazepam
Supplemental Drug: 11 mg/kg ketamine
Antagonist: None
References: Beck, 1976; Camburn and Stead, 1978; Schobert, 1987; Matthews, 1993; Lin snd Ko, 1997; Lin et al., 1997

RHEBOK, GREY, *Pelea capreolus*

Weight: 20–35 kg
Recommended Drug: 0.01 mg/kg thiafentanil plus 1 mg/kg azaperone
Supplemental Drug: 0.005 mg/kg thiafentanil
Antagonist: 1 mg/kg naltrexone
Alternative Drugs: 0.01 mg/kg etorphine plus 0.4 mg/kg xylazine; antagonize with 1 mg/kg naltrexone plus 0.25 mg/kg yohimbine
• 0.01 mg/kg carfentanil plus 0.4 mg/kg xylazine; antagonize with 1 mg/kg naltrexone plus 0.25 mg/kg yohimbine
• 0.2 mg/kg fentanyl plus 0.4 mg/kg xylazine
• 10 mg fentanyl plus 20 mg azaperone
Comments: Monitor for respiratory depression when using opioids. Long-acting tranquilizer doses: haloperidol (adult male, 20 mg; adult female, 15 mg; subadult, 10 mg; neonate, 5 mg); zuclopenthixol, 1 mg/kg; perphenazine (adults, 30 mg).
References: Van Niekerk et al., 1963a; IWVS, 1992; Burroughs, 1993d; Howard et al., 2003; 2004; Kock et al., 2006

RHINOCEROS, BLACK, *Diceros bicornis*

Weight: 800–1,400 kg
Recommended Drug: 4.5 mg etorphine plus 250 mg azaperone
Supplemental Drug: 2 mg etorphine
Antagonist: 2 mg diprenorphine per mg etorphine given
Alternative Drugs: 1 mg etorphine plus 30 mg fentanyl plus 200 mg azaperone; antagonize with 2 mg diprenorphine
• 4 mg etorphine plus 100 mg xylazine; antagonize with 8 mg diprenorphine
• 0.0015 mg/kg carfentanil plus 0.15 mg/kg azaperone; antagonize with 0.15 mg/kg naltrexone
Comments: Hyaluronidase (2,000 IU) should always be added to the drug mixture to hasten induction. Monitor for respiratory depression (< 4 breaths/min); administer 200 mg doxapram, if necessary. Oxygenation can be improved by titrating with 5–10 mg nalorphine IV; this will not cause complete antagonism of etorphine. Partial antagonism with 10 mg nalorphine may also assist in "walking" a rhino into a transport crate (Kock et al.,

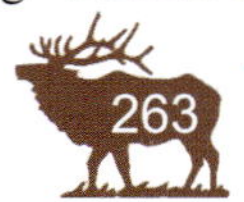

2006). Transport of rhino may be facilitated by using long-acting tranquilizers (Reuter and Winterbach, 1998). Change the animal's position every 20 minutes. If body temperature exceeds 41½ C (105.8½ F), consider giving the antagonist immediately. For calves (100-500 kg), use 2 mg etorphine plus 75 mg azaperone. Long-acting tranquilizer doses: zuclopenthixol (adults, 300 mg); perphenazine (adults, 300 mg; subadults, 100 mg; juveniles, 50 mg).
References: Buechner et al., 1960a; 1960c; Harthoorn, 1960; 1962b; 1963a; 1963d; 1965a; 1966; 1972a; 1973a; 1973b; Harthoorn and Lock, 1960; 1961; Larsen, 1963; Condy, 1964; King and Carter, 1965; Ebedes, 1966b; 1967; Jones, 1966; Jones and Roth, 1968; Wallach, 1968; 1969; Denney, 1969; Keep et al., 1969; King, 1969; Hitchins et al., 1972; Hofmeyr and de Bruine, 1973; Keep, 1973b; 1973c; Alford et al., 1974; De Vos, 1975; Eltringham, 1974; Manton and Jones, 1974; Hofmeyr, 1975; Röken, 1975; Haigh, 1976d; 1977b; Flamand et al., 1984; MacKintosh and Van Reenen, 1984b; Henwood, 1989; Morkel, 1989; Gaynor and Haigh, 1992; Kock et al., 1990a; 1990b; 1990c; Kock, 1992; IWVS, 1992; Kock and Morkel, 1993; Jessup et al., 1993; Rogers, 1993c; Reuter and Winterbach, 1998; Fahlman et al., 2004; Portas, 2004; Adams et al., 2005; Kock, M., et al., 2006

RHINOCEROS, INDIAN, *Rhinoceros unicornis*

Weight: 1,600–2,200 kg
Recommended Drug: 2.25 mg etorphine plus 10 mg acepromazine
Supplemental Drug: 2 mg etorphine
Antagonist: 2 mg diprenorphine per mg etorphine given
Alternative Drugs: 3.8 mg etorphine plus 14 mg detomidine plus 400 mg ketamine; antagonize with 300 mg naltrexone
References: Alford et al., 1974; Dinerstein et al., 1990; Atkinson et al., 2002; Portas, 2004

RHINOCEROS, SUMATRAN, *Dicerorhinus sumatrensis*

Weight: 800–1,000 kg
Recommended Drug: 0.3 mg/kg butorphanol plus 0.06 mg/kg detomidine
Antagonist: None reported, but naltrexone and atipamezole should be effective
References: Portas, 2004

RHINOCEROS, WHITE, *Ceratotherium simum*

Weight: 1,400–1,700 (f), 2,000–2,300 (m) kg
Recommended Drug: 3 mg etorphine plus 12 mg detomidine (f); 4 mg etorphine plus 20 mg detomidine (m)
Supplemental Drug: 1 mg etorphine
Antagonist: 150 mg naltrexone plus 60 mg atipamezole
Alternative Drugs: 0.001 mg/kg carfentanil plus 0.1 mg/kg azaperone; antagonize with 0.1 mg/kg naltrexone

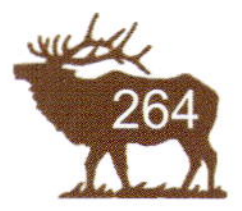

- 1.6 ml Large Animal Immobilon®; antagonize with 2 mg diprenorphine per mg etorphine given

Comments: Use large needles (45–60 mm length, ≥ 2 mm diam.) with minimal barb. The needle tip can be bent over the axis of the bore to prevent plugging or side port needles can be used. The dart injection site must be treated with antimicrobial agent to prevent abcesses. Hyaluronidase (1,500-3,000 IU) combined with immobilizing agent can speed induction. Prolonged recumbency may cause respiratory depression. Close monitoring is necessary, particularly if immobilization exceeds 40 minutes. Try to maintain the animal in sternal recumbency; however, if the animal ran some distance before induction, keeping it on its side for 5-10 minutes before rolling it on its sternum may decrease any lactic acid developed in the leg muscles (Kock et al., 2006). Oxygenation can be improved by giving 10–20 nalorphine or 20-40 nalbuphine IV immediately after induction; this will not cause complete antagonism of etorphine (Kock et al., 1995). Respirations may also be increased by administering 300-400 mg doxapram IV. The white rhino is particularly prone to renarcotization after carfentanil use; if at all possible use naltrexone to antagonize. Complications include hypoxia and hyperthermia. Oxygen insufflation may help to increase oxygen saturation (Bush et al., 2004). Muscle tremors can be reduced by giving 15 mg diazepam IV. Try to avoid darting at ambient temperatures >25½ C (77½ F). Cool the animal if body temperature >39½ C (102.2½ F). If hypoxia is evident, the pulse rate is >120 bpm, and body temperature is >39½ C, antagonize the immobilizing agent immediately. If the animal is being transported, it may be beneficial to antagonize the opioid anesthetic with diprenorphine instead of naltrexone because naltrexone can result in a fully alert animal that might fight the crate throughout transport (Rogers, 1993b). A combination of butorphanol (70 mg) plus azaperone (100 mg) has been shown effective for calm, captive rhinos (Radcliffe et al., 2000). Captive rhino can be immobilized with 1.5 mg etorphine. Long-acting tranquilizer doses: zuclopenthixol (adults, 300 mg); perphenazine (adults, 300 mg; subadults, 100 mg; juveniles, 50 mg).

References: Harthoorn, 1962a; 1962b; 1962c; 1963a; 1963d; 1965a; 1967; 1972a; 1973a; 1973b; Harthoorn and Player, 1963; Van Niekerk et al., 1963a; Ebedes, 1966b; Pienaar et al., 1966a; Wallach, 1966; Player, 1967; 1973; Wallach, 1968; 1969; Keep, 1969; 1971; 1972a; 1972b; 1973b; Pienaar, 1969a; York and Huggins, 1972; Alford et al., 1974; Manton and Jones, 1974; De Vos, 1975; Röken, 1975; Smuts, 1975; Haigh, 1976d; Jenkins, 1978; Wiesner et al., 1982; Flamand et al., 1984; LeBlanc et al., 1987; Allen et al., 1991; Heard et al., 1992; IWVS, 1992; Rogers, 1993b; Hattingh et al., 1994c; Raath, 1994; 1999; Kock, M., et al., 1995; 2006; Radcliffe et al., 2000; Walzer et al., 2000; Kock, 2001; Fahlman et al., 2004; Bush et al., 2004a; Portas, 2004

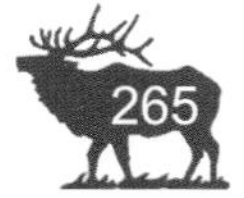

RINGTAIL, *Bassariscus astutus*

Weight: 0.8–1.3 kg
Recommended Drug: 10 mg/kg tiletamine-zolazepam
Supplemental Drug: 10 mg/kg ketamine
Antagonist: None
Alternative Drugs: 15 mg/kg ketamine plus 0.2 mg/kg acepromazine
References: Seal and Erickson, 1969; Seal et al., 1970; Gray et al., 1974; Jessup et al., 1980; Jessup, 1982b; Seal and Kreeger, 1987

ROAN - SEE ANTELOPE, ROAN

SABLE, *Hippotragus niger*

Weight: 150–260 kg
Recommended Drug: 0.03 mg/kg thiafentanil plus 0.4 mg/kg azaperone
Supplemental Drug: If not down in 15 minutes, repeat full dose
Antagonist: 0.6 mg/kg naltrexone
Alternative Drugs: 6 mg etorphine plus 20 mg xylazine; antagonize with 12 mg diprenorphine plus 0.125 mg/kg yohimbine

- 3 mg/kg tiletamine-zolazepam plus 0.2 mg/kg xylazine; antagonize with 0.15 mg/kg yohimbine
- 3 mg carfentanil plus 50 mg ketamine plus 50 mg xylazine; antagonize with 1 mg/kg naltrexone plus 0.125 mg/kg yohimbine
- 3 mg/kg xylazine; antagonize with 0.125 mg/kg yohimbine (calm animals only)

Comments: Prone to hyperthermia because of dark coat. Sable are very sensitive to xylazine or other alpha-adrenergic agonists; be sure to antagonize if used. Sable may not go down totally with etorphine; thiafentanil is drug of choice (Kock et al., 2006). Handle bulls separately to avoid intraspecific aggression. Semi-immobilized animals may be attacked by other sable, particularly from another herd. Restrain horns at all times. Long-acting tranquilizer doses: haloperidol (adults, 15 mg; subadult, 10 mg); zuclopenthixol (adult male, 300 mg; adult female, 225 mg; subadult, 125 mg); perphenazine (adults, 100 mg; subadults, 50 mg).
References: Pienaar et al., 1966a; Pienaar, 1968a; 1969b; 1973a; Göltenboth and Klös, 1970; Bauditz, 1972; Heck and Rivenburg, 1972; York and Huggins, 1972; Grobler and Van der Meulen, 1975; Röken, 1975; Smuts, 1975; York, 1975; Haigh, 1976d; Jones, 1977; Slee and Walker, 1977; Hofmeyr, 1981; Silvestris and Heck, 1984; Wiesner and von Hegel, 1985; Schobert, 1987; Strauss, 1987; Williams and Riedesel, 1987; Henwood and Keep, 1989; Bush et al., 1992; Snyder et al., 1992; Burroughs, 1993d; Kock, M., et al., 2006

SAIGA, RUSSIAN, *Saiga tatarica*

Weight: 29–69 kg
Recommended Drug: 2.1 mg carfentanil

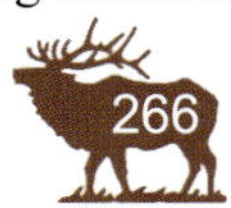

Supplemental Drug: If animal is not down in 15 minutes, repeat full dose
Antagonist: 4 mg/kg naltexone
Alternative Drugs: 7.4 mg/kg ketamine plus 4 mg/kg xylazine; antagonize with 1.2 mg/kg tolazoline
Comments: Prone to excessive running during induction with carfentanil. Monitor for hyperthermia and respiratory depression.
References: Jensen, 1982; Strauss, 1987; Allen et al., 1991

SAMBAR, *Cervus unicolor*

Weight: 109–260 kg
Recommended Drug: 2.1 mg carfentanil plus 30 mg xylazine (males); 1.2 mg carfentanil plus 15 mg xylazine (females)
Supplemental Drug: If animal is not down in 15 min, repeat full dose
Antagonist: 1 mg/kg naltrexone plus 0.125 mg/kg yohimbine
Alternative Drugs: 0.7 ml Large Animal Immobilon® plus 30 mg xylazine; antagonize with 2 mg diprenorphine per mg etorphine given plus 0.125 mg/kg yohimbine
- 6.6 mg/kg tiletamine-zolazepam
- 10 mg fentanyl plus 80 mg azaperone plus 100 mg xylazine (i.e., Fentaz® plus xylazine); antagonize with 0.2 mg/kg naloxone plus 2 mg/kg tolazoline

References: Rapley and Mehren, 1975; Wiesner, 1975; Nair, 1977; Keep, 1979; Wiesner et al., 1982; Arora et al., 1983; Jones, 1984; Wiesner and von Hegel, 1985; Mac Lentz et al., 1986; Schobert, 1987; Seal and Bush, 1987; Strauss, 1987; Arora, 1988; Van Mourik et al., 1988; Allen et al., 1991; Tung et al., 1993

SAMBAR, PHILLIPINE, *Cervus mariannus*

Weight: 40–60 kg
Recommended Drug: 6.6 mg/kg tiletamine-zolazepam
Supplemental Drug: 3.3 mg/kg ketamine
Antagonist: None
References: Gray et al., 1974; Schobert, 1987

SAMBAR, SUNDA, *Cervus timorensis*

Weight: 53–73 kg
Recommended Drug: 0.6 mg carfentanil plus 15 mg xylazine
Supplemental Drug: If animal is not down in 15 min, repeat full dose
Antagonist: 100 mg naltexone plus 0.125 mg/kg yohimbine
Alternative Drugs: 0.05 mg/kg etorphine plus 0.2 mg/kg acepromazine; antagonize with 0.1 mg/kg diprenorphine
References: Jones, 1972; 1978; 1984; Presidente et al., 1978b; Keep, 1979; Van Mourik and Stelmasiak, 1984; Seal and Bush, 1987; Allen et al., 1991

SEA LION, CALIFORNIA, *Zalophus californianus*

Weight: 50–110 (f), 200–400 (m) kg

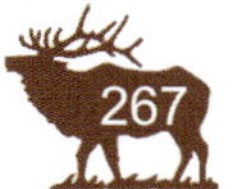

Recommended Drug: 2.5 mg/kg ketamine plus 0.14 mg/kg medetomidine
Supplemental Drug: 1.25 mg/kg ketamine (or isoflurane)
Antagonist: 0.2 mg/kg atipamezole
Alternative Drugs: 4 mg/kg ketamine plus 0.5 mg/kg xylazine
• 10 mg/kg ketamine plus 0.22 mg/kg midazolam or diazepam
• 1.0 mg/kg tiletamine-zolazepam plus 0.07 mg/kg medetomidine; antagonize with 2 mg/kg atipamezole
• Isoflurane
Comments: 0.02 mg/kg atropine may be added to the recommended dose to decrease secretions. For long procedures, you may wish to intubate the animal and use gas anesthesia. Isoflurane or halothane alone can be used to induce and anesthetize medium-sized females and pups using only physical restraint and a portable anesthesia machine (see Work et al., 1992; 1993; Heath et al., 1997; Paras et al., 1998). If seal becomes anoxic due to prolonged apnea, intubate with cuffed endotracheal tube and manually ventilate; doxapram IV may also be given.
References: Heuschele, 1961a; 1961b; Kroll, 1962; Ericksen, 1968; Ridgway and Simpson, 1969; Geraci, 1973; Beck, 1976; Gray et al., 1974; McGrath et al., 1979; Trillmich and Wiesner, 1979; Trillmich, 1983; Gage, 1984; 1993; Joseph and Cornell, 1988; Gales, 1989; Williams et al., 1990a; Work et al., 1992; 1993; Heard and Beusse, 1993; Heath et al., 1994; 1997; Paras et al., 1998; Haulena et al., 1998; 2000; Haulena and Gulland, 2001; Haulena and Heath, 2001; Spelman et al., 2004; Yamaya et al., 2006

SEA LION, NORTHERN (STELLER), *Eumetopias jubatus*

Weight: 270 (f), 1,000 (m) kg
Recommended Drug: 2.1 mg/kg ketamine
Supplemental Drug: 1 mg/kg ketamine
Antagonist: None
Alternative Drugs: 2 mg/kg Ttiletamine-zolazepam; do not give supplemental dose of tiletamine-zolazepam
Comments: 0.02 mg/kg atropine may be added to the recommended dose to decrease secretions. For extended immobilization times, induce with tiletamine-zolazepam then maintain on gas anesthesia. If induction with tiletamine-zolazepam is rapid (< 6 min), be prepared to stimulate respiration either chemically or manually.
References: Loughlin and Spraker, 1989; Gage, 1993; Heath et al., 1994; 1996; Haulena and Heath, 2001; Johnson et al., 2004

SEA LION, SOUTHERN, *Otaria flavescens*

Weight: 140 (f), 200–350 (m) kg
Recommended Drug: 2 mg/kg tiletamine-zolazepam
Supplemental Drug: 1 mg/kg ketamine
Antagonist: None
Comments: Monitor closely for hyperthermia, particularly when ambient

temperature >20½ C (68½ F). If seal becomes anoxic due to prolonged apnea, intubate with cuffed endotracheal tube and manually ventilate; doxapram IV may also be given.
References: Cárdenas and Cattan, 1986; IWVS, 1992; Haulena and Heath, 2001

SEAL, ANTARCTIC FUR, *Arctocephalus gazella*

Weight: 30–51 (f), 126–160 (m) kg
Recommended Drug: 5 mg/kg ketamine plus 1 mg/kg xylazine
Supplemental Drug: 2.5 mg/kg ketamine
Antagonist: None reported
Alternative Drugs: 1.7 mg/kg tiletamine-zolazepam; do not give supplemental dose of tiletamine-zolazepam
Comments: 0.02 mg/kg atropine may be added to the recommended dose to decrease secretions. For long procedures, you may wish to intubate the animal and use gas anesthesia. If seal becomes anoxic due to prolonged apnea, intubate with cuffed endotracheal tube and manually ventilate; doxapram IV may also be given.
References: Bester, 1988; Gales, 1989; Boyd et al., 1990; Williams et al., 1990a; Gage, 1993; Haulena and Heath, 2001

SEAL, CRABEATER, *Lobodon carcinophagus*

Weight: 200–300 kg
Recommended Drug: 6 mg/kg ketamine plus 0.2 mg/kg diazepam
Supplemental Drug: 3 mg/kg ketamine
Antagonist: None
Alternative Drugs: Isoflurane (see Gales et al., 2005)
Comments: If seal becomes anoxic due to prolonged apnea, intubate with cuffed endotracheal tube and manually ventilate; doxapram IV may also be given.
References: Cline et al., 1969; Vergani et al., 1986; Gales, 1989; Williams et al., 1990a; Shaughnessy, 1991; Gage, 1993; Lynch et al., 1999; Haulena and Heath, 2001; Tahmindjis et al., 2003; Gales et al., 2005

SEAL, GALAPAGOS FUR, *Arctocephalus galapagoensis*

Weight: 27 (f), 64 (m) kg
Recommended Drug: 4 mg/kg ketamine plus 0.5 mg/kg xylazine
Supplemental Drug: 2 mg/kg ketamine
Antagonist: None reported
Alternative Drugs: 1.7 mg/kg tiletamine-zolazepam; do not give supplemental dose of tiletamine-zolazepam
• 4.5 mg/kg ketamine plus 0.14 mg/kg diazepam
Comments: 0.02 mg/kg atropine may be added to the recommended dose to decrease secretions. Monitor continually for hyperthermia. The ketamine/diazepam dose may be given intravenously in restrained seals for a more

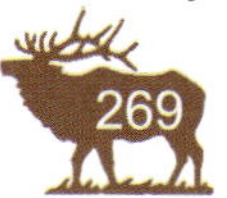

rapid induction. For long procedures, you may wish to intubate the animal and use gas anesthesia. If seal becomes anoxic due to prolonged apnea, intubate with cuffed endotracheal tube and manually ventilate; doxapram IV may also be given.
References: Trillmich, 1983; Cardenas and Cattan, 1986; Gales, 1989; Gage, 1993; Haulena and Heath, 2001; Páras et al., 2002b

SEAL, GRAY, *Halichoerus grypus*

Weight: 105–186 (f), 170–310 (m) kg
Recommended Drug: 1 mg/kg tiletamine-zolazepam
Supplemental Drug: 0.5 mg/kg ketamine only
Antagonist: None
Alternative Drugs: 4 mg/kg ketamine plus 0.75 mg/kg xylazine
• 6 mg/kg ketamine plus 0.2 mg/kg diazepam
Comments: Use needles over 60 mm long to penetrate blubber layer. Opioids are not recommended because they can cause prolonged apnea which must be antagonized to avoid death. If seal becomes anoxic due to prolonged apnea, intubate with cuffed endotracheal tube and manually ventilate; doxapram IV may also be given.
References: Jewell and Smith, 1965; Parry et al., 1981; Geraci et al., 1981; Baker and Gatesman, 1985; Baker et al., 1988; 1990; Gales, 1989; Williams et al., 1990a; Gage, 1993; Haulena and Heath, 2001

SEAL, GUADALUPE FUR, *Arctocephalus phillipi*

Weight: 50 (f), 140 (m) kg
Recommended Drug: 3.6 mg/kg ketamine plus 0.12 mg/kg diazepam
Supplemental Drug: 1.8 mg/kg ketamine
Antagonist: None
Comments: The recommended drug combination may be given IV, but the dose should be reduced by 50% and heart rate and core body temperature should be monitored throughout immobilization.
References: Cardenas and Cattan, 1986; Sepúlveda et al., 1994

SEAL, HARBOR (COMMON), *Phoca vitulina*

Weight: 50–150 (f), 70–170 (m) kg
Recommended Drug: 1.5 mg/kg tiletamine-zolazepam
Supplemental Drug: 1 mg/kg ketamine
Antagonist: None
Alternative Drugs: 1.5 mg/kg ketamine plus 0.05 mg/kg diazepam
Comments: 0.02 mg/kg atropine may be added to the recommended dose to decrease secretions. For long procedures, you may wish to intubate the animal and use gas anesthesia. If seal becomes anoxic due to prolonged apnea, intubate with cuffed endotracheal tube and manually ventilate; doxapram IV may also be given.
References: Finer, 1954; Kroll, 1962; Geraci, 1973; Hammond and Elsner,

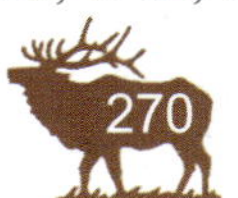

1977; Geraci et al., 1981; Sinnett et al., 1981; Gage, 1984; 1993; Joseph and Cornell, 1988; Gales, 1989; Williams et al., 1990a; Gulland et al., 1999; Tuomi et al., 2000; Haulena and Heath, 2001

SEAL, HARP, *Phoca groenlandica*

Weight: 120–135 kg
Recommended Drug: 6 mg/kg ketamine plus 0.2 mg/kg diazepam
Supplemental Drug: 3 mg/kg ketamine
Antagonist: None
Alternative Drugs: Isoflurane
Comments: If seal becomes anoxic due to prolonged apnea, intubate with cuffed endotracheal tube and manually ventilate; doxapram IV may also be given.
References: McDonell, 1972; Beck, 1976; Engelhardt, 1977; Gales, 1989; Williams et al., 1990a; Gage, 1993; Haulena and Heath, 2001; Pang et al., 2006

SEAL, HOODED, *Cystophora cristata*

Weight: 145–300 (f), 200–400 (m) kg
Recommended Drug: 6 mg/kg ketamine plus 0.2 mg/kg diazepam
Supplemental Drug: 3 mg/kg ketamine
Antagonist: None
Comments: If seal becomes anoxic due to prolonged apnea, intubate with cuffed endotracheal tube and manually ventilate; doxapram IV may also be given.
References: Haigh and Stewart, 1979; Gales, 1989; Williams et al., 1990a; Gage, 1993; Haulena and Heath, 2001

SEAL, LEOPARD, *Hydrurga leptonyx*

Weight: 500 (f), 270 (m) kg
Recommended Drug: 1.4 mg/kg tiletamine-zolazepam
Supplemental Drug: 0.7 mg/kg tiletamine-zolazepam
Antagonist: 0.006 flumazenil (optional)
Alternative Drugs: 8 mg/kg ketamine plus 0.22 mg/kg midazolam or diazepam
Comments: 0.02 mg/kg atropine may be added to the recommended dose to decrease secretions. If seal becomes anoxic due to prolonged apnea, intubate with cuffed endotracheal tube and manually ventilate; doxapram IV may also be given.
References: Gales, 1984; 1989; Williams et al., 1990a; Mitchell and Burton, 1991; Gage, 1993; Haulena and Heath, 2001; Higgins et al., 2002

SEAL, NORTHERN ELEPHANT, *Mirounga angustirostris*

Weight: 900 (f), 2,000–2,700 (m) kg

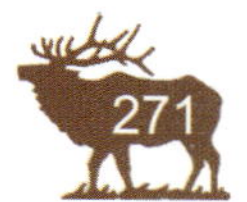

Recommended Drug: 10 mg/kg ketamine plus 0.22 mg/kg midazolam or diazepam
Supplemental Drug: 5 mg/kg ketamine
Antagonist: None
Alternative Drugs: 2.2 mg/kg tiletamine-zolazepam
Comments: If using ketamine/diazepam, give diazepam separately. 0.02 mg/kg atropine may be added to the recommended dose to decrease secretions.
References: Kroll, 1962; Ericksen, 1968; Cline et al., 1969; Gray et al., 1974; Briggs et al., 1975; Cornell, 1977; Hammond and Elsner, 1977; Gage, 1984; Sedgwick, 1986; Schobert, 1987; Joseph and Cornell, 1988; Gales, 1989; Nutter et al., 1998; Haulena and Heath, 2001

SEAL, NORTHERN FUR, *Callorhinus ursinus*

Weight: 43–50 (f), 181–272 (m) kg
Recommended Drug: 1.2 mg/kg tiletamine-zolazepam
Supplemental Drug: 1 mg/kg ketamine
Antagonist: None
Alternative Drugs: 7 mg/kg ketamine plus 0.22 mg/kg diazepam
Comments: If seal becomes anoxic due to prolonged apnea, intubate with cuffed endotracheal tube and manually ventilate; doxapram IV may also be given.
References: Kroll, 1962; Peterson, 1965; Keyes, 1965; Gage, 1984; Gales, 1989; Kiyota et al., 1992; Haulena and Heath, 2001

SEAL, RINGED, *Phoca hispida*

Weight: 61–142 kg
Recommended Drug: 5 mg/kg ketamine
Supplemental Drug: 2.5 mg/kg ketamine
Antagonist: None
Comments: If seal becomes anoxic due to prolonged apnea, intubate with cuffed endotracheal tube and manually ventilate; doxapram IV may also be given.
References: Geraci, 1973; Geraci et al., 1981; Gales, 1989; Williams et al., 1990a; Haulena and Heath, 2001

SEAL, SOUTHERN ELEPHANT, *Mirounga leonina*

Weight: 359–900 (f), 2,000–3,700 (m) kg
Recommended Drug: 1 mg/kg tiletamine-zolazepam
Supplemental Drug: 0.5 mg/kg ketamine
Antagonist: None
Alternative Drugs: 5 mg/kg ketamine plus 1 mg/kg xylazine
• 6 mg/kg ketamine plus 0.3 mg/kg diazepam
Comments: Tiletamine-zolazepam (0.5 mg/kg) may be given IV to physi-

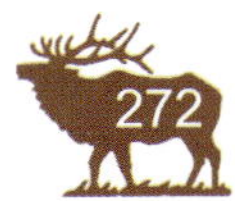

cally restrained seals (McMahon et al., 2000). If seal becomes anoxic give doxapram IV.
References: Ling and Nicholls, 1963; Ling et al., 1967; Cline et al., 1969; Ross and Saayman, 1970; Cornell, 1977; Hammond and Elsner, 1977; Ryding, 1982; Gales and Burton, 1987; Bester, 1988; Baker et al., 1988; 1990; Gales, 1989; Woods et al., 1989; Williams et al., 1990a; Mitchell and Burton, 1991; Gage, 1993; Woods et al., 1989; 1994a; 1994b; 1995; 1996a; 1996b; Slip and Woods, 1996; McMahon et al., 2000; Haulena and Heath, 2001; Ramdohr, et al., 2001; McMahon et al., 2005

SEAL, SOUTHERN (SOUTH AFRICAN) FUR, *Arctocephalus pusillus*

Weight: 36–122 (f), 134–363 (m) kg
Recommended Drug: 10 mg/kg ketamine plus 0.22 mg/kg midazolam or diazepam
Supplemental Drug: 5 mg/kg ketamine
Antagonist: None
Alternative Drugs: 1.7 mg/kg tiletamine-zolazepam; do not give supplemental dose of tiletamine-zolazepam
Comments: David et al. (1988) found no chemical immobilization suitable for the South African subspecies.
References: Thurman et al., 1982; Gage, 1984; 1993; David et al., 1988; Ferreira and Bester, 1999; Haulena and Heath, 2001

SEAL, SOUTHERN (SUBANTARCTIC) FUR, *Arctocephalus tropicalis*

Weight: 21–68 kg
Recommended Drug: 2 mg/kg ketamine
Supplemental Drug: 1 mg/kg ketamine
Antagonist: None
Alternative Drugs: 2 mg/kg tiletamine-zolazepam
Comments: Higher dosages may be required for seals in poor body condition.
References: Haulena and Heath, 2001; Dabin et al., 2002

SEAL, WEDDELL, *Leptonychotes weddelli*

Weight: 400–450 kg
Recommended Drug: 3 mg/kg ketamine plus 1 mg/kg xylazine
Supplemental Drug: 1 mg/kg ketamine plus 0.2 mg/kg xylazine
Antagonist: 0.2 mg/kg yohimbine
Alternative Drugs: 1 mg/kg tiletamine-zolazepam
Comments: Maintain anesthetized animals in lateral, as opposed to sternal, recumbency to assist respiration. If seal becomes anoxic due to prolonged apnea, intubate with cuffed endotracheal tube and manually ventilate; doxapram IV may also be given.
References: Flyger et al., 1965; Cline et al., 1969; Beck, 1972; 1976; Hammond and Elsner, 1977; Gales and Burton, 1988; Gales, 1989; Williams

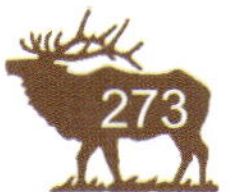

et al., 1990a; Phelan and Green, 1992; Bornemann and Plötz, 1993; Gage, 1993; Haulena and Heath, 2001; Kusagaya and Sato, 2001

SERVAL, *Felis serval*

Weight: 8.7–18 kg
Recommended Drug: 5 mg/kg tiletamine-zolazepam
Supplemental Drug: 2.5 mg/kg ketamine
Antagonist: None
Alternative Drugs: 1 mg/kg ketamine plus 0.05 mg/kg medetomidine plus 0.2 mg/kg butorphanol; antagonize with 0.25 mg/kg atipamezole

- 10 mg/kg ketamine plus 0.2 mg/kg acepromazine
- 15 mg/kg ketamine plus 0.5 mg/kg xylazine

Comments: Darting free-ranging serval is not recommended because they are lost easily before the drug takes effect; trapping is recommended (McKenzie and Burroughs, 1993). The ketamine-medetomidine-butorphanol dosage was based on captive servals (Erdtmann et al., 1998; Langan et al., 2000) .
References: Seal et al., 1970; Gray et al., 1974; Hime, 1974; Beck, 1976; Rowe-Rowe and Lowry, 1982; Genevois et al., 1984b; Wiesner and von Hegel, 1985; Schobert, 1987; McKenzie and Burroughs, 1993; Erdtmann et al., 1998; Ramsay et al., 1999; Langan et al., 2000a; Kock, M., et al., 2006

SHARKS, GENERAL

Weight: 10–180 kg
Recommended Drug: 20 mg/kg ketamine plus 10 mg/kg xylazine
Supplemental Drug: 10 mg/kg ketamine
Antagonist: None reported
Comments: Carfentanil or tiletamine-zolazepam were found unsuitable in four species of sharks. Propofol IV has been used successfully on bamboo sharks and presumably would would work as well on other species (see Miller, S. M. et al., 2005)
References: Gilbert and Wood, 1957; Stoskopf, 1986; 1993; Miller et al., 2005

SHEEP, BARBARY - SEE AOUDAD

SHEEP, BIGHORN, *Ovis canadensis*

Weight: 65–150 kg
Recommended Drug: 0.045 mg/kg carfentanil plus 0.2 mg/kg xylazine
Supplemental Drug: If animal is not down in 15 min, repeat full dose
Antagonist: 3 mg/kg naltrexone plus 0.125 mg/kg yohimbine
Alternative Drugs: 4.5 mg etorphine plus 50 mg xylazine; antagonize with 9 mg diprenorphine plus 0.125 mg/kg yohimbine
Comments: Bighorn sheep are very susceptible to capture myopathy and hyperthermia; careful monitoring of the animal is required. Sheep can be

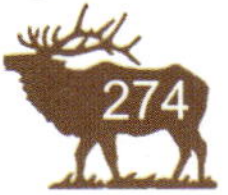

sensitive to xylazine; monitor carefully and always give an antagonist.
References: Franzmann and Thorne, 1970; Thorne, 1971; Alford et al., 1974; Gray et al., 1974; Stelfox and Robertson, 1976; Matthews, 1977; Winegardner et al., 1977; Jessup et al., 1980; 1982b; 1982c; 1984; 1985a; 1985b; 1988; De Vos and Remington, 1981; Thorne, 1982; Andryk et al., 1983; Carpenter and Lance, 1983; Bates et al., 1985; Festa-Bianchet and Jorgenson, 1985; Kock, M., et al., 1987a; 1987b; 1987c; Schobert, 1987; Williams and Riedesel, 1987; Jorgenson et al., 1990; Jessup, 1992a; Pond and O'Gara, 1994; Hunter, 1999; Jessup, 1999; Merwin et al., 1999; 2000; Shury and Caulkett, 2006

SHEEP, FERAL, *Ovis aries*

Weight: 40–100 kg
Recommended Drug: 2 mg/kg ketamine plus 0.05 mg/kg medetomidine
Supplemental Drug: If animal is not down in 15 min, repeat full dose
Antagonist: 0.25 mg/kg atipamezole

SIAMANG, *Hylobates syndactylus*

Weight: 8–13 kg
Recommended Drug: 10 mg/kg ketamine
Supplemental Drug: 5 mg/kg ketamine
Antagonist: None
References: Beck, 1972; 1976; Beck and Dresner, 1972

SITATUNGA, *Tragelaphus spekei*

Weight: 50–125 kg
Recommended Drug: 6.6 mg/kg ketamine plus 1.1 mg/kg xylazine
Supplemental Drug: 3.3 mg/kg ketamine
Antagonist: 0.125 mg/kg yohimbine
Alternative Drugs: 0.9 mg carfentanil; antagonize with 100 mg naltrexone

- 10 mg/kg tiletamine-zolazepam
- 5 mg etorphine; antagonize with 2 mg diprenorphine per mg etorphine given
- 5 mg/kg ketamine plus 1 mg/kg xylazine
- 3 mg/kg xylazine; antagonize with 0.125 mg/kg yohimbine (calm animals only)

Comments: Xylazine may produce rapid shallow respiration which may be improved by administration of doxapram (Densmore, 1979).
References: Hime and Jones, 1970; Göltenboth and Klös, 1970; Bauditz, 1972; Heck and Rivenburg, 1972; Jones, 1972; York and Huggins, 1972; Boever and Paluch, 1974; Mehren and Rapley, 1975; Rapley and Mehren, 1975; Röken, 1975; Densmore, 1979; Jensen, 1982; Göltenboth and Klös, 1987; Schobert, 1987; Kock et al., 1989; Allen et al., 1991

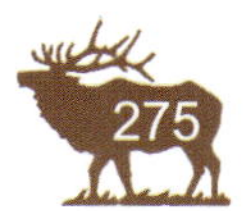

SKUNK, HOG-NOSED, *Conepatus leuconotus*

Weight: 2.3–4.5 kg
Recommended Drug: 10 mg/kg tiletamine-zolazepam
Supplemental Drug: 10 mg/kg ketamine
Antagonist: None
Alternative Drugs: 15 mg/kg ketamine plus 0.2 mg/kg acepromazine
References: Dyson, 1965; Seal and Erickson, 1969; Seal et al., 1970; Seal and Kreeger, 1987

SKUNK, HOODED, *Mephitis macroura*

Weight: 0.7–2.5 kg
Recommended Drug: 10 mg/kg tiletamine-zolazepam
Supplemental Drug: 10 mg/kg ketamine
Antagonist: None
Alternative Drugs: 15 mg/kg ketamine plus 0.2 mg/kg acepromazine
References: Seal and Erickson, 1969; Seal et al., 1970; Seal and Kreeger, 1987

SKUNK, SPOTTED, *Spilogale spp.*

Weight: 0.2–1 kg
Recommended Drug: 10 mg/kg tiletamine-zolazepam
Supplemental Drug: 10 mg/kg ketamine
Antagonist: None
Alternative Drugs: 16 mg/kg ketamine plus 8 mg/kg xylazine
• 15 mg/kg ketamine plus 0.2 mg/kg acepromazine
References: Seal and Erickson, 1969; Seal et al., 1970; Beck, 1976; Jessup et al., 1980; Jessup, 1982b; Seal and Kreeger, 1987; Pond and O'Gara, 1994; López González et al., 1998

SKUNK, STRIPED, *Mephitis mephitis*

Weight: 2–3 kg
Recommended Drug: 10 mg/kg tiletamine-zolazepam
Supplemental Drug: 10 mg/kg ketamine
Antagonist: None
Alternative Drugs: 15 mg/kg ketamine plus 0.2 mg/kg acepromazine
• Halothane (see Larivière and Messier, 2000)
References: Verts, 1960; Seal and Erickson, 1969; Seal et al., 1970; Beck, 1972; 1976; Gray et al., 1974; Haupert and Lindeen, 1974; Ramsden et al., 1976; Boever et al., 1977; Jessup et al., 1980; Hoilien and Oates, 1982; Jessup, 1982b; Rosatte and Hobson, 1983; Wright, 1983; Genevois et al., 1984b Schobert, 1987; Seal and Kreeger, 1987; Servin and Huxley, 1992; Pond and O'Gara, 1994; Larivière and Messier, 1996; 2000

SLOTH, THREE-TOED, *Bradypus variegatus*

Weight: 2–6 kg

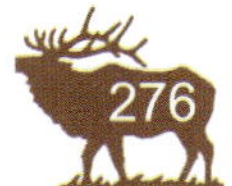

Recommended Drug: 2.5 mg/kg ketamine plus 0.02 mg/kg medetomidine
Supplemental Drug: 1.5 mg/kg ketamine
Antagonist: 0.1 mg/kg atipamezole, IM
Comments: Avoid hypothermia.
References: Hanley et al., 2006

SLOTH, TWO-TOED, *Choloepus spp.*

Weight: 4–8.5 kg
Recommended Drug: 3 mg/kg ketamine plus 0.04 mg/kg medetomidine
Supplemental Drug: 1.5 mg/kg ketamine
Antagonist: 0.2 mg/kg atipamezole, IM
Alternative Drugs: 10 mg/kg ketamine plus 1 mg/kg xylazine
• 10 mg/kg tiletamine-zolazepam
Comments: Avoid hypothermia.
References: Seal and Erickson, 1969; Seal et al., 1970; Schobert, 1987; Vogel et al., 1998; Hanley et al., 2006

SNAKES, GENERAL

Recommended Drug: 75 mg/kg ketamine
Supplemental Drug: 35 mg/kg ketamine
Antagonist: None
Alternative Drugs: 20 mg/kg tiletamine-zolazepam
Comments: Neither drug dose is completely satisfactory for snakes because they induce catalepsy. Expect prolonged recoveries.
References: Brazenor and Kaye, 1953; Karlstrom and Cook, 1955; Mosby and Cantner, 1956; Betz, 1962; Hackenbrock and Finster, 1963; Kraner et al., 1965; Gandal, 1968; Stemmler and Zingg, 1969; Burke and Wall, 1970; Jackson, 1970; Wallach and Hoessle, 1970; Calderwood, 1971; Beck, 1972; 1976; Glenn et al., 1972a; 1972b; Cooper, 1974; Gray et al., 1974; Stunkard and Miller, 1974; Hatori et al., 1975; Beck, 1976; Jones, 1977b; Wang et al., 1977; Calderwood and Jacobson, 1979; Jessup et al., 1980; Sedgwick, 1980b; Strond and Baxter, 1980; Amand, 1982b; Boever and Caputo, 1982; Gillingham et al., 1983; Mulder and Hauser, 1984; Garver and Jackson, 1985; Aird, 1986; Morris, 1986; Schobert, 1987; Johnson, 1991; Schumacher et al., 1992; Page, 1993; Nichols and Lamirande, 1994; Pratap et al., 2006

SPRINGBOK, *Antidorcas marsupialis*

Weight: 30–45 kg
Recommended Drug: 9 mg/kg ketamine plus 0.5 mg/kg xylazine
Supplemental Drug: 5 mg/kg ketamine only
Antagonist: 0.125 mg/kg yohimbine
Alternative Drugs: 0.03 mg/kg carfentanil; antagonize with 3 mg/kg naltrexone
• 10.6 mg/kg tiletamine-zolazepam
• 1.2 mg etorphine plus 10 mg xylazine; antagonize with 2.4 mg

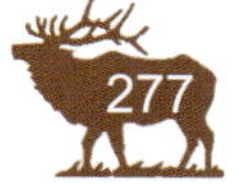

diprenorphine plus 0.125 mg/kg yohimbine

Comments: Springbok are difficult to approach and darts may cause injuries in these small antelope; physical capture may be safer and more effective (Kock et al., 2006). Long-acting tranquilizer doses: haloperidol (adult male, 20 mg; adult female, 15 mg, subadult, 7.5 mg; neonate, 5 mg); zuclopenthixol, 1 mg/kg; perphenazine (adult male, 100 mg; adult female, 70 mg; subadult, 50 mg; neonate, 20 mg).

References: Heuschele, 1961a; Ebedes, 1962; Van Niekerk et al., 1963a; Bigalke, 1965; Pienaar, 1969b; 1973a; Gauckler and Kraus, 1970; Bauditz, 1972; Heck and Rivenburg, 1972; De Vos, 1975; Rapley and Mehren, 1975; Röken, 1975; York, 1975; Haigh, 1976d; Hofmeyr et al., 1977; Wiesner et al., 1982; 1984; 1985; Jacobson, 1983; Jacobson and Kollias, 1984; Schobert, 1987; IWVS, 1992; Burroughs, 1993d; Kock, M., et al., 2006

SQUIRREL, BROWN, *Sciurus vulgaris*

Weight: 200–800 gm

Recommended Drug: 0.005 mg/gm ketamine plus 0.0001 mg/gm medetomidine

Supplemental Drug: 0.003 mg/gm ketamine

Antagonist: 0.0005 mg/gm atipamezole; give 1/2 dose IV, 1/2 IM

Comments: Ketamine-medetomidine may not induce complete immobilization; increase ketamine, if necessary

References: Jalanka and Roeken, 1990

SQUIRREL, AFRICAN GROUND, *Xerus inauris*

Weight: 375–800 gm

Recommended Drug: 0.080 mg/gm ketamine

Supplemental Drug: 0.040 mg/gm ketamine

Antagonist: None

References: Van Heerden, 1984; Van Heerden and Dauth, 1985

SQUIRREL, FLYING (NEW WORLD), *Glaucomys volans*

Weight: 50–185 gm

Recommended Drug: 0.005 mg/gm tiletamine-zolazepam

Supplemental Drug: 0.005 mg/gm ketamine

Antagonist: None

References: IWVS, 1992

SQUIRREL, FOX, *Sciurus niger*

Weight: 600–800 gm

Recommended Drug: 0.012 mg/gm tiletamine-zolazepam

Supplemental Drug: 0.012 mg/gm ketamine

Antagonist: None

Alternative Drugs: 0.036 mg/gm ketamine

References: IWVS, 1992; Arenz, 1997

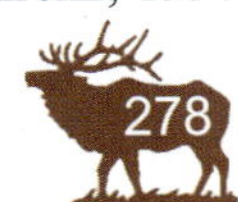

SQUIRREL, GRAY, *Sciurius carolinensis*

Weight: 300–700 gm
Recommended Drug: 0.0066 mg/gm tiletamine-zolazepam
Supplemental Drug: 0.0066 mg/gm ketamine
Antagonist: None
References: Murry and Dennett, 1963; Seal and Erickson, 1969; Seal et al., 1970; Barry, 1972; Beck, 1976; Moller, 1983; Schobert, 1987

SQUIRREL, RED, *Tamiasciurus hudsonicus*

Weight: 141–312 gm
Recommended Drug: 0.02 mg/gm ketamine plus 0.001 mg/gm xylazine
Supplemental Drug: 0.01 mg/gm ketamine
Antagonist: None reported
Alternative Drugs: Gas anesthesia such as isoflurane
References: Moller, 1983; Seal and Kreeger, 1987

SQUIRREL, RICHARDSON'S GROUND, *Spermophilus richardsonii*

Weight: 290–345 gm
Recommended Drug: 0.085 mg/gm ketamine plus 0.01 mg/gm xylazine
Supplemental Drug: 0.04 mg/gm ketamine
Antagonist: None reported
References: Love, 1970; Genevois et al., 1984a; Olson and McCabe, 1986; McColl and Boonstra, 1999

SQUIRREL, TRICOLORED, *Callosciurus erythraeus*

Weight: 150–500 gm
Recommended Drug: 0.012 mg/gm tiletamine-zolazepam
Supplemental Drug: 0.012 mg/gm ketamine
Antagonist: None
References: Gray et al., 1974; Schobert, 1987

STEENBOK, *Raphicerus campestris*

Weight: 7–16 kg
Recommended Drug: 0.4 mg/kg fentanyl plus 1 mg/kg azaperone
Supplemental Drug: 0.3 mg/kg fentanyl
Antagonist: 0.2 mg/kg naloxone
Alternative Drugs: 15 mg/kg tiletamine-zolazepam

- 0.04 mg/kg etorphine plus 0.4 mg/kg xylazine; antagonize with 0.04 mg/kg diprenorphine plus 0.15 mg/kg yohimbine
- 0.01 mg/kg carfentanil plus 0.1 mg/kg xylazine; antagonize with 1 mg/kg naltrexone plus 0.125 mg/kg yohimbine
- 0.04 mg/kg thiafentanil plus 1 mg/kg azaperone; antagonize with 1 mg/kg naltrexone
- 10 mg/kg ketamine plus 0.2 mg/kg xylazine
- 8 mg/gm tiletamine-zolazepam

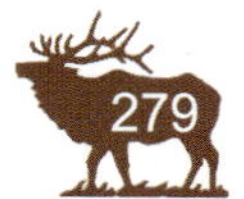

Comments: Monitor for respiratory depression when using opioids.
References: Van Niekerk et al., 1963a; De Vos, 1975; Smuts, 1975; Wiesner, 1975; 1977; Hofmeyr, 1981; IWVS, 1992; Burroughs, 1993d; Kock, 2001; Kock, M., et al., 2006

STOAT - SEE ERMINE

SUNI, *Neotragus moschatus*

Weight: 4–9 kg
Recommended Drug: 3 mg fentanyl plus 5 mg azaperone
Supplemental Drug: 1.5 mg fentanyl
Antagonist: 0.2 mg/kg naloxone
Alternative Drugs: 10 mg/kg tiletamine-zolazepam
• 0.2 mg/kg fentanyl plus 0.4 mg/kg xylazine
• 0.01 mg/kg etorphine plus 0.4 mg/kg xylazine; antagonize with 0.02 mg diprenorphine plus 0.125 mg/kg yohimbine
• 10 mg/kg ketamine IV after manual restraint
Comments: Monitor for respiratory depression when using opioids. Long-acting tranquilizer doses: haloperidol (adults 5 mg); zuclopenthixol (adults, 10-20 mg). Suni transport well in dark, individual crates when given 5 mg haloperidol.
References: Flamand and Lawson, 1986; Schobert, 1987; Burroughs, 1993d; Kock et al., 2006

SWAN, BLACK-NECKED, *Cygnus melanocoryphus*

Weight: 4–5.4 kg
Recommended Drug: 6.6 mg/kg tiletamine-zolazepam
Supplemental Drug: 6.6 mg/kg ketamine
Antagonist: None
References: Schobert, 1987

SWINE, WILD - SEE HOG, EUROPEAN WILD

TAHR, *Hemitragus jemlahicus*

Weight: 50–100 kg
Recommended Drug: 1.5 mg/kg ketamine plus 0.09 mg/kg medetomidine
Supplemental Drug: 1 mg/kg ketamine
Antagonist: 0.45 mg/kg atipamezole; give 1/2 dose IV, 1/2 IM
Alternative Drugs: 0.001 mg/kg carfentanil plus 0.01 mg/kg xylazine; antagonize with 1 mg/kg naltexone plus 0.125 mg/kg yohimbine
• 0.8 ml Large Animal Immobilon® plus 10 mg xylazine; antagonize with 2 mg diprenorphine per mg etorphine given
• 4.4 mg/kg tiletamine-zolazepam
• 3 mg/kg ketamine plus 1.7 mg/kg xylazine; antagonize with 0.1 mg/kg atipamezole

References: Jarvis and Morris, 1960; Heck and Rivenburg, 1972; Gray et al., 1974; Rapley and Mehren, 1975; Wiesner, 1975; 1977; Wiesner et al., 1982; 1984; Göltenboth and Klös, 1987; Schobert, 1987; Jalanka and Roeken, 1990; Allen et al., 1991; Dematteis et al., 2006

TAKIN, *Budorcas taxicolor*

Weight: 150–250 kg
Recommended Drug: 0.25 mg/kg butorphanol plus 0.03 mg/kg medetomidine
Supplemental Drug: 100 mg ketamine IV
Antagonist: 0.35 mg/kg naltrexone plus 0.15 mg/kg atipamezole
Alternative Drugs: 0.005 mg/kg carfentanil plus 0.1 mg/kg xylazine; antagonize with 0.5 mg/kg naltrexone plus 0.125 mg/kg yohimbine
Comments: Takin given carfentanil/xylazine tended to become laterally recumbent with increased probability of regurgitation than takin given butorphanol/medetomidine.
References: Morris et al., 2000

TALAPOIN, *Miopithecus talapoin*

Weight: 0.75–1.25 kg
Recommended Drug: 12 mg/kg ketamine
Supplemental Drug: 6 mg/kg ketamine
Antagonist: None
References: Beck, 1972; 1976; Beck and Dresner, 1972; Jessup et al., 1980

TAMARAW, *Bubalus mindorensis*

Weight: 700–1,200 kg
Recommended Drug: 0.02 mg/kg etorphine plus 0.1 mg/kg acepromazine
Supplemental Drug: 0.01 mg/kg etorphine
Antagonist: 2 mg diprenorphine per mg etorphine given
References: Roth and Montemayor-Taca, 1971; Masangkay et al., 1993

TAMARIN, COTTON-HEADED, *Saguinus oedipus*

Weight: 225–900 gm
Recommended Drug: 0.005 mg/gm ketamine plus 0.0001 mg/gm medetomidine
Supplemental Drug: 0.003 mg/gm ketamine
Antagonist: 0.0005 mg/gm atipamezole; give 1/2 dose IV, 1/2 IM
Alternative Drugs: 0.0022 mg/gm tiletamine-zolazepam
References: Kroll, 1962; Schobert, 1987; Jalanka and Roeken, 1990

TAMARIN, EMPEROR, *Saguinus imperator*

Weight: 225–900 gm
Recommended Drug: 0.005 mg/gm ketamine plus 0.0001 mg/gm medetomidine

Supplemental Drug: 0.003 mg/gm ketamine
Antagonist: 0.0005 mg/gm atipamezole; give 1/2 dose IV, 1/2 IM
Alternative Drugs: 0.0022 mg/gm tiletamine-zolazepam
References: Jalanka and Roeken, 1990

TAMARIN, GOLDEN LION, *Leontopithecus rosalia*

Weight: 0.6–0.8 kg
Recommended Drug: 10 mg/kg ketamine plus 0.02 mg/kg medetomidine
Supplemental Drug: 0.003 mg/gm ketamine
Antagonist: 0.1 mg/kg atipamezole
Alternative Drugs: 2.2 mg/kg tiletamine-zolazepam
References: Heuschele, 1961a; 1961b; Selmi et al., 2004b; 2004c

TAMARIN, RED-BELLIED, *Saguinus labiatus*

Weight: 225–900 gm
Recommended Drug: 0.005 mg/gm ketamine plus 0.0001 mg/gm medetomidine
Supplemental Drug: 0.003 mg/gm ketamine
Antagonist: 0.0005 mg/gm atipamezole; give 1/2 dose IV, 1/2 IM
Alternative Drugs: 0.0022 mg/gm tiletamine-zolazepam
References: Jalanka and Roeken, 1990

TAMARIN, WHITE-LIPPED, *Saguinus nigricollis*

Weight: 225–900 gm
Recommended Drug: 0.0088 mg/gm tiletamine-zolazepam
Supplemental Drug: 0.0088 mg/gm ketamine
Antagonist: None
References: Gray et al., 1974

TAPIR, BAIRD'S, *Tapirus bairdii*

Weight: 200–300 kg
Recommended Drug: 2 mg etorphine plus 8 mg acepromazine
Supplemental Drug: 1 mg etorphine
Antagonist: 0.2 mg/kg naltrexone
Alternative Drugs: 0.2 mg/kg butorphanol plus 0.4 mg/kg xylazine; antagonize with 0.2 mg/kg naltrexone plus 0.125 mg/kg yohimbine
Comments: The butorphanol/xylazine dose is only effective on calm animals. Sedation lasts for about 30 minutes. If additional down time is required, administer 1 mg/kg ketamine, preferably IV.
References: Paras-Garcia et al., 1996; Trim et al., 1998; Foerster et al., 1998; 2000

TAPIR, MALAYAN, *Tapirus indicus*

Weight: 180–320 kg
Recommended Drug: 0.5 ml Large Animal Immobilon® plus 10 mg

xylazine
Supplemental Drug: 0.25 ml Large Animal Immobilon®
Antagonist: 2 mg diprenorphine per mg etorphine given
References: Alford et al., 1974; Williams, 1979; Wiesner et al., 1982

TAPIR, MOUNTAIN, *Tapirus pinchaque*

Weight: 180–320 kg
Recommended Drug: 1 mg carfentanil plus 50 mg ketamine plus 20 mg xylazine
Supplemental Drug: If not down in 20 minutes, repeat full dose
Antagonist: 100 mg naltrexone plus 0.15 mg/kg yohimbine
References: Miller-Edge and Amsel, 1994

TAPIR, SOUTH AMERICAN, *Tapirus terrestris*

Weight: 180–320 kg
Recommended Drug: 2.8 mg/kg tiletamine-zolazepam
Supplemental Drug: 1.4 mg/kg ketamine
Antagonist: None
Alternative Drugs: 1.2 mg etorphine; antagonize with 2.4 mg diprenorphine
• 1.3 mg/kg xylazine
References: Kroll, 1962; Heck and Rivenburg, 1972; Alford et al., 1974; Gray et al., 1974; Hertzog, 1975; Mehren and Rapley, 1975; Rapley and Mehren, 1975; Hugues et al., 1986; Schobert, 1987; Pollock and Ramsay, 2003

TAYRA, *Eira barbara*

Weight: 4–5 kg
Recommended Drug: 3.3 mg/kg tiletamine-zolazepam
Supplemental Drug: 3.3 mg/kg ketamine
Antagonist: None
Alternative Drugs: 15 mg/kg ketamine
References: Seal et al., 1970; Beck, 1976; Schobert, 1987

TEAL, BLUE WING, *Anas discors*

Weight: 330–360 gm
Recommended Drug: 0.025 mg/gm tiletamine-zolazepam
Supplemental Drug: 0.025 mg/gm ketamine
Antagonist: None
References: Crider et al., 1968; Crider and McDaniel, 1968; Gray et al., 1974; Schobert, 1987

TEAL, GREEN WING, *Anas crecca*

Weight: 300–400 gm
Recommended Drug: 0.025 mg/gm tiletamine-zolazepam

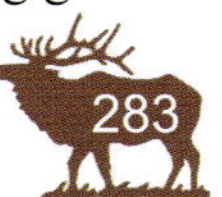

Supplemental Drug: 0.025 mg/gm ketamine
Antagonist: None
References: Crider et al., 1968; Schobert, 1987

TIGER, *Panthera tigris*

Weight: 100–160 (f), 140–300 (m) kg
Recommended Drug: 3 mg/kg ketamine plus 0.07 mg/kg medetomidine
Supplemental Drug: 1.5 mg/kg ketamine
Antagonist: 0.35 mg/kg atipamezole; give 1/2 dose IV, 1/2 IM
Alternative Drugs: 4 mg/kg tiletamine-zolazepam
• 11 mg/kg ketamine plus 0.8 mg/kg xylazine; antagonize with 0.125 mg/kg yohimbine
Comments: The ketamine/medetomidine dosage has been used on free-ranging Siberian tigers (Kreeger, unpubl. data), but lower doses may be effective in captive tigers (see Miller et al., 2003). The addition of 0.1 mg/kg midazolam to any of the above combinations may help to reduce convulsions.
References: Pistey and Wright, 1959; Jarvis and Morris, 1960; Heuschele, 1961a; Larsen, 1963; Ericksen, 1968; Seal and Erickson, 1969; Göltenboth and Klös, 1970; Seal et al., 1970; 1987; Bennet et al., 1971; Bauditz, 1972; Foster, 1974; Gray et al., 1974; Hime, 1974; Johnston, 1974; Seidensticker et al., 1974; Beck, 1976; Robinson, 1976; Kuntze, 1977; Wiesner, 1977; Chakrabarti, 1980; Arora et al., 1983; Genevois et al., 1984b; Smith et al., 1983; Wiesner and von Hegel, 1985; Gonzales and McDonnel, 1986; Hugues et al., 1986; Göltenboth and Klös, 1987; Röken, 1987; Schobert, 1987; Kock et al., 1989; Barnett and Lewis, 1990; Jalanka and Roeken, 1990; Vogelnest, 1999; Goodrich et al., 2001; Miller et al., 2003; Curro et al., 2004

TITI - SEE MARMOSET, SHORT-TUSKED

TOADS - SEE AMPHIBIANS, GENERAL

TOPI, *Damaliscus lunatus*

Weight: 120–140 kg
Recommended Drug: 0.03 mg/kg thiafentanil plus 0.6 mg/kg azaperone
Supplemental Drug: 0.015 mg/kg thiafentanil
Antagonist: 0.6 mg/kg naltrexone
Alternative Drugs: 4 mg etorphine plus 80 mg azaperone; antagonize with 8 mg diprenorphine
• 0.01 mg/kg carfentanil plus 0.1 mg/kg xylazine; antagonize with 1 mg/kg naltrexone plus 0.125 mg/kg yohimbine
Comments: Topi are susceptible to capture myopathy and will run long distances when darted from helicopters; net-gunning may be preferred. Hyaluronidase (1,500-3,000 IU) may be added to decrease induction time. Long-acting tranquilizer doses: haloperidol (adult male, 30 mg; adult female, 20 mg; subadult, 10 mg); zuclopenthixol, 1 mg/kg; perphenazine (adults,

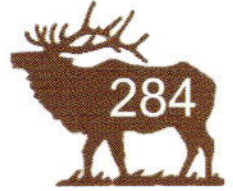

100-150 mg; subadults, 40 mg).

References: Talbot and Lamprey, 1961; Talbot and Talbot, 1962; Buck et al., 1963; Pienaar et al., 1966a; Pienaar, 1968a; 1969b; Patrick, 1971; Jones, 1972; De Vos, 1975; 1978a; York and Huggins, 1972; Röken, 1975; Smuts, 1975; York, 1975; Haigh, 1976d; Hofmeyr, 1981; Kock et al., 1989; 2006; IWVS, 1992; Burroughs, 1993d

TSESSEBE- SEE TOPI

TUAN - SEE MOUSE, BRUSH-TAILED MARSUPIAL

TURKEY, WILD, *Meleagris gallopavao*

Weight: 4–8 kg

Recommended Drug: Alpha-choralose given orally at a rate of 8 gm/liter cracked corn

Antagonist: None

Comments: Oral administration of immobilizing drugs is generally an ineffective method of capturing birds, but may be employed when no other alternatives exist. Be prepared for extreme variability of effects, ranging from little or no sedation to relatively high mortality.

References: Mosby and Cantner, 1956; Murry and Dennett, 1963; Williams, 1966; 1967; Williams et al., 1966; 1973a; 1973b; Bailey, 1972; Bailey and Doepker, 1977; Evans and Goertz, 1975; Donahue et al., 1982; Holbrook and Vaughan, 1985; Schumacher et al., 1997b

TURTLE, LOGGERHEAD, *Caretta caretta*

Weight: 100–500 kg

Recommended Drug: 5 mg/kg ketamine plus 0.05 mg/kg medetomidine

Supplemental Drug: maintain on 0.5-2% sevoflurane

Antagonist: 0.25 mg/kg atipamezole

Alternative Drugs: 5 mg/kg propofol, IV

Comments: The longer the turtle has been anesthetized, the less atipamezole needs to be given in order to avoid hyperexcitability upon recovery. For example, if the turtle has been anesthetized for 15-30 min, give 1/2 dose of atipamezole; 30-45 min., give 1/4 dose; and >45 min. give no atipameazole.

References: Chittick et al., 2002b; MacLean et al., 2005

TURTLE, SNAPPING, *Chelydra serpentina*

Weight: 5–30 kg

Recommended Drug: 40 mg/kg ketamine plus 2 mg/kg midazolam

Supplemental Drug: 20 mg/kg ketamine

Antagonist: None

Comments: Placing turtles/tortoises in dorsal recumbency (on their “backs”) may result in respiratory depression because the viscera will

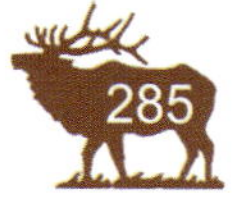

compress the lungs. Surgical anesthesia is achieved when the head is not retracted when pulled out, but the corneal reflex is still present.
References: Mosby and Cantner, 1956; Beck, 1972; Jessup et al., 1980; Bienzle et al., 1991; Bienzle and Boyd, 1992

TURTLES/TORTOISES: GENERAL

Recommended Drug: 44 mg/kg ketamine
Supplemental Drug: 22 mg/kg ketamine
Antagonist: None
Alternative Drugs: gas (sevoflurane) anesthesia
- 22 mg/kg tiletamine-zolazepam
- 5 mg/kg ketamine plus 0.1 mg/kg medetomidine; antagonize with 0.5 mg/kg atipamezole

Comments: Placing turtles/tortoises in dorsal recumbency (on their "backs") may result in respiratory depression because the viscera will compress the lungs. Surgical anesthesia is achieved when the head is not retracted when pulled out, but the corneal reflex is still present.
References: Mosby and Cantner, 1956; Kaplan and Taylor, 1957; Young and Kaplan, 1960; Hunt, 1964; Wallach and Hoessle, 1970; Calderwood, 1971; Beck, 1972; 1974; Gray et al., 1974; Kuehn, 1974; Calderwood and Jacobson, 1979; Jessup et al., 1980; Boever and Caputo, 1982; Wood et al., 1982; Garver and Jackson, 1985; Brannian et al., 1987; Schobert, 1987; Adest et al., 1988; Gyuris and Limpus, 1989; Bennett, 1991; Bienzle et al., 1991; Bienzle and Boyd, 1992; Page, 1993; Holz and Holz, 1994; Oppenheim and Moon, 1995; Moon and Stabenau, 1996; Lock et al., 1998; Pye and Carpenter, 1998; Norton et al., 1998; Rooney et al., 1999; Dennis et al., 2000; Sleeman et al., 2000; Greer et al., 2001; Dennis and Heard, 2002

UAKARI, *Cacajao spp.*

Weight: 5–10 kg
Recommended Drug: 3.2 mg/kg tiletamine-zolazepam
Supplemental Drug: 3.2 mg/kg ketamine
Antagonist: None
Alternative Drugs: 10 mg/kg ketamine
References: Beck, 1976; Bush et al., 1977; Schobert, 1987

URIAL, *Ovis vignei*

Weight: 50–100 kg
Recommended Drug: 1.2 mg carfentanil (males); 1 mg carfentanil (females)
Supplemental Drug: If animal is not down in 20 minutes, repeat full dose
Antagonist: 120 mg naltexone
References: Allen et al., 1991

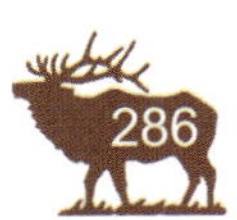

VERVET, *Cercopithecus pygerythrus*

Weight: 3–8 kg
Recommended Drug: 7 mg/kg tiletamine-zolazepam
Supplemental Drug: 7 mg/kg ketamine
Antagonist: None
Alternative Drugs: 12 mg/kg ketamine
References: Kroll, 1962; Graham-Jones, 1964; Beck, 1976; Eads, 1976; Schobert, 1987; Burroughs, 1993c

VICUÑA, *Vicugna vicugna*

Weight: 35–65 kg
Recommended Drug: 1 mg/kg ketamine plus 0.05 mg/kg medetomidine
Supplemental Drug: 1 mg/kg ketamine
Antagonist: 0.25 mg/kg atipamezole
Alternative Drugs: 2 mg/kg xylazine; antagonize with 0.125 mg/kg yohimbine
• 4 mg/kg tiletamine-zolazepam
Comments: Jones (1977a) stated that the use of opioids in llama was contraindicated; assume the same for vicuña.
References: Wiesner and von Hegel, 1985; Schiappacasse Faundes, 1991

VULTURE, CAPE, *Gyps coprotheres*

Weight: 5–7 kg
Recommended Drug: 10 mg/kg ketamine
Supplemental Drug: 5 mg/kg ketamine
Antagonist: None
References: Ebedes, 1973a; Van Heerden et al., 1987

VULTURE, TURKEY, *Cathartes aura*

Weight: 5–7 kg
Recommended Drug: 35 mg/kg ketamine plus 0.7 mg/kg diazepam, IV
Supplemental Drug: 5 mg/kg ketamine, IV
Antagonist: None
References: Redig and Diuke, 1976; Allen and Oosterhuis, 1986a

WALLABY, AGILE, *Macropus agilis*

Weight: 12–20 kg
Recommended Drug: 8 mg/kg ketamine plus 8 mg/kg xylazine
Supplemental Drug 4 mg/kg ketamine only
Antagonist: None
References: Kroll, 1962; Keep, 1973; Stirrat, 1997

WALLABY, BRUSH-TAILED ROCK, *Petrogale penicillata*

Weight: 3–9 kg
Recommended Drug: 6 mg/kg tiletamine-zolazepam

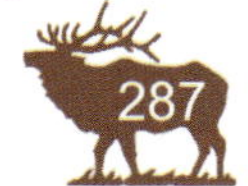

Supplemental Drug: 6 mg/kg ketamine
Antagonist: None
References: Holz, 1992; Shima et al., 1993

WALLABY, PARMA, *Macropus parma*

Weight: 2.6–5.9 kg
Recommended Drug: 6.5 mg/kg tiletamine-zolazepam
Supplemental Drug: 6.5 mg/kg ketamine
Antagonist: None
References: Bush et al., 1990

WALLABY, RED-NECKED, *Macropus rufogriseus*

Weight: 7–20 kg
Recommended Drug: 8 mg/kg ketamine plus 8 mg/kg xylazine
Supplemental Drug: 4 mg/kg ketamine only
Antagonist: None reported
Alternative Drugs: 5 mg/kg ketamine plus 0.1 mg/kg medetomidine; antagonize with 0.5 mg/kg atipamezole
• 10 mg/kg tiletamine-zolazepam
References: Seal and Erickson, 1969; Seal et al., 1970; Denny, 1974; Wiesner, 1977; England and Kock, 1988; Kock et al., 1989; Jalanka and Roeken, 1990; Holz, 1992; Shima et al., 1993; Holz and Barnett, 1996; vonDegerfeld, 2005

WALLABY, SWAMP, *Wallabia bicolor*

Weight: 10.3–15.4 (f), 12.3–20.5 (m) kg
Recommended Drug: 5 mg/kg tiletamine-zolazepam
Supplemental Drug: 5 mg/kg ketamine
Antagonist: None
References: Denny, 1974; Shima et al., 1993

WALLABY, TAMMAR, *Macropus eugenii*

Weight: 12–20 kg
Recommended Drug: 8 mg/kg ketamine plus 8 mg/kg xylazine
Supplemental Drug: 4 mg/kg ketamine only
Antagonist: None
References: Denny, 1974; Richardson and Cullen, 1981; 1984

WALLAROO, *Macropus robustus*

Weight: 20–40 kg
Recommended Drug: 19 mg/kg ketamine
Supplemental Drug: 10 mg/kg ketamine
Antagonist: None
References: Marlow, 1956; Denny, 1974; Finnie, 1976

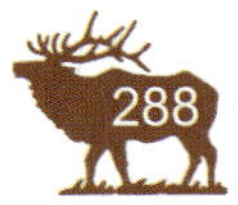

WALRUS, *Odobenus rosmarus*

Weight: 400–1,250 (f), 800–1,700 (m) kg

Recommended Drug: 2 mg/kg tiletamine-zolazepam

Supplemental Drug: 1 mg/kg ketamine

Antagonist: None

Alternative Drugs: 0.006 mg/kg etorphine; antagonize with 0.012 mg/kg diprenorphine

• 0.004 mg/kg carfentanil; antagonize with 0.8 mg/kg naltrexone

Comments: When using etorphine, monitor for apnea and be prepared to administer antagonist. Administer drugs as described in Stirling and Sjare (1988). Some workers have had increased mortality using tiletamine-zolazepam when working in higher ambient temperatures than Stirling and Sjare (1988). Consult Lanthier et al. (1999) prior to using carfentanil.

References: DeMaster et al., 1981; Ryding, 1982; Cornell and Antrim, 1987; Joseph and Cornell, 1988; Stirling and Sjare, 1988; Walsh et al., 1988; Gales, 1989; Born and Knutsen, 1990; Williams et al., 1990a; Griffiths et al., 1993; Tuomi et al., 1996; Lanthier et al., 1999

WAPITI - SEE ELK

WART HOG, *Phacochoerus aethiopicus*

Weight: 65–100 kg

Recommended Drug: 3 mg/kg tiletamine-zolazepam

Supplemental Drug: 2 mg/kg ketamine

Antagonist: None

Alternative Drugs: 200 mg ketamine plus 2 mg medetomidine

• 4 mg etorphine plus 20 mg xylazine; antagonize with 8 mg diprenorphine plus 0.125 mg/kg yohimbine

• 0.4 mg/kg butorphanol plus 0.125 mg/kg detomidine plus 0.4 mg/kg midazolam; antagonize with 5 mg/kg naltrexone plus 0.3 mg/kg yohimbine

• 3.5 mg/kg ketamine plus 0.2 mg/kg xylazine

Comments: Wart hogs are not easy to immobilize and they are highly susceptible to overheating. Do not overly stress before darting and keep cool after immobilization. High velocity darts may cause severe muscle damage; use low-impact darting systems, but maintain sufficient velocity to penetrate tough skin. Hindquarters are the preferred target area. Animals will run long distances after being darted and must be tracked. Overdose of etorphine can cause cardiac arrest. Ketamine combinations and Telazol® may result in light anesthesia, poor analgesia, and muscle spasms. Respiratory depression can be severe with opioids.

References: Bigalke, 1965; Pienaar et al., 1966a; Pienaar, 1969a; 1969b; Harthoorn, 1972a; 1973a; 1973b; Jones, 1972; De Vos, 1975; Röken, 1975; Smuts, 1975; Haigh, 1976d; IWVS, 1992; Burroughs, 1993e; Calle and Morris, 1999; Kock, M., et al., 2006

WATERBUCK, *Kobus ellipsiprymnus*

Weight: 225–260 kg

Recommended Drug: 0.03 mg/kg thiafentanil plus 0.6 mg/kg azaperone

Supplemental Drug: If animal is not down in 15 minutes, repeat full dose

Antagonist: 0.6 mg/kg naltrexone

Alternative Drugs: 0.01 mg/kg carfentanil plus 0.1 mg/kg xylazine; antagonize with 1 mg/kg naltrexone plus 0.125 mg/kg yohimbine

- 0.03 mg/kg etorphine plus 0.1 mg/kg xylazine; antagonize with 0.06 mg/kg diprenorphine plus 0.125 mg/kg yohimbine
- 50 mg fentanyl plus 300 mg azaperone
- 1.6 ml Large Animal Immobilon® plus 25 mg xylazine; antagonize with 2 mg diprenorphine per mg etorphine given

Comments: Difficult to immobilize. Prone to excessive running during induction with opioids; monitor for hyperthermia. Susceptible to capture myopathy. Carfentanil used without tranquilizers causes marked excitability. Long-acting tranquilizer doses: haloperidol (adult male, 20 mg; adult female, 15 mg; subadult, 8 mg); zuclopenthixol, 1 mg/kg; perphenazine (adults, 100-200 mg; subadults, 50 mg).

References: Buechner et al., 1960a; 1960c; Harthoorn and Bligh, 1965; Pienaar et al., 1966a; Hanks, 1967; Keep and Keep, 1967; Short and Spinage, 1967; Hanks and Dowsett, 1969; Pienaar, 1969b; Bauditz, 1972; Heck and Rivenburg, 1972; Jones, 1972; Pienaar, 1968a; 1973a; De Vos, 1975; Rapley and Mehren, 1975; Röken, 1975; York, 1975; Haigh, 1976d; De Vos, 1978a; Kupper et al., 1981; Wiesner et al., 1982; 1984; 1985; Janssen and Oosterhuis, 1984; Silvestris and Heck, 1984; Wiesner and von Hegel, 1985; Kock, R., et al., 1989; Allen et al., 1991; Janssen et al., 1991; IWVS, 1992; Burroughs, 1993d; Borkowski et al., 2004; Kock, M., et al., 2006

WATERFOWL, GENERAL

Recommended Drug: 25 mg/kg ketamine plus 1 mg/kg diazepam

Supplemental Drug: 15 mg/kg ketamine

Antagonist: None

References: Amand, 1982a; Langenberg et al., 1998; Machin and Caulkett, 1998a; 1998b; 1999; 2000

WEASEL LONG-TAILED, *Mustela frenata*

Weight: 85–200 gm

Recommended Drug: 0.005 mg/gm ketamine plus 0.0001 mg/gm medetomidine

Supplemental Drug: 0.0025 mg/gm ketamine

Antagonist: 0.0005 mg/gm atipamezole; give 1/2 dose IV, 1/2 IM

Alternative Drugs: 0.025 mg/gm ketamine plus 0.002 mg/gm xylazine

References: Seal et al., 1970; Jessup, 1982b; Seal and Kreeger, 1987; Gehring and Swihart, 2000

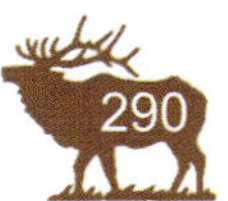

WEASEL-SHORT-TAILED - SEE ERMINE

WILDEBEEST, (BLACK, WHITE-TAILED), *Connochaetes gnou*

Weight: 120–180 kg

Recommended Drug: 0.007 mg/kg carfentanil plus 0.06 mg/kg xylazine

Supplemental Drug: 0.007 mg/kg carfentanil

Antagonist: 0.7 mg/kg naltrexone

Alternative Drugs: 0.025 mg/kg thiafentanil plus 0.5 mg/kg azaperone; antagonize with 0.5 mg/kg naltrexone

• 3 mg etorphine plus 15 mg xylazine; antagonize with 6 mg diprenorphine plus 0.125 mg/kg yohimbine

• 1 ml Large Animal Immobilon® plus 10 mg xylazine; antagonize with 2 mg diprenorphine per mg etorphine given plus 0.125 mg/kg yohimbine

• 3 mg/kg xylazine; antagonize with 0.125 mg yohimbine (calm animals only)

Comments: Wildebeest are susceptible to capture myopathy if over-exerted. Etorphine may not completely immobilize wildebeest and they may have to be finally captured by hand (Kock et el., 2006). Long-acting tranquilizer doses: haloperidol (adult male, 30 mg; adult female, 20 mg; subadult, neonate, 15 mg); zuclopenthixol, 1 mg/kg; perphenazine, 70-100 mg total dose.

References: Pienaar, 1969b; 1973; Gauckler and Kraus, 1970; Amand et al., 1972; Bauditz, 1972; Heck and Rivenburg, 1972; Keep, 1973a; Gray et al., 1974; De Vos, 1975; Rapley and Mehren, 1975; Röken, 1975; Haigh, 1976d; De Vos, 1978a; Wiesner et al., 1982; 1984; Silvestris and Heck, 1984; Wiesner et al., 1984; Wiesner and von Hegel, 1985; Hugues et al., 1986; Schobert, 1987; Williams and Riedesel, 1987; Allen et al., 1991; Berry, 1992; IWVS, 1992; Burroughs, 1993d; Kock et el., 2006

WILDEBEEST, (BLUE, BRINDLED, WHITE-BEARDED), *Connochaetes taurinus*

Weight: 118–275 kg

Recommended Drug: 0.03 mg/kg etorphine plus 0.15 mg/kg xylazine

Supplemental Drug: If animal is not down in 15 minutes, repeat full dose

Antagonist: 2 mg diprenorphine per mg etorphine given plus 0.125 mg/kg yohimbine

Alternative Drugs: 0.03 mg/kg thiafentanil plus 0.3 mg/kg azaperone; antagonize with 0.6 mg/kg naltrexone

• 0.008 mg/kg carfentanil plus 0.08 mg/kg xylazine; antagonize with 0.8 mg/kg naltrexone plus 0.125 mg/kg yohimbine

• 2.25 mg etorphine plus 5 mg detomidine plus 200 mg ketamine; antagonize with 4.5 mg diprenorphine

• 6.6 mg/kg tiletamine-zolazepam

• 3 mg/kg xylazine; antagonize with 0.125 mg yohimbine (calm animals)

Comments: Wildebeest are susceptible to capture myopathy if over-exerted.

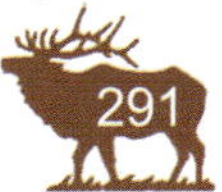

Monitor respiration rates closely. Wildebeest may not go down when given opioids, but can be approached. Much lower doses may be effective in captive animals (see Bertelsen et al., 2006). Long-acting tranquilizer doses: haloperidol (adults, 20 mg; subadult, 10 mg); zuclopenthixol, 1 mg/kg; perphenazine (adults, 100 mg; subadults, 50 mg).
References: Heuschele, 1961a; 1961b; Talbot and Lamprey, 1961; Talbot and Talbot, 1962; Harthoorn, 1962b; Van Niekerk et al., 1963a; 1963b; Orr and Moore-Gilbert, 1964; Harthoorn and Bligh, 1965; Hirst et al., 1965; Pienaar et al., 1966a; 1968a; Fenn and Sedgwick, 1969; Pienaar, 1969b; Harthoorn, 1971; Koci, 1971a; 1972; Bauditz, 1972; Jones, 1972; York and Huggins, 1972; Keep, 1973; Young and Whyte, 1973; De Vos, 1975; Röken, 1975; Smuts, 1975; Grootenhuis et al., 1976; Haigh, 1976d; Ebedes et al., 1977; Slee and Walker, 1977; De Vos, 1978a; Arora et al., 1983; Schobert, 1987; Williams and Riedesel, 1987; Kock, R., et al., 1989; Allen et al., 1991; IWVS, 1992; Burroughs, 1993d; Páras et al., 2002; Bertelsen et al., 2006; Kock, M., et al., 2006

WISENT - SEE BISON, EUROPEAN

WOLF, ETHIOPIAN - SEE JACKAL, SIMIEN

WOLF, GRAY, *Canis lupus*

Weight: 27–60 kg
Recommended Drug: 10 mg/kg tiletamine-zolazepam
Supplemental Drug: 5 mg/kg ketamine
Antagonist: None
Alternative Drugs: 10 mg/kg ketamine plus 2 mg/kg xylazine; antagonize with 0.15 mg/kg yohimbine
• 4 mg/kg ketamine plus 0.08 mg/kg medetomidine; antagonize with 0.4 mg/kg atipamezole
Comments: A standard dose of 500 mg tiletamine-zolazepam should be satisfactory for helicopter darting adult wolves. If using ketamine and xylazine, wait at least 45 min after last ketamine or tiletamine-zolazepam injection before administering yohimbine. Calm, captive wolves may be able to be immobilized with 4 mg/kg ketamine plus 2 mg/kg xylazine. This combination is more readily antagonized by yohimbine than when higher doses of ketamine are used. Atropine at 0.05 mg/kg can be given to decrease salivation, particularly when wolves are immobilized with tiletamine-zolazepam.
References: Kroll, 1962; Dyson, 1965; Seal and Erickson, 1969; Göltenboth and Klös, 1970; 1987; Seal et al., 1970a; Bauditz, 1972; Alford et al., 1974; Gray et al., 1974; Wentges, 1975; Wiesner, 1975; 1977; Haigh, 1976d; Boever et al., 1977b; Philo, 1978; Fuller and Keith, 1981; Ballard et al., 1982; 1991; Fuller and Kuehn, 1983; Genevois et al., 1984b; Wiesner et al., 1984; Duchamps, 1985; Hess and Knakal, 1985; Tobey and Ballard,

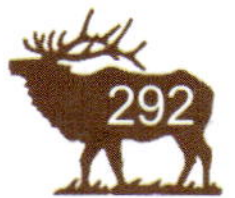

1985; Wiesner and von Hegel, 1985; Hugues et al., 1986; Kreeger and Seal, 1986a; 1990; Kreeger et al., 1986c; 1987a; 1988; 1989a; 1990c; 1990d; 1990e; 1995; 1996; Schobert, 1987; Seal and Kreeger, 1987; Strauss, 1987; Kock et al., 1989; Jalanka and Roeken, 1990; Mech and Gese, 1992; Chakraborty and Das, 1994; Holz et al., 1994; Pond and O'Gara, 1994; Vilà and Castroviejo, 1994; Sahr and Knowlton, 2000; Arnemo et al., 2003; Valerio et al., 2005; Arnemo, 2006

WOLF, MANED, *Chrysocyon brachturus*

Weight: 20–30 kg
Recommended Drug: 2.5 mg/kg ketamine plus 0.08 mg/kg medetomidine
Supplemental Drug: 2.5 mg/kg ketamine
Antagonist: 0.4 mg/kg atipamezole
Alternative Drugs: 3 mg/kg tiletamine-zolazepam
• 10 mg/kg ketamine plus 0.1 mg/kg acepromazine
References: Graham-Jones, 1964; Jalanka and Roenken, 1990; Furtado et al., 2006

WOLF, MEXICAN, *Canis lupus baileyi*

Weight: 23–28 kg
Recommended Drug: 4.2 mg/kg ketamine plus 2.3 mg/kg xylazine
Supplemental Drug: 2.3 mg/kg ketamine
Antagonist: 0.15 mg/kg yohimbine
Alternative Drugs: 10 mg/kg tiletamine-zolazepam
• 4 mg/kg ketamine plus 0.08 mg/kg medetomidine; antagonize with 0.4 mg/kg atipamezole
• 10 mg/kg ketamine plus 0.1 mg/kg acepromazine
References: Servin and Huxley, 1992

WOLF, RED, *Canis rufus*

Weight: 20–40 kg
Recommended Drug: 2 mg/kg ketamine plus 0.04 mg/kg medetomidine
Supplemental Drug: 2 mg/kg ketamine
Antagonist: 0.2 mg/kg atipamezole
Alternative Drugs: 10 mg/kg ketamine plus 2 mg/kg xylazine; antagonize with 0.15 mg/kg yohimbine
• 10 mg/kg tiletamine-zolazepam
• 10 mg/kg ketamine plus 0.1 mg/kg acepromazine
• 0.4 mg/kg butorphanol plus 0.04 mg/kg medetomidine; antagonize with 0.02 mg/kg naltrexone plus 0.2 mg/kg atipamezole (captive animals only)
Comments: If using xylazine, wait at least 45 min after last ketamine injection before administering yohimbine.
References: Seal et al., 1970; Seal and Kreeger, 1987; Sladky et al., 1999b; 2000; Larsen et al., 2001; 2002

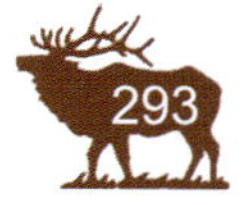

WOLVERINE, *Gulo gulo*

Weight: 7–32 kg

Recommended Drug: 7 mg/kg ketamine plus 0.3 mg/kg medetomidine

Supplemental Drug: If not down in 15 minutes, repeat full dose

Antagonist: 1.5 mg/kg atipamezole

Alternative Drugs: 15 mg/kg tiletamine-zolazepam

- 20 mg/kg ketamine plus 0.2 mg/kg acepromazine
- 0.1 mg/kg etorphine plus 1 mg/kg xylazine; antagonize with 0.2 mg/kg diprenorphine plus 0.15 mg/kg yohimbine

Comments: The ketamine-medetomidine and tiletamine-zolazepam dosages can be reduced by 50% in captive wolverines.

References: Seal and Erickson, 1969; Seal et al., 1970; Hash and Hornocker, 1980; Ballard et al., 1982; Wright, 1983; Wiesner and von Hegel, 1985; Röken, 1987; Seal and Kreeger, 1987; Jalanka and Roeken, 1990; Golden et al., 2002; Arnbemo et al., 2005b; Fahlman et al., 2005b; Arnemo, 2006

WOMBAT, *Vombatus ursinus*

Weight: 15–35 kg

Recommended Drug: 5 mg/kg tiletamine-zolazepam

Supplemental Drug: 5 mg/kg ketamine

Antagonist: None

References: Denny, 1974; Holz, 1992; Bush et al., 1990; Shima et al., 1993; Evans et al., 1998

WOMBAT, SOUTHERN HAIRY-NOSE, *Lasiorhinus latifrons*

Weight: 19–32 kg

Recommended Drug: 3 mg/kg tiletamine-zolazepam

Supplemental Drug: 3 mg/kg ketamine

Antagonist: None

References: Shima et al., 1993

WOODCHUCK, *Marmota monax*

Weight: 3–7.5 kg

Recommended Drug: 20 mg/kg ketamine plus 3 mg/kg xylazine

Supplemental Drug: 10 mg/kg ketamine

Antagonist: None

Alternative Drugs: 5 mg/kg tiletamine-zolazepam

References: Mosby and Cantner, 1956; Seal and Erickson, 1969; Seal et al., 1970; Noyes and Siekierski, 1975; Young and Sims, 1979; Wright, 1983; Genevois et al., 1984a

YAK, *Bos grunniens*

Weight: 250–400 (f), 800–1,000 (m) kg

Recommended Drug: 0.0075 mg/kg carfentanil plus 0.1 mg/kg xylazine

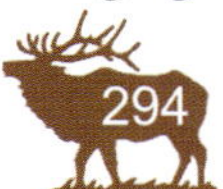

Supplemental Drug: 0.0075 mg/kg carfentanil
Antagonist: 0.7 mg/kg naltrexone plus 0.1 mg/kg yohimbine
Alternative Drugs: 0.006 mg/kg etorphine plus 0.04 mg/kg xylazine; antagonize with 0.012 mg/kg diprenorphine plus 0.125 mg/kg yohimbine
• 3 mg/kg ketamine plus 0.1 mg/kg medetomidine; antagonize with 0.5 mg/kg atipamezole
• 2.5 ml Large Animal Immobilon® plus 50 mg xylazine; antagonize with 2 mg diprenorphine per mg etorphine given plus 0.125 mg/kg yohimbine
• 1 mg/kg xylazine; antagonize with 0.125 mg/kg yohimbine
References: Bauditz, 1972; Heck and Rivenburg, 1972; Mehren and Rapley, 1975; Rapley and Mehren, 1975; Williams and Riedesel, 1987; Kock et al., 1989; Jalanka and Roeken, 1990; Kumar et al., 1998; 1999; Sharma et al., 1998; 2001

ZEBRA, BURCHELL'S (COMMON), *Equus burchelli*

Weight: 200–340 kg
Recommended Drug: 3 mg etorphine plus 150 mg ketamine plus 10 mg detomidine
Supplemental Drug: If not down in in 20 min, repeat full dose
Antagonist: 2 mg diprenorphine per mg etorphine given plus 50 mg atipamezole
Alternative Drugs: 5 mg etorphine plus 5 mg medetomidine; antagonize with 10 mg diprenorphine plus 0.1 mg/kg atipamezole
• 7 mg etorphine (male), 6 mg etorphine (female) plus 60 mg azaperone
• 2.5 ml Large Animal Immobilon® plus 50 mg xylazine; antagonize with 2 mg diprenorphine per mg etorphine given plus 0.125 mg/kg yohimbine
Comments: Complete muscle relaxation is difficult to obtain with wild equids; excessive leg movement is common. Detomidine (10 mg) or xylazine (60 mg) may be substituted for azaperone, but azaperone is preferred (Kock et al., 2006). Muscle relaxation appears better with detomidine than with xylazine. Opioids result in poor muscle relaxation; administer 10 mg diazepam to improve relaxation. Wild equids tend to overheat easily, particularly if there is a prolonged hyperexcitable state prior to anesthetic induction. Attempt to immobilize equids during the coolest part of the day. Etorphine may be more effective than carfentanil in zebras; thiafentanil *cannot* be used in zebras. Zebra skin is resilient sometimes making dart penetration difficult, but do not dart from behind because the skin of the perineum is soft and penetration of the abdomen can result. Dart wounds often bleed profusely; be sure to treat all dart wounds before release. Blindfolding is recommended. After recovery, zebraas often take off at a run, which may lead to stumbling and falling; choose a suitable release site. Long-acting tranquilizer doses: haloperidol (adults, 20-40 mg); zuclopenthixol, 1 mg/kg; perphenazine (adults, 100 mg). Zebras from different family units cannot be mixed in one compartment during transport because they will fight even when tranquillized.

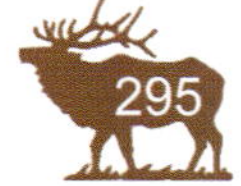

References: Talbot and Lamprey, 1961; Talbot and Talbot, 1962; Lanphear, 1963; Van Niekerk et al., 1963a; Wright, 1963; Bigalke, 1965; Harthoorn, 1965a; 1971; 1972a; 1973b; Harthoorn and Bligh, 1965; King and Klingel, 1965; Ebedes, 1966a; 1971a; Pienaar et al., 1966a; Ericksen, 1968; Klingel, 1968; Wallach, 1968; 1969; Pienaar, 1968a; 1969b; Taylor and Chandler, 1971; Bauditz, 1972; Heck and Rivenburg, 1972; Higgins, 1973; Harthoorn and Young, 1974; Hertzog, 1975; Rapley and Mehren, 1975; Röken, 1975; Jones, 1976; Oosterhuis, 1979; Hofmeyr, 1981; Wiesner et al., 1982; Silvestris and Heck, 1984; Kock and Pearce, 1985; Wiesner and von Hegel, 1985; Fukumoto and Nisshiyama, 1989; IWVS, 1992; Burroughs, 1993f; Lin et al., 1993a; Vitaud, 1993; Wiesner, 1993; Hashizaki et al., 1996; Arnemo, 2004b; Kock, M., et al., 2006

ZEBRA, GREVY, *Equus grevyi*

Weight: 352–450 kg
Recommended Drug: 6 mg etorphine plus 25 mg acepromazine
Supplemental Drug: If not down in in 20 min, repeat full dose
Antagonist: 2 mg diprenorphine per mg etorphine given
Alternative Drugs: 6 mg etorphine plus 100 mg xylazine; antagonize with 2 mg diprenorphine per mg etorphine given plus 0.125 mg/kg yohimbine
• 12 mg carfentanil plus 13 mg detomidine; antagonize with 100 mg naltrexone per mg carfentanil given
Comments: Complete muscle relaxation is difficult to obtain with wild equids; excessive leg movement is common. Muscle relaxation appears better with detomidine than with xylazine. Opioids result in poor muscle relaxation; administer 10 mg diazepam to improve relaxation. Wild equids tend to overheat easily, particularly if there is a prolonged hyperexcitable state prior to anesthetic induction. Attempt to immobilize equids during the coolest part of the day. Etorphine may be more effective than carfentanil in zebras; thiafentanil *cannot* be used in zebras. The carfentanil dosage given is based on repeated immobilizations of a captive female zebra (Renner, 1998). Zebra skin is resilient sometimes making dart penetration difficult, but do not dart from behind because the skin of the perineum is soft and penetration of the abdomen can result. Dart wounds often bleed profusely; be sure to treat all dart wounds before release. Blindfolding is recommended. After recovery, zebraas often take off at a run, which may lead to stumbling and falling; choose a suitable release site. Long-acting tranquilizer doses: haloperidol (adults, 20-40 mg); zuclopenthixol, 1 mg/kg; perphenazine (adults, 100 mg). Zebras from different family units cannot be mixed in one compartment during transport because they will fight even when tranquillized.
References: Lock and Harthoorn, 1959; Buechner et al., 1960a; 1960c; Lanphear, 1963; Wright, 1963; Heck and Rivenburg, 1972; Alford et al., 1974; Rapley and Mehren, 1975; Röken, 1975; Jones, 1976; Oosterhuis, 1979; Jessup et al., 1980; Wiesner et al., 1982; Bristol et al., 1984; Kock and

Pearce, 1985; Wiesner and von Hegel, 1985; Pospisil et al., 1989; Allen, 1990a; Klein and Citino, 1995; Chaduc, 1996; Renner, 1998

ZEBRA, MOUNTAIN, *Equus zebra*

Weight: 150–350 kg

Recommended Drug: 6 mg etorphine (male), 4 mg etorphine (female) plus 80 mg azaperone

Supplemental Drug: If not down in in 20 min, repeat full dose

Antagonist: 2.4 mg diprenorphine per mg etorphine given

Alternative Drugs: 6 mg etorphine plus 100 mg xylazine; antagonize with 2 mg diprenorphine per mg etorphine given plus 0.125 mg/kg yohimbine • 2.5 ml Large Animal Immobilon® plus 50 mg xylazine; antagonize with 2 mg diprenorphine per mg etorphine given plus 0.125 mg/kg yohimbine • 0.011 mg/kg carfentanil; antagonize with 1 mg/kg naltexone

Comments: Complete muscle relaxation is difficult to obtain with wild equids; excessive leg movement is common. Muscle relaxation appears better with detomidine than with xylazine. Opioids result in poor muscle relaxation; administer 10 mg diazepam to improve relaxation. Wild equids tend to overheat easily, particularly if there is a prolonged hyperexcitable state prior to anesthetic induction. Attempt to immobilize equids during the coolest part of the day. Etorphine may be more effective than carfentanil in zebras; thiafentanil *cannot* be used in zebras. Zebra skin is resilient sometimes making dart penetration difficult, but do not dart from behind because the skin of the perineum is soft and penetration of the abdomen can result. Dart wounds often bleed profusely; be sure to treat all dart wounds before release. Blindfolding is recommended. After recovery, zebras often take off at a run, which may lead to stumbling and falling; choose a suitable release site. Long-acting tranquilizer doses: haloperidol (adults, 20-40 mg); zuclopenthixol, 1 mg/kg; perphenazine (adults, 100 mg). Zebras from different family units cannot be mixed in one compartment during transport because they will fight even when tranquillized.

References: Heck and Rivenburg, 1972; Young and Penzhorn, 1972; Röken, 1975; Jones, 1976; Oosterhuis, 1979; Shalka, 1979; Hofmeyr, 1981; Wiesner et al., 1982; Silvestris and Heck, 1984; Kuttner and Wiesner, 1987; Burroughs, 1993f; Allen, 1990a; 1994; Kock, M., et al., 2006

ZEBU, *Bos taurus*

Weight: 800–1,000 kg

Recommended Drug: 3.6 mg/kg tiletamine-zolazepam

Supplemental Drug: 1 mg/kg ketamine

Antagonist: None

Alternative Drugs: 8 mg etorphine; antagonize with 16 mg diprenorphine

References: Jarvis and Morris, 1960; Beck, 1972; Woolf et al., 1973; Wiesner, 1975; Wiesner and von Hegel, 1985; Schobert, 1987

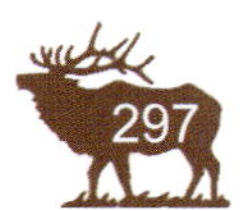

References

Abbott, C. W. 1973. Reactions of eland to immobilising drugs. Lammergeyer. 18: 30-38.

Ables, E. D. 1969. Field immobilization of free ranging impala in northern Kenya. E. Afr. Wildl. J. 7: 61-66.

Adams, W. A., K. J. Robinson, R. S. Jones, and S. Sanderson. 2003. Isoflurane to prolong medetomidine/ketamine anaesthesia in six adult female chimpanzees (*Pan troglodytes*). Vet. Rec. 152: 18-20.

Adams, W. A., K. J. Robinson, R. S. Jones, and G. B. Edwards. 2005. Overdose during chemical restraint in a black rhinoceros (*Diceros bicornis*). Vet. Anaesth. Analg. 32: 53-57.

Addison, E. M., G. B. Kolenosky. 1979. Use of ketamine hydrochloride and xylazine hydrochloride to immobilize black bears (*Ursus americanus*). J. Wildl. Dis. 15: 253-258.

Adest, G. A., J. Jarchow, and B. Brydolf. 1988. A method for manual ventilation of tranquilized tortoises. Herpetol. Rev. 19: 80.

Aird, S. D. 1986. Methoxyflurane anesthesia in Crotalus: Comparisons with other gas anesthetics. Herpetol. Rev. 17: 82-84.

Agoramoorthy, G, and R. Rudran. 1994. Field application of Telazol (tiletamine hydrochloride and zolazepam hydrochloride) to immobilize wild red howler monkeys (*Alouatta seniculus*) in Venezuela. J. Wildl. Dis. 30: 417-420.

Aguilar, R. F., V. E. Smith, P. Ogburn, and P. T. Redig. 1996. Arrhythmias associated with isoflurane anesthesia in bald eagles (*Haliaeetus leucocephalus*). J. Zoo Wildl. Med. 26: 508-516.

Aguirre, A. A., B. Zimmerman, M. Tannerfeldt, A. Angerbjörn, and T. Mörner. 1998. Medetomidine-ketamine/atipamezole anesthesia/reversal in wild arctic fox pups in Swedish Lapland. Proc. Joint Conf. Am. Assoc. Zoo Vet. and Am. Assoc. Wildl. Vet. P. 49.

Aguirre, A. A., B. Principe, M. Tannerfeldt, A. Angerbjörn, and T. Mörner. 2000. Field anestheisa ofwild arctic fox (*Alopex lagopus*) cubs in the Swedish Lapland using medetomidine-ketamine-atipamezole. J. Zoo Wildl. Med. 31: 244-246.

Akhari, S., and S. Dehghani. 1993. Introduction of a recirculator for longterm anaesthesia applicable in the surgery of fishes. J. Vet. Faculty U. Tehran. 47: 15-22.

Al Busadah, K. A., and T. E. A. Osman. 2001. Failure of yohimbine to reverse the haematological changes associated with xylazine anesthesia in the camel (*Camelus dromedarius*). J. Camel. Pract. Res. 8: 43-46.

Alford, B. T., L. Burkhart, W. P. Johnson. 1974. Etorphine and diprenorphine as immobilizing and reversing agents in captive and free-ranging mammals. J. Am. Vet. Med. Assoc. 154: 701-705.

Alkon, P. U. 1984. Chemical restraint of Indian crested porcupines (*Hysterix indica*). Mammalia. 48: 150-152.

Allen, J. L. 1986a. Use of tolazoline as an antagonist to xylazine-ketamine-induced immobilization in African elephants. Am. J. Vet. Res. 47: 781-783.

Allen, J. L. 1986b. Tolazoline antagonism of xylazine-ketamine immobilization in selected non-domestic hoofstock. Proc. Am. Assoc. Zoo Vet. Pp. 3-4.

Allen, J. L. 1989. Renarcotization following carfentanil immobilization of nondomestic ungulates. J. Zoo An. Med. 20: 423-426.

Allen, J. L. 1990a. Renarcotization following etorphine immobilization of nondomestic Equidae. J. Zoo An. Med. 21: 292-294.

Allen, J. L. 1990b. Pulse oximetry: clinical applications in zoological medicine. Proc. Am. Assoc. Zoo Vet. 163-164.

Allen, J. L. 1992a. Immobilization of Mongolian wild horses (*Equus przewalskii przewalskii*) with carfentanil and antagonism with naltrexone. J. Zoo Wildl. Med. 23: 422-425.

Allen, J. L. 1992b. Immobilization of giant Chacoan peccaries (*Catagonus wagneri*) with a tiletamine hydrochloride/zolazepam hydrochloride combination. J. Wildl. Dis. 28: 499-501.

Allen, J. L. 1994. Immobilization of Hartmann's mountain zebras (*Equus zebra hartmannae*) with carfentanil and antagonism with naltrexone or nalmefene. J. Zoo Wildl. Med. 25: 205-208.

Allen, J. L. 1996. A comparison of nalmafene and naltrexone for the prevention of renarcotization following carfentanil immobilization of nondomestic ungulates. J. Zoo Wildl. Med. 27: 496-500.

Allen, J. L. 1997. Anesthesia of non-domestic horses with carfentanil and antagonism with naltrexone or

nalmefene. Proc. Am. Assoc. Zoo Vet. P. 126.
Allen, J. L. 1999. Use of pulse oximetry in monitoring anesthesia. *In* Fowler, M. E., and R. E. Miller (eds.). Zoo & Wild Animal Medicine. Current Therapy 4. W. B. Saunders Company, Philadelphia, Pennsylvania. Pp. 2-3.
Allen, J. L., and J. E. Oosterhuis. 1986a. Effect of tolazoline on xylazine-ketamine-induced anesthesia in turkey vultures. J. Am. Vet. Med. Assoc. 189: 1011-1012.
Allen, J. L., and J. E. Oosterhuis. 1986b. Use of tolazoline as an antagonist to xylazine-ketamine anesthesia in selected avian species. Proc. Annu. Meet. Assoc. Avian Vet. 1986: 281-282.
Allen, J. L., D. L. Janssen, J. E. Oosterhuis, and T. H. Stanley. 1991. Immobilization of captive non-domestic hoofstock with carfentanil. Proc. Am. Assoc. Zoo Vet. Pp. 343-353.
Allen, K. E. 1965. Immobilizing beaver with succinylcholine chloride. Game Res. Ohio. 3: 215-220.
Allen, T. J. 1970. Immobilization of white-tailed deer with succinylcholine chloride and hyaluronidase. J. Wildl. Manage. 34: 207-209.
Allsup, F. C. 1977. Accidental self injection. Vet. Rec. 100: 499.
Althouse, G. C., C. M. Hodges, S. J. Magyar, T. G. Biediger, and S. W. J. Seager. 1987. Immobilization of a pregnant nilgai (*Boselaphus tragocamelus*) using a combination of etorphine, xylazine, and acepromazine with reversal using yohimbine and diprenorphine. Southwest Vet. 38: 47-50.
Altman, R. B., and M. S. Miller. 1979. Effects of anesthesia on the temperature and electrocardiogram of birds. Proc. Am. Assoc. Zoo Vet. Pp. 61-62.
Amand, W. B. 1980. Avian anesthetic agents and techniques – a review. Proc. Am. Assoc. Zoo Vet. 8: 68-72.
Amand, W. B., H. W. Calderwood, C. E. Harvey, G. W. McConnel, and A. M. Klide. 1972. Chemical restraint of a black gnu (*Connachaetes gnou*) with BAY-VA 1470. J. Zoo An. Med. 2: 22-25.
Amand, W. B. 1982a. Chemical immobilization of birds. *In* Nielsen, L., J. C. Haigh, and M. E. Fowler (eds.). Chemical Immobilization of North American Wildlife. Milwaukee, Wisconsin: Wisconsin Humane Society, Inc. Pp. 199-213.
Amand, W. B. 1982b. Chemical immobilization of reptiles. *In* Nielsen, L, J. C. Haigh, and M. E. Fowler (eds.). Chemical Immobilization of North American Wildlife. Milwaukee, Wisconsin: Wisconsin Humane Society, Inc. Pp. 199-213.
Amass, K., and M. Drew. 2006. How much Telazol® is really in the bottle? Inaccurate labeling of Telazol® from 1987-1998 and the impact on published literature. Proc. Am. Assoc. Zoo Vet. Pp. 298-302.
Amstrup, S. C., and T. B. Segerstrom. 1981. Immobilizing free-ranging pronghorns with powdered succinylcholine chloride. J. Wildl. Manage. 45: 740-745.
Amstrup, S. C., B. W. O'Gara, and H. Musgrave. 1982. Immobilizing elk with powdered succinylcholine chloride. Wildl. Soc. Bull. 10: 333-340.
Ancrenaz, M. 1994. Use of atipamezole to reverse xylazine tranquilization in captive Arabian oryx (*Oryx leucoryx*). J. Wildl. Dis. 30: 592-595.
Ancrenaz, M., S. Ostrowski, A. Delhomme, and A. Greth. 1995. Latest developments in translocation techniques of the Arabian Oryx, *Oryx leucoryx*. Proc. Joint Conf. Am. Assoc. Zoo Vet., Wildl. Dis. Assoc., Am. Assoc. Wildl. Vet. East Lansing, Michigan. Pp. 184-189.
Ancrenaz, M., S. Ostrowski, S. Anagariyah, and A. Delhomme. 1996. Long-duration anesthesia in Arabian oryx (*Oryx leucoryx*) using a medetomidine-etorphine combination. J. Zoo Wildl. Med. 27: 209-216.
Andau, P. M., L. K. Hiong, and J. B. Sale. 1994. Translocation of pocketed orang-utans in Sabah. Oryx 28: 263-268.
Anderson, C. F. 1961. Anesthetizing deer by arrow. J. Wildl. Manage. 25: 202-203.
Anderson, M. D., and P. R. K. Richardson. 1992. Remote immobilization of the aardwolf. So. Afr. J. Wildl. Res. 22: 26-28.
Andryk, T. A., L. R. Irby, D. L. Hook, J. J. McCarthy, and G. Olson. 1983. Comparison of mountain sheep capture techniques: helicopter darting versus net-gunning. Wildl. Soc. Bull. 11: 184-187.
Anonymous. 1976. Veterinary surgeon's Immobilon death "accidental." Vet. Rec. 98: 414-415.
Apelt, H. J. 1993. Use of tiletamine-zolazepam combination as an injectable anaesthetic and as a premedication for isoflurane anaesthesia in tortoises. Tierarztliche Hochscule, Hannover. 111 pp.
April, M., E. Tabor, and R. J. Gerety. 1982. Combination of ketamine and xylazine for effective anesthesia of juvenile chimpanzees (*Pan troglodytes*). Lab. An. 16: 116-118.

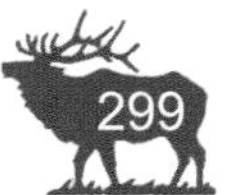

Arena, P. C., K. C. Richardson, and L. K. Cullen. 1988. Anaesthesia in two species of large Australian skink. Vet. Rec. 123: 155-158.

Arenz, C. L. 1997. Handling fox squirrels: ketamine hydrochloride versus a simple restraint. Wildl. Soc. Bull. 25: 107-109.

Armstrong, D. L. 1989. An evaluation of carfentanil as an immobilizing agent for gaur (*Bos gaurus*). Proc. Am. Assoc. Zoo Vet. P. 8.

Arnemo, J. M. 1989. Surgical implantation of intraperitoneal radiotelemetry devices in European river otters (*Lutra lutra*). Proc. V Int. Otter Colloquium - Habitat 7, Hankensbüttel.

Arnemo, J. M. 1990. Chemical immobilization of European river otter (*Lutra lutra*). Norsk Veterinaertidsskrift 102: 767-770.

Arnemo, J. M. 1995. Immobilization of free-ranging moose (*Alces alces*) with medetomidine-ketamine and remobilization with atipamezole. Rangifer 15:19-25.

Arnemo, J. M. 2004a. Chemical immobilization and anaesthesia of wild boars. Orion Pharma Newsletter DDA News 1: 4.

Arnemo, J. M. 2004b. Chemical immobilization of zebras. Orion Pharma Newsletter DDA News 2: 3-4.

Arnemo, J. M. (ed.). 2006. Biomedical protocols for free-ranging brown bears, gray wolves, wolverines, and lynx. Norwegian School of Veterinary Science, TromsØ, Norway. 18 pp.

Arnemo, J. M. 2005. Sedation and anaesthesia of llamas. The role of medetomidine and atipamezole. Orion Pharma Newsletter DDA News 2: 4-5.

Arnemo, J. M., and N. E. SØli. 1992. Immobilization of mink (*Mustela vison*) with medetomidine-ketamine and remobilization with atipamezole. Vet. Res. Comm. 16: 281-292.

Arnemo, J. M., and N. E. SØli. 1993. Chemical capture of free-ranging cattle: immobilization with xylazine or medetomidine, and reversal with atipamezole. Vet. Res. Comm. 17: 469-477.

Arnemo, J. M., and N. E. SØli. 1994. Injection darts containing drugs - a potential health hazard for several years? Norsk Veterinaer. 106: 306-308.

Arnemo, J. M., and N. E. SØli. 1995a. Chemical immobilization of free-ranging European hedgehogs (*Erinaceus europaeus*). J. Zoo Wildl. Med. 26: 246-251.

Arnemo, J. M., and N. E. SØli. 1995b. Immobilization of free-ranging cattle with medetomidine and its reversal by atipamezole. Vet. res. Comm. 19: 59-62.

Arnemo, J. M., and B. Ranheim. 1999. Effects of medetomidine and atipamezole on serum glucose and cortisol levels in captive reindeer (*Rangifer tarandus tarandus*). Rangifer 19: 85-89.

Arnemo, J. M., R. Moe, and A. J. Smith. 1993a. Immobilization of captive raccoon dogs (*Nyctereutes procyonoides*) with medetomidine-ketamine and remobilization with atipamezole. J. Zoo Wildl. Med. 24: 102-108.

Arnemo, J. M., T. Negard, and N. E. SØli 1993b. Deer farming in Norway. A review of the currently available drugs that can be used for immobilization, pain relief, and anaesthesia. Norsk Veterinaer. 105: 517-521.

Arnemo, J. M., R. Moe, and N. E. SØli. 1993c. Xylazine-induced sedation in axis deer (*Axis axis*) and its reversal by atipamezole. Vet. Res. Comm. 17: 123-128.

Arnemo, J. M., T. Soveri, Ø. Os, and N. E. SØli. 1994a. Immobilization of free-ranging moose (*Alces alces*) with medetomidine-ketamine and reversal with atipamezole. Joint Conf. Am. Assoc. Zoo Vet. Assoc. Reptil. Amphib. Vet. Pp. 197-199.

Arnemo, J. M., T. Negard, and N. E. SØli. 1994b. Chemical capture of free-ranging red deer (*Cervus elaphus*) with medetomidine-ketamine. Rangifer 14: 123-127.

Arnemo, J. M., R. O. Moe, and N. E. SØli. 1994c. Immobilization of captive pine martens (*Martes martes*) with medetomidine-ketamine and reversal with atipamezole. J. Zoo Wildl. Med. 25: 548-554.

Arnemo, J. M., J. D. C. Linnell, S. J. Wedule, B. Ranheim, J. Odden, and R. Andersen. 1999. Use of intraperitoneal radio-transmitters in lynx *Lynx lynx* kittens: anaesthesia, surgery and behaviour. Wildl. Biol. 5: 245-250.

Arnemo, J. M., S. Brunberg, R. Franzén, A. Friebe, P. Segerström, A. Söderberg, and J. E. Swenson. 2001. Reversible immobilization and anesthesia of free-ranging brown bears (*Ursus arctos*) with medetomidine-tiletamine-zolazepam and atipamezole: a review of 575 captures. Proc. Am. Assoc. Zoo Vet. Pp. 234-236.

Arnemo, J. M., T. J. Kreeger, and T. Soveri. 2003. Chemical immobilization of free-ranging moose. Alces 39: 243-253.

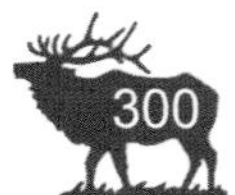

Arnemo, J. M., G. Ericsson, E. O. Øen, E. Broman, K. Wallin, and J. Ball. 2004. Immobilization of free-ranging moose (*Alces alces*) with etorphine or etorphine-acepromazine-xylazine in Scandinavia 1994-2003: a review of 2,754 captures. Proc. Am. Assoc. Zoo Vet. Pp. 515-516.

Arnemo, J. M., T. Storass, C. B. Khadka, and P. Wegge. 2005a. Use of medetomidine-ketamine and atipamezole for reversible immobilization of free-ranging hog deer (*Axi porcinus*) captured in drive nets. J. Wildl. Dis. 41: 467-470.

Arnemo, J. M., Å. Fahlman, J. Persson, and P. Segerström. 2005b. Anaesthetic and surgical protocols for implantation of intraperitoneal radiotransmitters in free-ranging wolverines (*Gulo gulo*). Proc. 1st Intl. Symp. Wolverine Res. Mgmt., Jokkmokk, Sweden. Pp. 17-18.

Arnemo, J. M., P. Ahlqvist, R. Andersen, F. Berntsen, G. Ericsson, J. Odden, S. Brunberg, P. Segerstrom, and J. E. Swenson. 2006. Risk of capture-related mortality in large free-ranging mammals: experiences in Scandinavia. Wildl. Biol. 1: 109-113.

Arnold, G. W., D. Steven, J. Weeldenburg, and O. E. Brown. 1986. The use of alpha-chloralose for the repeated capture of Western grey kangaroos, *Macropus fuliginosus*. Aust. Wildl. Res. 13: 527-533.

Arora, B. M. 1988. Chemical immobilization of deer and antelopes. Tigerpaper. 15: 8-14.

Arora, B. M., H. Wiesner, and A. K. Malhotra. 1983. A note on chemical immobilization of zoo animals with blow pipe. Indian J. Vet. Surg. 4: 78-81.

Arthur, S. M. 1988. An evaluation of techniques for capturing and radiocollaring fishers. Wildl. Soc. Bull. 16: 417-421.

Atkinson, M. W., B. Hull, A. R. Gandolf, and E. S. Blumer. 2002. Repeated chemical immobilization of captive greater one-horned rhinoceros (*Rhinoceros unicornis*), using a combination of etorphine, detomidine, and ketamine. J. Zoo Wildl. Med. 33: 157-162.

Austin, D. H., and J. H. Peoples. 1967. Capturing hogs with alpha-chloralose. Proc. Ann. Conf. Southeast. Assoc. Game Fish Comm. 21: 201- 203.

Autenrieth, R. E., G. L. Copeland, and T. D. Reynolds. 1981. Capturing pronghorn using a helicopter and etorphine hydrochloride. Wildl. Soc. Bull. 9: 314-319.

Baber, D. W., and E. C. Bruce. 1982. Immobilization of feral pigs with a combination of ketamine and xylazine. J. Wildl. Manage 46: 557-559.

Bacher, J. D., S. Potkay, and E. J. Baas. 1976. An evaluation of sedatives and anesthetics in the agouti (*Dasyprocta sp.*). Lab. An. Sci. 26: 195-197.

Backhouse, K. M. 1964. The anesthesia of marine mammals. *In* Jones, G. (ed.). Small Animal Anesthesia. Pergamon Press, London. Pp. 79-82.

Baer, C. H., R. E. Severson, and S. B. Linhart. 1978. Live capture of coyotes from a helicopter with ketamine hydrochloride. J. Wildl. Manage. 42: 452-454.

Baharav, D. and A. Tadmor. 1981. Immobilization of mountain gazelles with M99. Mammalia. 45: 391-393.

Bailey, P. L., J. D. Port, N. L. Pace, T. H. Stanley, and J. Kimball. 1985. The ED_{50} of carfentanil for elk immobilization with and without the tranquilizer R51703. J. Wildl. Manage. 49: 931-934.

Bailey, P. L., D. Port, S. McJames, L. Reinersman, and T. H. Stanley. 1987. Is fentanyl an anesthetic in the dog? Anesth. Analg. 66: 542-548.

Bailey, R. W. 1972. Use of stimulants in reducing mortality in narcotized wild turkeys. Proc. Ann. Conf. Southeast. Assoc. Game Fish Comm. 26: 212-213.

Bailey, R. W., and R. V. Doepker. 1977. Problems in capturing wild turkeys with trichloroethanol. Proc. Ann. Conf. Southeast. Assoc. Game Fish Comm. 31: 283-284.

Bailey, T. A., C. A. Baker, P. K. Nicholls, and K. Wilson. 1995. Reversible anesthesia of the blue duiker (*Cephalophus monticola*) with medetomidine and ketamine. J. Zoo Wildl. Med. 26: 237-239.

Bailey, T. A., A. Toosi, and J. H. Samour. 1999. Anaesthesia of cranes with alphaxolone-alphadolone. Vet. Rec. 145: 84-85.

Bailey, T. N. 1971. Immobilization of bobcats, coyotes, and badgers with phencyclidine hydrochloride. J. Wildl. Manage. 35: 847-849.

Baker, J. R., and T. J. Gatesman. 1985. Use of carfentanil and a ketamine-xylazine mixture to immobilise wild grey seals (*Halichoerus grypus*). Vet. Rec. 116: 208-210.

Baker, J. R., S. S. Anderson, and M. A. Fedak. 1988. The use of ketamine-diazepam mixture to immobilise wild grey seals (*Halichoerus grypus*) and southern elephant seals (*Mirounga leonina*). Vet. Rec. 123: 287-289.

Baker, J. R., M. A. Fedak, S. S. Anderson, T. Arnborn, and R. Baker. 1990. The use of tiletamine/zolazepam

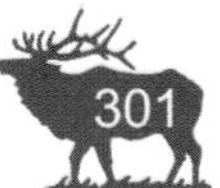

mixture to immobilize wild grey seals and southern elephant seals. Vet. Rec. 126: 75-77.
Ballard, W. B., and R. W. Tobey. 1981. Decreased calf production of moose immobilized with anectine administered from helicopter. Wildl. Soc. Bull. 9: 207-209.
Ballard, W. B., A. W. Franzmann, and C. L. Gardner. 1982. Comparison and assessment of drugs used to immobilize Alaskan gray wolves (*Canis lupus*) and wolverines (*Gulo gulo*) from a helicopter. J. Wildl. Dis. 18: 339-342.
Ballard, W. B., L. A. Ayres, K. E. Roney, and T. H. Spraker. 1991. Immobilization of gray wolves with a combination of tiletamine hydrochloride and zolazepam hydrochloride. J. Wildl. Manage. 55: 71-74.
Ballard, W. B., H. A. Whitlaw, D. L. Sabine, R. A. Jenkins, S. J. Young, and G. F. Forbes. 1998. White-tailed deer, *Odocoileus virginianus*, capture techniques in yarding and non-yarding populations in New-Brunswick. Can. Field Natur. 112: 254-261.
Balser, D. S. 1965. Tranquilizer tabs for capturing wild carnivores. J. Wildl. Manage. 29: 438-442.
Banknieder, A. R., J. M. Phillips, K. T. Jackson, and S. I. Vinal. 1978. Comparison of ketamine with the combination of ketamine and xylazine for effective anesthesia in the rhesus monkey (*Macaca mulatta*). Lab. An. Sci. 28: 742-745.
Barkhuizen, G. F. 1972. Notes on the use of azaperone and fentanyl in the immobilization of the bontebok (*Damaliscus dorcas dorcas*) in the Bontebok National Park. Koedoe 15: 101-105.
Barnard, S. M., and J. S. Dobbs. 1980. A handmade blowgun dart: it's preparation and application in a zoological park. J. Am. Vet. Med. Assoc. 177: 953-955.
Barnes, D. M., and L. L. Rogers. 1980. Clostridial myonecrosis in a black bear associated with drug administration. J. Wildl. Dis. 17: 95-110.
Barnett, J. E. F., and J. C. M. Lewis. 1990. Medetomidine and ketamine anaesthesia in zoo animals and its reversal with atipamezole: a review and update with specific reference to work in British zoos. Proc. Am. Assoc. Zoo Vet. Pp. 207-214.
Barrett, M., J. W. Nolan, and L. D. Roy. 1982. Evaluation of a hand-held net-gun to capture large mammals. Wildl. Soc. Bull. 10: 108-114.
Barry, W. J. 1972. Methoxyflurane: an anesthetic for field and laboratory use on squirrels. J. Wildl. Manage. 36: 992-993.
Bartels, P., N. Grobler, and N. Rauch. 1992. The adaptation of the wild blesbok to captive conditions. Use of Tranquilizers in wildlife. *In* Ebedes, H. (ed.). Proceedings of the Wildlife Tranquilizer Symposium, National Zoological Gardens, Pretoria, South Africa, 17-18 March 1989. pp. 17-18.
Barter, L. S., M. G. Hawkins, R. J. Brosnan, J. E. Antognini, and B. H. Pypendop. 2006. Median effective dose of isoflurane, sevoflurane, and desflurane in green iguanas. Amer. J. Vet. Res. 67: 392-397.
Bartmann, W. 1972. Korrekturmassnahmen nach spontaner Gehörndeformation beim Jacksons Hartebeest (*Alcelaphus busephalus jacksoni*). Zool. Garten. 42: 159-165.
Bartsch, R. C., E. E. McConnell, G. D. Imes, and J. M. Schmidt. 1977. A review of exertional rhabdomyolysis in wild and domestic animals and man. Vet. Path. 14: 214-324.
Bassett, J. E. 1987. Hemodilution with anesthesia in the bat, *Antrozous pallidus*. J. Mammal. 68: 378-381.
Basson, P. A., and J. M. Hofmeyr. 1972. Mortalities associated with wildlife capture operations. Specialized University Course on Wildlife Capture Techniques and General Husbandry. Onderstpoort (South Africa).
Bates, J. W., and J. G. Guymon. 1985. Comparison of drive nets and darting for capture of desert bighorn sheep. Wildl. Soc. Bull. 13: 73-76.
Bauditz, R. 1972. Sedation, immobilization and anesthesia with Rompun in captive and free-living wild animals. Vet. Med. Rev. 3: 204-226.
Baumgardner, D. J., and D. A. Dewsbury. 1979. Surgical anesthesia of seven rodent species with chloral hydrate. Physiol. Beh. 23: 609-610.
Baumgartner, L. L. 1940. Trapping, handling, and marking fox squirrels. J. Wildl. Manage. 4: 444-450.
Beale, D. M., and A. D. Smith. 1967. Immobilization of pronghorn antelopes with succinylcholine chloride. J. Wildl. Manage. 31: 840-842.
Beck, C. C. 1971. Chemical restraint of exotic species. Proc. Am. Assoc. Zoo Vet. Pp. 1-81.
Beck, C. C. 1972. Chemical restraint of exotic species. J. Zoo An. Med. 3: 3-66.
Beck, C. C. 1974. Ketamine anesthesia. J. Zoo An. Med. 5: 6.
Beck, C. C. 1976. Vetalar (ketamine hydrochloride) a unique cataleptoid anesthetic agent for multispecies

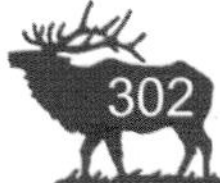

usage. J. Zoo An. Med. 7: 11-38.

Beck, C. C., and A. J. Dresner. 1972. Vetalar® (ketamine HCL): a cataleptoid anesthetic agent for primate species. Vet. Med. Sm. An. Clin. 67: 1082-1084.

Beck, S. W., and J. S. Gaynor. 2003. Comparison of isoflurane and sevoflurane for anesthesia in beaver. J. Wildl. Dis. 39: 387-392.

Beeman, L. E., M. R. Pelton, and L. C. Marcum. 1974. Use of M99 etorphine for immobilizing black bears. J. Wildl. Manage. 38: 568-569.

Behrend, D. F. 1965. Notes on field immobilization of white-tailed deer with nicotine. J. Wildl. Manage. 29: 889-890.

Beiglböck, C., and W. Zenker. 2003. Evaluation of three combinations of anesthetics for use in free-ranging alpine marmots (*Marmota marmota*). J. Wildl. Dis. 39: 665-674.

Belant, J. L. 1991. Immobilization of fishers (*Martes pennanti*) with ketamine hydrochloride and xylazine hydrochloride. J. Wildl. Dis. 27: 328-330.

Belant, J. L. 1992. Field immobilization of American martens (*Martes americana*) and short-tailed weasels (*Mustela erminea*). J. Wildl. Dis. 28: 662-665.

Belant, J. L. 1995a. Field Immobilization of raccoons with ketamine-hydrochloride and xylazine hydrochloride. Acta Theriol. 40: 327-330.

Belant, J. L. 1995b. Isoflurane as an inhalation anesthetic for muskrats (*Ondatra zibethicus*). J. Wildl. Dis. 31: 573-575.

Belant, J. L. 1996. Immobilization of muskrats (*Ondatra zibethicus*) with ketamine and xylazine. J. Wildl. Dis. 32: 152-155.

Belant, J. L. 2004. Field immobilization of raccoons (*Procyon lotor*) with Telazol® and xylazine. J. Wildl. Dis. 40: 787-790.

Belant, J. L. 2005. Tiletamine-zolazepam-xylazine immobilization of American marten (*Martes americana*). J. Wildl. Dis. 41: 659-663.

Belant, J. L., and T. W. Seamans. 1997. Comparison of three formulations of alpha-chloralose for immobilization of Canada geese. J. Wildl. Dis. 33: 606-610.

Belant, J. L., and T. W. Seamans. 1999. Alpha-chloralose immobilization of rock doves in Ohio. J. Wildl. Dis. 35: 239-242.

Belant, J. L., L. A. Tyson, and T. W. Seamans. 1999. Use of alpha-chlorolose by the Wildlife Services program to capture nuisance birds. Wildl. Soc. Bull. 27:938-942.

Bell, R. H. V., and G. L. Van Rooyen. 1985. A range-finder sight for use with capture guns. So. Afr. J. Wildl. Res. 15: 37-38.

Beltrán, J. F., M. Delibes, and C. Ibáñez. 1985. Immobilization and marking the Egyptian mongoose, *Herpestes ichneumon* (L.), in Spain. Zeitschrift für Säugertierkunde 50: 243-244.

Beltrán, J. F., and M. E. Tewes. 1995. Immobilization of oceolots and bobcats with ketamine hydrochloride and xylazine hydrochloride. J. Wildl. Dis. 31: 43-48.

Bengis, R. 1993. Chemical capture of the African buffalo *Syncerus caffer*. *In* McKenzie, A. A. (ed.). The Capture and Care Manual. Wildlife Decision Support Services and The South African Veterinary Foundation, Pretoria. Pp. 583-589.

Bengis, R. G., V. de Vos,, and J. van Niekerk. 1985. Immobilization of the African elephant. Proc. 2nd Int. Congr. Vet. Anesth. Pp. 142-143.

Bengis, R. G., and D. F. Keet. 2000. Chemical capture of free-ranging lions(*Panthera leo*). Proc. N. Am. Vet. Conf. 14: 1029-1031.

Bennett, R. A. 1991. A review of anesthesia and chemical restraint in reptiles. J. Zoo Wildl. Med. 22: 282-303.

Bennett, R. A. 1993a. Current techniques in reptile anesthesia. Proc. No. Am. Vet. Conf. Orlando, Florida. Pp. 767-768.

Bennett, R. A. 1993b. Basic anesthesia and surgery in avian patients. Proc. No. Am. Vet. Conf. Orlando, Florida. Pp. 701-703.

Bennet, R. A. 1994. Current techniques in reptile anesthesia and surgery. Joint Conf. Am. Assoc. Zoo Vet. Assoc. Reptil. Amphib. Vet. Pp. 36-44.

Bennett, R. A. 1998. Reptile Anesthesia. Semin. Avian Exotic. Pet. Med. 7: 30-40.

Bennett, R. A., J. Schumacher, K. Hedjazi-Haring, and S. Newell. 1998a. Cardiopulmonary and anesthetic effects of propofol administered intraosseously to green iguanas, *Iguana iguana*. J. Am. Vet. Med. Assoc. 212:93-98.

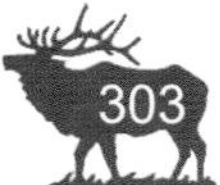

Bennett, R. A., J. Schumacher, K. Hedjazi-Haring, and S. Newell. 1998b. Cardiopulmonary and anesthetic effects of propofol for induction and maintenance of anesthesia in green iguanas (*Iguana iguana*). Proc. Joint Conf. Am. Assoc. Zoo Vet. and Am. Assoc. Wildl. Vet. Pp. 272-273.

Bennett, R. R., and P. J. Tillotson. 1969. Cyclohexanone as an anesthetic for the leopard and the bengal tiger. J. Am. Vet. Med. Assoc. 155: 1098.

Bennett, R. R., F. O. Zydeck, and R. Wilson. 1971. Tiletamine anesthesia of a Siberian tiger and a lion. J. Am. Vet. Med. Assoc. 159: 620-621.

Berger, J., and M. D. Kock. 1988. Overwinter survival of carfentanil-immobilized male bison. J. Wildl. Dis. 24: 555-556.

Berger, J., M. Kock, C. Cunningham, and N. Dodson. 1983. Chemical restraint of wild horses: effects of reproduction and social structure. J. Wildl. Dis. 19: 265-268.

Bergerud, A. T., A. Butt, H. L. Russell, and H. Whalen. 1964. Immobilization of Newfoundland caribou and moose with succinylcholine chloride and Cap-Chur equipment. J. Wildl. Manage. 28: 49-53.

Berrie, P. M. 1972. Sex differences in response to phencyclidine hydrochloride in lynx. J. Wildl. Manage. 36: 994-996.

Berry, M. P. S. 1992. The tranquillization of captive red hartebeest, black wildebeest and gemsbok. *In* Ebedes, H. (ed.) The Use of Tranquillizers in Wildlife. Dept. Ag. Develop., Pretoria. Bull. No. 423. Pp. 40-43.

Bertelsen, M. F., C. Mosley, G. J. Crawshaw, D. Dyson, and D. A. Smith. 2004. Evaluation of isoflurane, sevoflurane and nitrous oxide anesthesia in Dumeril's monitor (*Varanus dumerili*). Proc. Am. Assoc. Zoo Vet. Pp. 505-507.

Bertelsen, M. F., C. Mosley, G. J. Crawshaw, D. Dyson, and D. A. Smith. 2005. Inhalation anesthesia in Dumeril's monitor (*Varanus dumerili*) with isoflurane, sevoflurane, and nitrous oxide: effects of inspired gases on induction and recovery. J. Zoo Wildl. Med. 36: 62-68.

Bertelsen, M., T. Møller, and B. Röken. 2006. Chemical immobilization of blue wildebeest (*Connochaetes taurinus*) with etorphine-xylazine or fentanyl-azaperone-xylazine. Proc. Am. Assoc. Zoo Vet. Pp. 325.

Bertnsen, F., T. Kvam, O. J. Sorensen, and K. Knutsen. 1994. Drug immobilization of brown bears (*Ursus arctos*). Field experience. Norsk Veterinaer. 106: 120-124.

Bertram, B. C. R. 1976. Lion immobilization using phencyclidine (Sernylan). E. Afr. Wildl. J. 14: 233-235.

Bertram, B. C. R., and J. M. King. 1976. Lion and leopard immobilization using CI-744. E. Afr. Wildl. J. 14: 237-239.

Bester, M. N. 1988. Chemical restraint of Antarctic fur seals and Southern elephant seals. So. Afr. J. Wild. Res. 18: 57-60.

Betz, T. W. 1962. Surgical anesthesia in reptiles, with special reference to the water snake, *Natrix rhombifera*. Copeia 284-287.

Beynon, P. H., and J. E. Cooper (eds.). 1991. Manual of Exotic Pets. Brit. Sm. An. Vet. Assoc., Cheltenham. 312 pp.

Bhargava, A. K., R. B. Heath, R. L. Rudy, and A. A. Gabel. 1969. Clinical trials of halothane anaesthesia in a camel (*Camelus dromedarius*). Ind. Vet. J. 46: 999-1001.

Bienzle, D., C. J. Boyd, A. Valverde, and D. A. Smith. 1991. Sedative effects of ketamine and midazolam in snapping turtles (*Chelydra serpentina*). Vet. Surg. 20: 154.

Bienzle, D., and C. J. Boyd. 1992. Sedative effects of ketamine and midazolam in snapping turtles (*Chelydra serpentina*). J. Zoo Wildl. Med. 23: 201-204.

Bigalke, R. C. 1965. Experiments in immobilizing ungulate mammals. 1: 239-247.

Bigler, W. J., and G. L. Hoff. 1974. Anesthesia of raccoons with ketamine hydrochloride. J. Wildl. Manage. 38: 364-366.

Birnbaum, C., R. Gabler, J. Hartung, E. Schimke, and U. D. Wenzel. 1969. Halothannarkose bei Musteliden. Arch. Exp. Vet. 23: 561- 565.

Black, H. C., O. H. Hewitt, and C. W. Severinghaus. 1959. Use of drugs in handling black bears. New York Fish Game J. 6: 179-203.

Black, S. R., and D. P. Whiteside. 2005. Immobilization of captive sloth bear (*Melursus ursinus*), spectacled bear (*Tremarctos ornatus*), black bear (*Ursus americanus*) and polar bear (*Ursus maritimus*) with a medetomidine, ketamine, and midazolam combination. Proc. Am. Assoc. Zoo Vet. Pp. 104-105.

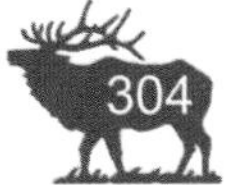

Blackshaw, G. D., and B. Wakeman. 1972. Immobilization of an adult ostrich for surgery. J. Zoo An. Med. 2: 11-12.

Blake, D. K. 1993. The Nile crocodile *Crocodylus niloticus*: capture, care, accommodation, and transportation. *In* McKenzie, A. A. (ed.). The Capture and Care Manual. Wildlife Decision Support Services and The South African Veterinary Foundation, Pretoria. Pp. 654-676.

Blanchette, P. 1989. Use of halothane to anesthetize muskrats in the field. J. Wildl. Manage. 53: 172-174.

Blazhis, A. S., A. V. Mitskus, and P. P. Bluzma. 1972. [Experience of using the myorelaxant lysthenon (succinylbischoline chloride) for roe immobilization]. Liet. TSR Moksiu Akad. Darb. Ser. C. 2: 77-81.

Blumer, E. S. 1991. A review of the use of selected neuroleptic drugs in the management of nondomestic hoofstock. Proc. Am. Assoc. Zoo Vet. Pp. 333-339.

Bó, R. F., F. Palomares, J. F. Beltrán, G. de Villafañe, and S. Moreno. 1994. Immobilization of coypus (*Myocastor coypus*) with ketamine hydrochloride and xylazine hydrochloride. J. Wildl. Dis. 30: 596-598.

Boch, J., W. Nerl, P. Hunl, F. Feig. 1961. The present state of experience in the use of nicotine salicylate for capturing chamois, ibex, and red deer. Z. Jagdwiss 7: 18-25.

Böer, M., J. Schöne, M. A. Schneider,and C. Hackenbroich. 2002. Medetomidine-ketamine-remote anaesthesia of the Asiatic wild dog (*Cuon alpinus* Hodgson 1838): Effects on cardiopulmonary and metabolic parameters. Tierarztl. Prax. Aus. Klein. Heim. 30: 63-69.

Boever, W. J. 1974. Injectable anesthetics in wild ruminants. Vet. Med. Sm. An. Clin. Pp. 548-550.

Boever, W. J. 1977. Restraint of exotic animals. Mod. Vet. Pract. 58: 229-232.

Boever, W. J. 1979. The restraint of non-domestic pets. Vet. Clin. North Amer. (Small Anim. Pract.). 9: 391-403.

Boever, W. J. 1986. Artiodactylids: restraint, handling, and anesthesia. *In* Fowler, M. E. (ed.). Zoo and Wild Animal Medicine. W. B. Saunders, Philadelphia. Pp. 940-952.

Boever, W. J., and H. Paluch. 1974. Injectable anesthetics in wild ruminants. Vet. Med. Small An. Clin. 69: 548-551.

Boever, W. J., and W. Wright. 1975. Use of ketamine for restraint and anesthesia of birds. Vet. Med. Small An. Clin. 70: 86-88.

Boever, W. J., and F. Caputo. 1982. Tilazol (sic)(CI 744) as an anesthetic agent in reptiles. J. Zoo An. Med. 13: 59-61.

Boever, W. J., D. Stuppy, and K. Kane. 1977a. Clinical experience with Telazol™ (CI-744) as a new agent for chemical restraint and anesthesia in the red kangaroo (*Macropus rufus*). J. Zoo An. Med. 8: 14-17.

Boever, W. J., J. Holden, and K. K. Kane. 1977b. Use of Telazol™ (CI-744) for chemical restraint and anesthesia in wild and exotic carnivores. Vet. Med. Small An. Clin. 72: 1722-1725.

Bolz, W. 1962. Neuroleptica und potenzierte Narkose speziell bei Zootieren. Nord. Vet. Med. 14, Suppl. 1: 17-29.

Bonath, K. 1979. Halothane inhalation anesthesia in reptiles and its clinical control. Int. Zoo Yb. 19: 112-115.

Bonath, K. H. 1995. Xylazine-anaesthesia and antagonism in dromedaries. *In:* Evans, J. O., S. P. Simpkins, and D. J. Atkins (eds.). Camel Keeping in Kenya. Republic of Kenya, Ministry of Agriculture, Livestock Development and Marketing, Nairobi, Kenya. Pp. 7:20-7:21.

Bonath, K. H., I. Bonath, R. D. Haller, J. Bonath, and D. Amelang. 1991. Medicamentous immobilization of Nile crocodile by means of anaesthesia and muscle relaxation, with reference to some cardiovascular and respiratory parameters. Erkrankungen Der Zootiere 33: 191-194.

Bonath, K. H., P. Hauck, and D. Amelang. 1992. Die Tiletamin-Zolazepam-Immobilisation beim Wildschwein (*Sus scrofa*) und ihre bedeutung fur Gatterwild. Erkr. Zootiere 34: 179-184.

Bonath, K. H., R. D. Haller, J. Bonath, and D. Amelang. 1990. Tiletamine-zolazepam-acepromazine anesthesia in *Crocodylus niloticus* with regard to the respiratory and cardiovascular systems. Proc. 10th Work. Meet. Crocodile Spec. Group Species Survival Comm. IUCN-World Conserv. Union. 1: 8-12.

Bongso, T. A. 1979. Sedation of the Asian elephant (*Elephas maximus*) with xylazine. Vet. Rec. 105: 442-443.

Bongso, T. A. 1980. Use of xylazine for the transport of elephants by air. Vet. Rec. 107: 492.

Bongso, T. A., and B. M. A. O. Perera. 1978. Observations on the use of etorphine alone and in combina-

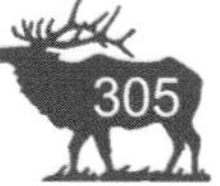

tion with acepromazine maleate for immobilization of aggressive Asian elephants (*Elephas maximus*). Vet. Rec. 102: 339-340.

Bonner, W. B., M. E. Keeling, E. T. Van Ormer, and J. E. Haynie. 1972. Ketamine anesthesia in chimpanzees and other great ape species. Chimpanzee 5: 255-268.

Booth, V. R., and A. M. Coetzee. 1988. The capture and relocation of black and white rhinoceros in Zimbawe. *In* Nielsen, L., and R. D. Brown (eds.). Translocation of Wild Animals. Wisconsin Humane Society, Inc., and Cesar Kleberg Wildlife Research Institute, Milwaukee, Wisconsin. Pp. 191-209.

Borchard, R. E. 1980. Evaluation of chemical restraint methods for potential use in wild, free roaming horses. Report to Bureau of Land Management , contract YA-512-CT8-116. Pullman, Wash. 16 pp.

Borg, K. 1955. Chloralose and its use for catching crows, gulls, pigeons, etc. Viltrevy Jakbiologisk Tidskrift 1: 88-121.

Borkowski, R., B. Irvine, and P. Wollenman. 2004. Rapid immobilization of hoofstock in large herds. Proc. Am. Assoc. Zoo Vet. Pp. 509-513.

Born, E. W., and L. Ø. Knutsen. 1990. Immobilization of Atlantic walrus (*Odobenus rosmarus rosmarus*) by use of etorphine hydrochloride reversed by diprenorphine hydrochloride. Teknisk rapport - Greenlands Hjemmestyre. Milj-og Naturforvaltning. 14.

Bornemann, H., and J. Plötz. 1993. A field method for immobilizing Weddell seals. Wildl. Soc. Bull. 21: 437-441.

Borzio, F. 1973. Ketamine hydrochloride as an anesthetic for wildfowl. Vet. Med. Small An. Clin. 68: 1364-1365.

Bose, A. S., O. Ramakrishna, N. T. Krishna Murthy, and M. Kalyanam. 1982. Anaesthesia in a porcupine during minor surgical intervention. Vet. Med. Rev. 1982: 100-103.

Boyd, I. L., N. J. Lunn, C. D. Duck, and T. Barton. 1990. Response of Antarctic fur seals to immobilization with ketamine, a ketamine-diazepam or ketamine-xylazine mixture, and Zoletil®. Marine Mamm. Sci. 6: 135-145.

Boyd, R. J. 1962. Succinylcholine chloride for immobilization of Colorado mule deer. J. Wildl. Manage. 26: 332-333.

Boyer, T. H. 1992. Clinical anesthesia of reptiles. Bull. Assoc. Amphib. Reptil. Vet. 2: 10-13.

Bradshaw, C. J. A., L. W. Traill, K. L. Wertz, W. H. White, and I. M. Gurry. 2005. Chemical immobilisation of wild banteng (*Bos javanicus*) in northern Australia using detomidine, tiletamine, and zolazepam. Aust. Vet. J. 83: 616-617.

Brannian, R. E., C. Kirk, and D. Williams. 1987. Anesthetic induction of kinosternid turtles with halothane. J. Zoo An. Med. 18: 115-117.

Brass, W. 1983. [Clinical use of psychotropic drugs in pet animals as well as in zoo and wild animals]. DTW. 90: 46-47.

Brazenor, C. W., and G. Kaye. 1953. Anaesthesia for reptiles. Copeia 1953: 165-170.

Bree, M. M. 1972. Dissociative anesthesia in *Macaca mulatta*. Clinical evaluation of CI-744. J. Med. Primatol. 1: 256-260.

Bressler, K., and B. Ron. 2004. Effect of anesthetics on stress and innate immune system of gilthead seabream (*Sparus aurata*). Isr. J. Aquacult. Bamidgeh. 56: 5-13.

Briggs, G. D., R. V. Henrickson, and B. J. Le Boeuf. 1975. Ketamine immobilization of northern elephant seals. J. Am. Vet. Med. Assoc. 167: 546-548.

Brisbin, I. L. 1966. Reactions of the American alligator to several immobilizing drugs. Copeia 1966: 129-130.

Bristol, D. G., J. Smith, and M. S. Silberman. 1984. Acepromazine and etorphine for prolonged anesthesia of a zebra. J. Am. Vet. Med. Assoc. 185: 1439-1440.

Brockelman, W. Y., and N. K. Kobayashi. 1971. Live capture of free-ranging primates with a blowgun. J. Wildl. Manage. 35: 852-855.

Brooks, C., and K. D. Morris. 1979. Blood values and the use of ketamine HCL in the fox. Vet. Med. Sm. An. Clin. 74: 1179-1180.

Brown, D. C., R. O. Mulhausen, D. J. Andrew, and U. S. Seal. 1971. Renal function in anesthetized dormant and active bears. Am. J. Phsyiol. 220: 293.

Brown, L. A. 1993. Anesthesia and restraint. *In* Stoskopf, M. K. (ed.). Fish Medicine. Saunders, Philadelphia. Pp. 79-80.

Brunson, D. B. 1998. Evaluating published immobilization and anesthesia information. Proc. Joint Conf.

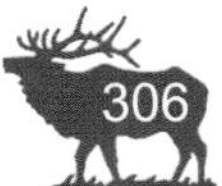

Am. Assoc. Zoo Vet. and Am. Assoc. Wildl. Vet. Pp. 5-10.
Brunson, D. B., T. K. Rowles, F. Gulland, M. Walsh, J. L. Dunn, T. Hammer, and M. Moore. 2002. Technique for drug delivery and sedation of free-ranging north Atlantic right whale. (*Balenea glacialis*). Proc. Am. Assoc. Zoo Vet. Pp. 320-322.
Bryon, H. T., J. F. Copeland, M. J. Schmidt, J. Olsen, and R. Hauck. 1985. Surgical approach to the abdomen of the elephant. Proc. Am. Assoc. Zoo Vet. P. 2.
Bryson, P. D. 1989. Narcotic antagonists. *In* Comprehensive Review in Toxicology. Aspen Publications, Rockville, Maryland. Pp. 339-343.
Bubenik, A. B., I. Gajic, V. Jovic, and R. Tachezy. 1967. Traitment de perdrix et de faisans par des tranquillisants du groupe des benzodiazepines. [Treatment of partridges and pheasants with benzodiazepine group tranquilizers]. Int. Congr. Game Biol. 7: 261-265.
Bubenik, A. B., and G. A. Bubenik. 1976. New, non-traumatic, disposable, automatic injection dart. Proc. Can. Assoc. Lab. An. Sci. Pp. 48-53.
Bubenik, G. A. 1982. Chemical immobilization of captive white-tailed deer and the use of automatic blood samplers. *In* Nielsen, L., J. C. Haigh, and M. E. Fowler (eds.). Chemical Immobilization of North American Wildlife. Milwaukee, Wisconsin: Wisconsin Humane Society, Inc. Pp. 335-354.
Bubenik, G. A., and R. D. Brown. 1989. The effect of yohimbine on plasma levels of T-3, T-4, and cortisol in xylazine-immobilized white-tailed deer. J. Zoo Wildl. Med. 92: 315-318.
Buck, N., F. Fry, C. Green, R. Gwynn, and P. Keen. 1963. The use of thiambutene, phencyclidine, hyoscine mixture for the immobilisation of the topi and the hippopotamus. Vet. Rec. 75: 630-633.
Buechner, H. K., A. M. Harthoorn, and J. A. Lock. 1959. Using drugs to control game. Wild Life 1: 49-52.
Buechner, H. K., A. M. Harthoorn, and J. A. Lock. 1960a. A new method of control of African wild animals. Nature. 185: 47-48.
Buechner, H. K., A. M. Harthoorn, and J. A. Lock. 1960b. Immobilizing Uganda kob with succinylcholine chloride. Can. J. Comp. Med. 24: 317-325.
Buechner, H. K., A. M. Harthoorn, and J. A. Lock. 1960c. Recent advances in field immobilization of large animals with drugs. Trans. North Am. Wildl. Nat. Res. Conf. 25: 415-422.
Buechner, H. K., A. M. Harthoorn, and J. A. Lock. 1960d. The immobilization of African animals in the field, with special references to their transfer to other areas. Proc. Zool. Soc. London 135: 261-268.
Buechner, H. K., A. M. Harthoorn, and J. A. Lock. 1960e. The immobilization of wild animals as an aid to management and control. Oryx 5: 346-351.
Bull, E. L., T. W. Heater, and F. G. Culver. 1996. Live-trapping and immobilizing American martens. Wildl. Soc. Bull. 24: 555-558.
Burger, H. 1980. Modified .22 rifle ammunition for capture purposes. Br. Vet. Zool. Soc. March: 9-10.
Burke, T. J. 1986. Reptile anesthesia. *In* Fowler, M. E. (ed.). Zoo and Wild Animal Medicine. W. B. Saunders Co., Philadelphia, Pennsylvania. Pp. 153-155.
Burke, T. J., and B. E. Wall. 1970. Anesthetic deaths in cobras (*Naja naja* and *Ophiophagus hannah*) with methoxyflurane. J. Am. Vet. Med. Assoc. 157: 620-621.
Burroughs, R. E. J. 1992. The opiates - a review of narcotics used for immobilization. *In* Ebedes, H. (ed.) The Use of Tranquillizers in Wildlife. Dept. Ag. Develop., Pretoria. Bull. No. 423. Pp. 54-57.
Burroughs, R. E. J. 1993a. A summary of the practical aspects of drugs commonly used for the restraint of wild animals. *In* McKenzie, A. A. (ed.). The Capture and Care Manual. Wildlife Decision Support Services and The South African Veterinary Foundation, Pretoria. Pp. 65-70.
Burroughs, R. E. J. 1993b. Principles of darting antelope and other herbivores. *In* McKenzie, A. A. (ed.). The Capture and Care Manual. Wildlife Decision Support Services and The South African Veterinary Foundation, Pretoria. Pp. 131-137.
Burroughs, R. E. J. 1993c. Chemical capture of primates. *In* McKenzie, A. A. (ed.). The Capture and Care Manual. Wildlife Decision Support Services and The South African Veterinary Foundation, Pretoria. Pp. 328-331.
Burroughs, R. E. J. 1993d. Chemical capture of antelope. *In* McKenzie, A. A. (ed.). The Capture and Care Manual. Wildlife Decision Support Services and The South African Veterinary Foundation, Pretoria. Pp. 348-380.
Burroughs, R. E. J. 1993e. Chemical capture of the warthog *Phacochoerus aethiopicus*. *In* McKenzie, A. A. (ed.). The Capture and Care Manual. Wildlife Decision Support Services and The South African Veterinary Foundation, Pretoria. Pp. 621-622.
Burroughs, R. E. J. 1993f. Chemical capture of Burchell's zebra *Equus burchelli* and the mountain zebra

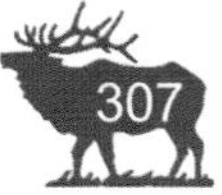

Equus zebra. *In* McKenzie, A. A. (ed.). The Capture and Care Manual. Wildlife Decision Support Services and The South African Veterinary Foundation, Pretoria. Pp. 627-629.

Burroughs, R. 1996. Capture and immobilization of ostriches. Am. J. Vet. Res. 51: 391-398.

Burroughs, R. E. J., and A. A. McKenzie. 1993a. Handling, care, and loading of immobilized carnivores. *In* McKenzie, A. A. (ed.). The Capture and Care Manual. Wildlife Decision Support Services and The South African Veterinary Foundation, Pretoria. Pp. 178-183.

Burroughs, R. E. J., and A. A. McKenzie. 1993b. Handling, care, and loading of immobilized herbivores. *In* McKenzie, A. A. (ed.). The Capture and Care Manual. Wildlife Decision Support Services and The South African Veterinary Foundation, Pretoria. Pp. 184-193.

Bush, M. 1976. Giraffe restraint and immobilization. Proc. Am. Assoc. Zoo Vet. Pp. 151-154.

Bush, M. 1982. Chemical immobilization. *In* Beck, B, C. M. Wemmer, (eds.). Biology and Management of an Extinct Species, Pere David's deer. Noyes Publications. Park Ridge, New Jersey. pp. 36-38.

Bush, M. 1992. Remote drug delivery systems. J. Zoo Wildl. Med. 23: 159-180.

Bush, M. 1993. Anesthesia of high-risk animals: giraffe. *In* Fowler, M. E. (ed.). Zoo & Wild Animal Medicine: Current Therapy 3. W. B. Saunders Co., Philadelphia, Pennsylvania. Pp. 545-547.

Bush, M., and C. W. Gray. 1972. Sterilization of projectile syringes. J. Am. Vet. Med. Assoc. 161: 672-673.

Bush, M, and V. De Vos. 1987. Observations on field immobilization of free-ranging giraffe (*Giraffa camelopardalis*) using carfentanil and xylazine. J. Zoo An. Med. 18: 135-140.

Bush, M., J. A. Moore, and L. M. Neeley. 1971. Sedation for transportation of a lowland gorilla. J. Am. Vet. Med. Assoc. 159: 546-548.

Bush, M., P. K. Ensley, K. Mehren, and W. Rapley. 1976. Immobilization of giraffes with xylazine and etorphine hydrochloride. J. Am. Vet. Med. Assoc. 169: 884-885.

Bush, M., R. Custer, J. Smeller, and L. M. Bush. 1977. Physiological measures of nonhuman primates during physical restraint and chemical immobilization. J. Am. Vet. Med. Assoc. 171: 866-869.

Bush, M., R. Custer, J. Smeller, L. M. Bush, U. S. Seal, and R. Barton. 1978. The acid-base status of lions, *Panthera leo*, immobilized with four drug combinations. J. Wildl. Dis. 4: 102-109.

Bush, M., R. S. Custer, and E. E. Smith. 1980a. Use of dissociative anesthetics for the immobilization of captive bears: blood gas, hematology and biochemical values. J. Wildl. Dis. 16: 481-489.

Bush, M., R. Custer, and J. C. Whitla. 1980b. Hematology and serum chemistry profiles for giraffes (*Giraffa camelopardalis*): variations with age, sex, and restraint. J. Zoo An. Med. 11: 122-129.

Bush, M. J., A. M. Graves, S. J. O'Brien, and D. E. Wildt. 1990. Dissociative anaesthesia in free-ranging male koalas and selected marsupials in captivity. Austr. Vet. J. 67: 449-451.

Bush, M., S. B. Citino, and L. Tell. 1992. Telazol and Telazol/Rompun anesthesia in non-domestic cervids and bovids. Proc. Joint Conf. Am. Assoc. Zoo Vet. and Am. Assoc. Wildl. Vet. Pp. 252-252.

Bush, M., D. G. Grobler, J. P. Raath, L. G. Phillips, M. A. Stamper, and W. R. Lance. 2001. Use of medetomidine and ketamine for immobilization of free-ranging giraffes. J. Am. Vet. Med. Assoc. 218: 245-249.

Bush, M., J. P. Raath, D. Grobler, and L. Klein. 2004a. Severe hypoxaemia in field-anaesthetized white rhinoceros (*Ceratotherium simum*) and effects of using tracheal insufflation of oxygen. J. S. Afr. Vet. Assn. 75: 79-84.

Bush, M., J. P. Raath, L. G. Phillips, and W. Lance. 2004b. Immobilisation of impala (*Aepyceros melampus*) with ketamine hydrochloride/medetomidine hydrochloride combination, and reversal with atipamezole hydrochloride. J. S. Afr. Vet. Assoc. 75: 14-18.

Button, C., D. G. A. Meltzer, and M. S. G. Mülders. 1981. Saffan induced poikilothermia in cheetah (*Acinonyx jubatus*). J. So. Afr. Vet. Assoc. 52: 237-238.

Cakir, Y., and S. M. Strauch. 2005. Tricaine (MS-222) is a safe anesthetic compound compared to benzocaine and pentobarbital to induce anesthesia in leopard frogs (*Rana pipiens*). Pharmacol. Rep. 57: 467-474.

Calderwood, H. W. 1971. Anesthesia for reptiles. J. Am. Vet. Med. Assoc. 159: 1618-1625.

Calderwood, H. W., and E. Jacobson. 1979a. Anesthesia for reptiles. J. Am. Vet. Med. Assoc. 159: 1618-1625.

Calderwood, H. W., and E. Jacobson. 1979b. Preliminary report on the use of saffan on reptiles. Proc. Am. Assoc. Zoo Vet. Pp. 23-26.

Calle, P. P., and J. C. Bornmann. 1988. Giraffe restraint, habituation, and desensitization at the Cheyenne Mountain Zoo. Zoo Biol. 7: 243-252.

Calle, P. P., and P. J. Morris. 1999. Anesthesia for nondomestic suids. *In* Fowler, M. E., and R. E. Miller (eds.). Zoo & Wild Animal Medicine. Current Therapy 4. W. B. Saunders Company, Philadelphia, Pennsylvania. Pp. 639-646.

Camburn, M. A., and A. C. Stead. 1978. Anaesethesia in wild and aviary birds. J. Small An. Pract. 19: 395-400.

Campbell, H., and A. M. Harthoorn. 1963. The capture and anesthesia of the African lion in his natural environment. Vet. Rec. 75: 275-276.

Campbell, J. A. 1950. Use of anaesthesia in treatment of zoo inmates. Can. J. Comp. Med. 14: 39-41.

Cárdenas, J. C., and P. E. Cattan. 1986. Acción de xilacina como agente inmovilizante en lobos marinos (*Otaria flavescens, Arctocephalus philippi*)(Xylazine as an immobilizing agent for wild pinnipeds). Avances en Ciencias Veterinarias 1: 116-121.

Carpenter, J. W., and C. N. Hillman. 1978. Husbandry, reproduction, and veterinary care of captive ferrets. Proc. Am. Assoc. Zoo Vet. Pp. 36-47.

Carpenter, L. H., and W. R. Lance. 1983. Approved use of etorphine (M99®) in North American game animals. Rpt. Colorado Div. Wildl. 25 pp.

Carpenter, N. A. 1998. Anesthetic apnea in two black and white colobus monkeys (*Colobus guereza*) postulated to have resulted from butorphanol tartrate administration. Proc. Joint Conf. Am. Assoc. Zoo Vet. and Am. Assoc. Wildl. Vet. Pp. 193-195.

Carr, H. D. 1989. Immobilization of grizzlies with ketamine-xylazine and morphometrics of the bear drugged in Kananaskis Country, Alberta. Alberta Forestry-Lands-Wildlife, Fish and Wildlife Division, Wildlife Research Series 3a, 25 pp.

Carruthers, S. G., H. R. Wexler, and C. R. Stiller. 1979. Xylazine hydrochloride (Rompun) overdose in man. Clin. Toxicol. 15: 281-285.

Carter, N. 1961. Progress in drugging techniques. Wild Life 2: 9-10.

Casteel, D. A., and W. R. Edwards. 1965. Surgical anesthesia for cottontails. J. Wildl. Manage. 29:196.

Castro, M. I., J. Rose, W. Green, N. Lehner, D. Peterson, and D. Taub. 1981. Ketamine-HCl as a suitable anesthetic for endocrine, metabolic and cardiovascular studies in *Macaca fascicularis* monkeys. Proc. Soc. Exp. Biol. Med. 168: 389-394.

Cathers, T., G. A. Lewbart, M. Correa, and J. B. Stevens. 1997. Serum chemistry and hematology values for anesthetized American bullfrogs (*Rana catesbeiana*). J. Zoo Wildl. Med. 28: 171-174.

Cattet, M. R. L., N. A. Caulkett, S. C. Polischuk, and M. A. Ramsay. 1997. Reversible immobilization of free-ranging polar bears with medetomidine-zolazepam-tiletamine and atipamezole. J. Wildl. Dis. 33: 611-617.

Cattet, M. R. L., N. A. Caulkett, M. A. Ramsay, K. A. Streib, and K. E. Torske. 1998. Cardiopulmonary response of anesthetized polar bears (*Ursus maritimus*) to restraint and suspension by net. Proc. Joint Conf. Am. Assoc. Zoo Vet and Am. Assoc. Wildl. Vet. Pp. 320-324.

Cattet, M. R. L., N. A. Caulkett, S. C. Polischuk, and M. A. Ramsay. 1999a. Anesthesia of polar bears (*Ursus maritimus*) with zolazepam-tiletamine, medetomidine-ketamine, and medetomidine-zolazepam-tiletamine. J. Zoo Wildl. Med. 30: 354-360.

Cattet, M. R. L., N. A. Caulkett, K. A. Streib, K. E. Torske, and M. A. Ramsay. 1999b. Cardiopulmonary response of anesthetized polar bears to suspension by net and sling. J. Wildl. Dis. 35: 548-556.

Cattet, M. R., N. A. Caulkett, and N. J. Lunn. 2003a. Anesthesia of polar bears using xylazine-zolazepam-tiletamine or zolazepam-tiletamine. J. Wildl. Dis. 39: 655-664.

Cattet, M. R., N. A. Caulkett, and G. B. Stenhouse. 2003b. Anesthesia of grizzly bears using xylazine-zolazepam-tiletamine or zolazepam-tiletamine. Ursus 14: 88-93.

Cattet, M. R. L., K. Christison, N. A. Caulkett, and G. B. Stenhouse. 2003c. Physiologic responses of grizzly bears to different methods of capture. J. Wildl. Dis. 39: 649-654.

Cattet, M. R., N. A. Caulkett, C. Wilson, T. Vanderbrink, and R. K. Brook. 2004. Intranasal administration of xylazine to reduce stress in elk captured by net gun. J. Wildl. Dis. 40: 562-565.

Cattet, M., T. Shury, and R. Patenaude (eds.). 2005. The chemical immobilization of wildlife - 2nd edition. Canadian Association of Zoo and Wildlife Veterinarians, 231 pp.

Caulkett, N. A. 1997. Anesthesia for North American cervids. Can. Vet. J. 38: 389-390.

Caulkett, N. A., and M. R. L. Cattet. 1997. Physiological effects of medetomidine-zolazepam-tiletamine immobilization in black bears. J. Wildl. Dis. 33: 618-622.

Caulkett, N. A., and J. M. Arnemo. 2007. Chemical immobilization of free-ranging terrestrial mammals. *In* Tranquilli, W. J., J. C. Thurmon, and K. Grimm (eds.). Lumb and Jones' veterinary anesthesia and

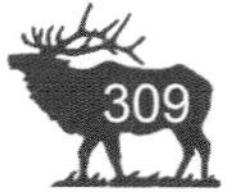

analgesia. 4th ed. Blackwell Publications.

Caulkett, N. A., J. C. Haigh, and P. H. Cribb. 1995. Medetomidine-ketamine and carfentanil-xylazine in mule deer and mule deer hybrids. Proc. Am. Coll. Vet. Anesthesiol. P. 43

Caulkett, N. A., W. J. Rettie, and J. C. Haigh. 1996a. Immobilization of free-ranging woodland caribou (*Rangifer tarandus caribou*) with medetomidine-ketamine and reversal with atipamezole. Proc. Am. Assoc. Zoo Vet. Pp. 389-393.

Caulkett, N. A., J. C. Haigh, and P. H. Cribb. 1996b. Medetomidine-ketamine and carfentanil-xylazine in mule deer and mule deer hybrids. Vet. Surg. 25: 179.

Caulkett, N. A., M. R. L. Cattet, and S. C. Polischuk. 1996c. Comparative cardiopulmonary effects of medetomidine-ketamine and Telazol® in polar bears (*Ursus maritimus*). Proc. Am. Assoc. Zoo Vet. Pp. 394-400.

Caulkett, N. A., M. R. L. Cattet, S. Cantwell, N. Cool, and W. Olsen. 1998a. Anesthesia of wood bison (*Bison bison athabascae*) with medetomidine-Telazol and xylazine-Telazol combinations. Proc. Joint Conf. Am. Assoc. Zoo Vet and Am. Assoc. Wildl. Vet. Pp. 342-349.

Caulkett, N. A., M. R. L. Cattet, J. M. Caulkett, and S. C. Polischuk. 1998b. Comparative cardiopulmonary effects of medetomidine-zolazepam-tiletamine and Telazol® in polar bears (*Ursus maritimus*). Proc. Joint Conf. Am. Assoc. Zoo Vet and Am. Assoc. Wildl. Vet. Pp. 314-319.

Caulkett, N. A., M. R. L. Cattet, J. M. Caulkett, and S. C. Polischuk. 1999. Comparative physiologic effects of Telazol®, medetomidine-ketamine, and medetomidine-Telazol® in captive polar bears (*Ursus maritimus*). J. Zoo Wildl. Med. 30:504-509.

Caulkett, N. A., M. R. L. Cattet, S. Cantwell, N. Cool, and W. Olsen. 2000a. Anesthesia of wood bison with medetomidine-zolazepam/tiletamine and xylazine-zolazepam/tiletamine combinations. Can. Vet. J. 41: 49-53.

Caulkett, N. A., P. H. Cribb, and J. C. Haigh. 2000b. Comparative cardiopulmonary effects of carfentanil-xylazine and medetomidine-ketamine used for immobilization of mule deer and mule deer/white-tailed deer hybrids. Can. J. Vet. Res. 64: 64-68.

Caulkett, N., J. Paterson, J. C. Haigh, and L. Siefert. 2006. Comparative physiologic effects of thiafentanil-azaperone and thiafentanil-medetomidine-ketamine in free-ranging Uganda kob (*Kobus kob thomasi*). Proc. Am. Assoc. Zoo Vet. Pp. 216-219.

Celly, C. S., W. N. McDonell, S. S. Young, and W. D. Black. 1997. The comparative hypoxemic effect of four α_2 adrenoceptor agonists (xylazine, romfidine, detomidine and medetomidine) in sheep. J. Vet. Pharmacol. Ther. 20: 464-471.

Chaduc, Y. 1996. Use of Zalopin for anesthetization of zebras at Touroparc. Point. Vet. 27: 8.

Chakrabarti, K. 1980. Successful tranquilization of a sundarbans tiger. Tigerpaper. 7: 10.

Chakraborty, G. 1993. Xylazine-ketamine anaesthesia in a red panda (*Ailurus fulkgens*). Zoo's Print 8: 11.

Chakraborty, G., and A. K. Das. 1994. Xylazine-ketamine anesthesia in a Tibetan wolf (*Canis lupus* Chanco). Indian Vet. J. 71: 1047.

Chalmers, G. A., and M. W. Barrett. 1977. Capture myopathy in pronghorns in Alberta, Canada. J. Am. Vet. Med. Assoc. 171: 918-923.

Chandrasekara Pillai, K. 1992. Record of behaviour of Asiatic lion on being immobilised at Nehru Zoological Park, Hyderabad. Zoo's Print 7: 18.

Channing, C. P., S. Fowler, B. Engel, and K. Vitek. 1977. Failure of daily injections of ketamine HCL to adversely alter menstrual cycle length, blood estrogen, and progesterone levels in the Rhesus monkey. Proc. Soc. Exp. Biol. Med. 155: 615-619.

Chao, C. C., R. D. Brown, and L. J. Deftos. 1984. Effects of xylazine immobilization on biochemical and endocrine values in white-tailed deer. J. Wildl. Dis. 20: 328-332.

Chapman, D. 1973. Immobilon and deer. Vet. Rec. 92: 711.

Cheney, C. S., and J. Hattingh. 1988. Effects of chemical immobilisation on the blood composition of impala (*Aepyceros melampus* Lichtenstein). J. So. Afr. Vet. Assoc. 59: 13-18.

Chittick, E. J., G. A. Lewbart, and C. Swanson. 2000. Post-anesthetic hypoxemia in freshwater fish. Proc. Joint Conf. Am. Assoc. Zoo Vet. and Intl. Assoc. Aquatic An. Med. Pp. 372-373.

Chittick, E., W. Horne, B. Wolfe, K. Sladky, and M. Loomis. 2002a. Cardiopulmonary assessment of medetomidine, ketamine, and butorphanol in captive Thomson's gazelles (*Gazella thomsoni*). J. Zoo Wildl. Med. 32: 168-175.

Chittick, E. J., M. A. Stamper, J. F. Beasley, G. A. Lewbart, and W. A. Horne. 2002b. Medetomidine,

ketamine, and sevoflurane for anesthesia for injured loggerhead sea turtles: 13 cases. J. Amer. Vet. Med. Assoc. 221: 1019-1025.

Chung, H., H. Choi, E. Kim, W. Jin, H. Lee, and Y. Yoo. 2000. A fatality due to injection of tiletamine and zolazepam. J. Analyt. Toxicol. 24: 305-308.

Citino, S. B., M. Bush, and L. G. Phillips. 1984. Dystocia and fatal hyperthermic episode in a giraffe. J. Am. Vet. Med. Assoc. 185: 1440-1442.

Citino, S. B., M. Bush, D. Grobler, and W. Lance. 2001. Anaesthesia of roan antelope (*Hippotragus equinus*) with a combination of A3080, medetomidine and ketamine. J. So. Afr. Vet. Assoc. 72: 29-32.

Citino, S. B., M. Bush, D. Grobler, and W. Lance. 2002. Anesthesia of boma-captured Lichtenstein's hartebeest (*Sigmoceros lichtensteinii*) with a combination of thiafentanil, medetomidine, and ketamine. J. Wildl. Dis. 38: 457-462.

Citino, S. B., M. Bush, W. Lance, M. Hofmeyr, and D. Grobler. 2006. Use of thiafentanil (A3080), medetomidine, and ketamine for anesthesia of captive and free-ranging giraffe (*Giraffa camelopardalis*). Proc. Am. Assoc. Zoo Vet. Pp. 211-213.

Clarke, C. M. H., and R. J. Henderson. 1979. Evaluation of a helicopter/dart-gun technique for capturing chamois and attaching radio telemetry collars. N. Z. J. Zool. 6: 493-498.

Clarke, N. P., M. J. Huheey, and W. M. Martin. 1963. Pentobarbital anesthesia in bears. J. Am. Vet. Med. Assoc. 143: 47-51.

Clausen, B. 1994. The use of trilafon during translocation of muskoxen in west Greenland. IUCN Veterinary Specialist Group Newsletter 8: 5.

Clausen, B., P. Hjort, H. Strandgaard, and P. L. Soerensen. 1984. Immobilization and tagging of muskoxen (*Ovibus moschatus*) in Jameson Land, Northeastern Greenland. J. Wildl. Dis. 20: 141-145.

Clifford, D. H. 1958. Effect of preanesthetic medication with meperidine and promazine on barbiturate anesthesia in an ocelot and leopard. J. Am. Vet. Med. Assoc. 133: 459-463.

Clifford, D. H., C. M. Stowe, and A. L Good. 1960. Pentobarbital anesthesia in lions with special reference to preanesthetic medication. J. Am. Vet. Med. Assoc. 139: 111-116.

Clifford, D. H., A. L Good, and C. M. Stowe. 1962. Observations on the use of ataractic and narcotic preanesthesia and pentobarbital anesthesia in bears. J. Am. Vet. Med. Assoc. 140: 464-470.

Cline, D. R., and R. J. Greenwood. 1972. Effect of certain anesthetic agents on mallard ducks. J. Am. Vet. Med. Assoc. 161: 624-633.

Cline, D. R., D. B. Siniff, and A. W. Erickson. 1969. Immobilizing and collecting blood from Antarctic seals. J. Wildl. Manage. 33: 138-144.

Clippinger, T. L., S. B. Citino, and S. Wade. 1998. Behavioral and physiologic response to an intermediate-acting tranquilizer, zuclopenthixol, in captive Nile lechwe (*Kobus megaceros*). Proc. Joint Conf. Am. Assoc. Zoo Vet. and Am. Assoc. Wildl. Vet. Pp. 38-40.

Clutton, R. E. 1986. Prolonged isoflurane anesthesia in the golden eagle. J. Zoo An. Med. 17: 103-105.

Clutton, R. E. 1987. Anesthesia in an epileptic black bear (*Ursus americanus*): A case report and discussion of dilemma. J. Zoo An. Med. 18: 66-69.

Clutton, R. E. 1988. Inefficacy of oral ketamine for chemical restraint in turkeys. J. Wildl. Dis. 24: 380-381.

Clutton, R. E., and L. B. Duggan. 1986. Saffan anesthesia in the raccoon: a preliminary report. J. Zoo An. Med. 17: 91-99.

Clyde, V. L., P. Cardeilhac, and E. Jacobson. 1990. Chemical restraint of American alligators (*Alligator mississipiensis*) with atacurium and tiletamine-zolazepam. Proc. Am. Assoc. Zoo Vet. P. 288.

Clyde, V. L., P. Cardeilhac, and E. R. Jacobson. 1994. Chemical restraint of American alligators (*Alligator mississipiensis*) with atacurium or tiletamine-zolazepam. J. Zoo Wildl. Med. 25: 525-530.

Coetzee, H. G. J. 1964. The use of phencyclidine for immobilization of the chimpanzee. J. So. Afr. Vet. Assoc. 35: 97.

Coggins, V. L. 1975. Immobilization of Rocky Mountain elk with M99. J. Wildl. Manage. 39: 814-816.

Cohen, B. J., and M. M. Bree. 1978. Chemical and physical restraint of nonhuman primates. J. Med. Primatol. 7: 193-201.

Cole, A., A. Mutlow, R. Isaza, J. W. Carpenter, D. E. Koch, R. P. Hunter, and B. L. Dresser. 2005. Pharmacokinetics of carfentanil and naltrexone in the common eland (*Taurotragus oryx*). Proc. Am. Assoc. Zoo Vet. Pp. 263.

Cole, A., A. Mutlow, R. Isaza, J. W. Carpenter, D. E. Koch, R. P. Hunter, and B. L. Dresser. 2006. Pharma-

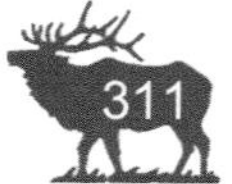

cokinetics and pharmacodynamics of carfentanil and naltrexone in female common eland (*Taurotragus oryx*). J. Zoo Wildl. Med. 37: 318-326.
Condy, J. B. 1964. The capture of black rhinoreros (*Diceros bicornis*) and buffalo (*Syncerus caffer*) on Lake Kariba. Rhodesian J. Agri. Res. 2: 1.
Condy, J. C. 1987. Practical aspects in the handling of African buffalo (*Syncerus caffer*). J. So. Afr. Vet. Assoc. 3: 158-159.
Conroy, P. J. 1986. Immobilizing gaur with an etorphine and tranquilizer mixture. J. Bombay Nat. Hist. Soc. 83: 499-504.
Cook, B. 1984. Chemical immobilization of black bears in Great Smoky Mountains National Park. Proc. East. Conf. Black Bear Res. Manage. 7: 79-81.
Cook, C. S., and K. K. Kane. 1980. Apparent suppression of gastrointestinal motility due to xylazine - a comparative study. J. Zoo An. Med. 11: 46-48.
Cook, R. A., and D. A. Clarke. 1984. The use of isoflurane as a general anesthetic in the Western lowland gorilla (*Gorilla g. gorilla*). Proc. Am. Assoc. Zoo Vet. Pp. 83-85.
Cook, R. A., and D. A. Clarke. 1985. The use of isoflurane as a general anesthetic in the Western lowland gorilla (*Gorilla g. gorilla*). J. Zoo An. Med. 16: 122-124.
Cooke, S. W. 1995. Swan anesthesia. Vet. Rec. 136: 476.
Cooper, D. V., D. Grobler, M. Bush, D. Jessup, and W. Lance. 2005. Anaesthesia of nyala (*Tragelaphus angasi*) with a combination of thiafentanil (A3080), medetomidine, and ketamine. J. S. Afr. Vet. Assn. 76: 18-21.
Cooper, J. E. 1971. Surgery on a captive iguana (*Iguana iguana*). J. Zoo An. Med. 2: 29-31.
Cooper, J. E. 1974. Ketamine hydrochloride as an anaesthetic for East African reptiles. Vet. Rec. 95: 37-41.
Cooper, J. E. 1984. Anaesthesia of exotic animals. An. Technol. 35: 13-20.
Cooper, J. E. 1987. Veterinary work with non-domesticated pets. IV. Lower vertebrates. Br. Vet. J. 143: 193-202.
Cooper, J. E., and L. G. Frank. 1973. Use of the steroid anaesthetic CT 1341 in birds. Vet. Rec. 92: 474-479.
Cooper, J. E., and P. T. Redig. 1975. Unexpected reactions to the use of CT 1341 by red-tailed hawks. Vet. Rec. 97: 352.
Cooper, J. E., A. Forbes, S. Harris, and N. Chapman. 1984. Chemical restraint of deer. Vet. Rec. 114: 483.
Cooper, J. E., S. Harris, A. Forbes, N. G. Chapman, and D. I. Chapman. 1986. A comparison of xylazine and methohexitone for the chemical immobilization of Reeves' muntjac (*Muntiacus reevesi*). Br. J. Vet. 142: 350-357.
Cooper, R. M., S. R. Black, and V. Honeyman. 1992. On the use of succinycholine in elk. J. Wildl. Dis. 28: 684 (letter).
Copeland, G. L., R. E. Autenrieth, L. E. Oldenburg, and T. P. Kistner. 1978. Tranquilizing pronghorns with M-99 from a helicopter. Proc. Pronghorn Antelope Workshop 8: 94-112.
Cording, C. J., R. DeLuca, T. Camporese, and E. Spratt. 1999. A fatality related to the veterinary anesthetic Telazol. J. Analyt. Toxicol. 23: 552-555.
Cornell, L. 1977. Sedation of elephant seals. J. Zoo An. Med. 8: 39.
Cornell, L. H., and J. E. Antrim. 1987. Anesthesia and tusk extraction in walrus. J. Zoo An. Med. 18: 3-6.
Cornely, J. E. 1979. Anesthesia of coyotes with ketamine hydrochloride and xylazine. J. Wildl. Manage. 43: 577-579.
Cornick, J. L., and J. Jensen. 1992. Anesthetic management of ostriches. J. Am. Vet. Med. Assoc. 200: 1661-1666.
Corson, I. D., P. F. Fennessy, and J. M. Suttie. 1984. An improved design for home-made projectile syringe. N. Z. Vet. J. 32: 74-75.
Côté, S. D., M. Festa-Bianchet, and F. Fournier. 1998. Life-history effects of chemical immobilization and radiocollars on mountain goats. J. Wildl. Manage. 62: 745-752.
Counsilman, J. W. 1954. Demorol hydrochloride as an anaesthetic for an elephant. No. Am. Vet. 35: 835-836.
Cowan, I., A. J. Wood, and H. C. Nordan. 1962. Studies in the tranquilization and immobilization of deer (*Odocoileus*). Can. J. Comp. Med. 26: 57-61.
Craighead, J. J., M. Hornocker, W. Woodgerd, and F. C. Craighead. 1960. Trapping, immobilizing and color-marking grizzly bears. Trans. No. Am. Wildl. Nat. Res. Conf. 25: 347-363.

Craigmill, A. L., M. Rangel-Lugo, P. Damian, and J. E. Riviere. 1997. Extralabel use of tranquilizers and general anesthetics. J. Am. Vet. Med. Assoc. 211: 302-304.
Crawshaw, G. J., and K. G. Mehren. 1986. Use of idazoxan as an antagonist to xylazine and ketamine/ xylazine sedation. *In* Scott, P. W., and A. G. Greenwood (eds.). Proc. 25th Anniv. Symp. Br. Vet. Zool. Soc. London, UK. 155 pp.
Crawshaw, G. J., K. G. Mehren, S. Black. 1986. Antagonism of xylazine and ketamine/xylazine combinations in exotic species by idazoxan and RX821002A. Proc. Am. Assoc. Zoo Vet. Pp. 1-2.
Crawshaw, P. G., and H. B. Quigley. 1989. Notes on oceolot movement and activity in the Pantanal region, Brazil. Biotropica 21: 377-379.
Cribb, P. H., and J. C. Haigh. 1977. Anaesthetics for avian species. Vet. Rec. 100: 472.
Crider, E. D., and J. C. McDaniel. 1966. Technique for capturing Canada geese with alpha-chloralose. Proc. Ann. Conf. Southeast. Assoc. Game Fish Comm. Pp. 206-233.
Crider, E. D., and J. C. McDaniel. 1967. Alpha-chloralose used to capture Canada geese. J. Wildl. Manage. 31: 258-264.
Crider, E. D., and J. C. McDaniel. 1968. Oral drugs used to capture waterfowl. Proc. Annu. Conf. Southeast. Assoc. Game and Fish Comm. 22: 156-161.
Crider, E. D., V. D. Stotts, and J. C. McDaniel. 1968. Diazepam and alpha-chloralose mixtures to capture waterfowl. Proc. Ann. Conf. Southeast. Assoc. Game Fish Comm. 22: 133-141.
Crittal, J. W., and J. R. Smith. 1972. Darting of pigtail macaques (*Macaca menoestrina*) using an etorphine mixture. Vet. Rec. 14: 409-410.
Crockford, J. A., F. A. Hayes, J. H. Jenkins, S. D. Feurt. 1957a. Nicotine salicylate for capturing deer. J. Wildl. Manage. 21: 213-220.
Crockford, J. A., F. A. Hayes, J. H. Jenkins, and S. D. Feurt. 1957b. Field application of nicotine salicylate for capturing deer. Trans. No. Am. Wildl. Nat. Res. Conf. 22: 579-583.
Crockford, J. A., F. A. Hayes, J. H. Jenkins, and S. D. Feurt. 1958. An automatic projectile type syringe. Vet. Med. 53: 115-119.
Cross, J. P., C. G. MacKintosh, and J. F. T. Griffin. 1988. Effect of physical restraint and xylazine sedation on haematological values in red deer (*Cervus elephus*). Res. Vet. Sci. 45: 281-286.
Cross, J. P., Griffin, J. F. T., and C. G. MacKintosh. 1992. Influence of xylazine on hematology values in farmed red deer. *In* Brown, R. D. (ed.). The Biology of Deer. New York, Springer-Verlag. Pp. 136-140.
Cullingham, T. J. 1970. The owl monkey (*Aotus trivirgatus*) as a research animal. J. Inst. Anim. Techn. 21: 84.
Cummins, F. H. 2005. Accidental human poisoning with a veterinary tranquilliser. Emerg. Med. J. 22: 524-525.
Curro, T. G. 1998. Anesthesia of pet birds. Semin. Avian Exotic. Pet. Med. 7: 10-21.
Curro, T. G., D. Okeson, D. Zimmerman, D. L. Armstrong, and L. G. Simmons. 2004. Xylazine-midazolam-ketamine versus medetomidine-midazolam-ketamine anesthesia in captive Siberian tigers (*Panthera tigris altaica*). J. Zoo Wildl. Med. 35: 320-327.
Custer, R. S., and M. Bush. 1980. Physiologic and acid-base measures of gopher snakes during ketamine or halothane-nitrous oxide anesthesia. J. Am. Vet. Med. Assoc. 177: 870-874.
Custer, R. S., L. Kramer, S. Kennedy, and M. Bush. 1977. Hematologic effects of xylazine when used for restraint of Bactrian camels. J. Am. Vet. Med. Assoc. 171: 899-901.
Custer, R. S., M. Bush, J. M. Smeller, amd E. E. Smith. 1978. Clinical experience with dissociative anesthetics in lesser pandas (*Ailurus fulgens*): Hematology and blood chemistry values. J. Zoo An. Med. 9: 22-28.
Cyr, A., and R. Brunet. 1992. Anesthetization of captive red-winged blackbirds with mixtures of alpha-chloralose and secobarbital. J. Wildl. Manage. 56: 806-809.
Dabin, W., G. Beauplet, and C. Guinet. 2002. Response of wild subantarctic fur seal (*Arctocephalus tropicalis*) females to ketamine and tiletamine-zolazepam anesthesia. J. Wildl. Dis. 38: 846-850.
Dangolla, A., I. Silva, and V. Y. Kuruwita. 2004. Neuroleptanalgesia in wild Asian elephants (*Elephas maximus maximus*). Vet. Anaesth. Analg. 31: 276-279.
Davis, J. L., C-L. B. Chetkiewicz, V. C. Bleich, G. Raygorodetsky, B. M. Pierce, J. W. Ostergard, and J. D. Wehausen. 1996. A device to safely remove immobilized mountain lions from trees and cliffs. Wildl. Soc. Bull. 24: 537-539.
Davis, J. R., D. C. Guynn, Jr., and B. D. Hyder. 1994. Feasibility of using tribromoethanol to recapture

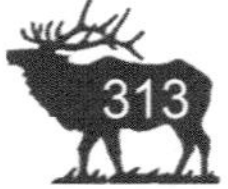

wild turkeys. Wildl. Soc. Bull. 22: 496-500.

David, J. M. H., J. M. Hofmyer, P. B. Best, M. A. Meyer, and P. D. Shaughnessy. 1988. Chemical immobilization of free-ranging African (Cape) fur seals. So. Afr. J. Wildl. Res. 18: 154-157.

Davis, K. B., and B. R. Griffin. 2004. Physiological reponses of hybrid striped bass under sedation by several anesthestics. Aquaculture 233: 531-548.

Davy, C. W., P. N. Trennery, J. G. Edmunds, J. F. B. Altman, and D. A. Eichler. 1987. Local myotoxicity of ketamine in the marmoset. Lab. An. 21: 61-67.

Day, G. I., R. F. Dyson, and F. H. Landeen. 1965. A portable resuscitator for use on large game animals. J. Wildl. Manage. 29: 511-515.

Day, G. I., S. D. Schemnitz, and R. D. Taber. 1980. Capturing and marking wild animals. *In* Shemnitz, S. D. (ed.). Wildlife Management Techniques Manual, The Wildlife Society, Washington, D. C. Pp. 61-88.

Day, J. 1969a. Cap-chur problems and remedies. Wildlife Digest, Arizona Game and Fish Department. 2.

Day, J. 1969b. Drug use for capturing and restraining animals. Wildlife Digest, Arizona Game and Fish Department. 4: 1.

Day, P. W. 1965. Techniques of bear anesthesia applicable to research. *In* Sawyer, D. C. (ed.). Symposium on Experimental Animal Anesthesiology. Brooks Air Force Base, Texas.

Day, T. K., and C. K. Roge. 1996. Evaluation of sedation in quail induced by use of midazolam and reversed by use of flumazenil. J. Am. Vet. Med. Assoc. 209: 969.

De Lamo, D. A., and J. L. Garrido. 1983. [Immobilization of guanacos *Lama guanicoe* Muller]. Cent. Nac. Patagonico Contrib. 77: 1-9.

De Maar, T. W. J., H. van Bolhuis, and M. J. Mugo. 1998. Field anesthesia of camels (*Camelus dromedarius*) and the use of medetomidine/ketamine with atipamezole reversal. Proc. Joint Conf. Am. Assoc. Zoo Vet. and Am. Assoc. Wildl. Vet. Pp. 54-57.

De Meneghi, D., P. G. Meneguz, O. Abate, G. Quaranta, L. Rossi, and P. Lafranchi. 1987. Blood serum analyses of chemically captured alpine ibex, I: Values at the onset of anaesthesia. Trans. Congr. Int. Union Game Biol. Suppl. 18: 1.

De Vos, J. C., and T. Remington. 1981. A summary of capture efforts in Arizona since 1977. Desert Bighorn Council Trans. Pp. 57-59.

De Vos, V. 1978a. Immobilization of free-ranging wild animals using a new drug. Vet. Rec. 103: 64-68.

De Vos, V. 1978b. A new potent analgesic for chemical immobilization of gemsbok (*Oryx gazella gazella*). Koedoe. 21: 173-180.

De Vos, V. 1979. Do-it-yourself remote chemical immobilization equipment. Koedoe. 22: 177-186.

De Vos, V. 1985. Remote chemical immobilization of African buffalo (*Syncerus caffer*). Proc. Buffalo Symp., Pretoria, So. Afr. P. 157. (abstr.)

De Vos, V., G. L. Van Rooyen, and J. J. Kloppers. Anthrax immunization of free-ranging roan antelope *Hippotragus equinus* in the Kruger Narional Park. Koedoe 16: 11-25.

Dean, R., W. W. Hines, and D. C. Church. 1973. Immobilizing free-ranging and captive deer with phencyclidine hydrochloride. J. Wildl. Manage. 37: 82-86.

Deem, S. L., J. C. H. Ko, and S. B. Citino. 1998. Anesthetic and cardiorespiratory effects of tiletamine-zolazepam-medetomidine in cheetahs. J. Am. Vet. Med. Assoc. 213: 1022-1026.

Degernes, L. A., T. J. Kreeger, R. Mandsager, and P. T. Redig. 1988. Ketamine-xylazine anesthesia in red-tailed hawks with antagonism by yohimbine. J. Wildl. Dis. 24: 322-326.

DelGiudice, G. D., L. D. Mech, W. J. Paul, and P. D. Karns. 1986. Effects on fawn survival of multiple immobilizations of captive pregnant white-tailed deer. J. Wildl. Dis. 22: 245-248.

DelGiudice, G. D., U. S. Seal, and T. J. Kreeger. 1988. Xylazine and ketamine-induced glycosuria in white-tailed deer. J. Wildl. Dis. 24: 317-321.

DelGiudice, G. D., P. R. Krausman, E. S. Bellantioni, R. C. Etchberger, and U. S. Seal. 1989. Reversal by tolazoline hydrochloride of xylazine hydrochloride-ketamine hydrochloride immobilizations in free-ranging desert mule deer. J. Wildl. Dis. 25: 347-352.

DelGiudice, G. D., B. A. Mangipane, B. A. Sampson, and C. O. Kochanny. 2001. Chemical immobilization, body temperature, and post-release mortality of white-tailed deer captured by Clover trap and net-gun. Wildl. Soc. Bull. 29: 1147-1157.

DelGiudice, G. D., B. A. Sampson, D. W. Kuehn, M. C. Powell, and J. Fieberg. 2005. Understanding margins of safe capture, chemical immobilization, and handling of free-ranging white-tailed deer. Wildl. Soc. Bull. 33: 677-687.

DeLeeuw, A. N. S., G. J. Forrester, P. D. Spyvee, M. G. I. Brash, and R. J. Delahay. 2004. Experimental comparison of ketamine with a combination of ketamine, butorphanol and medetomidine for general anaesthesia of the Eurasian badger (*Meles meles* L.). Vet. J. 167: 186-193.

Delvaux, H., R. Courtois, L. Breton, and R. Patenaude. 1999. Relative efficiency of succinycholine, xylazine, and carfentanil/xylazine mixtures to immobilize free-ranging moose. J. Wildl. Dis. 35: 38-48.

Demaster, D. P., J. B. Faro, J. A. Estes, J. Taggart, and C. Zabel. 1981. Drug immobilization of walrus (*Odobenus rosmarus*). Can. J. Fish. Aquat. Sci. 38: 365-367.

Dematteis, A., A. Menzano, P. Tizzani, B. Karmacharya, P. G. Meneguz, and S. Lovari. 2006. Immobilization of Himalayan tahr with a xylazine-ketamine mixture and reversal with atipamezole under field conditions. J. Wildl. Dis. 42: 633-639.

DeNicola, A. J., and R. K. Swihart. 1997. Capture-induced stress in white-tailed deer. Wildl. Soc. Bull. 25: 500-503.

DeNicola, A. J., D. J. Kesler, and R. K. Swihart. 1996. Ballistics of a biobullet delivery system. Wildl. Soc. Bull. 24: 301-305.

Dennig, H. K. 1972. The use of Rompun in the Dromedary in diagnostic splenectomy. Vet. Med. Rev. 4

Dennis, P. M., and D. J. Heard. 2002. Cardiopulmonary effects of medetomidine-ketamine combination administered intravenously in gopher tortoises. J. Amer. Vet. Med. Assoc. 220: 1516-1519.

Denney, R. N. 1965. Immobilization and tranquilization studies on Colorado deer and elk. Colorado Game, Fish and Parks Department Job Completion Report, W-38-R18. Part I: 5-22.

Denney, R. N. 1966. Neckbanding techniques (elk) with the helicopter. Trans. W. Assoc. Game Fish Comm. 46: 134-138.

Denney, R. N. 1969. Black rhinoceros immobilization utilizing a new tranquilizing agent. E. Afr. Wildl. J. 7: 159-165.

Denney, R. N. and B. R. Gill. 1970. Annotated bibliography on mammal immobilization with drugs. Colorado Division of Game, Fish and Parks Special Report. 15. 27 pp.

Dennis, P. M., D. J. Heard, and J. S. Davidson. 2000. Cardiopulmonary effects of medetomidine and ketamine in the gopher tortoise (*Gopherus polyphemus*). Proc. Joint Conf. Am. Assoc. Zoo Vet. and Intl. Assoc. Aquatic An. Med. P. 54.

Denny, M. J. S. 1973. The use of ketamine hydrochloride as a safe short duration anaesthetic in kangaroos. Br. Vet. J. 129: 362-365.

Denny, M. J. S. 1974. Anaesthesia in kangaroos and a list of anaesthetics used in monotremes and marsupials. Austral. Mammal. 1: 294-298.

Densmore, M. A. 1979. A survey of immobilization techniques used in captive sitatunga (*Tragelaphus spekei*). J. Zoo An. Med. 10: 98-102.

Densmore, M. A., M. J. Bowen, R. M. Robinson, P. G. Harms, and D. C. Kraemer. 1987. Hematologic and serum chemistry profiles of four male addax (*Addax nasomaculatus*) immobilized with etorphine and xylazine. J. Zoo An. Med. 18: 123-130.

Deresienski, D. T., and C. E. Rupprecht. 1989. Yohimbine reversal of ketamine-xylazine immobilization of raccoons (*Procyon lotor*). J. Wildl. Dis. 25: 169-174.

Des Meules, P., B. R. Simard, and J. M. Brassard. 1971. A technique for the capture of caribou, *Rangifer tarandus*, in winter. Can. Fld. Nat. 85: 221-229.

Devilliers, M. S., A. S. Vanjaarsveld, D. G. A. Meltzer, and P. R. K. Richardson. 1997. Social dynamics and the cortisol response to immobilization stress of the African wild dog, *Lycaon pictus*. Hormon. Behav. 31: 3-14.

Dew, T. L. 1988. Use of tolazoline hydrochloride to reverse multiple anesthetic episodes induced with xylazine hydrochloride and ketamine hydrochloride in white-tailed deer and goats. J. Zoo An. Med. 19: 8-13.

Dewey, R. W., and A. Rudnick. 1973. An Orang Asli blowpipe with a syringe-type dart for the live capture of wild primates in Malaysia. S.E. Asian J. Trop. Med. Publ. Health 4: 285.

Dhungel, S. K. 1985. Use of Rompun (xylazine) to immobilize hog deer in Royal Chitwan National Park, Nepal. Tigerpaper. 12: 18-20.

Dickson, S. J., H. M. Stone, and E. A. Queree. 1983. Xylazine (Rompun) levels in deer antler velvet. N. Z. J. Agric. Res. 26: 93-94.

Diehl, S. R. 1988. The translocation of urban white-tailed deer. *In* Nielsen, L. and R. D. Brown (eds.). Translocation of Wild Animals. Wisconsin Humane Society, Inc., and Cesar Kleberg Wildlife Research Institute, Milwaukee, Wisconsin. Pp. 239-249.

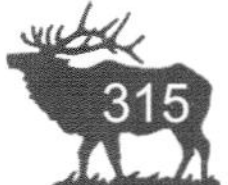

Dieterich, R. A. 1968. The use of M-99 etorphine and its antagonist, M-285 cyprenorphine, for immobilization of wild animals. Proc. 19th Alaskan Science Conf. Abstract No. 37: 22-23.
Dieterich, R. A. 1984. Muskox medical practices. Biol. Pap. Univ. Alaska Spec. Rep. No. 4: 167-169.
Dinerstein, E., S. Shrestha, and H. Mishra. 1990. Capture, chemical immobilization, and radio-collar life for greater one-horned rhinoceros. Wildl. Soc. Bull. 18: 36-41.
Dinnes, M. R. 1982. Use of the blowpipe as an instrument for remote injection of animals. *In* Nielsen, L., J. C. Haigh, and M. E. Fowler (eds.). Chemical Immobilization of North American Wildlife. Wisconsin Humane Society, Inc. Milwaukee, Wisconsin. Pp. 188-193.
Dioli, M., H. J. Schwartz, and R. Stimmelmayr. 1992. Management and handling of the camel. *In* Schwartz, M., and M. Dioli (eds.). *Camelus dromedarius* in Eastern Africa: a pictorial guide to diseases, health care, and management. Verlag Josef Margraf, Weikersheim, Germany. Pp. 62-154.
Ditman, K. S. 1964. Drug immobilization of wild animals. Mind-Psychiatry Gen. Prac. 2: 103-113, 124.
Diverio, S., P. J. Goddard, I. J. Gordon, and D. A. Elston. 1993. The effect of management practices on stress in farmed red deer (*Cervus elaphus*) and its modulation by long-acting neuroleptics (LANs): behavioural responses. Appl. Anim. Beh. Sci. 36: 363-376.
Diverio, S., P. J. Goddard, and I. J. Gordon. 1996. Use of long-acting neuroleptics to reduce the stress response to management practices in red deer. Appl. Anim. Beh. Sci. 49: 83-88.
Divers, S. J. 1996. The use of propofol in reptile anesthesia. Proc. Ann. Conf. Assoc. Reptil. Amphib. Vet. Sacramento, Calif. Pp. 57-59.
Dixon, R., J. Howes, J. Gentile, H. B. Hsu, J. Hsiao, D. Gar, D. Weidler, M. Meyer, and R. Tuttle. 1986. Nalmefene: intravenous safety and kinetics of a new opioid antagonist. Clin. Pharmacol. Ther. 39: 49-52.
Dobbs, H. E. 1968. Effects of cypronophine (M-285), a morphine antagonist, on the distribution and excretion of etorphine (M.99) a potent morphine like drug. J. Pharmacol. Exp. Therap. 160: 407-411.
Dodman, N. H. 1980. Chemical restraint in the horse. Equine Vet. J. 12: 166-170.
Doherty, T. J., and D. P. R. Tweedie. 1989. Evaluation of xylazine hydrochloride as the sole immobilizing agent in moose and caribou and its subsequent reversal with idazoxan. J. Wildl. Dis. 25: 95-98.
Dolensek, E. P. 1971. Anesthesia of exotic felines with ketamine HCl. J. Zoo An. Med. 2: 16-19.
Donahue, M. A., M. E. Lisano, and J. K. Kennamer. 1982. Effects of alpha-chloralose drugging on blood constituents in the eastern wild turkey. J. Wildl. Manage. 46: 468-474.
Done, S. H., P. Lees, O Dansie, and L. W. Watkins. 1975. Sedation and restraint of fallow deer with diazepam. Brit. Vet. J. 131: 545-548.
Dräger, N. 1974. Immobilisation von Afrikanischen Büffeln im Rahmen der Maul- und Klauenseuchebekämpfung in Botswana. Berl. Münch. Tierärztl. Wschr. 87: 328-329.
Dräger, N., L. Patterson, and D. Breton. 1976. Immobilization of African buffaloes (*Syncerus caffer caffer*) in large numbers for veterinary research. E. Afr. Wildl. J. 14: 113-120.
Drevemo, S., and L. Karstad. 1974. The effect of xylazine and xylazine-etorphine-acepromazine combination of some clinical and hematological parameters in impala and eland. J. Wildl. Dis. 10: 377-383.
Drevemo, S., J. G. Grootenhuis, and L. Karstad. 1974. Blood parameters in wild ruminants in Kenya. J. Wildl. Dis. 10: 327-334.
Duchamps, A. 1985. [Immobilization of wild animals in practice]. Trans. Congr. Int. Union Game Biol. 17: 795-802.
Dugdale, A. 2001. Anaesthesia of a pregnant alpaca (*Lama pacos*). Vet. Rec. 149: 28.
Duke, T., C. M. Egger, J. G. Ferguson, and M. M. Frketic. 1997. Cardiopulmonary effects of propofol infusion in llamas. Am. J. Vet. Res. 58: 153-156.
Dunlop, C. I., D. S. Hodgson, and E. P. Steffy. 1984. Observations during anesthetic management of an adult elephant. Proc. Ann. Meeting Am. Coll. Vet. Anesthesiol. Pp. 1-2.
Dyson, R. F. 1965. Experience with succinylcholine chloride in zoo animals. Intl. Zoo Yb. 5: 205-206.
Dzialak, M. R., and T. L. Serfass. 2003. Effects of flumazenil on fishers, *Martes pennanti*, restrained with tiletamine-zolazepam. Wildl. Biol. 9: 235-239.
Dzialak, M. R., T. L. Serfass, and T. L. Blankenship. 2001. Reversible chemical restraint of fishers with medetomidine-ketamine and atipamezole. J. Wildl. Manage. 65: 157-163.
Dzialak, M. R., T. L. Serfass, D. L. Shumway, L. M. Hegde, and T. L. Blankenship. 2002. Chemical restraint of fishers (*Martes pennanti*) with ketamine and medetomidine-ketamine. J. Zoo Wildl. Med. 33: 45-51.

Eads, F. E. 1976. Tilazol™ (CI-744): a new agent for chemical restraint and anesthesia in nonhuman primates. Vet. Med. Small An. Clin. 71: 648-652.

Ebedes, H. 1962. Practical experience in the use of the Cap-Chur gun. J. So. Afr. Vet. Assoc. 33: 87-91.

Ebedes, H. 1966a. Notes on the immobilization and biology of zebra (*Equus burchelli antiquorum*) in the Etosha Game Park, S.W. Africa. J. So. Afr. Vet. Assoc. 37: 299-303.

Ebedes, H. 1966b. Gemsbok and black rhinoceros immobilization with M99. M-series, Vet. Appl. Rpt. No. 48, Reckitt and Sons, Hull, England.

Ebedes, H. 1967. Gemsbok and black rhinoceros immobilization with etorphine. M-series, Vet. Appl. Rpt. No. 57, Reckitt and Sons, Hull, England.

Ebedes, H. 1969. Notes on the immobilization of gemsbock (*Oryx gazella*) in South West Africa using etorphine hydrochloride (M99). Madoqua. 1: 35-45.

Ebedes, H. 1970. The use of sernylan as an immobilizing agent and anesthesic for wild carnivorous mammals in South West Africa. Madoqua. 2: 19-25.

Ebedes, H. 1971a. The capture of plains zebra (*Equus burchelli antiquorum*, Smith) with M.99 (Reckitt) and tranquilizers in Etosha National Park. Madoqua 3: 67-76.

Ebedes, H. 1971b. The use of sernylan to immobilize South West Africa Felidae. J. Zoo An. Med. 2: 12.

Ebedes, H. 1972. Drug immobilization of wild carnivorous animals. Onderstport (Afrique du Sud). Pp. 24-28.

Ebedes, H. 1973a. The capture of free-living vultures in the Etosha National Park with phencyclidine. J. So. Afr. Wildl. Manage. Assoc. 3: 105-107.

Ebedes, H. 1973b. The drug immobilization of carnivorous animals. *In* E. Young (ed.). The Capture and Care of Wild Animals. Human and Rouseau, Cape Town, South Africa. Pp. 62-68.

Ebedes, H. 1975a. The capture and translocation of gemsbok *Oryx gazella gazella* in the Namib Desert with the aid of fentanyl, etorphine and tranquilizers. J. So. Afr. Vet. Assoc. 46: 359-362.

Ebedes, H. 1975b. The immobilization of adult male and female elephant *Loxodonta africana* Blumenbach with etorphine and observation on the action of diprenorphine. Madoqua. 9: 19-24.

Ebedes, H. 1991. Reduce deaths with drugs. Natura 23: 15-17.

Ebedes, H. 1992a. The use of long-acting neuroleptics for translocating some South African wild animals. J. So. Afr. Vet. Assoc.

Ebedes, H. 1992b. A note on haloperidol for translocation. *In* Ebedes, H. (ed.) The Use of Tranquillizers in Wildlife. Dept. Ag. Develop., Pretoria. Bull. No. 423. Pp. 21-22.

Ebedes, H. 1993. The use of long-acting tranquilizers in captive wild animals. *In* McKenzie, A. A. (ed.). The Capture and Care Manual. Wildlife Decision Support Services and The South African Veterinary Foundation, Pretoria. Pp. 71-99.

Ebedes, H., and M Grobler. 1979. The restraint of the Cape Hunting dog *Lycaon pictus* with phencyclidine hydrochloride and ketamíne hydrochloride. J. So. Afr. Vet. Assoc. 50: 113-114.

Ebedes, H., and J. P. Raath. 1995. The use of long term neuroleptics in the confinement and transport of wild animals. Proc. Joint Conf. Am. Assoc. Zoo Vet., Wildl. Dis. Assoc., Am. Assoc. Wildl. Vet. East Lansing, Michigan. Pp. 173-176.

Ebedes, H., and J. P. Raath. 1999. Use of tranquilizers in wild herbivores. *In* Fowler, M. E., and R. E. Miller (eds.). Zoo & Wild Animal Medicine. Current Therapy 4. W. B. Saunders Company, Philadelphia, Pennsylvania. Pp. 575-585.

Ebedes, H., E. Leibnitz, and J. Joubert. 1977. The immobilisation of wildebeest (*Connochaetes taurinus*) with etorphine and the use of diphrenorphine as an etorphine antagonist. Madoqua. 10: 71-73.

Ebedes, H., J. G. du Toit, and J. Van Rooyen. 1989. Game capture. *In* Bothma, J. du P. (ed.). Game Ranch Management. J. L. Schaik, Pretoria, South Africa. Pp. 409-483.

Ebedes, H., and R. E. J. Burroughs. 1992. Long-acting neuroleptics in wildlife. *In* Ebedes, H. (ed.) The Use of Tranquillizers in Wildlife. Dept. Ag. Develop., Pretoria. Bull. No. 423. Pp. 31-37.

Eisele, P. H., T. L. Faith, P. M. Menth, J. C. Parker, and D. H. Vanvuren. 1997. Ketamine-isoflurane combination anesthesia for surgical implantation of intraperitoneal radio transmitters in the beaver. Contemp. Top. Lab. Anim. Sci. 36: 97-99.

Elder, W. H., and D. H. Rodgers. 1974. Immobilization and marking of African elephants and the prediction of body weight from foot circumference. Mammalia. 38: 33-53.

El Maghraby, H. M., and K. Al Qudah. 2005. Sedative and analgesic effects of detomidine in camels (*Camelus dromedarius*). J. Camel. Pract. Res. 12: 41-45.

Elmore, R. G., D. K. Hardin, J. M. E. Balke, R. S. Younquist, and D. W. Erickson. 1985. Analyzing the

effects of diazepam used in combination with ketamine. Vet. Med. Sm. An. Clin. 80: 55-57.

Eltringham, S. K. 1974. The rescue of distressed large mammals in national parks using drug immobilization. E. Afr. Wildl. J. 12: 233-238.

Engelhardt, F. R. 1977. Immobilization of harp seals, *Phoca groenlandica*, by intravenous injection of ketamine. Comp. Biochem. Physiol. 56: 75-76.

England, G. C., and R. A. Kock. 1988. The use of two mixtures of ketamine and xylazine to immobilise free ranging Bennetts wallabies. Vet. Rec. 122: 11-14.

English, A. W. 1984. Chemical restraint of deer. *In* Deer Refresher Course. Proc. Vet. Univ. Sydney, Sydney, Australia 72: 325-350.

Enqvist, K. E., J. M. Arnemo, J. P. Lemel, and J. Truvé. 2000. Medetomidine/tiletamine-zolazepam and medetomidine/butorphanol/tiletamine-zolazepam: a comparison of two anesthetic regimens for surgical implantation on intraperitoneal radiotransmitters in free-ranging juvenile European wild boars (*Sus scrofa scrofa*). Proc. Joint Conf. Am. Assoc. Zoo Vet. and Intl. Assoc. Aquatic An. Med. Pp. 261-263.

Ensley, P. K., D. P. Launer, and J. P. Blasingame. 1984. General anesthesia and surgical removal of a tumor-like growth from the foot of a double-wattled cassowary. J. Zoo An. Med. 15: 35-37.

Enzhu, Z. 1990. Anaesthesia of cranes with ketamine hydrochloride. Chin. J. Vet. Med. 16: 28.

Epstein, A., R. White, I. H. Horowitz, P. H. Kass, and R. Ofri. 2002. Effects of propofol as an anaesthetic agent in adult lions (*Panthera leo*): a comparison with two established protocols. Res. Vet. Sci. 72: 137-140.

Erdtmann, J. N., J. Schumacher, C. Pollock, S. E. Orosz, M. P. Jones, and R. C. Harvey. 1998. Cardiopulmonary and anesthetic effects of medetomidine-ketamine-butorphanol and antagonism with atipamezole in servals (*Felis serval*). Proc. Joint Conf. Am. Assoc. Zoo Vet. and Am. Assoc. Wildl. Vet. P. 135.

Erickson, A. W. 1957. Techniques for live-trapping and handling black bears. Trans. No. Am. Wildl. Nat. Res. Conf. 22: 520-543.

Eriksen, E. 1963. Om Cap-chur instrumentariet. Medlemsbl. Danske Dyrlaegeforen. 3: 53-72.

Eriksen, E. 1968a. Medikamentel immobilisering og faengsling af dyr. I. Teknik og medikamenter. Nord. Vet. Med. 20: 499-510

Eriksen, E. 1968b. Medikamentel immobilisering og faengsling af dyr. II. Indgangning af vilde knjer og hjorte. Nord. Vet. Med. 20: 576-591.

Eriksen, E. 1968c. Medikamentel immobilisering og faengsling af dyr. III. Indgangning af vilde knjer og hjorte. Nord. Vet. Med. 20: 657-679.

Eriksen, E. 1970. Indfangning af hjortevildt ved immobilisering med neuroleptika. [Capture of cervidae by immobilization with neuroleptics]. Nord. Vet. Med. 22: 385-400.

Eriksen, E. 1976. Capture and investigation of 42 polar bears in northeast Greenland, April-May 1974. Proc. Polar Bear Spec. Group. 5: 37-47.

Eriksen, E. 1978. Medicamentous immobilization and capture of wild animals and deer. Kongelige Veterinaer. og Landbohojskole. Cophenhagen, Denmark. 198 pp.

Eriksen, E., and J. F. Hansen. 1966. Erfolge und Misserfolge bei der Anwendung von Phencylidine bei einigen Wiederkäuern und einem Elefanten. VIII Int. Symp. Erkrank. Zootiere. Leipsig. Pp. 182-188.

Escos, J., and C. L. Alados. 1993. Immobilization of Spanish ibex with etorphine plus acepromazine. Mammalia 57: 601-605.

Evans, M., S. Atkinson, and A. Horsup. 1998. Combination of zolazepam and tiletamine as a sedative and anesthetic for wombats. Aust. Vet. J. 76: 355-356.

Evans, R. R., and J. W. Goertz. 1975. Capturing wild turkeys with tribromoethanol. J. Wildl. Manage. 39: 630-634.

Fabry, M., S. Celis, R. León, S. Jiménez, and P. Morris. 2001. Immobilization of captive pudu (*Pudu puda*) with ketamine-medetomidine-butorphanol and reversal with atipamezole and naloxone. Proc. Am. Assoc. Zoo Vet. Pp. 232-233.

Faggella, A. M., and M. R. Raffe. 1987. The use of isoflurane anesthesia in a water monitor lizard and a rhino iguana. Comp. Anim. Pract. 1: 52-53.

Faggella, A. M., T. J. Kreeger, and U. S. Seal. 1986. Cardiovascular effects of xylazine HCL and ketamine HCL anesthesia in dogs and wolves. Midwest Anesthesia Conference, Univ. of Illinois, Urbana.

Fahlman, Å., E. J. Bosi, and G. Nyman. 1999. Immobilization of southeast Asian primates with

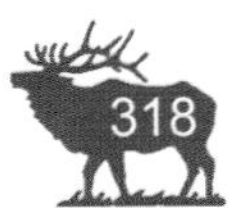

medetomidine, zolazepam, and tiletamine, and reversal with atipamezole. Proc. Am. Assoc. Zoo Vet. P. 334.

Fahlman, Å., C. Foggin, and G. Nyman. 2004. Pulmonary gas exchange and acid-base status in immobilized black rhinoceros (*Diceros bicornis*) and white rhinoceros (*Ceratotherium simum*) in Zimbabwe. Proc. Am. Assoc. Zoo Vet. Pp. 519-521.

Fahlman, Å., A. Loveridge, C. Wenham, C. Foggin, J. M. Arnemo, and G. Nyman. 2005a. Reversible anesthesia of free-ranging lions (*Panthera leo*) in Zimbabwe. J. So. Afr. Vet. Assoc. 76: 187-192.

Fahlman, Å., J. M. Arnemo, J. Persson, P. Segerström, and G. Nyman. 2005b. Physiological parameters during anaesthesia of free-ranging wolverines (*Gulo gulo*). Proc. 1st Intl. Symp. Wolverine Res. Mgmt. Jokkmokk, Sweden. P. 18.

Fan, Z., Y. Ou, and Y. Chao. 1987. A discussion on anesthesia of the giant panda with the injection ketamine. *In* Proceedings of Therapeutics of the Giant Panda. China Forestry Publishing House. Pp. 61-65. (Chinese)

Fanton, J. W., G. B. Hubbard, and K. C. Fletcher. 1984. Halothane induced hepatic necrosis in a snow leopard. J. Zoo An. Med. 15: 108-111.

Farnsworth, R. J., and C. M. Stowe. 1976. Depression of a newborn elk calf associated with the prepartum use of etorphine hydrochloride in the dam. J. Am. Vet. Med. Assoc. 169: 888-889.

Faulkner, J. E., and A. Archambault. 1993. Anesthesia and surgery in the green iguana. Seminars in Avian Exotic Pet Med. 2: 103-108.

Feldman, D. B., and J. L. Self. 1971. Sedation and anesthesia of the Virginia opossum, *Didelphis virginiana*. Lab. An. Sci. 21: 717-720.

Felkai, F. 1993. Anaesthetization of the budgerigar by ketamine-xylazine. Magyar Allatorvosok Lapja 48: 154-155. (Hungarian)

Fenn, H. S., and C. J. Sedgwick. 1969. Immobilization and removal of retained placenta in the wild gnu (wildebeest). Clif. Vet. 23: 17-18.

Ferin, M., P. W. Carmel, M. P. Warren, R. L. Himsworth, A. G. Frantz, and M. R. Nocenti. 1976. Phencyclidine sedation as a technique for handling rhesus monkeys: effects on LH, GH, and prolactin secretions. Proc. Soc. Exp. Biol. Med. 151: 428-433.

Fernández-Morán, J., and V. I. Peinado. 1996. Comparison of two methods of chemical immobilization in fallow deer (*Cervus dama*): medetomidine-tiletamine-zolazepam versus xylazine-tiletamine-zolazepam. Proc. Am. Assoc. Zoo Vet. Pp. 382-388.

Fernández-Morán, J., J. Palomeque, and V. I. Peinado. 2000. Medetomidine/tiletamine/zolazepam and xylazine/tiletamine/zolazepam combinations for immobilization of fallow deer (*Cervus dama*). J. Zoo Wildl. Med. 31: 62-64.

Fernández-Morán, J., E. Perez, M. Sanmartin, D. Saavedra, and X. Manteca-Vilanova. 2001. Reversible immobilization of Eurasian otters with a combination of ketamine and medetomidine. J. Wildl. Dis. 37: 561-565.

Fernández-Morán, J., D. Saavedra, and X. Manteca-Vilanova. 2002. Reintroduction of the Eurasian otter (*Lutra lutra*) in northeastern Spain: trapping, handling, and medical management. J. Zoo Wildl. Med. 33: 222-227.

Fernández-Morán, J., D. Saavedra, J. L. R. DeLaTorre, and X. Manteca-Vilanova. 2004. Stress in wild-caught Eurasian otters (*Lutra lutra*): effects of a long-acting neuroleptic and time in captivity. Anim. Welfare. 13: 143-149.

Ferney, J. 1966. Del'emploi de la carabine Cap-shur Palmer pour les injections a distance chez les animaux. Bull. Soc. Sci. Vet. et Med. comparee, Lyon. 68: 7-426.

Ferreira, S. M., and M. N. Bester. 1999. Chemical immobilization, physical restraint and stomach lavaging of fur seals at Marion Island. S. Afr. J. Wildl. Res. 29: 55-61.

Ferreras, P., J. J. Aldama, J. F. Beltràn, and M. Delibes. 1994. Immobilization of the endangered Iberian lynx with xylazine- and ketamine-hydrochloride. J. Wildl. Dis. 30: 65-68.

Fessel, L. 1971. Zur Sedation und Immobilisation von Wildtieren. Wien. Tierärztl. Mschr. 58: 179-185.

Fessel, L. 1972. Zur medikamentoesen immobilisation von Wildtieren. [On the medical immobilization of wild animals]. Z. Jagdwiss. 18: 15-23.

Festa-Bianchet, M., and J. T. Jorgenson. 1985. Use of xylazine and ketamine to immobilize bighorn sheep in Alberta. J. Wildl. Manage. 49: 162-165.

Feurt, S. D., J. H. Jenkins, F. A. Hayes, and J. A. Crockford. 1958. Pharmacology and toxicology of nicotine with special reference to species variation. Science 127: 1054-1055.

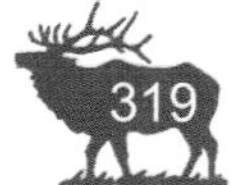

Fiala, L., P. Guba, and M. Hojovcova. 1984. [Controlled respiration of exotic animals - its use in anaesthesia]. Proc. Int. Symp. Dis. Zoo. Anim. 26: 205-206.

Field, W. E., J. Yelnosky, J. Mundy, and J. Mitchell. 1966. Use of droperidol and fentanyl for analgesia and sedation in primates. J. Am. Vet. Med. Assoc. 149: 896-901.

Finer, B. L. 1954. Anaesthesia of the common seal. Anaesthesia 9: 34.

Finnie, E. P. 1976. Restraint and anaesthesia in monotremes and marsupials. Proc. Post-Grad. Committee in Vet. Sci., U. Sydney. 29: 49-52.

Finnie, E. P. 1986. Restraint: monotremes and marsupials. *In* Fowler, M. E. (ed.). Zoo and Wild Animal Medicine, 2nd ed. W. B. Saunders Co., Philadelphia, Pennsylvania. Pp 570-572.

Firn, S. 1973. Accidental poisoning by an animal immobilizing agent. The Lancet 2: 95-96.

Fischer, M. T., R. E. Miller, and E. W. Houston. 1997. Serial tranquilization of a reticulated giraffe (*Giraffa camelopardalis reticulata*) using xylazine. J. Zoo Wildl. Med. 28: 182-184.

Fisher, L. E. 1965. General and chemical restraint technics used in a zoological garden. *In* Sawyer, D. C. (ed.). Symposium on Experimental Animal Anesthesiology. Brooks Air Force Base, Texas.

Fitzgerald, G. 1993. Effect of nitrous oxide on the minimal anaesthetic dose of isoflurane in the pigeon and red-tailed hawk. Med. Vet. Quebec. 23: 132.

Fitzgerald, J. P. 1973. Four immobilizing agents used on badgers under field conditions. J. Wildl. Manage. 37: 8-421.

Flamand, J. R. B. 1999. Medical aspects of Arabian oryx reintroduction. *In* Fowler, M. E., and R. E. Miller (eds.). Zoo & Wild Animal Medicine. Current Therapy 4. W. B. Saunders Company, Philadelphia, Pennsylvania. Pp. 687-698.

Flamand, J. R. B., and D. Lawson. 1986. Capture and care of suni (*Neotragus moschatus*) in Natal. Lammergeyer. 37: 36-39.

Flamand, J. R. B., and P. S. Rogers. 1992. The tranquillization of reedbuck and nyala. *In* Ebedes, H. (ed.) The Use of Tranquillizers in Wildlife. Dept. Ag. Develop., Pretoria. Bull. No. 423. Pp. 47-48.

Flamand, J. R. B., K. Rochat, and M. E. Keep. 1984. Instruction guide to the most commonly and most successfully used methods in rhino capture, handling, transport, and release. *In* Corfield, T. (ed.). The Wilderness Guardian. Nairobi Space Publishers, Nairobi. Pp. 546-584.

Flamand, J. R. B., P. S. Rogers, and D. K. Blake. 1992. Immobilization of crocodiles. *In* Ebedes, H. (ed.) The Use of Tranquillizers in Wildlife. Dept. Ag. Develop., Pretoria. Bull. No. 423. Pp. 61-65.

Flecknell, P. A., M. John, M. Mitchell, and C. Shurey. 1983. Injectable anaesthetic techniques in two species of gerbil (*Meriones libycus* and *Meriones unguiculatus*). Lab. An. 17: 118-128.

Flecknell, P. A., I. J. Cruz, J. H. Liles, and G. Whelan. 1996. Induction of anesthesia with halothane and isoflurane in the rabbit - a comparison of the use of a face-mask or an anesthetic chamber. Lab An. 30: 67-74.

Flecknell, P. A., J. V. Roughan, and P. Hedenqvist. 1999. Induction of anaesthesia with sevoflurane and isoflurane in the rabbit. Lab An. 33: 41-46.

Fleming, G. J. 1996. Capture and chemical immobilization of the Nile crocodile (*Crocodylus niloticus*) in South Africa. Proc. Ann. Conf. Assoc. Reptil. Amphib. Vet. Sacramento, Calif. Pp. 63-66.

Fleming, G. J., D. J. Heard, R. F. Floyd, and A. Riggs. 2003. Evaluation of propofol and medetomidine-ketamine for short-term immobilization of Gulf of Mexico sturgeon (*Acipenser oxyrinchus de soti*). J. Zoo Wildl. Med. 34: 153-158.

Fleming, G. J., S. B. Citino, and M. Bush. 2006. Reversible anesthetic combination using medetomidine-butorphanol-midazolam in in-situ African wild dogs (*Lycaon pictus*). Proc. Am. Assoc. Zoo Vet. Pp. 214-215.

Fletch, A. L., G. Wobeser, and L. Karstad. 1967. The use of etorphine (M.99) and cyprenorphine (M.285) for immobilizing of white-tailed deer (*Odocoileus virginianus*). Unpublished report F.A.O.

Fletcher, J. 1974. Hypersensitivity of an isolated population of red deer (*Cervus elaphus*) to xylazine. Vet. Rec. 94: 85-86.

Fletcher, J. 1995. Handling farmed deer. In Practice 17: 30-37.

Fletcher, K. C. 1980. Needle reinforcement of butane powered darts. J. Zoo An. Med. 11: 44-46.

Fletcher, K. C., L. Boyce, and D. Florence. 1979. Butane powered injection by pole syringe. J. Zoo An. Med. 10: 106-112.

Fletcher, T. J. 1986. Sedation and immobilization. *In* Alexander, T. L. (ed.). Management and Diseases of Deer. Veterinary Deer Society, London, U.K. Pp. 57-59.

Flook, D. R., J. R. Robertson, O. R. Hermanrude, and H. K. Buechner. 1962. Succinylcholine chloride for

immobilization of North American elk. J. Wildl. Manage. 26: 334-336.

Flyger, V., M. S. R. Smith, R. L. Damm, and R. S. Peterson. 1965. Effects of three immobilizing drugs on Weddell seals. J. Mammal. 46: 345-347.

Flyger, V., M. W. Schein, A. W. Erickson, and I. Larsen. 1967. Capturing and handling polar bears: a progress report on polar bear ecological research. Trans. No. Am. Wildl. Nat. Res. Conf. Pp. 107-119.

Flynn, R. W., and T. Schumacher. 1994. Ecology of martens in southeast Alaska. Alaska Dept. Fish and Game, Fed. Aid in Wildl. Restor., Res. Prog. Rep. 38 pp.

Fong, D. W. 1982. Immobilization of caribou with etorphine plus acepromazine. J. Wildl. Manage. 46: 560-562.

Foerster, S. H., J. E. Bailey, R. Aguilar, D. L. Loria, and C. R. Foerster. 1998. Cardiopulmonary effects and utility of a butorphanol/xylazine/ketamine anesthetic protocol for immobilization of free-ranging Baird's tapir (*Tapirus bairdii*) in Costa Rica. Proc. Joint Conf. Am. Assoc. Zoo Vet. and Am. Assoc. Wildl. Vet. Pp. 41-48.

Foerster, S. H., J. E. Bailey, R. Aguilar, D. L. Loria, and C. R. Foerster. 2000. Butorphanol/xylazine/ketamine immobilization of free-ranging Baird's tapir in Costa Rica. J. Wildl. Dis. 36: 335-341.

Forsythe, D. B., A. J. Payton, D. Dixon, P. H. Myers, J. A. Clark, and J. R. Snipe. 1992. Evaluation of Telazol-xylazine as an anesthetic combination for use in Syrian hamsters. Lab. An. Sci. 42: 497-502.

Foster, C. A. 1999. Immobilization of goitred gazelles (*Gazella subgutterosa*) and Arabian mountain gazelles (*Gazella gazella*) with xylazine-ketamine. J. Zoo Wildl. Med. 30: 448-450.

Foster, J. W. 1974. Case reports from preliminary investigations of a new tranquilizer. World's Cats. 2: 228-236.

Foster, P. A. 1973. Immobilization and anaesthesia of primates. *In* E. Young (ed.). The Capture and Care of Wild Animals. Human and Rouseau, Cape Town, South Africa. Pp. 69-76.

Fournier-Chambrillon, C., P. Fournier, and J.-C. Vie´. 1997. Immobilization of wild collared anteaters with ketamine and xylazine hydrochloride. J. Wildl. Dis. 33: 795-800.

Fournier-Chambrillon, C., I. Vogel, P. Fournier, B. de Thoisy, and J.-C. Vie´. 2000. Immobilization of free-ranging nine-banded and great long-nosed armadillos with three anesthetic combinations. J. Wildl. Dis. 36:131-140.

Fournier, P., C. Fournier-Chambrillon, and J.-C. Vie´. 1998. Immobilization of wild kinkajous (*Potos flavus*) with medetomidine-ketamine and reversal by atipamezole. J. Zoo Wildl. Med. 29: 190-194.

Fournier-Chambrillon, C., J.-P. Chusseau, J. Dupuch, C. Maizeret, and P. Fournier. 2003. Immobilization of free-ranging European mink (*Mustela lutreola*) and polecat (*Mustela putorius*) with medetomidine-ketamine and reversal by atipamezole. J. Wildl. Dis. 39: 393-399.

Fowler, M. E. 1978a. Restraint and handling of wild and domestic animals. Iowa State University Press, Ames Iowa.

Fowler, M. E. (ed.). 1978b. Zoo & Wild Animal Medicine. W. B. Saunders Company, Philadelphia, Pennsylvania. 951 pp.

Fowler, M. E. 1981a. Immobilization of caribou with etorphine plus acepromazine. Proc. Am. Assoc. Zoo Vet. Pp. 87-91.

Fowler, M. E. 1981b. Problems with immobilizing and anesthetizing elephants. Proc. Am. Assoc. Zoo Vet. Pp. 87-91.

Fowler, M. E. 1982. Delivery systems for chemical immobilization. *In* Nielsen, L., J. C. Haigh, and M. E. Fowler (eds.). Chemical Immobilization of North American Wildlife. Wisconsin Human Society Inc., Milwaukee, Wisconsin. Pp. 18-45.

Fowler, M. E. (ed.). 1986. Zoo & Wild Animal Medicine. Second edition. W. B. Saunders Company, Philadelphia, Pennsylvania. 1127 pp.

Fowler, M. E. 1988. Medicine and Surgery of South American Camelids. Iowa State University Press, Ames Iowa.

Fowler, M. E. (ed.). 1993. Zoo & Wild Animal Medicine. Current Therapy 3. W. B. Saunders Company, Philadelphia, Pennsylvania. 617 pp.

Fowler, M. E. 1995. Restraint and handling of wild and domestic animals. 2nd ed. Iowa State University Press, Ames Iowa.

Fowler, M. E., and R. Hart. 1973. Castration of the Asian elephant using etorphine anesthesia. J. Am. Vet. Med. Assoc. 163: 539-541.

Fowler, M. E., E. P. Steffey, L. Galuppo, and J. R. Pascoe. 1999. Standing immobilization and anesthesia

in an Asian elephant (*Elephas maximus*). Proc. Am. Assoc. Zoo Vet. Pp. 107-110.

Fowler, M. E., E. P. Steffey, L. Galuppo, and J. R. Pascoe. 2000. Facilitation of Asian elephant (*Elephas maximus*) standing immobilization and anesthesia with a sling. J. Zoo Wildl. Med. 31: 118-123.

Frahm, M. W. 1999. Medical management of duikers. *In* Fowler, M. E., and R. E. Miller (eds.). Zoo & Wild Animal Medicine. Current Therapy 4. W. B. Saunders Company, Philadelphia, Pennsylvania. Pp. 668-681.

Frank, L. G., and J. E. Cooper. 1974. Further notes on the use of CT 1341 in birds of prey. Raptor Res. 8: 29-32.

Franzmann, A. W. 1982. An assessment of chemical immobilization of North American moose. *In* Nielsen, L., J. C. Haigh, and M. E. Fowler (eds.). Chemical Immobilization of North American Wildlife. Wisconsin Humane Society, Inc., Milwaukee, Wisconsin. Pp. 393-407.

Franzmann, A. W., and E. T. Thorne. 1970. Physiological values in wild bighorn sheep (*Ovis canadensis canadensis*) at capture, after handling, and after captivity. J. Am. Vet. Med. Assoc. 157: 647-650.

Franzmann, A. W., and P. D. Arneson. 1974. Immobilization of Alaskan moose. J. Zoo An. Med. 5: 26-32.

Franzmann, A. W., and W. R. Lance. 1988. Chemical immobilization of wildlife: recent advances. *In* Nielsen, L., and R. D. Brown (eds.). Translocation of Wild Animals. Wisconsin Humane Society, Inc., and Cesar Kleberg Wildlife Research Institute, Milwaukee, Wisconsin. Pp. 99-109.

Franzmann, A. W., A. Flynn, and P. D. Arneson. 1975. Serum corticoid levels relative to handling stress in Alaskan moose. Can. J. Zool. 53: 1424-1426.

Franzmann, A. W., C. C. Schwartz, and D. C. Johnson. 1982. Chemical immobilization of moose at the Moose Research Center, Alaska (1968-1981). Alces. 18: 94-115.

Franzmann, A. W., C. C. Schwartz, D. C. Johnson, and J. B. Faro. 1984. Immobilization of moose with carfentanil. Alces. 20: 259-281.

Franzmann, A. W., C. C. Schwartz, and D. C. Johnson. 1987. Anesthesia of moose for vasectomy using carfentanil/xylazine and reversal with naloxone/ yohimbine. Alces. 23: 221-226.

Frase, B. A., and D. Van Vuren. 1989. Techniques for immobilizing and bleeding marmots and woodrats. J. Wildl. Dis. 25: 444-445.

Fredrickson, L. F., and C. G. Trautman. 1974. Use of stupefacient and tranquilizer drugs for capturing and handling pheasants, 1967-1973, South Dakota. South Dakota Dept. Game, Fish, and Parks, P-R Project W-75-R-16, Study No. P-10.2-16-I, Pierre, So. Dakota. 31 pp.

Fredrickson, L. F., and C. G. Trautman. 1978. Use of drugs for capturing and handling pheasants. J. Wildl. Manage. 42: 690-693.

Freed, D., and B. Baker. 1989. Antagonism of xylazine hydrochloride sedation in raptors by yohimbine hydrochloride. J. Wildl. Dis. 25: 136-138.

Freeman, R. R. 1986. Pre-anesthetic, anesthetic and post-anesthetic care for raptors. Wildl. J. 9: 3-6.

Frye, F. L. 1981. Biomedical and Surgical Aspects of Captive Reptile Husbandry. Vet. Med. Publ. Co., Edwardsville, Kansas. Pp. 241-246.

Frye, F. L. 1991. Anesthesia. *In* Frye, F. L. (ed.). Biomedical and Surgical Aspects of Captive Reptile Husbandry. Krieger, Malabar, Florida. Pp. 421-437.

Fuglei, E., J. B. Mercer, and J. M. Arnemo. 2002. Surgical implantation of radio transmitters in arctic foxes (*Alopex lagopus*) on Svalbard, Norway. J. Zoo Wildl. Med. 33: 342-349.

Fuhrman, F. A., and E. T. Stuhr. 1941. Pentobarbital sodium as an anesthetic for minks. J. Am. Vet. Med. Assoc. 98: 43-44.

Fukumoto, Y., and Y. Nisshiyama. 1989. *Equus burchelli boehmi*, sedation-immobilization with diazepam, ketamine hydrochloride and xylazine. J. Japan. Assoc. Zool. Gard. Aquar. 31: 63-65.

Fuller, G. B., W. C. Hobson, F. I. Reyes, J. S. D. Winter, and C. Faiman. 1984. Influence of restraint and ketamine anesthesia on adrenal steroids, progesterone, and gonadotropins in rhesus monkeys. Proc. Soc. Exp. Biol. Med. 175: 487-490.

Fuller, T. K., and L. B. Keith. 1981. Immobilization of wolves in winter with etorphine. J. Wildl. Manage. 45: 271-273.

Fuller, T. K., and D. W. Kuehn. 1983. Immobilization of wolves using ketamine in combination with xylazine or promazine. J. Wildl. Dis. 19: 69-72.

Fuller, T. K., K. D. Kerr, and P. D. Karns. 1985. Hematology and serum chemistry of bobcats in north central Minnesota. J. Wildl. Dis. 21: 29-32.

Fuller, T. K., A. R. Biknevicus, and P. Kat. 1990. Movements and behavior of large spotted genets (*Genetta maculata* Gray 1830) near Elmenteita, Kenya (Mammalia Viverridae). Trop. Zool. 3: 13-19.

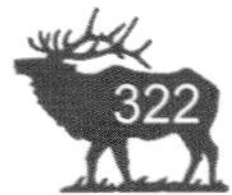

Furley, C. W. 1986. Effect of chemical immobilisation on the heart rate and haematological values in captive gazelles. Vet. Rec. 118: 178-180.

Furtado, M. M., C. K. Kashivakura, C. Ferro, A. T. de Almeida Jácomo, L. Silveira, and S. Astete. 2006. Immobilization of free-ranging maned wolf (*Chrysocyon brachyurus*) with tiletamine and zolazepam in central Brazil. J. Zoo Wildl. Med. 37: 68-70.

Fyffe, J. J. 1994. Effects of xylazine on humans - a review. Aust. Vet. J. 71: 294-295.

Gabor, T. M., E. C. Hellgren, and N. J. Silvy. 1997. Immobilization of collared peccaries (*Tayasu tajacu*) and feral hogs (*Sus scrofa*) with Telazol® and xylazine. J. Wildl. Dis. 33: 161-164.

Gage, L. J. 1984. Restraint and anesthesia in pinnipeds. Proc. Am. Assoc. Zoo Vet. P. 31.

Gage, L. J. 1993. Pinniped anesthesia. *In* Fowler, M. E. (ed.). Zoo & Wild Animal Medicine: Current Therapy 3. W. B. Saunders Co., Philadelphia, Pennsylvania. Pp. 412-413.

Gales, N. J. 1984. Ketamine HCl and diazepam anesthesia of a leopard seal (*Hydrurga leptonyx*) for the biopsy of multiple fibromatous epulis. Aust. Vet. J. 61: 295-296.

Gales, N. J. 1989. Chemical restraint and anesthesia of pinnipeds: a review. Mar. Mamm. Sci. 5: 228-256.

Gales, N. J., and H. R. Burton. 1987. Prolonged and multiple immobilizations of the Southern elephant seal using ketamine hydrochloride-xylazine hydrochloride or ketamine hydrochloride-diazepam combinations. J. Wildl. Dis. 23: 614-618.

Gales, N. J., and H. R. Burton. 1988. Use of emetics and anaesthesia for dietary assessment of Weddell Seals. Austr. Wildl. Res. 15: 423-433.

Gales, N. J., and R. H. Mattlin. 1998. Fast, safe, field-portable gas anesthesia for otariids. Mar. Mam. Sci. 14: 355-361.

Gales, N., J. Barnes, B. Chittick, M. Gray, S. Robinson, J. Burns, and D. Costa. 2005. Effective, field-based inhalation anesthesia for ice seals. Mar. Mammal Sci. 21: 717-727.

Galka, M. E., J. M. Aguilar, M. A. Guevedo, J. M. Santisteban, and R. J. Gómez-Villamandos. 1999. Alpha-2 agonist dissociative anesthetic combinations in fallow deer (*Cervus dama*). J. Zoo Wildl. Med. 30: 451-453.

Gallagher, J. F., R. L. Lochmiller, and W. E. Grant. 1985. Immobilization of collared peccaries with ketamine hydrochloride. J. Wildl. Manage. 49: 356-357.

Gallanosa, A. C., D. A. Spyker, J. R. Shipe, and D. L. Morris. 1981. Human xylazine overdose: a comparative review with clonidine, phenothiazines, and tricyclic antidepressants. Clin. Toxicol. 18: 663-678.

Gandal, C. P. 1967. Drugs used in the zoo. Fed. Proc. 26: 1247-1250.

Gandal, C. P. 1968. A practical anesthetic technique in snakes, utilizing methoxyflurane. J. Am. Anim. Hosp. 4: 258-260.

Gandini, G. C. M., R. H. Keffen, R. E. J. Burroughs, and H. Ebedes. 1986. An anaesthetic combination of ketamine, xylazine and alphaxalone-alphadolone in ostriches. Vet. Rec. 118: 729-730.

Gandini, G. C. M., H. Ebedes, and R. E. J. Burroughs. 1989. The use of long-acting neuroleptics in impala (*Epicures melampus*). J. So. Afr. Vet. Assoc. 60: 206-207.

Ganhao, M. F., J. Hatting, N. Pitts, C. Raath, B. De Klerk, and V. De Vos. 1988. Physiological responses of blesbok, eland and red hartebeest to different capture methods. S. Afr. J. Wildl. Res. 18: 134-136.

Garcia-Villar, R., P. L. Toutain, M. Alvinerie, and Y. Ruckebusch. 1981. The pharmacokinetics of xylazine hydrochloride: an interspecific study. J. Vet. Pharmacol. Therap. 4: 87-92.

Garner, D. L., and E. M. Addison. 1994a. Postpartum immobilization of adult female moose using xylazine, ketamine, and yohimbine hydrochloride. J. Wildl. Dis. 30: 123-125.

Garner, D. L., and E. M. Addison. 1994b. Postpartum immobilization of adult female moose using xylazine, ketamine, and yohimbine hydrochloride. Joint Conf. Am. Assoc. Zoo Vet. Assoc. Reptil. Amphib. Vet. Pp. 123-125.

Garruthers, S. C., M. Nelson, C. R. Stiller, and H. R. Stiller. 1979. Xylazine hydrochloride (Rompun) overdose in man. Clin. Toxicol. 15: 281-285.

Garshelis, D. L., K. V. Noyce, and P. D. Karns. 1987. Yohimbine as an antagonist to ketamine-xylazine immobilization of black bears. Int. Conf. Bear Res. and Manage. 6.

Garver, B. H., and L. L. Jackson. 1985. Restraint and anaesthesia of uncommon veterinary patients. Iowa State Univ. Vet. 47: 46-53.

Gasaway, W. C., A. W. Franzmann, and J. B. Faro. 1978. Immobilizing moose with a mixture of etrophine and xylazine hydrochloride. J. Wildl. Manage. 42: 686-690.

Gass, H. 1970. Parke-Sernyl (Phencyclidine) used in lions. Kleintier-Praxis 15: 66.

Gates, J. B. 1972. A report of halothane anesthesia in a camel. J. Zoo An. Med. 2: 26-27.

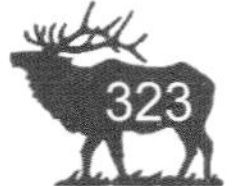

Gatesman, T., and H. Wiesner. 1982. Immobilization of polar (*Thalarctos maritimus*) and brown (*Ursus arctos*) bears using etorphine and xylazine. J. Zoo An. Med. 13: 11-18.

Gaukler, A., and M. Kraus. 1970. Zur immobilization von Wildwiederkäuern mit Xylazin (Bay Va 1470). Der Zoologische Garten. 38: 37-46.

Gavier, M. D., M. Kittleson, M. E. Fowler, L. Johnson, G. Hall, and D. Nearenberg. 1986. Evaluation of xylazine, ketamine hydrochloride and halothane for anaesthesia in llamas. Proc. Am. Assoc. Zoo Vet. P. 127.

Gaynor, B., and S. Haigh. 1992. Rhinoceros anaesthesia. Austral. Reg. Assoc. Zool. Parks Aquaria. 7: 3-4.

Gaynor, J. S., J. Wimsatt, C. Mallinckrodt, and D. Biggins. 1997. A comparison of sevoflurane and isoflurane for short-term anesthesia of polecats (*Mustela eversmanni*). J. Zoo Wildl. Med. 28: 274-279.

Gehring, T. M., and R. K. Swihart. 2000. Field immobilization and use of radiocollars on long-tailed weasels. Wildl. Soc. Bull. 28: 579-585.

Gehrt, S. D., L. L. Hungerford, and S. Hatten. 2001. Drug effects on recaptures of raccoons. Wildl. Soc. Bull. 29: 833-837.

Geiger, G. 1976. Combination of Rompun (xylazine) and Valium (diazepam) for the immobilization of fallow deer. Praktische Tierarzt. 57: 830-833.

Geiser, D. R., P. J. Morris, and H. S. Adair. 1992. Multiple anesthetic events in a reticulated giraffe (*Giraffa camelopardalis*). J. Zoo Wildl. Med. 23: 189-196.

Genevois, J. P., A. Autefage, P. Fayolle, A. Cazieux, and P. Bonnemaison. 1983a. [Anaesthesia of unusual species in common veterinary practice. Note 1. Fishes and reptiles anaesthesia]. Rev. Med. Vet. (Toulouse). 134: 471-479.

Genevois, J. P., A. Autefage, P. Fayolle, A. Cazieux, and P. Bonnemaison. 1983b. [Anaesthesia of unusual species in common veterinary practice. Note 2. Birds anaesthesia]. Rev. Med. Vet. (Toulouse). 134: 601-607.

Genevois, J. P., A. Autefage, P. Fayolle, A. Cazieux, and P. Bonnemaison. 1984a. [Anaesthesia of unusual species in common veterinary practice. Note 3. Rabbit and rodents anaesthesia]. Rev. Med. Vet. (Toulouse). 135: 273-279.

Genevois, J. P., P. Fayolle, A. Autefage, P. Bonnemaison, and A. Cazieux. 1984b. [Anaesthesia of unusual species in common veterinary practice. Note 4. Wild carnivora anaesthesia]. Rev. Med. Vet. (Toulouse). 135: 379-384.

Gentry, R. L., and J. H. Johnson. 1978. Physical restraint for immobilizing fur seals. J. Wildl. Manage. 42: 944-946.

Gentry, R. L., and J. R. Holt. 1982. Equipment and techniques for handling northern fur seals. U.S. Dept. Commerce, NOAA Tech. Rpt., NMFS SSRF-758.

Georoff, T. A., D. Boon, E. E. Hammond, S. T. Ferrell, and R. W. Radcliffe. 2004. Preliminary results of medetomidine-ketamine-butorphanol for anesthetic management of captive white-nosed coati (*Nasua narica*). Proc. Am. Assoc. Zoo Vet. Pp. 384-387.

Geraci, J. R. 1973. An appraisal of ketamine as an immobilizing agent in wild and captive pinnipeds. J. Am. Vet. Med. Assoc. 163: 574-577.

Geraci, J. R., K. Skirnisson, and D. J. St. Aubin. 1981. A safe method for repeatedly immobilizing seals. J. Am. Vet. Med. Assoc. 179: 1192-1193.

Giacometti, M. 1994. Projektoren, Injektionssysteme und Medikamente bei der medikamentellen Immobilisation von ausgewaehlten Schalenwildarten: eine Uebersicht. Wiener Tieraerztliche Monatsschrift 81: 141- 144.

Gibeau, M. L., and P. C. Paquet. 1991. Evaluation of Telazol® for immobilization of black bears. Wildl. Soc. Bull. 19: 400-402.

Gibson, D. F., A. Oelschlaeger, P. F. Scanlon, and R. L. Kirkpatrick. 1979. Some reactions of white-tailed deer to xylazine hydrochloride. Va. J. Sci. 30: 48.

Gibson, D. F., P. F. Scanlon, R. J. Warren, A. Oelschlaeger, and R. L. Kirkpatrick. 1980a. Dose rates of xylazine hydrochloride (Rompun) for the immobilization of white-tailed deer. Va. J. Sci. 31: 99.

Gibson, D. F., P. F. Scanlon, and R. L. Kirkpatrick. 1980b. Effects of xylazine hydrochloride (Rompun) on respiration rates and rectal temperatures of white-tailed deer. Va. J. Sci. 31: 98.

Gibson, D. F., P. F. Scanlon, and R. J. Warren. 1982. Xylazine hydrochloride for immobilizing captive white-tailed deer (*Odocoileus virginianus*). Zoo Biol. 1: 311-322.

Gilbert, F. F. 1976. Impact energy thresholds for anesthetized raccoons, mink, muskrats, and beavers. J.

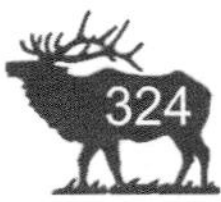

Wildl. Manage. 40: 669-676.
Gilbert, P. W., and F. G. Wood. 1957. Method of anesthetizing large sharks and rays safely and rapidly. Science. 126: 212-213.
Gillespie, D., and C. Adams. 1985. Anatomy, husbandry, and anesthesia of the giant anteater (*Myrmecophaga tridactyla*). Proc. Am. Assoc. Zoo Vet. Pp. 35-36.
Gillingham, J. C., D. L. Clark, and G. R. Ten Eyck. 1983. Venomous snake immobilization: a new technique. Herpetol. Rev. 14: 40.
Gilroy, B. A., and J. S. Varga. 1980. Use of ketamine-diazepam and ketamine-xylazine combinations in guinea pigs. Vet. Med. Sm. An. Clin. 75: 508-509.
Glander, K. E., L. M. Fedigan, L. Fedigan, and C. Chapman. 1991. Capture techniques for three species of monkeys in Costa Rica. Folia Primatologica 57: 70-82.
Glenn, J. L., R. Straight, and C. C. Snyder. 1972a. Clinical use of ketamine hydrochloride as an anesthesic agent for snakes. Am. J. Vet. Res. 33: 1901-1903.
Glenn, J. L., R. Straight, and C. C. Snyder. 1972b. Ketalar - a new anaesthetic for use in snakes. Int. Zoo Yb. 12: 224-226.
Glover, G. J., D. G. Larson, and J. C. Haigh. No Date. Immobilization of moose (*Alces alces*) using combinations of carfentanil, fentanyl, and xylazine. Glover Wildlife Veterinary Services, Box 880, Stonewall, Manitoba.
Goetz, R. H. 1955. Curare "spiked" bullet in giraffe. Time. 66: 65.
Golden, H. N., B. S. Shults, and K. E. Kunkel. 2002. Immobilization of wolverines with Telazol® from a helicopter. Wildl. Soc. Bull. 30: 492-497.
Golightly, R. T. Jr., and T. D. Hofstra. 1989. Immobilization of elk with a ketamine-xylazine mix and rapid reversal with yohimbine hydrochloride. Wildl. Soc. Bull. 17: 53-58.
Göltenboth, R. 1988. Zum aktuellen Stand der Immobilisation der Zootiere. Deutsche Tierärztliche Wochenschrift 95: 402-403.
Göltenboth, R., and H.-G. Klös. 1970. Application of Rompun for the immobilization of zoo animals. Berliner Muenchener Tierarztliche Wochenschrift. 83: 147-151.
Göltenboth, R., and H.-G. Klös. 1976. Zur Immobilisation von Zootieren mit Vetelar und Rompun. 18th Int. Symp. Dis. Zoo and Wild An. Innsbruck. Pp. 287-293.
Göltenboth, R., and H.-G. Klös. 1987. Versuche mit Yohimbin als Antidot bei durch Xylazin (Rompun®) Immobilisierten Zootieren im Zoo Berlin. 29th Int. Symp. Dis. Zoo and Wild An. Pp 143-149.
Gonzales, B. J., and T. McDonnel. 1986. The effects of yohimbine on xylazine-ketamine anesthesia in exotic felidae. Proc. Am. Assoc. Zoo Vet. Pp. 142-143
Goodrich, J. M., L. L. Kerley, B. O. Schleyer, D. G. Miquelle, K. S. Quigley, Y. N. Smirnov, I. G. Nikolaev, H. B. Quigley, and M. G. Hornocker. 2001. Capture and chemical anesthesia of Amur (Siberian) tigers. Wildl. Soc. Bull. 29: 533-542.
Goodrich, P. G. E. 1977. Accidental self injection. Vet. Rec. 100: 458-459.
Goosen, D. J., J. H. Davies, M. Maree, and I. C. Dormehl. 1984. The influence of physical and chemical restraint on the physiology of the chacma baboon (*Papi ursinus*). J. Med. Primatol. 13: 339-351.
Gordon, B. 1977. The use of sodium amobarbital for waterfowl capture. J. Zoo An. Med. 8: 34-35.
Gordon, D. F. 1966. A brief history of drug capture. Colorado Game, Fish and Parks. 36: 4 pp.
Graham, D. L., R. H. Dunlop, and H. F. Travis. 1967. Barbiturate anesthesia in ranch mink (*Mustela vison*). Am. J. Vet. Res. 28: 293-296.
Graham-Jones, O. 1964. Restraint and anesthesia of some captive wild animals. Vet. Rec. 76: 1216-1248.
Grassman, L. I., S. C. Austin, M. E. Tewes, and N. J. Silvy. 2004. Comparative immobilization of wild felids in Thailand. J. Wildl. Dis. 40: 575-578.
Gray, C. W. 1974. Immobilization of the bongo (*Boocercus eurycerus*). J. Zoo An. Med. 5: 19-20.
Gray, C. W., and A. P. W. Nettashinghe. 1970. A preliminary study on the immobilization of the Asiatic elephant (*Elephas maximus*) utilizing etorphine (M-99). Zoologica. 55: 51-54.
Gray, C. W., M. Bush, and C. C. Beck. 1974. Clinical experience using CI-744 in chemical restraint and anesthesia of exotic specimens. J. Zoo An. Med. 5: 12-21.
Green, B. 1976. The use of etorphine hydrochloride (M99) in the capture and immobilization of wild dingoes, *Canis familiaris dingo*. Austral. Wildl. Res. 3: 123-128.
Green, C. J. 1978. Anesthetizing ferrets. Vet. Rec. 102: 269.
Green, C. J., J. Knight, S. Precious, and S. Simpkin. 1981. Ketamine alone and combined with diazepam or xylazine in laboratory animals: a 10-year experience. Lab. An. 15: 163-170.

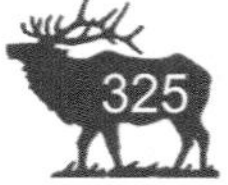

Green, H. 1963. New technique for using the Cap-Chur gun. J. Wildl. Manage. 27: 292-296.
Green, M. J. B. 1986. Immobilization of Himalayan musk deer, *Moschus chrysogaster*, in captivity using ketamine and xylazine. J. Zoo An. Med. 17: 56-58.
Greene, S. A. 1988. Capture and anesthetic techniques for deer and elk. Southwest Vet. 38: 11-15.
Greene, S. A., and J. C. Thurmon. 1988. Xylazine – a review of its pharmacology and use in veterinary medicine. J. Vet. Pharmacol. Ther. 11: 295-313.
Greenwood, A. G., and D. C. Taylor. 1983. Anesthesia in seals. Vet. Rec. 113: 303.
Greer, L. L., K. J. Jenne, and H. E. Diggs. 2001. Medetomidine-ketamine anesthesia in red-eared slider turtles (*Trachemys scripta elegans*). Contemp. Lab. Anim. Sci. 40: 8-11.
Gregg, D. A., and L. D. Olson. 1975. The use of ketamine hydrochloride as an anesthetic for raccoons. J. Wildl. Dis. 11: 335-337.
Greth, A., M. Vassart, and S. Anagariyah. 1993. Evaluation of medetomidine-induced immobilization in Arabian oryx (*Oryx leucoryx*): clinical, hematologic and biochemical effects. J. Zoo Wildl. Med. 24: 445-453.
Greth, A., M. Vassart, and S. Anagariyah. 1993. Chemical immobilization in gazelles, *Gazell sp*, with fentanyl and azaperone. Afr. J. Ecol. 31: 6674.
Griesemer, S. J., M. O. Hale, U. Roze, and T. K. Fuller. 1999. Capturing and marking adult North American porcupines. Wildl. Soc. Bull. 27: 310-313.
Griffiths, D., Ø. Wiig, and I. Gjertz. 1993. Immobilization of walrus with etorphine hydrochloride and Zoletil. Mar. Mamm. Sci. 9: 250-257.
Grobler, D., M. Bush, D. Jessup, and W. Lance. 2001. Anaesthesia of gemsbok (*Oryx gazella*) with a combination of A-3080, medetomidine and ketamine. J. So. Afr. Vet. Assoc. 72: 81-83.
Grobler, J. H., and J. H. Van der Meulen. 1975. The capture of sable, *Hippotragus niger niger* (Harris, 1838), using etorphine hydrochloride (M99), Rompun (VA 1470) and chlorpromazine hydrochloride. Arnoldia (Rhod.). 7: 1-14.
Grootenhuis, J. G., L. Karstad, and S. A. Drevemo. 1976. Experience with drugs for capture and restraint of wildebeest, impala, eland and hartebeest in Kenya. J. Wildl. Dis. 12: 435-443.
Gulland, F. M. D., M. Haulena, S. Elliott, and L. Gage. 1999. Anesthesia of juvenile Pacific harbor seals using propofol alone and in combination with isoflurane. Mar. Mammal. Sci. 15: 234-238.
Gullett, P. A. 1984. Use of yohimbine to reverse chemical immobilization in selected California ungulates. Proc. Am. Assoc. Zoo Vet. P. 58.
Gyuris, E., and C. J. Limpus. 1989. Rapid method for immobilization and collection of sea turtle muscle biopsies for electrophoresis. Aust. Wildl. Res. 13: 333-334.
Hackenbrock, C. R., and M. Finster. 1963. Fluothane: a rapid and safe inhalation anesthetic for poisonous snakes. Copeia 2: 440-441.
Hagenbeck, C. C., H. Linder, and D. Weber. 1975. Fiberoptic gastroscopy in an anaesthetized walrus (*Odobenus rosmarus*). Aquat. Mamm. 3: 20-22.
Haager, G. V., and D. S. Reynolds. 1992. Preliminary observations on the use of zolitil for the immobilization of captive Nile crocodiles (*Crocodylus niloticus lauranti*). Herp. Assoc. Africa J. 41: 25-27.
Haefele, H. J., J. R. Zuba, E. E. Hammond, and R. W. Radcliffe. 2005. Immobilization of captive free-ranging fallow deer (*Dama dama*) with a carfentanil, xylazine, and butorphanol combination. Proc. Am. Assoc. Zoo Vet. Pp. 261-262.
Hahn, N., R. J. Eisen, L. Eisen, and R. S. Lane. 2005. Ketamine-medetomidine anesthesia with atipamezole reversal: practical anesthesia for rodents under field conditions. Lab Animal 34: 48-51.
Haigh, J. C. 1976a. Some mechanical faults associated with dart immobilization. J. Zoo An. Med. 7: 12-14.
Haigh, J. C. 1976b The immobilisation of the bongo (*Boocercus eurycus*) and other African antelopes in captivity. Vet. Rec. 98: 237-239.
Haigh, J. C. 1976c. The use of CT1341 for surgical anesthesia in a pelican. J. Zoo An. Med. 7: 39.
Haigh, J. C. 1976d. Fentanyl-based mixtures in exotic animal neuroleptanalgesia. Proc. Am. Assoc. Zoo Vet. Pp. 164-180.
Haigh, J. C. 1976e. An extra tool for medication of exotic or dangerous animals. Proc. Am. Assoc. Zoo Vet. Pp. 249-260.
Haigh, J. C. 1977a. Fallow deer immobilisation with fentanyl and a neuroleptic. Vet. Rec. 100: 386-387.
Haigh, J. C. 1977b. The capture of wild black rhinoceros using fentanyl and azaperone. So. Afr. J. Wildl. Res. 7: 11-14.

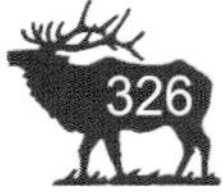

Haigh, J. C. 1978a. Freeze-dried ketamine and Rompun for use in exotic species. Proc. Am. Assoc. Zoo Vet. Pp. 21-23.

Haigh, J. C. 1978b. Use and abuse of drugs for chemical restraint of wildlife. Vet. Clin. North Am. 8: 343-352.

Haigh, J. C. 1978c. Capture of woodland caribou in Canada. Proc. Am. Assoc. Zoo Vet. Pp. 110-115.

Haigh, J. C. 1979. Hyaluronidase as an adjunct in an immobilizing mixture for moose. J. Am. Vet. Med. Assoc. 175: 916-917.

Haigh, J. C. 1981. Anaesthesia of raptorial birds. 1980. *In* Cooper, J. E., A. G. Greenwood (eds.). Recent Advances in the Study of Raptor Diseases. Proceedings of the International Symposium on Diseases of Birds of Prey. London. Pp. 61-66.

Haigh, J. C. 1982. Mammalian immobilizing drugs: their pharmacology and effects. *In* Nielsen, L., J. C. Haigh, and M. E. Fowler (eds.). Chemical Immobilization of North American Wildlife. Wisconsin Humane Society, Inc. Milwaukee, Wisconsin. Pp. 46-62.

Haigh, J. C. 1987a. Yohimbine and physostigmine as antidotes to xylazine in elk (*Cervus elaphus*). J. Zoo An. Med. 18: 70-72.

Haigh, J. C. 1987b. Naltrexone HCL in zoological medicine–a preliminary report. Proc. 1st Int. Conf. Zool Avian Med., Oahu, Hawaii. Omnipress, Madison, Wisconsin. P. 529.

Haigh, J. C. 1988. Misuse of xylazine. Can. Vet. J. 29: 782-784.

Haigh, J. C. 1989. Hazardous drugs in zoo and wildlife medicine. Proc. Am. Assoc. Zoo Vet. Pp. 69-71.

Haigh, J. C. 1990a. Opioids in zoological medicine. J. Zoo Wildl. Med. 21: 391-413.

Haigh, J. C. 1990b. Immobilization of wapiti with carfentanil and xylazine. 2nd Intl. Wildl. Ranching Symp., Edmonton, Alberta, Canada.

Haigh, J. C. 1991. Immobilization of wapiti with carfentanil and xylazine and opioid antagonism with diprenorphine, naloxone, and naltrexone. J. Zoo Wildl. Med. 22: 318-323.

Haigh, J. C. 1993. Low-dose carfentanil together with xylazine in wapiti. Proc. Am. Assoc. Zoo Vet. P. 146.

Haigh, J. C., and H. C. Hopf. 1976. The blowgun in veterinary practice: its uses and preparation. J. Am. Vet. Med. Assoc. 169: 881-883.

Haigh, J. C., and R. E. A. Stewart. 1979. Narcotics in hooded seals (*Cystophora cristata*): a preliminary report. Can. J. Zool. 57: 946-949.

Haigh, J. C., and J. M. Haigh. 1980. Immobilizing drug emergencies in humans. Vet. Human Toxicol. 22: 94-98.

Haigh, J. C., and R. Alsager. 1987. Yohimbine and physostigmine as antidotes to xylazine in elk (*Cervus elaphus*) J. Zoo Anim. Med. 18: 70-72.

Haigh, J. C., and R. J. Hudson. 1993. Farming Wapiti and Red Deer. Mosby, St. Louis. Pp. 83-98.

Haigh, J. C., and C. C. Gates. 1995. Capture of wood bison (*Bison bison athabascae*) using carfentanil-based mixtures. J. Wildl. Dis. 31: 37-42.

Haigh, J. C., R. F. Stewart, G. Wobeser, and P. S. MacWilliams. 1977. Capture myopathy in moose. J. Am. Vet. Med. Assoc. 171: 924-926.

Haigh, J. C., R. Stewart, R. Frokjer, and T. Hauge. 1977. Capture of moose with fentanyl and xylazine. J. Zoo An. Med. 8: 22-29.

Haigh, J. C., I. S. C. Parker, D. A. Parkinson, and A. L. Archer. 1979. An elephant extermination. Environ. Conserv. 6: 305-310.

Haigh, J. C., L. J. Lee, and R. E. Schweinsburg. 1983. Immobilization of polar bears with carfentanil. J. Wildl. Dis. 19: 140-144.

Haigh, J. C., I. Stirling, and E. Broughton. 1984. Clinical experiences with Telazol for polar bear (*Ursus maritimus*) immobilization. Proc. Am. Assoc. Zoo Vet. Pp. 130-131.

Haigh, J. C., I. Stirling, and E. Broughton. 1985. Immobilization of polar bears (*Ursus maritimus*) with a mixture of tiletamine hydrochloride and zolazepam hydrochloride. J. Wildl. Dis. 21: 43-47.

Haigh, J. C., A. S. Dradjat, A. W. English. 1993. Comparison of two extenders for the cryopreservation of chital (*Axis axis*) semen. J. Zoo Wildl. Med. 24: 454-458.

Hale, M. B., S. J. Griesemer, and T. K. Fuller. 1994. Immobilization of porcupines with tiletamine hydrochloride and zolazepam hydrochloride (Telazol®). J. Wildl. Dis. 30: 429-431.

Hall, L. W., and K. W. Clarke. 1991. Anaesthesia of birds, laoboratory animals and wild animals. *In* L. W. Hall and K. W. Clarke (eds). Veterinary Anaesthesia. London, Bailliere Tindall Ltd. Pp. 339-351.

Hall, L. W., K. W. Clarke, and C. M. Trim. 2001. Veterinary anaesthesia. London, W. B. Saunders, 561 pp.

Hall, T. C., E. B. Taft, W. H. Baker, and J. C. Aub. 1953. A preliminary report on the use of Flaxedil to produce paralysis in the white-tailed deer. J. Wildl. Manage. 17: 516-520.
Hallett, D. L., J. D. Rhoades, and R. R. Paddleford. 1979. Immobilization of coyotes with ketamine and propiomazine. J. Am. Vet. Med. Assoc. 175: 1007-1008.
Halloran, D. W., and A. M. Pearson. 1972. Blood chemistry of the brown bear (*Ursus arctos*) from southwestern Yukon Territory, Canada. Can. J. Zool. 50: 827-833.
Hamilton, R. (No date). Capture of deer in Indiana with nicotine salicylate. Research Report of the Indiana Department of Conservation.
Hammond, O., and R. Elsner. 1977. Anesthesia in phocid seals. J. Zoo An. Med. 8: 7-13.
Hanks, J. 1967a. The use of M.99 for the immobilisation of Defassa waterbuck (*Kobus defassa penricei*). E. Afr. Wildl. J. 5: 96-105.
Hanks, J. 1967b. Crossbow darting. Animals – The International Wildlife Magazine. No. 248.
Hanks, J. 1967c. The use of the new "hypodart" for animal immobilization. Puku 5: 228-231.
Hanks, J. 1967d. The capture of young elephants in the Zambesi Valley. Puku 5: 87-90.
Hanks, J., and R. J. Dowsett. 1969. The use of etorphine (M.99) for the immobilisation and translocation of the Puku (*Kobus vardonie*). Puku 5: 123-130.
Hanley, C. S., J. Siudak-Campfield, J. Paul-Murphy, C. Vaughan, O. Ramirez, and K. K. Sladky. 2006. Immobilization of free-ranging Hoffman's two-toed (*Choloepus hoffmanni*) and brown-throated three-toed (*Bradypus variegates*) sloths using medetomidine-ketamine: a comparison of physiologic parameters. Proc. Am. Assoc. Zoo Vet. Pp. 224-225.
Hansen, M. K., U. Nymoen, and T. E. Horsberg. 2003. Pharmacokinetic and pharmacodynamic properties of metomidate in turbot (*Scopthalmus maximus*) and halibut (*Hippoglossus hippoglossus*). J. Vet. Pharmacol. Ther. 26: 95-103.
Harms, C. A. 1999. Anesthesia in fish. *In* Fowler, M. E., and R. E. Miller (eds.). Zoo & Wild Animal Medicine. Current Therapy 4. W. B. Saunders Company, Philadelphia, Pennsylvania. Pp. 158-163.
Harms, C. A., and R. S. Bakal. 1994. Techniques in fish anesthesia. Joint Conf. Am. Assoc. Zoo Vet. Assoc. Reptil. Amphib. Vet. Pp. 202-209.
Harper, J. A. 1964. Succinylcholine chloride for immobilization of Roosevelt Elk in southern Oregon. Oregon State Game Comm. 17 pp.
Harper, J. A. 1965. Immobilization of Roosevelt elk by succinylcholine chloride. J. Wildl. Manage. 29: 339-345.
Harper, R. C. 1984. Anaesthetising reptiles. Vet. Rec. 115: 475-476.
Harrington, R. 1974. Immobilon-Rompun in deer. Vet. Rec. 94: 362.
Harthoorn, A. M. 1960. Methods of control of wild animals with the use of drugs with special reference to therapeutic and veterinary aspects. Int. Zoo Yb. 2: 302-307.
Harthoorn, A. M. 1962a. The capture and relocation of the white (square- lipped) rhinoceros (*Cerathoteium simum simum*) using drug immobilizing techniques, at the Umfolozi Game Reserve, Zululan, Natal. Lammergeyer 2: 1-9.
Harthoorn, A. M. 1962b. Capture of the white (square-lipped) rhinoceros, *Ceratotherium simum simum* (Burchell) with the use of drug immobilisation techniques. Can. J. Comp. Med. 26: 203-208.
Harthoorn, A. M. 1962c. On the use of phencyclidine for narcosis in larger animals. Vet. Rec. 74: 410-411.
Harthoorn, A. M. 1962d. Producing "twilight sleep" in large wild animals. J. Am. Vet. Med. Assoc. 141: 1473.
Harthoorn, A. M. 1962e. Translocation as a means of preserving wild animals. Oryx 6: 215-227.
Harthoorn, A. M. 1963a. Modern trends in animal health and husbandry: ataractic, hypnotic and narcotic mixtures for the capture and handling of large wild animals. Brit. Vet. J. 119: 47-63.
Harthoorn, A. M. 1963b. Neuroleptic narcosis: approach to anesthesia in large animals. Nature. 198: 1116.
Harthoorn, A. M. 1963c. The value of neuroleptic narcosis in restraint, compared with that of anesthesia, sedation or paralysis. Proc. Symposium of African Mammals Zool. Soc. South Africa, Capetown.
Harthoorn, A. M. 1963d. Techniques of handling large animals such as elephant, rhinoceros, and hippopotamus etc. by use of drugs. World Vet. Cong. 1: 183-187.
Harthoorn, A. M. 1965a. Application of pharmacological and physiological principles in restraint of wild animals. Wildl. Mon. 14: 1-78.
Harthoorn, A. M. 1965b. The use of a new oripavine derivative for restraint of domestic hoofed animals. J. So. Afr. Vet. Assoc. 36: 45-50.

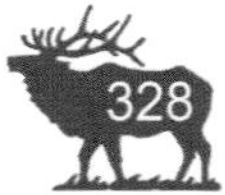

Harthoorn, A. M. 1965c. The use of a new oripavine derivative with potent morphine-like activity for the restraint of hoofed wild animals. Res. Vet. Science. 6: 290-299.

Harthoorn, A. M. 1966a. Large animals restraint - a prerequisite for conservation and research. African. 2: 19-21.

Harthoorn, A. M. 1966b. The use of drugs in conservation. Oryx 8: 223-227.

Harthoorn, A. M. 1966c. Restraint of undomesticated animals. J. Am. Vet. Med. Assoc. 149: 875-880.

Harthoorn, A. M. 1967a. Comparative pharmacological reactions of certain wild and domestic mammals to thebaine derivatives in the M-series of compounds. Fed. Proc. 26: 1251-1261.

Harthoorn, A. M. 1967b. Problems and hazards of chemical restraint in wild animals. Int. Zoo Yb. 8: 215-220.

Harthoorn, A. M. 1970. The flying syringe. Geoffrey Bles, London, U. K.

Harthoorn, A. M. 1971a. Advances in anesthesiology in zoo and wild animals: a review of recent advances. XIX Congres mondial Medec. Vet. Mexico. 2: 509.

Harthoorn, A. M. 1971b. The capture and restraint of wild animals. *In* Soma, L. R. (ed.). Textbook of Veterinary Anesthesia. Williams and Wilkins, Baltimore. Pp. 404-437.

Harthoorn, A. M. 1972a. Classification and properties of drugs in common use. Communication for the Specialised University Course on Wildlife Capture Techniques and General Husbandry. Onderstport, South Africa. 45 pp.

Harthoorn, A. M. 1972b. Drug immobilisation of other large wild herbivores (i.e. buffalo, hippo, rhino, elephant, zebra, etc.). Communication for the Specialised University Course on Wildlife Capture Techniques and General Husbandry. Onderstport, South Africa. 17 pp.

Harthoorn, A. M. 1972c. Restraint and neuroleptanalgesia in ungulates. Vet. Rec. 91: 63-66.

Harthoorn, A. M. 1973a. Review of wildlife capture drugs in common use. *In* E. Young (ed.). The Capture and Care of Wild Animals. Human and Rouseau, Cape Town, South Africa. Pp. 14-34.

Harthoorn, A. M. 1973b. The drug immobilization of large wild herbivores other than antelopes. *In* E. Young (ed.). The Capture and Care of Wild Animals. Human and Rouseau, Cape Town, South Africa. Pp. 51-61.

Harthoorn, A. M. 1974. The effects of immobilizing drugs on different species of game animals. Fauna Flora. 25: 12-13.

Harthoorn, A. M. 1976a. The Chemical Capture of Animals. London: Bailliere Tindall. 416 pp.

Harthoorn, A. M. 1976b. Use of Immobilon. Vet. Rec. 99: 240.

Harthoorn, A. M. 1977. Problems relating to capture. Animal Regulation Studies. 1: 23-46.

Harthoorn, A. M. 1980. Exercise as a necessary preliminary to disturbance, restraint or handling of captive wild animals. Communication-Pretoria. 67

Harthoorn, A. M. 1982a. Mechanical capture as a preliminary to chemical immobilization and the use of taming and training to prevent post capture stress. *In* Nielsen, L., J. C. Haigh, and M. E. Fowler (eds.). Chemical Immobilization of North American Wildlife. Wisconsin Humane Society, Inc. Milwaukee, Wisconsin. Pp. 150-164.

Harthoorn, A. M. 1982b. Physical aspects of both mechanical and chemical capture. *In* Nielsen, L., J. C. Haigh, and M. E. Fowler (eds.). Chemical Immobilization of North American Wildlife. Wisconsin Human Society, Inc. Milwaukee, Wisconsin. Pp. 63-71.

Harthoorn, A. M., and J. A. Lock. 1960. The rescue of rhinoceros from Kariba Dam. Oryx 5: 352-355.

Harthoorn, A. M., and J. A. Lock. 1961. Advances in the use of muscle relaxing drugs for immobilization and handling of larger land animals. J. Sm. An. Prac. 2: 163-169.

Harthoorn, A. M., and L. P. Luck. 1962. The handling and marking of the wild East African elephant (*Loxondonta africana*) with the use of drug immobilizing technique - second preliminary report. Brit. Vet. J. 118: 526-530.

Harthoorn, A. M., and H. Campbell. 1963. The capture and anesthesia of the African lion in his natural environment. Vet. Rec. 75: 275-276.

Harthoorn, A. M., and I. C. Player. 1963. The narcosis of the white rhinoceros. A series of eighteen case histories. 5th Int. Symp. Dis. Zoo and Wild An., Amsterdam, Tidjdschr. Diergin. 89: 225.

Harthoorn, A. M., and J. Bligh. 1965. The use of a new oripavine derivative with potent morphine-like activity for the restraint of hoofed wild animals. Res. Vet. Sci. 6: 290-299.

Harthoorn, A. M., and I. C. Player. 1967. The pharmacology and chemistry of the M-series of compounds. 9th Int. Symp. Dis. Zoo and Wild An., Prague. 1967: 135-139.

Harthoorn, A. M., and E. Young. 1974. A relationship between acid-base balance and capture myopathy in

zebra (*Equus burchelli*) and an apparent therapy. Vet. Rec. 95: 337-342.

Harthoorn, A. M., and K. Van der Walt. 1974. Physiological aspects of forced exercise in wild ungulates with special reference to (so-called) over-straining disease. I. Acid-base balance and pO_2 levels in Blesbok (*Damaliscus dorcas phillipsi*). J. So. Afr. Wildl. Manage. Assoc. 4: 25-28.

Harthoorn, A. M., J. A. Lock, and L. P. Luck. 1961a. Immobilization of wild elephants in Africa. Br. Vet. J. 117: 87.

Harthoorn, A. M., J. A. Lock, and L. P. Luck. 1961b. Handling and marking of wild African elephants (*Loxodonta africana*) with the use of the drug immobilizing technique - a preliminary report. Br. Vet. J. 117: 87-91.

Harthoorn, A. M., S. Harthoorn, and P. D. Sayer. 1971. Two field operations on the African lion (*Felis leo*). Vet. Rec. 89: 159-164.

Hartsfield, S. M. 1982. A review of avian anesthesia. Southwest. Vet. 35: 117-126.

Harvey, B., C. Denny, S. Kaiser, and J. Young. 1988. Remote intramuscular injection of immobilising drugs into fish using a laser-aimed underwater dart gun. Vet. Rec. 122: 174-177.

Hash, H. S., and M. G. Hornocker. 1980. Immobilizing wolverines with ketamine hydrochloride. J. Wildl. Manage. 44: 713-715.

Hashizaki, F., H. Tajima, K. Saito, Y. Miyoshi, S. Shichiri, J. Sato, K. Kanaya, K. Tanabe, K. Tashiro, M. Saito, and T. Nakayama. 1996. Immobilization of Grant's zebra, *Equus burchelli bohmi*, with etorphine hydrochloride (M99R). J. Japan. Assoc. Zool. Gard. Aquar. 37: 3-4.

Hastings, B. E., S. G. Stadler, and R. A. Kock. 1989. Reversible immobilization of Chinese water deer (*Hydropotes inermis*) with ketamine and xylazine. J. Zoo Wildl. Med. 20: 427-433.

Hatlapa, H. H. M., and H. Wiesner. 1982. Die Praxis der Wildtierimmobilisation. Verlag Paul Parey, Hamburg und Berlin. 1982: 1-96.

Hattingh, J., P. G. Wright, V. de Vos, L. Levine, M. Ganhao, S. McNairn, A. Russell, C. Knox, S. T. Cornelius, and J. Bar-Noy. 1984. Effects of etorphine and succinyldicholine on blood composition in elephant and buffalo. So. Afr. J. Zool. 19: 286-290.

Hattingh, J. 1985. Remote controlled blood sampling. So. Afr. J. Sci. 81: 644.

Hattingh, J., M. F. Ganhao, F. J. N. Kruger, V. De Vos, and G. W. Kay. 1985. Remote controlled sampling of cattle and buffalo blood. Comp. Biochem. Physiol. 89A: 231-235.

Hattingh, J., N. I. Pitts, and M. F. Ganhao. 1988. Immediate response to repeated capture and handling of wild impala. J. Exp. Zool. 248: 109-112.

Hattingh, J., N. I. Pitts, V. de Vos, D. G. Moyes, and M. F. Ganhao. 1991. The response of animals to suxamethonium (succinyldicholine) and succinylmonocholine. J. So. Afr. Vet. Assoc. 62: 126-129.

Hattingh, J., C. M. Knox, and J. P. Raath. 1994a. Arterial blood pressure of the African elephant (*Loxodonta africana*) under etorphine anaesthesia and after remobilisation with diprenorphine. Vet. Rec. 135: 458-459.

Hattingh, J., C. M. Knox, J. P. Raath, and D. F. Keet. 1994b. Arterial blood pressure in anaesthetized African elephants. So. Afr. J. Wildl. Res. 24: 15-17.

Hattingh, J., C. M. Knox, and J. P. Raath. 1994c. Arterial blood pressure and blood gas composition of white rhinoceroses under etorphine anaesthesia. So. Afr. J. Wildl. Res. 24: 12-14.

Hattori, Z., N. Kitano, T. Okonogi, Y. Sawai, Y. Kawamura, and S. Yamasato. 1975. [Anesthetic effect of ketamine hydrochloride for snakes]. Snake. 7: 33-37.

Haugen, A. O., M. J. Swenson, M. J. Shult, and S. J. Petersburg. 1976. Immobilization of adult bull bison with etorphine. Proc. Iowa Acdy. Sci. 83: 67-70.

Haulena, M., and F. M. D. Gulland. 2001. Use of medetomidine-zolazepam-tiletamine with and without atipamezole reversal to immobilize captive California sea lions. J. Wildl. Dis. 37: 566-573.

Haulena, M., and R. B. Heath. 2001. Marine mammal anesthesia. *In* Dierauf, L. A., and F. M. D. Gulland (eds.). CRC handbook of marine mammal medicine. CRC Press, Boca Raton, Florida. Pp. 655-688.

Haulena, M., F. M. D. Gulland, D. G. Calkins, and T. R. Spraker. 1998. Immobilization of California sea lions (*Zalophus californianus*) using medetomidine and ketamine and reversal with atipamezole. Proc. Joint Conf. Am. Assoc. Zoo Vet and Am. Assoc. Wildl. Vet. Pp. 370-371.

Haulena, M., F. M. D. Gulland, D. G. Calkins, and T. R. Spraker. 2000. Immobilization of California sea lions using medetomidine plus ketamine with and without isoflurane and reversal with atipamezole. J. Wildl. Dis. 36:124-130.

Haulten, S. M., W. F. Porter, and B. A. Rudolph. 2001. Evaluating 4 methods to capture white-tailed deer. Wildl. Soc. Bull. 29: 255-264.

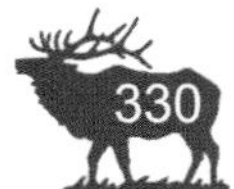

Haupert, J., and M. Lindeen. 1974. The use of ketamine hydrochloride in wild birds, mammals, and reptiles. Iowa St. U. Vet. 36: 21-22.

Haviernick, M., S. D. Côté, and M. Festa-Bianchet. 1998. Immobilization of mountain goats with xylazine and reversal with idazoxan. J.Wildl. Dis. 34: 342-347.

Hawkey, C. M., T. Frankel, D. Jones, D. Ashton, G. Nevill, M. Hart, C. Alderson, and P. Bircher. 1980. Preliminary report of a study of changes in red blood cells of zoo animals during sedation. *In* Montali, R. J., and G. Migaki (eds.). The Comparative Pathology of Zoo Animals. Smithsonian Institution Press, Washington, D. C. Pp. 625-632.

Hawkey, C. M. 1985. Changes in blood count during sedation and anaesthesia. Brit. Vet. Zool. Soc. Newsletter. 19: 27-31.

Hawkins, M. G., B. D. Wright, P. J. Pascoe, P. H. Kass, L. K. Maxwell, and L. A. Tell. 2003. Pharmacokinetics and anesthetic and cardiopulmonary effects of propofol in red-tailed hawks (*Buteo jamaicensis*) and great horned owls (*Bubo virginianus*). Amer. J. Vet. res. 64: 677-683.

Hawkins, R. E., D. C. Autry, and W. D. Klimstra. 1967. Comparison of methods used to capture white-tailed deer. J. Wildl. Manage. 31: 460-464.

Hawkins, R. E., L. D. Martoglio, and G. F. Montgomery. 1968. Cannon-netting deer. J. Wildl. Manage. 32: 191-195.

Hawkins, R. E., W. D. Klimstra, L. W. Lamely, and D. C Autry. 1979. A new remote capture method for free-ranging deer. J. Mammal. 51: 392-394.

Hayes, F. A., J. H. Jenkins, S. D. Feurt, and J. A. Crockford. 1957. Observations on the use of nicotine for immobilizing semiwild goats. J. Am. Vet. Med. Assoc. 130: 479-482.

Hayes, F. A., J. H. Jenkins, S. D. Feurt, and J. A. Crockford. 1959. The propulsive administration of nicotine as a new approach for capturing and restraining cattle. J. Am. Vet. Med. Assoc. 134: 283-286.

Hayes, M. A., B. K. Hartup, J. M. Pittman, and J. A. Barzen. 2003. Capture of sandhill cranes using alpha-chloralose. J. Wildl. Dis. 39: 859-868.

Heard, D. J. 2001. Reptile anesthesia. Vet. Clin. North Am.: Exotic Anim. Pract. 4: 83-117.

Heard, D. J., and D. O. Beusse. 1993. Combination detomidine, ketamine, and isoflurane anesthesia in California sea lions, *Zalophus californianus*. J. Zoo Wildl. Med. 24: 168-170.

Heard, D. J., and V. J. Huft. 1998. The effects of short-term physical restraint and isoflurane anesthesia on hematology and plasma biochemistry in the island flying fox (*Pteropus hypomelanus*). J. Zoo Wildl. Med. 29: 14-17.

Heard, D. J., E. R. Jacobson, and K. A. Brock. 1986. Effects of oxygen supplementation on blood gas values in chemically restrained juvenile African elephants. J. Am. Vet. Med. Assoc. 189: 1071-1074.

Heard, D. J., G. V. Kollias, A. I. Webb, E. R. Jacobson, and K. A. Brock. 1988. Use of halothane to maintain anesthesia induced with etorphine in juvenile African elephants. J. Am. Vet. Med. Assoc. 193: 254-256.

Heard, D. J., J. H. Olsen, and J. Stover. 1992. Cardiopulmonary changes associated with chemical immobilization and recumbency in a white rhinoceros (*Ceratotherium simum*). J. Zoo Wildl. Med. 23: 197-200.

Heard, D. J., C. Beale, and J. Owens. 1996. Ketamine and ketamine:xylazine ED_{50} for short-term immobilization of the island flying fox (*Pteropus hypomelanus*). J. Zoo Wildl. Med. 27: 44-48.

Heard, D., J. Towles, and D. LeBlanc. 2006. Evaluation of medetomidine/ketamine for short-term immobilization of variable flying foxes (*Pteropus hypomelanus*). J. Wildl. Dis. 42: 437-441.

Heath, R. B., D. Calkins, W. Taylor, D. McAllister, and T. Spraker. 1994. Isoflurane field anesthesia in sea lions. Vet. Surg. 23: 80.

Heath, R. B., D. Calkins, D. McAllister, W. Taylor, and T. Spraker. 1996. Telazol and isoflurane field anesthesia in free-ranging Steller's sea lions (*Eumetopias jubatus*). J. Zoo Wildl. Med. 27: 35-43.

Heath, R. B., R. DeLong, V. Jameson, D. Bradley, and T. Spraker. 1997. Isoflurane anesthesia in free ranging sea lion pups. J. Wildl. Dis. 33: 206-210.

Heaton, J. T., and S. E. Brauth. 1992. Effects of yohimbine as a reversing agent for ketamine-xylazine anesthesia in budgerigars. Lab. An. Sci. 42: 54-56.

Heaton-Jones, T. G. 1996. Development of anesthesia in crocodilians. Proc. Ann. Conf. Assoc. Reptil. Amphib. Vet. Sacramento, Calif. P. 61.

Heaton-Jones, T. G., J. C.-H. Ho, and D. L. Heaton-Jones. 2002. Evaluation of medetomidine-ketamine anesthesia with atipamezole reversal in American alligators (*Alligator mississippiensis*). J. Zoo

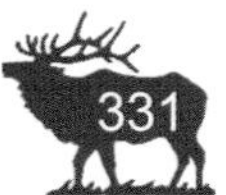

Wildl. Med. 33: 36-44.
Hebert, D. M. 1982. Philosophy, stratification and training courses for the use of drugs by various levels of personnel. *In* Nielsen, L., J. C. Haigh, and M. E. Fowler (eds.). Chemical Immobilization of North American Wildlife. Wisconsin Human Society, Inc. Milwaukee, Wisconsin. 137-149.
Hebert, D. M., and I. M. Cowen. 1971. White muscle disease in the mountain goat. J. Wildl. Manage. 35: 752-756.
Hebert, D. M., and R. J. McFetridge. 1976. Chemical immobilization of North American wildlife. Alberta Parks, Recreation and Wildlife, Edmonton, Alberta, Canada 84 pp.
Hebert, D. M., and R. J. McFetridge. 1982. Chemical immobilization of North American wildlife. Alberta Parks, Recreation and Wildlife, Edmonton, Alberta, Canada 250 pp.
Hebert, D. M., D. W. Lay, and W. G. Turnbull. 1980. Immobilization of coastal grizzly bears with etorphine hydrochloride. J. Wildl. Dis. 16: 339-342.
Hebert, D. M., D. W. Janz, K. Brunt, and J. Youds. 1982. Chemical immobilization of North American elk. *In* Nielsen, L., J. C. Haigh, and M. E. Fowler (eds.). Chemical Immobilization of North American Wildlife. Wisconsin Humane Society, Inc. Milwaukee, Wisconsin. Pp. 380-392.
Heck, H., and F. Dovigh. 1967. The immobilization of various ungulates with Anectine at Catskill Game Farm. D. Zool. Garten 33: 182-185.
Heck, H., and E. Rivenburg. 1972. Dosages of M99 used in hoofed mammals at Catskill Game Farm. D. Zool. Garten 42: 282-287.
Heck, L. 1965. Narcosis of a polar bear using the projectile gun. Int. Zoo Yb. 5: 193-194.
Heck, L. 1966. Immobilisation einer Hartmann-Bergzebrastute mit Hife des Cap Chur Gun in Tierpark Hellabrunn, München. D. Zool. Garten 32: 312-316.
Heidt, G. A. 1978. A portable anesthesia chamber for intractable small mammals. Lab. An. Sci. 28: 212-213.
Held, J. P., and R. R. Paddleford. 1982. Clinical use of succinylcholine and gallamine in the camel (*Camelus bactrianus*) during general anesthesia. J. Zoo An. Med. 13: 84-87.
Hellebrekers, L. J., E. J. W. Deboer, M. A. Vanzuylen, and H. Vosmeer. 1997. A comparison between medetomidine-ketamine and medetomidine-propofol anesthesia in rabbits. Lab An. 31: 58-69.
Hellgren, E. C., and M. R. Vaughn. 1989. Rectal temperatures of immobilized, snare-trapped black bears in Great Dismal Swamp. J. Wildl. Dis. 25: 440-443.
Hellgren, E. C., R. L. Lochmiller, M. S. Amoss, and W. E. Grant. 1985. Endocrine and metabolic responses of the collared peccary (*Tayassu tajacu*) to immobilization with ketamine hydrochloride. J. Wildl. Dis. 21: 417-425.
Henke, J., U. Roberts, K. Otto, C. Lendl, U. Matis, T. Brill, and W. Erhardt. 1996. Clinical investigations of an intramuscularly administered combination anesthesia with fentanyl -climazolaml-xylazine and its postoperative intravenous antagonisation by naloxone-sarmazenil-yohimbine in the guinea pig. Tierarztl. Prax. 24: 85-87.
Henry, V. G., and G. H. Matschke. 1968. Immobilizing trapped European wild hogs with Cap-Chur-Barb. J. Wildl. Manage. 32: 970-972.
Henry, V. G., and G. H. Matschke. 1972. Immobilizing European wild hogs with sernylan. J. Tennessee Acdy Sci. 47: 81-84.
Henwood, R. R. 1989. Black rhinoceros (*Diceros bicornis*) capture, transportation and boma management by Natal Parks Board. Koedoe 32: 43.
Henwood, R. R., and M. E. Keep. 1989. The capture and translocation of hippopotamus by means of chemical immobilization. Lammergeyer 40: 30-38.
Hepp, G. R., and C. A, Manlove. 2001. A comparison of methoxyflurane and propofol to reduce nest abandonment by wood ducks. Wildl. Soc. Bull. 29: 546-550.
Herbst, L. H., C. Packer, and U. S. Seal. 1985. Immobilization of free-ranging African lions (*Panthera leo*) with a combination of xylazine hydrochloride and ketamine hydrochloride. J. Wildl. Dis. 21: 401-404.
Herman, M. F., J. F. Pepper, and L. A. Herman. 1982. Field and laboratory techniques for anesthetizing marten with halothane gas. Wildl. Soc. Bull. 10: 275-277.
Hernandez-Divers, S. M., J. Schumacher, M. R. Read, S. Stahl, and S. Hernandez-Divers. 2003. Comparison of isoflurane anesthesia following premedication with butorphanol in the green iguana (*Iguana iguana*). Proc. Am. Assoc. Zoo Vet. Pp. 1.
Hernandez-Divers, S. M., J. Schumacher, S. Stahl, and S. J. Hernandez-Divers. 2005. Comparison of

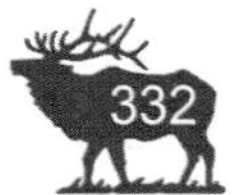

isoflurane and sevoflurane anesthesia after premedication with butorphanol in the green iguana (*Iguana iguana*). J. Zoo Wildl. Med. 36: 169-175.

Hertzog, R. E. 1975. Xylazine in exotic animal practice. Proc. Am. Assoc. Zoo Vet. Pp. 40-42.

Hess, L., and J. Knakal. 1985. [First experience with the immobilization with carfentanyl at Zoo Prague]. Gazella. 3: 87-91.

Hess, L., I. Dvoracek, J. Knakal, J. Chlupaty, J. Svobodnik, Z. Vranova, and M. Vrana. 1987. Use of opiates in primates with special emphasis on etorphine and carfentanyl. D. Zool. Garten. 57: 49.

Heuschele, W. P. 1959. Experiences with promazine in captive wild animals. Biochem. Rev. 29: 3-4.

Heuschele, W. P. 1960. Immobilization of captive wild animals with succinylcholine chloride using the projectile type syringe. Int. Zoo Yb. 2: 308-309.

Heuschele, W. P. 1961a. Immobilization of captive wild animals. Vet. Med. 56: 348-351.

Heuschele, W. P. 1961b. Chlordiazepoxide for calming zoo animals. J. Am. Vet. Med. Assoc. 139: 996-998.

Heuschele, W. P. 1961c. Librium (chlordiazepoxide) Roche in some wild animals. Int. Zoo Yb. 3: 116.

Higgins, D., P., T. L. Rogers, A. D. Irvine, and S. A. Hall-Aspland. 2002. Use of midazolam/pethidine and tiletamine/zolazepam combinations for the chemical restraint of leopard seals (*Hydrurga leptonyx*). Mar. Mamm. Sci. 18: 483-499.

Higgins, A. J., and R. A. Kock. 1984. A guide to the clinical examination, chemical restraint and medication of the camel. Br. Vet. J. 140: 485-492.

Higgins, W. Y. 1972. Zebra immobilization at Lion Country Safari. Proc. Am. Assoc. Zoo Vet. P. 237.

Hildebrand, S. V., and T. Hill. 1993. Neuromuscular blockade by use of atracurium in anesthetized llamas. Am. J. Vet. Res. 54: 429-433.

Hill, F. W. G., and D. A. Smith. 1990. Clinical chemistry values for free-ranging elephants (*Loxodonta africana*) in Hwange National Park, Zimbabwe. Zimb. Vet. J. 21: 33-42.

Hime, J. M. 1974. The use of ketamine hydrochloride in non-domesticated cats. Vet. Rec. 95: 193-195.

Hime, J. M., and D. M. Jones. 1970. The use of xylazine in captive wild ruminants. 12th Int. Symp. Dis. Zoo and Wild An. Budapest. Pp. 143-146.

Hinsch, H., and C. P. Gandal. 1969. The effects of etorphine (M-99), oxymorphone hydrochloride and meperidine hydrochloride in reptiles. Copeia 1969: 404-405.

Hiramatsu, H. 1993. Using anesthesia. An. Zoos 45: 14-17.

Hirst, S. M. 1966. Immobilization of the transvaal giraffe (*Giraffa camelopardalis geraffa*) using an oripovine derivative. J. So. Afr. Vet. Assoc. 37: 85-89.

Hirst, S. M., W. K. Kettlitz, and G. P. Visagie. 1963. The use of Ro 5-2807 (Roche) as a tranquilliser in wild ungulates. Zool. Afr. 1: 231-238.

Hitchins, P. M., M. E. Keep, and K. Rochat. 1972. The capture of black rhinoceros in Hluhluwe Game Reserve and their translocation to the Kruger National Park. Lammergeyer 17: 9: 18-22.

Hochleithner, M. 1992. Erfahrungen mit der Isofluran (Forane) Narkose bei Vogeln und Reptilien. Erkr. Zootiere. 34: 171-177.

Hochleithner, M. 1993. Isoflurane anaesthesia in birds and reptiles. Wiener Tierarztliche Monatsschrift 80: 100, 102-105.

Hoekstra, T. W. 1968. Cap-Chur syringes modified for easier locating. J. Wildl. Manage. 32: 626-628.

Hofman, D. E., and H. Weaver. 1980. Immobilization of captive mallards and pintails with alpha-chloralose. Wildl. Soc. Bull. 8: 156-158.

Hofmeyr, J. M. 1974. Developments in the capture and airlift of roan antelope *Hippotragus equinus equinus* under narcosis to the Etosha National Park. Madoqua Ser. 1. 8: 37-48.

Hofmeyr, J. M. 1977. The introduction of R 33799 in game immobilization procedures. Etosha Ecological Institute. Pp. 1-9.

Hofmeyr, J. M. 1978. Immobilisation of black rhinos, eland and roan antelope with R 33799. Etosha Ecological Institute.

Hofmeyr, J. M. 1981. The use of haloperidol as a long-acting neuroleptic in game capture operations. J. So. Afr. Vet. Assoc. 52: 273-282.

Hofmeyr, J. M., and J. R. de Bruine. 1973. The problems associated with the capture, translocation and keeping of wild ungulates in South West Africa. Lammergeyer 18: 21-29.

Hofmeyr, J. M., H. Ebedes, R. E. M. Fryer, and J. R. de Bruine. 1975. The capture and translocation of the black rhinoceros *Diceros bicornis* Linn. in South West Africa. Madoqua. 9: 35-44.

Hofmeyr, J. M., H. G. Luchtenstein, and P. K. N. Mostert. 1977. Capture, handling and transport of spring-

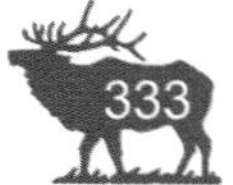

bok and the application of haloperidol as a long-acting neuroleptic. Madoqua. 10: 123-130.
Hoilien, J., and D. Oates. 1982. Tranquilizer use in wildlife damage control. Proc. Great Plains Wildl. Damage Control Workshop. 5: 71-77.
Holbrook, H. T., and M. R. Vaughan. 1985. Capturing adult and juvenile wild turkeys with adult doses of alpha-chloralose. Wildl. Soc. Bull. 13: 160-163.
Holmes, A. A. 1974. Immobilon in the otter. Vet. Rec. 95: 574.
Holmes, R. G., and S. Ngethe. 1973. Restraint of captive and wild lion (*Panthera leo*), leopard (*Panthera pardus*), and cheetah (*Acinonyx jubatus*). Vet. Rec. 92: 290-291.
Holt, G., J. J. Nygard, and A. Tevik. 1971. Bruk av injeksjonsgevaer til innfanging av ville eller forvillede. [The use of injection guns for catching wild or wild-running animals]. Nor. Vet. Tidsskr. 83: 3-10.
Holt, K., and S. P. Manning. 1978. The Missouri stabbing stick. Vet. Rec. 103: 186.
Holz, P. 1992. Immobilization of marsupials with tiletamine and zolazepam. J. Zoo Wildl. Med. 23: 426-428.
Holz, P., and J. E. F. Barnett. 1996. Long-acting tranquilizers: their use as a management tool in the confinement of free-ranging red-necked wallabies (*Macropus rufogriseus*). J. Zoo Wildl. Med. 27: 54-60.
Holz, P., and R. M. Holz. 1994. Evaluation of ketamine, ketamine/xylazine, and ketamine/midazolam anesthesia in red-eared sliders (*Trachemys scripta elegans*). J. Zoo Wildl. Med. 25: 531-537.
Holz, P., R. M. Holz, and J. E. F. Barnett. 1994. Effects of atropine on medetomidine/ketamine immobilization in the gray wolf (*Canis lupus*). J. Zoo Wildl. Med. 25: 209-213.
Hönich, M. 1970. Untersuchungen über die Wirkung von Bay Va 1470 beim Wild. 12th Int. Symp. Dis. Zoo and Wild An. Budapest. Pp. 153-154.
Hoover, J. P. 1984. Surgical implantation of radiotelemetry devices in American river otters. J. Am. Vet. Med. Assoc. 185: 1317-1320.
Hoover, J. P. 1985. Electrocardiograms of American river otters (*Lutra canadensis*) during immobilization. J. Wildl. Dis. 21: 331-334.
Hoover, J. P., and E. M. Jones. 1986. Physiologic and electrocardiographic responses of American river otters (*Lutra canadensis*) during chemical immobilization and inhalation anesthesia. J. Wildl. Dis. 22: 557-563.
Hoover, J. P., C. R. Root, and M. A. Zimmer. 1984. Clinical evaluation of American river otters in a reintroduction study. J. Am. Vet. Med. Assoc. 185: 1321-1326.
Horne, W. A., T. M. Norton, and M. R. Loomis. 1997. Cardiopulmonary effects of medetomidine-ketamine-isoflurane anesthesia in the gorilla (*Gorilla gorilla*) and chimpanzee (*Pan troglodytes*). Proc. Am. Assoc. Zoo Vet. Pp. 140-142.
Horne, W. A., B. A. Wolfe, T. N. Norton, and M. R. Loomis. 1998. Comparison of the cardiopulmonary effects of medetomidine-ketamine and medetomidine-Telazol induction on maintenance isoflurane anesthesia in the chimpanzee (*Pan troglodytes*). Proc. Am. Assoc. Zoo Vet. and Am. Assoc. Wildl. Vet. Pp. 22-25.
Horne, W. A., M. N. Tchamba, and M. R. Loomis. 2001. A simple method for providing intermittent positive pressure ventilation to etorphine-immobilized elephants (*Loxodonta africana*) in the field. J. Zoo Wildl. Med. 32: 519-522.
Hornocker, M. G., and W. V. Wiles. 1972. Immobilizing pumas (*Felis concolor*)with phencyclidine hydrochloride. Int. Zoo Yb. 12: 220-222.
Hornocker, M. G., J. J. Craighead, and E. W. Pfeiffer. 1965. Immobilizing mountain lions with succinylcholine chloride and pentobarbital sodium. J. Wildl. Manage. 29: 880-883.
Houston, A. H., J. A. Madden, R. J. Woods, and H. M. Miles. 1971. Some physiological effects of handling and tricaine methanesulphonate anesthetization upon brook trout, *Slavelinus fontinalis*. J. Fish. Res. Bd. Canada 28: 625-633.
Houston, D. B. 1969. Immobilization of the Shiras moose. J. Wildl. Manage. 33: 534-537.
Houston, D. B. 1970. Immobilization of moose with M99 etorphine. J. Mammal. 51: 396-399.
Houston, D. C., and J. E. Cooper. 1973. Use of the drug metomidate to facilitate the handling of vultures. Int. Zoo Yb. 13: 269-271.
Howard, L. L., K. S. Kearns, T. L. Clippinger, R. S. Larsen, and P. J. Morris. 2003. Immobilization of rhebok (*Pelea capreolus*) with carfentanil-xylazine and etorphine-xylazine. Proc. Am. Assoc. Zoo Vet. Pp. 285.
Howard, L. L., K. S. Kearns, T. L. Clippinger, R. S. Larsen, and P. J. Morris. 2004. Chemical immobiliza-

tion of rhebok (*Pelea capreolus*) with carfentanil-xylazine or etorphine-xylazine. J. Zoo Wildl. Med. 35: 312-319.
Howe, D. L. 1966. Investigation of tranquilizing, anesthetizing and immobilizing drugs when used on game animals. Wyoming Job Completion Report FW-3-R-13. WP9-J3W. 15 pp.
Hsu, W. H., and W. P. Shulaw. 1984. Effect of yohimbine on xylazine-induced immobilization in white-tailed deer. J. Am. Vet. Med. Assoc. 185: 1301-1303.
Huber, C., C. Walzer, and L. Bachmayr. 1999. A potential method of stress reduction in cheetah (*Acinonyx jubatus*) translocations using perphenazine enanthate and zuclopenthixol acetate. Erkrankugen Der Zootiere 39: 369-375.
Huber, C., C. Walzer, and L. Slotta-Bachmayr. 2001. Evaluation of long-term sedation in cheetah (*Acinonyx jubatus*) with perphenazine enanthate and zuclopenthixol acetate. J. Zoo Wildl. Med. 32: 329-335.
Hubbell, G. L. 1965. Capture and restraint of zoo animals. J. Am. Vet. Med. Assoc. 147: 1044-1048.
Hughes, H. C., W. J. White, and C. M. Lang. 1975. Guidelines for the use of tranquilizers, anesthetics, and analgesics in laboratory animals. Vet. Anesth. 3: 19-23.
Hugie, R. D. 1977. Use of chemical restraints in handling wildlife. Parks 2: 19-22.
Hugie, R. D., J. Landry, and J. Hermes. 1977. The use of ketamine hydrochloride as an anesthetic in black bears (*Ursus americanus*) in Maine. Trans. Northeast Sect. Wildl. Soc. 33: 83-86.
Hugues, F., M. Leclerc-Cassan, and J. P. Marc. 1986. [Anaesthesia of untamed animals. The attempted use of a new anaesthetic: the combination tiletamine-zolazepam (Zoletil N.D.)]. Recl. Med. Vet. Ec. Alfort. 162: 427-431.
Hunt, P. S. 1976. Anaesthesia of the European badger using ketamine hydrochloride. Vet. Rec. 98: 94.
Hunt, T. J. 1964. Anesthesia of the tortoise. *In* Graham-Jones, O. (ed.). Small Animal Anesthesia. Pergamon Press, Macmillan Co., New York.
Hunter, D. 1999. Chemical immobilization of wild sheep - history and cautions. Trans. 2nd No. Am. Wild Sheep Conf. Pp. 265-267.
Hunter, R. P., R. Isaza, J. W. Carpenter, and D. E. Koch. 2004. Clinical effects and plasma concentrations of fentanyl after transmucosal administration in three species of great ape. 35: 162-166.
Hyman, W. B. 1992. Veterinary restraint drugs with special reference to detomidine. *In* Ebedes, H. (ed.) The Use of Tranquillizers in Wildlife. Dept. Ag. Develop., Pretoria. Bull. No. 423. Pp. 25-30.
Idowu, A. L., and J. F. Akinrinmade. 1986. Xylazine and ketamine anaesthesia in captive Nile crocodiles (*Crocodylus niloticus*). Trop. Vet. 4: 139-142.
IndrebØ, A. 1989. Anestesi av blarev med Ketelar® og Rompun® [Anesthesia of blue foxes using ketamine and xylazine). Nor. Veterinäeridsskr. 101: 767-770.
International Zoo Yearbook. 1960. Doses and effects of succinylcholine chloride delivered with projectile syringe to immobilize several species of wild animals at the San Diego Zoo. Int. Zoo Yb. 2: 319-321.
International Zoo Yearbook. 1961. A table of paralytic drugs used to restrain animals at the Bloemfontein zoo, South Africa. Int. Zoo Yb. 3: 121.
Iversen, M., B. Finstad, R. S. McKinley, and R. A. Eliassen. 2003. The efficacy of metomidate, clove oil, Aqui-S™ and Benzoak® as anaesthetics in Atlantic salmon (*Salmo salar* L.) smolts, and their potential stress-reducing capacity. Aquaculture 221: 549-566.
IWVS. 1992. Wildlife Restraint Series. International Wildlife Veterinary Services, Salinas, California.
Jackson, O. F. 1970. Snake anesthesia. Br. J. Herpetol. 4: 172-175.
Jackson, O. F., and J. E. Cooper. 1981. Anesthesia and surgery. *In* Cooper, J. E., and O. F. Jackson (eds.). Diseases of the Reptilia, Vol. 2. New York, Academic Press. Pp. 535-549.
Jackson, R., A. Gary, and B. S. Karan. 1990. Capture and immobilization of wild snow leopards. Int. Pedigree Book Snow Leopard. 6: 93-102.
Jacobsen, N. K. 1983. Effects of age and behavior of black-tailed deer on dosages of xylazine. J. Wildl. Manage. 47: 252-255.
Jacobsen, N. K., S. P. Armstrong, and A. N. Moen. 1976. Seasonal variation in succinylcholine immobilization of captive white-tailed deer. J. Wildl. Manage. 40: 447-453.
Jacobson, E. R. 1983. Hematologic and serum chemical effects of a ketamine/xylazine combination when used for immobilizing springbok. J. Am. Vet. Med. Assoc. 183: 1260-1262.
Jacobson, E. R. 1984. Immobilization, blood sampling, necropsy techniques and diseases of crocodilians: a review. J. Zoo An. Med. 15: 38-45.
Jacobson, E. R., and G. V. Kollias. 1984. Yohimbine antagonism of ketamine/ xylazine tranquillization and immobilization in hoofstock. Proc. Am. Assoc. Zoo Vet. P. 57.

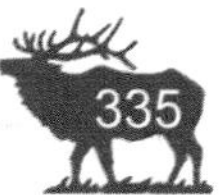

Jacobson, E. R., and J. Lukas. 1988. Immobilization of dama gazelle (*Gazella dama*) with carfentanil citrate. Chinkara 1: 12-18.

Jacobson, E. R., J. Allen, H. Martin, and G. V. Kollias. 1985. Effects of yohimbine on combined xylazine-ketamine-induced sedation and immobilization in juvenile African elephants. J. Am. Vet. Med. Assoc. 187: 1195-1198.

Jacobson, E. R., C.-L. Chen, R. Gronwall, and A. Tiller. 1986. Serum concentrations of etorphine in juvenile African elephants. J. Am. Vet. Med. Assoc. 189: 1079-1081.

Jacobson, E. R., D. J. Heard, R. Caligiuri, and G. V. Kollias. 1987. Physiological effects of etorphine and carfentanil in African elephants. Proc. Int. Conf. Zool. Avian Med. 1: 525-527.

Jacobson, E. R., G. V. Kollias, D. J. Heard, and R. Caliguiri. 1988. Immobilization of African elephants with carfentanil and antagonism with nalmefene and diprenorphine. J. Zoo An. Med. 19: 1-7.

Jacquier, M., P. Aarhaug, J. M. Arnemo, H. Bauer, and B. Enriquez. 2006. Reversible immobilization of free-ranging African lions (*Panthera leo*) with medetomidine-tiletamine-zolazepam and atipamezole. J. Wildl. Dis. 42: 432-436.

Jaczewski, Z. and K. Swierzynski. 1955. Anaesthesia in the European bison (*Bison bonasus* L.) by chloralum hydratum. Zool. Pol. 6: 80-87.

Jainudeen, M. R. 1970. The use of etorphine hydrochloride for restraint of a domesticated elephant. J. Am. Vet. Med. Assoc. 157: 624-626.

Jainudeen, M. R., and M. Khan. 1977. The immobilization and translocation of wild Asian elephant, *Elephas maximus*, in peninsular Malaysia. Kajian Vet. 9: 1-7.

Jainudeen, M. R., T. A. Bongso, and B. M. O. A. Perera. 1971. Immobilisation of aggressive working elephants (*Elaphus maximus*). Vet. Rec. 89: 686-688.

Jalanka, H. H. 1986. The chemical restraint and anesthesia of Finnish wildlife species and some other species kept in Helsinki Zoo. Br. Vet. Zool. Soc. Newsl. 21: 31-37.

Jalanka, H. H. 1987. Clinical-pharmacological properties of a new sedative—medetomidine—and its antagonist, MPV-1248. Proc. Int. Conf. Zool. Avian Med. 1: 530-534.

Jalanka, H. H. 1988. Evaluation of medetomidine- and ketamine-induced immobilization in markhors (*Capra falconeri megaceros*) and its reversal by atipamezole. J. Zoo An. Med. 19: 95-105.

Jalanka, H. H. 1989a. Chemical restraint and reversal in captive markhors (*Capra falconeri megaceros*): a comparison of two methods. J. Zoo An. Med. 20: 413-422.

Jalanka, H. H. 1989b. Evaluation and comparison of two ketamine-based immobilization techniques in snow leopards (*Panthera uncia*). J. Zoo An. Med. 20: 163-169.

Jalanka, H. H. 1989c. Medetomidine- and ketamine-induced immobilization of snow leopards (*Panthera uncia)*: doses, evaluation, and reversal by atipamezole. J. Zoo An. Med. 20: 154-162.

Jalanka, H. H. 1989d. Medetomidine- and ketamine-induced immobilization in forest reindeer (*Rangifer tarandus fennicus)* and its reversal by atipamezole. Proc. Am. Assoc. Zoo Vet. Pp. 1-7.

Jalanka, H. H. 1989e. The use of medetomidine, medetomidine-ketamine combinations, and atipamezole at Helsinki Zoo—a review of 240 cases. Acta Vet. Scand. 85: 193-197.

Jalanka, H. H. 1990. Medetomidine- and medetomidine-ketamine-induced immobilization in blue foxes (*Alopex lagopus*) and its reversal by atipamezole. Acta Vet. Scand. 31: 63-71.

Jalanka, H. H. 1992. Physiologic responses to medetomidine, medetomidine-ketamine combinations, and atipamezole in nondomestic animals. *In* Short, C. E. (ed.). Animal Pain. Churchill Livingston, New York. Pp. 220-223.

Jalanka, H. H. 1993. New α_2-adrenoceptor agonists and antagonists. *In* Fowler, M. E. (ed.). Zoo & Wild Animal Medicine: Current Therapy 3. W. B. Saunders Co., Philadelphia, Pennsylvania. Pp. 477-481.

Jalanka, H. H., and B. O. Roeken. 1990. The use of medetomidine, medetomidine-ketamine combinations, and atipamezole in nondomestic animals: a review. J. Zoo Wildl. Med. 21: 259-282.

Jalanka, H. H. , and E. Teräväinen. 1992. Propofol - a potentially useful intravenous anesthetic agent in non-domestic ruminants and camelids. Proc. Joint Conf. Am. Assoc. Zoo Vet. and Am. Assoc. Wildl. Vet. Pp. 264-270.

James, S. B., R. A. Cook, B. L. Raphael, M. D. Stetter, P. Kalk, K. MacLaughlin, and P. P. Calle. 1998. Immobilization of babirusa (*Babyrousa babyrussa*) with xylazine and tiletamine/zolazepam and reversal with yohimbine and flumazenil. Proc. Joint Conf. Am. Assoc. Zoo Vet. and Am. Assoc. Wildl. Vet. Pp. 204-206.

James, S. B., R. A. Cook, B. L. Raphael, M. D. Stetter, P. Kalk, K. MacLaughlin, and P. P. Calle. 1999.

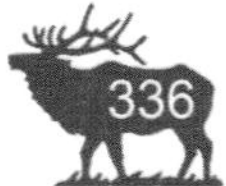

Immobilization of babirusa (*Babyrousa babyrussa*) with xylazine and tiletamine/zolazepam and reversal with yohimbine and flumazenil. J. Zoo Wildl. Med. 30:521-525.

Janovsky, M., F. Tataruch, M. Ambuehl, and M. Giacometti. 2000. A Zoletil®-Rompun® mixture as an alternative to the use of opioids for immobilization of feral red deer. J. Wildl. Dis. 36: 663-669.

Janovsky, M., T. Ruf, and W. Zenker. 2002. Oral administration of tiletamine/zolazepam for the immobilization of the common buzzard (*Buteo buteo*). J. Raptor Res. 36: 188-193.

Janssen, D. L., and J. E. Oosterhuis. 1984. Guaifenesin for muscle relaxation in immobilized hoofstock. Proc. Am. Assoc. Zoo Vet. P. 59.

Janssen, D. L., J. E. Oosterhuis, J. L. Allen, and T. H. Stanley. 1987. Carfentanil immobilization of non-domestic livestock. Proc. 1st Int. Conf. Zool. Avian Med. Omnipress, Madison, Wisconsin. 1: 582.

Janssen, D. L., J. P. Raath, G. E. Swan, D. Jessup, and T. H. Stanley. 1991. Field studies with the narcotic immobilizing agent A3080. Proc. Am. Assoc. Zoo Vet. Pp. 340-342.

Janssen, D. L., G. E. Swan, J. P. Raath, S. W. McJames, J. L. Allen. V. de Vos, K. E. Williams, J. M. Anderson, and T. H. Stanley. 1993. Immobilization and physiological effects of the narcotic A-3080 in impala (*Aepyceros melampus*). J. Zoo Wildl. Med. 24: 11-18.

Janssen, P. 1969. Immobilization and restraint of large wild mammals with azaperone and fentanyl. Janssen Pharmaceutica, Beerse, Belgium.16 pp.

Janssen, P. A. J. 1981. Potent new analgesics, tailor-made for different purposes. Janssen Res. News 6: 2-15.

Jarofke, C. D. 1980. Cervidae. *In* Klos, H. G., E. M. Lang (eds.). Handbook of Zoo Medicine. Van Nostrand Reinhold Company New York. Pp. 223-247.

Jarofke, D. 1978. Improvements of the distance-injection systems and the successful application of a variable-length blow-gun. Proc. Am. Assoc. Zoo Vet. Pp. 24-25.

Jarofke, D. 1981a. Use of halothane-oxygen anesthesia in elephants (*Elephas maximus*). J. Zoo An. Med. 12: 93-95.

Jarofke, D. 1981b. Etorphine anesthesia in the elephant. J. Zoo An. Med. 11: 90-92

Jarofke, D., and H.-G. Klos. 1983. Immobilisierung und Krankenheiten von Flusspferden (*Hippopotamus amphibius*) Auswertung einer Umfrage bei mehr als 100 Zoologischen Garten. Verh. Ber. Erkg. Zoot. 25: 389-403.

Jarvis, C., and D. Morris (eds.). 1960. Animal Restraint Technique Survey. Int. Zoo Yb. 2: 300-327.

Jasinski, D. R., J. D. Griffith, and C. B. Carr. 1975. Etorphine in man I. Subjective effects and suppression of morphine abstinence. Clin. Pharmacol. Ther. 17: 267-272.

Jenkins, D. H. 1978. The use of etorphine (M99) and diprenorphine (M5050) for anesthesia in a white rhinoceros for the removal of growths on the third eyelid. Auburn Vet. 34: 39-43.

Jenkins, D., and M. L. Gorman. 1981. Anaesthsia of the European otter *Lutra lutra* using ketamine hydrochloride. J. Zool. 194: 265-267.

Jenkins, J. H., S. D. Feurt, F. A. Hayes, and J. A. Crockford. 1955. A preliminary report on the use of drugs for capturing deer. Proc. Ann. Conf. Southeast. Assoc. Game Fish Comm. 9: 41-43.

Jenkins, J. H., F. A. Hayes, S. D. Feurt, and J. A. Crockford. 1961. A new method for the live capture of canines with applications to rabies control. Am. J. Public Health. 51: 902-908.

Jensen, J. M. 1982. Fentanyl citrate immobilization of zoo ungulates. J. Zoo An. Med. 13: 101-103.

Jensen, J. M., N. S. Matthews, and S. M. Hartsfield. 1994. Metabolic scaling of ketamine in ostriches and emus. Joint Conf. Am. Assoc. Zoo Vet. Assoc. Reptil. Amphib. Vet. Pp. 134-137.

Jensen, J., P. Tamas, B. and McNeil. 1983. Antagonism of xylazine/atropine immobilization by yohimbine and 4-aminopyridine. Proc. Am. Assoc. Zoo Vet. Pp. 65-66.

Jepsen, O. R., G. Dirch-Paulson, and G. Jorgensen. 1981. Collection of blood, sedation and anaesthesia in mink. A haematological and clinical-chemical study. Nord. Vet-Med. Suppl. Pp. 1-99.

Jessup, D. A. 1982a. Chemical capture of upland game birds and waterfowl: Oral anesthetics. *In* Nielsen, L., J. C. Haigh, and M. E. Fowler (eds.). Chemical Immobilization of North American Wildlife. Wisconsin Humane Society, Inc. Milwaukee, Wisconsin. Pp. 214-226.

Jessup, D. A. 1982b. Restraint and chemical immobilization of carnivores and furbearers. *In* Nielsen, L., J. C. Haigh, and M. E. Fowler (eds.). Chemical Immobilization of North American Wildlife. Wisconsin Humane Society, Inc., Milwaukee, Wisconsin. Pp. 227-244.

Jessup, D. A. 1992a. On capturing bighorn sheep. J. Wildl. Dis. 28: 512-513.

Jessup, D. A. 1992b. Veterinary contributions toward improving capture, medical management, and anesthesia of free-ranging wildlife. J. Am. Vet. Med. Assoc. 200: 653-658.

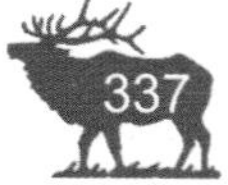

Jessup, D. A. 1993. Remote treatment and monitoring of wildlife. *In* Fowler, M. E. (ed.). Zoo & Wild Animal Medicine: Current Therapy 3. W. B. Saunders Co., Philadelphia, Pennsylvania. Pp. 499-504.

Jessup, D. A. 1999. Capture and handling of mountain sheep and goats. *In* Fowler, M. E., and R. E. Miller (eds.). Zoo & Wild Animal Medicine. Current Therapy 4. W. B. Saunders Company, Philadelphia, Pennsylvania. Pp. 681-687.

Jessup, D. 2001. Reducing capture-related mortality and dart injury. Wildl. Soc. Bull. 29: 751-753.

Jessup, D., B. Hunter, and W. Clark. 1980. Wildlife restraint handbook. California Dept. Fish and Game, Rancho Cordova, Cal. 160 pp.

Jessup, D. A., J. W. Foster, and W. E. Clark. 1982a. An electronic means of immobilizing deer: Taser. California Vet. 36: 31-34.

Jessup, D. A., R. Mohr, and B. Feldman. 1982b. A comparison of four methods for capturing bighorn. Desert Bighorn Council Trans. P. 21-25.

Jessup, D. A., R. Mohr, and B. Feldman. 1982c. Comparing methods of capturing bighorn sheep: a preliminary report. *In* Nielsen, L., J. C. Haigh, and M. E. Fowler (eds.). Chemical Immobilization of North American Wildlife. Wisconsin Humane Society, Inc. Milwaukee, Wisconsin. Pp. 422-438.

Jessup, D. A., W. E. Clark, P. A. Gullett, and K. R. Jones. 1983. Immobilization of mule deer with ketamine and xylazine, and reversal of immobilization with yohimbine. J. Am. Vet. Med. Assoc. 183: 1339-1340.

Jessup, D. A., W. E. Clark, and K. R. Jones. 1984a. Immobilization of captive mule deer with carfentanil. J. Zoo An. Med. 15: 8-10.

Jessup, D. A., W. E. Clark, and R. C. Mohr. 1984b. Capture of bighorn sheep: management recommendations. Wildlife Management Branch Administrative Report 84-1, Pp. 1-29.

Jessup, D. A., K. Jones, R. Mohr, and T. Kucera. 1985a. Yohimbine antagonism to xylazine in free-ranging mule deer and desert bighorn sheep. J. Am. Vet. Med. Assoc. 187: 1251-1253.

Jessup, D. A., W. E. Clark, K. R. Jones, R. Clark, and W. R. Lance. 1985b. Immobilization of free-ranging desert bighorn sheep, tule elk, and wild horses, using carfentanil and xylazine: reversal with naloxone, diprenorphine, and yohimbine. J. Am. Vet. Med. Assoc. 187: 1253-1254.

Jessup, D. A., R. K. Clark, R. A. Weaver, and M. D. Kock. 1988. The safety and cost-effectiveness of net-gun capture of desert bighorn sheep (*Ovis canadensis nelsoni*). J. Zoo An. Med. 19: 208-213.

Jessup, D. A., M. D. Kock, and P. Morkel. 1993. Health data gained from black rhino immobilized for relocation. *In* Ryder, O. A. (ed.). Rhinoceros Biology and Conservation. Zoological Society of San Diego, San Diego. Pp. 311-314.

Jessup, D. A., E. T. Thorne, M. W. Miller, and D. L. Hunter. 1996. Capture and translocation of wild ungulates in North America. Suppl. Ric. Biol. Selvaggina XXIV: 355-365.

Jewell, P. A., and E. A. Smith. 1965. Immobilization of grey seals. J. Wildl. Manage. 29: 316-318.

Jewell, P. A., and V. P. W. Lowe. 1965. A trial with the projectile-syringe rifle to capture wild red deer on Rhum. J. Zool. 146: 2672-277.

Jewell, P. A., P. Keen, and E. H. Tong. 1965. The use of the muscle relaxant suxethonium to immobilize captive animals with the projectile syringe rifle. J. Zool. 146: 263-271.

Jingfors, K., and A. Gunn. 1989. The use of snowmobiles in the drug immobilization of muskoxen. Can. J. Zool. 67: 1120-1121.

Johnsingh, A. J. T., J. Joshua, R. Chellam, N. V. K. Ashraf, V. Krishnamurthy, and D. V. S. Khati. 1993. Etorphine and acepromazine combination for immobilising wild Indian elephants, *Elephas maximus*. J. Bombay Nat. Hist. Soc. 90: 45-49.

Johnson, C. B., P. R. Wilson, M. R. Woodbury, and N. A. Caulkett. 2005. Comparison of analgesic techniques for antler removal in halothane-anaesthetized red deer (*Cervus elaphus*): electroencephalographic responses. Vet. Anaesth. Analg. 32: 61-71.

Johnson, J. H. 1991. Anesthesia, analgesia and euthanasia of reptiles and amphibians. Proc. Am. Assoc. Zoo Vet. Pp. 132-138.

Johnson, S. P., T. Gelatt, R. B. Heath, and W. Taylor. 2004. Field inhalation anesthesia in free-ranging juvenile Steller sea lions (*Eumetopias jubatus*). Proc. Am. Assoc. Zoo Vet. Pp. 502-504.

Johnston, N. L. 1974. Techniques for anesthetizing and vaccinating exotic Felidae. Vet. Med. Small An. Clin. 69: 1243-1247.

Jolly, D. W., L. E. Mawdsley-Thomas, and D. Bucke. 1972. Anaesthesia in fish. Vet. Rec. 91: 424-426.

Jones, D. M. 1971a. Sedation of a bull musk ox (*Ovibos moschatus*). D. Zool. Garten 40: 138-142.

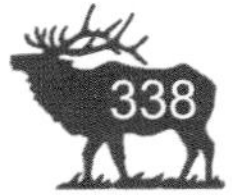

Jones, D. M. 1971b. Sedation of a bull musk ox *Ovibos moschatus* using xylazine. Int. Zoo Yb. 11: 242-244.

Jones, D. M. 1972. The use of drugs for immobilization, capture and translocation of non-domestic animals. Vet. Ann. 13: 320-352.

Jones, D. M. 1976a. An assessment of weapons and projectile syringes used for capturing mammals. Vet. Rec. 99: 250-253.

Jones, D. M. 1976b. The husbandry and veterinary care of wild horses in captivity. Equine Vet. J. 8: 140-146.

Jones, D. M. 1977a. Immobilising exotic animals. Vet. Rec. 101: 352-353.

Jones, D. M. 1977b. The sedation and anaesthesia of birds and reptiles. Vet. Rec. 101: 340-342.

Jones, D. M. 1978. A short analysis of 2000 ungulate immobilizations involving 71 species mainly from the collection of the Zoological Society of London. *In* Sonderdruck aus Verhandlungsbericht des XX Internationalen Symposiums über die Erkrankungen der Zootiere Kralove 1978, Berlin, Akafemie-Verlag. Pp. 173-178.

Jones, D. M. 1983. The capture and handling of deer. *In* Rudge, A. J. B. (ed.). The Capture and Handling of Deer. Nature Conservancy Council, Peterborough, England. Pp. 1-136.

Jones, D. M. 1984. Physical and chemical methods of capturing deer. Vet. Rec. 114: 109-112.

Jones, R. D. 1966. A comparison between morphine and M99 for the immobilization of the black rhinoceros. M-series Vet. Appl. Rpt. No. 46, Reckitt and Sons, Hull, England.

Jones, R. D., and H. H. Roth. 1968. Cooperative study of the efficiency of morphine and etorphine (M.99) in the immobilisation of black rhinoceros (*Diceros bicornis* L.). Wildlife National Parks, Rhodesia. 16 pp.

Jones, W. T., and B. B. Bush. 1988. Darting and marking techniques for an arboreal forest monkey, *Cercopithecus ascanius*. Am. J. Primatol. 14: 83-89.

Jonkel, C. J., and R. P. Weckwerth. 1963. Sexual maturity and implantation of blastocysts in the wild pine marten. J. Wildl. Manage. 27: 93-98.

Jonkel, C. J., D. R. Gray, and B. Hubert. 1975. Immobilizing and marking wild muskoxen in arctic Canada. J. Wildl. Manage. 39: 112-117.

Jonsson, N. N., S. D. Johnston, H. Field, C. de Jong, and C. Smith. 2004. Field anaesthesia of three Australian species of flying fox. Vet. Rec. 154: 664.

Jorgenson, J. T., J. Samson, and M. Festa-Bianchet. 1990. Field immobilization of bighorn sheep with xylazine hydrochloride and antagonism with idazoxan. J. Wildl. Dis. 26: 522-527.

Joseph, B. E., and L. H. Cornell. 1987. The use of meperidine hydrochloride in cetaceans and pinnipeds. Proc. 1st Int. Conf. Zool. Avian Med. 1: 400.

Joseph, B. E., and L. H. Cornell. 1988. The use of meperidine hydrochloride for chemical restraint in certain cetaceans and pinnipeds. J. Wildl. Dis. 24: 691-694.

Joseph, B. E., L. H. Cornell, and T. Williams. 1987. Chemical sedation of sea otters. J. Zoo An. Med. 18: 7-13.

Joshi, B. P. 1991. Wild Animal Medicine. Oxford and IBH Publishing Co., New Delhi, India. 279 pp.

Joubert, F. G., and P. E. Stander. 1990. Capture myopathy in an African lion. Madoqua 17: 51-52.

Joyal, R., G. Rivard, and J. Vallee. 1978. L'evaluation de methodes d'immobilisation d'orignaux en liberte pour etudes telemetriques. [Evaluation of methods of moose immobilization for telemetric studies]. Nat. Can. (Que.). 105: 451-456.

Joyner, P. H., M. P. Jones, N. Zagaya, D. Ward, R. E. Gompf, and J. M. Sleeman. 2006. Comparison of induction and recovery characteristics and cardiopulmonary effects of sevoflurane and isoflurane in bald eagles (*Haliaeetus leucocephalus*). Proc. Am. Assoc. Zoo Vet. Pp. 231-232.

Ju Guichun et al. 1992. Mian nai ning (MNN) - a new anesthetic used for black bear and brown bear. Acta Agric. Univ. Jilinensis 14: 64-66.

Jurczynski, K., M. Flügger, and M. McClean. 2006. Comparison of anesthesia of aoudads (*Ammotragus lervia*) in a city zoo enclosure in Germany with a free-ranging group of aoudads in a safari park in the United States and reference hematologic data values of one of the parks. Proc. Am. Assoc. Zoo Vet. Pp. 336-341.

Kalema-Zikusoka, G., W. A. Horne, J. Levine, and M. R. Loomis. 2003. Comparison of the cardiorespiratory effects of medetomidine-butorphanol-ketamine and medetomidine-butorphanol-midazolam in patas monkeys (*Erythrocebus patas*). J. Zoo Wildl. Med. 34: 47-52.

Kane, K. K. 1979. Medical management of the otter. Proc. Am. Assoc. Zoo Vet. Pp. 100-103.

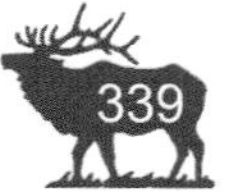

Kania, B. F. 1985. Neurochemical changes in the brain and spinal cord of sheep: a basis for the immobilizing action of etorphine. J. So. Afr. Vet. Assoc. 56: 89-92.

Kania, B. F., and J. K. Teuchmann. 1975. The use of etorphine hydrochloride (M99) as an immobilizing agent in the European bison (*Bison bonasus* L.). Zool. Pol. 25: 85-98.

Kania, B. F., E. Suminski, and J. Kossakowski. 1985. An effective immobilizing agent for hybrids of European bison and domestic cattle. Acta Theriol. 30: 435-444.

Kania, B. F., J. K. Teuchmann, S. Piwowarczyk, and Z. Krasinski. 1973. Badania nad immobilizujacym dzialaniem chlorowodorkiem cyprenorfiny (M 285). [Pharmacological aspects of immobilizing effects of M 99 in *Bison bonasus* L. and attempts to antagonize these effects with M 285]. Przegl. Zool. 17: 242-247.

Kaplan, H. M. 1969. Anesthesia in amphibians and reptiles. Fed. Proc. 28: 1541-1546.

Kaplan, H. M., and R. Taylor. 1957. Anesthesia in turtles. Herpetologica 13: 43-45.

Kaplan, H. M., and M. Kaplan. 1961. Anesthesia of frogs with ethyl alcohol. Proc. An. Care Panel 11: 31-35.

Kaplan, H. M., N. R. Brewer, and M. R. Kaplan. 1962. Comparative value of some barbiturates for anesthesia in the frog. Proc. An. Care Panel. 12: 141.

Karesh, W. B., D. L. Janssen, and J. E. Oosterhuis. 1986. A comparison of carfentanil and etorphine/xylazine immobilization of axis deer. J. Zoo An. Med. 17: 58-61.

Karesh, W. B., R. B. Wallace, R. E. Painter, D. Rumiz, W. E. Braselton, E. S. Dierenfeld, and H. Puche. 1998a. Immobilization and health assessment of free-ranging black spider monkeys (*Ateles paniscus chamek*). Am. J. Primatol. 44: 107-123.

Karesh, W. B., M. M. Uhart, E. S. Dierenfeld, W. E. Braselton, A. Torres, C. House, H. Puche, and R. A. Cook. 1998b. Health evaluation of free-ranging guanaco (*Lama guanicoe*). J. Zoo. Wildl. Med. 29: 134-141.

Karhuvaara, S., A. Kallio, M. Salonen, J. Tuominen, and M. Scheinin. 1991. Rapid reversal of α_2-adrenoceptor agonist effects by atipamezole in human volunteers. Brit. J. Clin. Pharmacol. 31: 160-165.

Karlstrom, E. L., and S. F. Cook. 1955. Notes on snake anesthesia. Copeia 1: 57-58.

Karns, P. D., and V. F. J. Crichton. 1978. Effects of handling and physical restraint on blood parameters of woodland caribou. J. Wildl. Manage. 42: 904-908.

Kato, H., and M. Seino. 1996. Obervations on chemical immobilization of a reticulated giraffe, *Giraffa camelopardalis reticulata*, using etorphine (M99R) and xylazine. J. Japan. Assoc. Zool. Gard. Aquar. 37: 3-4.

Kaufman, P. L., and R. Hahnenberger. 1975. CI-744 anesthesia for opthamological examination and surgery in monkeys. Invest. Opthalmol. 14: 788-791.

Kaunda, S. S. K. 2001. Capture and chemical immobilization of black backed jackals at Mokolodi Nature Reserve, Botswana. Mammal Res. Inst., U. Pretoria 002.

Kattel, B., and A. W. Alldredge. 1991. Capturing and handling of the Himalayan musk deer. Wildl. Soc. Bull. 19: 397-399.

Kearns, K. S., E. C. Ramsay, and B. Swenson. 1996. Oral anesthetic induction of chimpanzees (*Pan troglodytes*) with droperidol and carfentanil citrate. Proc. Am. Assoc. Zoo Vet. Pp. 401-403.

Kearns, K. S., J. Afema, and A. Duncan. 1998. Dosage trials using medetomidine as an oral preanesthetic agent in chimpanzees (*Pan troglodytes*). Proc. Joint Conf. Am. Assoc. Zoo Vet. and Am. Assoc. Wildl. Vet. Omaha, Nebraska. P. 511.

Kearns, K. S., B. Swenson, and E. C. Ramsay. 1999. Dosage trials with transmucosal carfentanil citrate in non-human primates. Zoo. Biol. 18: 397-402.

Kearns, K. S., B. Swenson, and E. C. Ramsay. 2000. Oral induction of anesthesia with droperidol and transmucosal carfentanil citrate in chimpanzees (*Pan troglodytes*). J. Zoo Wildl. Med. 31: 185-189.

Keep, J. M. 1971. Some observations on the use of drugs for the capture of feral beffalo. Austral. Vet. J. 47: 553-556.

Keep, J. M. 1973. Notes on the field capture of the agile wallaby (*Macropus agilis*). Austral. Vet. J. 49: 385-387.

Keep, J. M. 1978. Marsupials - anaesthesia. Proc. Post-Grad. Committee in Vet. Sci., U. Sydney. 36: 123-124.

Keep, J. M., and A. M. Fox. 1971. The capture, restraint, and translocation of kangaroos in the wild. Austral. Vet. J. 47: 141.

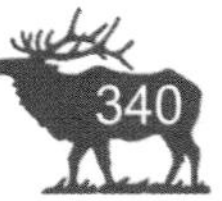

Keep, M. E. 1969. Report on the immobilization of white rhinoceros using fentanyl (R4263). Janssen Pharmaceutica, Beerse.

Keep, M. E. 1971. Etorphine hydrochloride antagonists used in the capture of the white rhinoceros *Ceratotherium simum simum*. Lammergeyer. 3: 60-68.

Keep, M. E. 1972a. The use of "Rompun" (Va 1470) Bayer on the white rhinoceros. Lammergeyer. 17: 31-35.

Keep, M. E. 1972b. The use of "Rompun" (Va 1470) Bayer on the white rhinoceros. J. Zoo An. Med. 4: 21-24.

Keep, M. E. 1972c. Capturing lions on the loose. Vet. Clin. 9: 2-3.

Keep, M. E. 1973a. The immobilization and translocation of black wildebeest. Lammergeyer 18: 39-43.

Keep, M. E. 1973b. The use of etorphine hydrochloride (M99) (Reckitt), fentanyl (Janssen) and hyoscine hydrobromide combination for field capture of white rhinoceros. Lammergeyer 19: 28-30.

Keep, M. E. 1973c. The problems associated with the capture and translocation of the black rhinoceros in Zululand, Republic of South Africa. Lammergeyer 18: 15-20.

Keep, M. E. 1979. The sedation and immobilisation of deer. Proc. Refresher Course for Veterinarians, The Australian Museum, Sydney. 49: 21-28.

Keep, M. E. 1992. The immobilization and tranquillization of rhino. *In* Ebedes, H. (ed.) The Use of Tranquillizers in Wildlife. Dept. Ag. Develop., Pretoria. Bull. No. 423. Pp. 44-46.

Keep, M. E., and P. J. Keep. 1967. Immobilization of waterbuck. Vet. Rec. 81: 552.

Keep, M. E., and P. J. Keep. 1968. The immobilization of eland using new drug combinations. Lammergeyer 9: 18-23.

Keep, M. E., J. L. Tinley, K. Rochat, and J. V. Clark. 1969. The immobilization and translocation of black rhinoceros *Diceros bicornis* using etorphine hydrochloride (M99). Lammergeyer 10: 4-11.

Keffen, R. H. 1993. The ostrich *Strurhio camelus*: capture, care, accommodation, and transportation. *In* McKenzie, A. A. (ed.). The Capture and Care Manual. Wildlife Decision Support Services and The South African Veterinary Foundation, Pretoria. Pp. 634-653.

Keller, G. L., D. H. Bauman, and L. Abbott. 1988. Yohimbine antagonism of ketamine and xylazine anesthesia in rabbits. Lab An. Pp. 28-30.

Keyes, M. 1965. Immobilizing, tranquilizing and anesthetizing drugs used for fur seals, *Callorhinus ursinus*. Conf. Biol. Sonar Diving Mammals. Pp. 74-79.

Khamis, Y., K. Fouad, and A. Sayed. 1973. Vergleichende Untersuchungen von Tranquilizern/Sedativa beim Dromedar. Vet. Med. Nachr. 4: 335-344.

Kilde, A. M., and L. V. Klein. 1973. Restraint of two fallow deer with xylazine. J. Zoo An. Med. 4: 21.

Kilpatrick, H. J., and S. M. Spohr. 1999. Telazol®-xylazine versus ketamine-xylazine: a field evaluation for immobilizing white-tailed deer. Wildl. Soc. Bull. 27: 566-570.

Kilpatrick, H. J., A. J. DeNicola, and M. R. Ellingwood. 1996. Comparison of standard and transmitter-equipped darts for capturing white-tailed deer. Wildl. Soc. Bull. 24: 306-310.

Kilpatrick, H. J., S. M. Spohr, and A. J. DeNicola. 1997. Darting urban deer: techniques and technology. Wildl. Soc. Bull. 25: 542-546.

Kim, C-Y, H-S Lee, S-C Han, J-D Heo, M-S Kwon, C-S Ha, and S-S Han. 2005. Hematological and serum biochemical values in cynomolgus monkeys anesthetized with ketamine hydrochloride. J. Med. Primatol. 34: 96-100.

King, J. M. 1969. The capture and translocation of the black rhinoceros. E. Afr. Wildl. J. 7: 115-130.

King, J. M., and B. M. Carter. 1965. The use of oripavine derivative M.99, for the immobilisation of the black rhinoceros (*Diceros bicornis*) and its antagonism with the related compound M.285, or nalorphine.E. Afr. Wildl. J. 3: 19-26.

King, J. M., and H. Klingel. 1965. The use of the oripavine derivative M99 for the restraint of equine animals and its antagonism with the related compound M285. Res. Vet. Sci. 6: 447-455.

King, J. M., B. C. Bertram, and P. H. Hamilton. 1977. Tiletamine and zolazepam for immobilization of wild lions and leopards. J. Am. Vet. Med. Assoc. 171: 894-898.

Kisloff, B. 1975. Ketamine-paraldehyde anesthesia for rabbits. Am. J. Vet. Res. 36: 1033-1034.

Kistchinski, A. A., and S. M. Uspenski. 1970. Immobilization and tagging of polar bears in maternity dens. *In* Herrero, S. (ed.). Bears - Their Biology and Management. IUCN publ. 23: 172-180.

Kitchen, H. 1966. Handling and restraint in deer and other wild animals. Lab. An. Digest 4: 3-7.

Kitchen, H. 1976. The use of succinylcholine in deer. Proc. Am. Assoc. Zoo Vet. Pp. 185-194.

Kittle, E. L. 1971. Ketamine HCL as an anesthetic for birds. Mod. Vet. Pract. 52: 40-41.

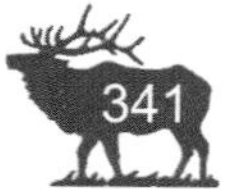

Kittle, E. L. 1972. Ketamine hydrochloride as an anesthetic for birds. Raptor Res. 6: 49-50.

Kiyota, M., T. R. Loughlin, N. Baba, M. Nakajima, and K. Kohyama. 1992. Use of a tiletamine hydrochloride zolazepam hydrochloride mixture as an immobilizing agent for northern fur seals *Callorhinus ursinus*. Honyurui Kagaku 32: 1-7 (Japanese).

Klein, L. 1980. Clinical pharmacology of agents used in the restraint of felidae and hoofed stock. Proc. Am. Assoc. Zoo Vet. Pp. 7-12.

Klein, L. V., and A. M. Klide. 1989. Central α_2-adrenergic and benzodiazepine agonists and their antagonists. J. Zoo Wildl. Med. 20: 138-153.

Klein, L., and J. Stover. 1993. Medetomidine-ketamine-isoflurane anesthesia in captive cheetah (*Acinonyx jubatus*) and antagonism with atipamezole. Proc. Am. Assoc. Zoo Vet. Pp. 144-145.

Klein, L., and S. B. Citino. 1995. Comparison of detomidine/carfentanil/ketamine and medetomidine/ketamine anesthesia in Grevy's zebra. Proc. Joint Conf. Am. Assoc. Zoo Vet., Wildl. Dis. Assoc., Am. Assoc. Wildl. Vet. East Lansing, Michigan. Pp. 290-293.

Klein, L., E. Blumer, and T. DeMaar. 1994. Cardiopulmonary and acid-base status in captive addax anesthetized with carfentanil-acetylpromazine-ketamine. Joint Conf. Am. Assoc. Zoo Vet. Assoc. Reptil. Amphib. Vet. Pp. 200-201.

Klein, L., B. L. Raphael, P. Kalk, and R. A. Cook. 1996. Immobilization of Eld's deer (*Cervus eldi*): medetomidine-ketamine versus carfentanil. Proc. Am. Assoc. Zoo Vet. Pp. 376-381.

Klide, A. M., and L. V. Klein. 1971. Chemical restraint of three reptilean species. J. Zoo An. Med. 4: 8-11.

Klide, A. M., and L. V. Klein. 1971. Restraint of two fallow deer with xylazine. J. Zoo An. Med. 4: 21.

Klingel, H. 1968. Die Immobilisation von Steppenzebras (*Equus quagga bohmi*). D. Zool. Garten. 35: 54-66.

Klöppel, G. 1962. Schwergeburt bei einem See-Elephanten. Nord. Vet. Med. 14 (Suppl. 1): 161-163.

Klöppel, G. 1965. Immobilisation und Narkode bei Zoo und Wildtieren. Berl. Münch. Tierärztl. Wochenschr. 88: 295-298.

Klöppel, G. 1969. Zur Immobilisation von Zoo- und Wildtieren. Die Kleintier-Praxis 14: 203-207.

Klos, H. G., and E. M. Lang (eds.). 1980. Handbook of Zoo Medicine. Van Nostrand Reinhold Company, New York.

Knakal, J., J. Svobodnik, and L. Hess. 1988. Initial experiences with the use of carfentanil at Prague Zoo. Veterinarstvi 38: 40-41.

Knight, A. P. 1980. Xylazine. J. Am. Vet. Med. Assoc. 176: 454-455.

Knox, C. M., J. Hattingh, and J. P. Raath. 1989. The effects of Trilafon enanthate on boma stress in the impala, *Aepyceros melampus* (Lichstenstein). S. Afr. J. Sci. 85: 335.

Knox, C. M., J. Hattingh, and J. P. Raath. 1990. The effect of tranquilizers on the immediate responses to repeated capture and handling of boma-kept impala. Comp. Biochem. Physiol. 95: 247-251.

Knox, C. M., J. Hattingh, and J. P. Raath. 1991. The effect of zeranol on body mass and physiological responses to repeated capture in boma-confined impala. So. Afr. J. Wildl. Res. 21: 38-42.

Kocan, A. A., T. R. Thedford, B. L. Glenn, M. G. Shaw, and R. Wood. 1980. Myopathy associated with immobilization in captive white-tailed deer. J. Am. Vet. Med. Assoc. 177: 879-881.

Kocan, A. A., B. L. Glenn, T. R. Thedford, R. Doyle, K. Waldrup, G. Kubat, and M. G. Shaw. 1981. Effects of chemical immobilization on hematologic and serum chemical values in captive white-tailed deer. J. Am. Vet. Med. Assoc. 179: 1153-1156.

Kocan, A. A., E. F. Blouin, and B. L. Glenn. 1985. Hematologic and serum chemical values for free-ranging bobcats, *Felis rufus* (Schreber), with reference to animals with natural infections of *Cytauxzoon felis* Kier, 1979. J. Wildl. Dis. 21: 190-192.

Koci, P. 1970. Application of injection preparations to animals with Cap-Chur pistol. Veterinarstvi 20: 568-570. (Czech)

Koci, P. 1971a. Use of Bay Va 1470, 10% Rompun preparation (Bayer, Leverkusen) for immobilization of white bearded gnus (*Connochaetes taurinus albojubatus*). Veterinarstvi 21: 132-134. (Czech)

Koci, P. 1971b. Practical results with the application of BAY Va 1470 10% (Rompun) for the immobilisation of *Hippotragus equinus*. Veterinarstvi 21: 565-567. (Czech)

Koci, P. 1972. Bay Va 1470, 10% (Rompun) its use to immobilize white bearded gnus and roan antelopes. Verhandlungsber. XIV. Internat. Symp. Erkankungen Zootiere, Wroclaw. Pp. 375-384.

Kock, M. D. 1992. Use of hyaluronidase and increased etorphine (M99) doses to improve induction times and reduce capture related stress in the chemical immobilization of free ranging black rhinoceros (*Diceros bicornis*) in Zimbabwe. J. Zoo Wildl. Med. 23: 181-188.

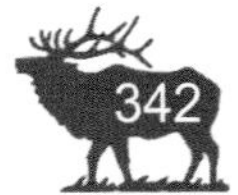

Kock, M. D. (ed.). 2001. Chemical and Physical Restraint of Wild Animals: A Course Manual. Zimbabwe Vet. Assoc. Wildl. Grp. 237 pp.

Kock, M. D., and J. Berger. 1987. Chemical immobilization of free-ranging North American bison (*Bison bison*) in Badlands National Park, South Dakota. J. Wildl. Dis. 23: 625-633.

Kock, M. D., and P. Morkel. 1993. Capture and translocation of the free-ranging black rhinoceros: medical and management problems. *In* Fowler, M. E. (ed.). Zoo & Wild Animal Medicine: Current Therapy 3. W. B. Saunders Co., Philadelphia, Pennsylvania. Pp. 466-475.

Kock, M. D., N. Kock, and A. Arif. 1984. Immobilization techniques and complications associated with bull Indian elephant (*Elephus maximus*) in musth. Proc. Am. Assoc. Zoo Vet. P. 68.

Kock, M. D., D. A. Jessup, R. K. Clark, C. E. Franti, and R. A. Weaver. 1987a. Capture methods in five subspecies of free-ranging bighorn sheep: an evaluation of drop-net, drive-net, chemical immobilization and the net gun. J. Wildl. Dis. 23: 634-640.

Kock, M. D., D. A. Jessup, R. K. Clark, and C. E. Franti. 1987b. Effects of capture on biological parameters in free-ranging bighorn sheep (*Ovis canadensis*): Evaluation of drop-net, drive-net, chemical immobilization and the net-gun. J. Wildl. Dis. 23: 641-651.

Kock, M. D., R. K. Clark, C. E. Franti, D. A. Jessup, and J. D. Wehausen. 1987c. Effects of capture on biological parameters in free-ranging bighorn sheep (*Ovis canadensis*): evaluation of normal, stressed and mortality outcomes and documentation of postcapture survival. J. Wildl. Dis. 23: 652-662.

Kock, M. D., M. la Grange, and R. du Toit. 1990a. Chemical immobilization of free-ranging black rhinoceros (*Diceros bicornis*) using combinations of etorphine (M99), fentanyl and xylazine. J. Zoo Wildl. Med. 21: 155-165.

Kock, M. D., R. du Toit, N. Kock, D. Morton, C. Foggin, M. la Grange, and B. Paul. 1990b. Effects of capture and translocation on biological parameters in free-ranging black rhinoceros (*Diceros bicornis*) in Zimbabwe. J. Zoo Wildl. Med. 21: 414-424.

Kock, M. D., R. du Toit, D. Morton, N. Kock, and B. Paul. 1990c. Baseline biological data collected from chemically immobilized free-ranging black rhinoceros (*Diceros bicornis*) in Zimbabwe. J. Zoo Wildl. Med. 21: 283-291.

Kock, M. D., R. B. Martin, and N. Kock. 1993. Chemical immobilization of free-ranging African elephants (*Loxodonta africana*) in Zimbabwe, using etorphine (M99) mixed with hyaluronidase, and evaluation of biological data collected soon after immobilization. J. Zoo Wildl. Med. 24: 1-10.

Kock, M. D., P. Morkel, M. Atkinson, and C. Foggin. 1995. Chemical immobilization of free-ranging white rhinoceros (*Ceratotherium simum simum*) in Hwange and Matobo National Parks, Zimbabwe, using combinations of etorphine (M99), fentanyl, xylazine, and detomidine. J. Zoo Wildl. Med. 26: 207-217.

Kock, M. D., D. Meltzer, and R. Burroughs. 2006. Chemical and physical restraint of wild animals. Zimbabwe Veterinary Association Wildlife Group and International Wildlife Veterinary Services (Africa). 292 pp.

Kock, R. A. 1987. Remote injection systems: science and art. Vet. Rec. 121: 76-80.

Kock, R. A., and P. C. Pearce. 1985. Anaesthesia in zoo ungulates. J. Assoc. Vet. Anaesth. 13: 59-88.

Kock, R. A., J. P. P. Harwood, P. C. Pearce, and R. N. Cinderey. 1987. Chemical immobilization of Formosan sixa deer (*Cervus nippon*): a physiological study. J. Assoc. Vet. Anaesth. 14: 120-151.

Kock, R. A., P. C. Pearce, and P. Taylor. 1988. The use of detomidine and butorphanol in zoo equids. Proc. Joint Mtg. Am. Assoc. Zoo Vet. Am. Assoc. Wildl. Vet. Pp. 188-191.

Kock, R. A., M. Jago, F. M. D. Gulland, and J. Lewis. 1989. The use of two novel alpha$_2$-adrenoceptor antagonists, idazoxan and its analogue RX821002A in zoo and wild animals. J. Assoc. Vet. Anaesth. 16: 4-10.

Kock, R. A., P. Morkel, and M. D. Kock. 1993. Current immobilization procedures used in elephants. *In* Fowler, M. E. (ed.). Zoo & Wild Animal Medicine: Current Therapy 3. W. B. Saunders Co., Philadelphia, Pennsylvania. Pp. 436-440.

Kodituwakku, G. E., K. Dissanayake, and D. Seneviratna. 1961. General anaesthesia in an elephant. Ceylon Vet. J. 9: 75-76.

Kok, O. B. 1973. Etorphine (M-99) immobilisation and associated behaviour of the red hartebeest (*Alcelaphus buselaphus caama*). J. So. Afri. Wildl. Manage. Assoc. 3: 9-15.

Kollias, G. V. Jr., and I. McLeish. 1978. Effects of ketamine hydrochloride in red-tailed hawks (*Buteo jamaicensis*) I - arterial blood gas and acid-base. Comp. Biochem. Physiol. 60C: 57-59.

Kopf, V. E., D. F. Gibson, A. Oelschlaeger, P. F. Scanlon, R. L. Kirkpatrick, and F. C. Gwazdauskas.

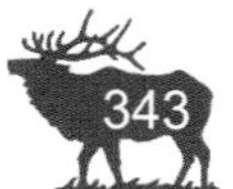

1981a. Effects of xylazine hydrochloride on thyroxine and triiodothyronine in white-tailed deer. Va. J. Sci. 32: 94.

Kopf, V. E., D. F. Gibson, T. J. Dietrick, P. F. Scanlon, and R. L. Kirkpatrick. 1981b. Xylazine hydrochloride for restraint of white-tailed deer. Va. J. Sci. 32: 94.

Koubek, P., and V. Mrlik. 1988. [Immobilization of red deer stags (*Cervus elaphus* L.) using etorphine]. Veterinarni Medicina (Czeck). 123: 375-380.

Kozlowski. J., and K. 1972. Pharmacological immobilization and anaesthesia in the lion (*Panthera leo*) for surgery. Medycyna-Weterynaryjna 28: 303–304.

Krahwinkel, D. J. 1970. The use of tiletamine hydrochloride as an incapacitating agent for a lion. J. Am. Vet. Med. Assoc. 157: 622-623.

Krahwinkel, D. J. 1970. Primate anesthesiology. J. Zoo Anim. Med. 1: 4-12.

Kraner, K. L., A. M. Silverstein, and C. J. Parshall Jr. 1965. Anesthesia in snakes. *In* Sawyer, D. C. (ed.). Symposium on Experimental Animal Anesthesiology. Brooks Air Force Base, Texas. Pp. 374-378.

Krapu, G. L. 1976. Experimental responses of mallards and Canada geese to tribromoethanol. J. Wildl. Manage. 40: 180-183.

Krasinski, Z. A., K. Cabon-Raczynska, and M. Krasinska. 1982. Immobilizing and marking of the European bison. Acta Theriol. 27: 181-190.

Krausman, P. R., J. J. Hervert, L. L. Ordway, K. Rautenstrauch, and T. Remington. 1984. Immobilization of desert mule deer with etorphine plus azaperone. *In* Krausman, P. R., and N. S. Smith (eds.). Deer in the Southwest: A Workshop. New Mexico State University, Las Cruces. Pp. 103-105.

Krausman, P. R., K. R. Rautenstrauch, J. J. Hervert, R. Remington, and L. L. Ordway. 1986. Immobilization of desert mule deer with etorphine plus azaperone. Southwest. Nat. 31: 411-414.

Krechetov, Y. N. 1980. [Catching of corvid birds with the help of narcotics]. Ornitologiya. 15: 211-212.

Kreeger, T. J. 1992. A review of chemical immobilization of wild canids. Proc. Joint Conf. Am. Assoc. Zoo Vet. and Am. Assoc. Wildl. Vet. Pp. 271-283.

Kreeger, T. J. 1999. Chemical restraint and immobilization of wild canids. *In* Fowler, M. E., and R. E. Miller (eds.). Zoo & Wild Animal Medicine. Current Therapy 4. W. B. Saunders Company, Philadelphia, Pennsylvania. Pp. 429-435.

Kreeger, T. J. 2000. Xylazine-induced aspiration pneumonia in Shira's moose. Wildl. Soc. Bull. 28: 751-753.

Kreeger, T. J. 2002. Analyses of immobilizing dart characteristics. Wildl. Soc. Bull. 30: 968-970

Kreeger, T. J., and U. S. Seal. 1986a. Failure of yohimbine hydrochloride to antagonize ketamine hydrochloride immobilization in gray wolves. J. Wildl. Dis. 22: 600-603.

Kreeger, T. J., and U. S. Seal. 1986b. Immobilization of coyotes with xylazine hydrochloride-ketamine hydrochloride and antagonism by yohimbine hydrochloride. J. Wildl. Dis. 22: 604-606.

Kreeger, T. J., and U. S. Seal. 1990. Immobilization of captive gray wolves (*Canis lupus*) with sufentanil citrate. J. Wildl. Dis. 26: 561-563.

Kreeger, T. J., G. D. Del Giudice, U. S. Seal, and P. D. Karns. 1986a. Immobilization of white-tailed deer with xylazine hydrochloride and ketamine hydrochloride and antagonism by tolazoline hydrochloride. J. Wildl. Dis. 22: 407-412.

Kreeger, T. J., G. D. Del Giudice, U. S. Seal, and P. D. Karns. 1986b. Methods of urine collection for male white-tailed deer. J. Wildl. Dis. 22: 442-445.

Kreeger, T. J., U. S. Seal, and A. M. Faggella. 1986c. Xylazine hydrochloride-ketamine hydrochloride immobilization of wolves and its antagonism by tolazoline hydrochloride. J. Wildl. Dis. 22: 397-402.

Kreeger, T. J., A. M. Faggella, U. S. Seal, L. D. Mech, M. Callahan, and B. Hall. 1987a. Cardiovascular and behavioral responses of gray wolves to ketamine-xylazine immobilization and antagonism by yohimbine. J. Wildl. Dis. 23: 463-470.

Kreeger, T. J., E. D. Plotka, and U. S. Seal. 1987b. Immobilization of white-tailed deer by etorphine and xylazine and its antagonism by nalmefene and yohimbine. J. Wildl. Dis. 23: 619-624.

Kreeger, T. J., U. S. Seal, M. Callahan, and M. Beckel. 1988. Use of xylazine sedation with yohimbine antagonism in captive gray wolves. J. Wildl. Dis. 24: 688-690.

Kreeger, T. J., R. E. Mandsager, U. S. Seal, M. Callahan, M. Beckel. 1989a. Physiological response of gray wolves to butorphanol-xylazine immobilization and antagonism by naloxone and yohimbine. J. Wildl. Dis. 25: 89-94.

Kreeger, T. J., D. Monson, V. B. Kuechle, U. S. Seal, and J. R. Tester. 1989b. Monitoring heart rate and

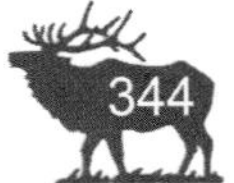

body temperature via radio telemetry in red foxes (*Vulpes vulpes*). Can. J. Zool. 67: 2455-2458.
Kreeger, T. J., U. S. Seal, and J. R. Tester. 1990a. Chemical immobilization of red foxes (*Vulpes vulpes*). J. Wildl. Dis. 26: 95-98.
Kreeger, T. J., P. J. White, U. S. Seal, and J. R. Tester. 1990b. Pathological responses of red foxes to foothold traps. J. Wildl. Manage. 54: 147-160.
Kreeger, T. J., U. S. Seal, M. Callahan, and M. Beckel. 1990c. Physiological and behavioral responses of gray wolves to immobilization with tiletamine and zolazepam (Telazol). J. Wildl. Dis. 26: 90-94.
Kreeger, T. J., U. S. Seal, J. R. Tester, M. Callahan, and M. Beckel. 1990d. Physiological responses of red foxes (*Vulpes vulpes*) to surgery. J. Wildl. Dis. 26: 162-174.
Kreeger, T. J., V. B. Kuechle, L. D. Mech, J. R. Tester, and U. S. Seal. 1990e. Physiological monitoring of gray wolves (*Canis lupus*) by radiotelemetry. J. Mammal. 71: 258-261.
Kreeger, T. J., A. S. Levine, U. S. Seal, M. Callahan, and M. Beckel. 1991. Diazepam-induced feeding in captive gray wolves (*Canis lupus*). Pharmacol. Biochem. Behav. 39: 559-561.
Kreeger, T. J., L. A. Degernes, J. S. Kreeger, and P. T. Redig. 1993. Immobilization of raptors with tiletamine and zolazepam (Telazol®). *In* Redig, P. T., J. E. Cooper, J. D. Remple, and D. Bruce Hunter (eds.). Raptor Biomedicine. University of Minnesota Press, Minneapolis. Pp. 141-144.
Kreeger, T. J., D. L. Hunter, and M. R. Johnson. 1995. Immobilization protocol for free-ranging gray wolves (*Canis lupus*) translocated to Yellowstone National Park and central Idaho. Proc. Joint Conf. Am. Assoc. Zoo Vet., Wildl. Dis. Assoc., Am. Assoc. Wildl. Vet. East Lansing, Michigan. Pp. 529-530.
Kreeger, T. J., M. Callahan, and M. Beckel. 1996. Use of medetomidine for chemical restraint of captive gray wolves (*Canis lupus*). J. Zoo Wildl. Med. 27: 507-512.
Kreeger, T. J., A. Vargas, G. E. Plumb, and E. T. Thorne. 1998. Ketamine-medetomidine or isoflurane immobilization of black-footed ferrets. J. Wildl. Manage. 62: 654-662.
Kreeger, T. J., R. Lanka, T. Smith, and T. Smeltzer. 1999. Anesthesia of pronghorn in an urban environment using carfentanil and xylazine. 18th Biennial Pronghorn Antelope Workshop 18: 69-73.
Kreeger, T. J., W. E. Cook, C. Piché, and T. Smith. 2001. Anesthesia of pronghorns with thiafentanil or thiafentanil plus xylazine. J. Wildl. Manage. 65: 25-28.
Kriek, J. C. 1992. Post-darting tranquillization of game. *In* Ebedes, H. (ed.) The Use of Tranquillizers in Wildlife. Dept. Ag. Develop., Pretoria. Bull. No. 423. Pp. 52-53.
Kroll, W. R. 1962. Experience with Sernylan in zoo animals. Int. Zoo Yb. 4: 131-141.
Kuehn, G. 1974. Anesthesia in turtles. J. Zoo An. Med. 5: 35.
Kuiken, T. 1988. Anaesthesia in the European otter (*Lutra lutra*). Vet. Rec. 123: 59.
Kumar, A., J. M. Nigam, and S. K. Sharma. 1998. Clinico-biochemical effects of xylazine in yaks. Indian J. Anim Sci. 68: 1175-1176.
Kumar, A., J. M. Nigam, and S. K. Sharma. 1999. Diazepam sedation in yaks. Indian Vet. J. 76: 211-213.
Kuntze, A. 1967. Neuroleptanalgesia in bears. Vet. Rec. 80: 278-280.
Kuntze, A. 1967. Klinische Beiträge zur Anästhesie und Medikamentellen Immobilisation der Zootiere (Ursiden, Feliden, Ruminantier). Zentralblatt für Veterinärmedizin, Beiheft 6. Pp. 1-144.
Kuntze, A. 1976. Vergleichende Betrachtungen über Phenzyklidin-Propionylpromazin und Ketaminhydrochlorid zur Narkose oder Immobilisation von Raubtieren (Löwe, Tiger, Leopard, Puma, Eisbär). 18th Int. Symp. Dis.
Zoo and Wild An. Innsbrück. Pp. 295-301.
Kuntze, A. 1977. Kritische Analyse der Erfahrungen mit Ketamin-Xylazin bei der Immobilisation oder Narkose von Grosskatzen. 19th Int. Symp. Dis. Zoo and Wild An. Pp. 399-405.
Küpper, W., N. Drager, D. Mehlitz, and U. Zillmann. 1981. On the immobilization of hartebeest and kob in Upper Volta. Tropenmed. Parasitol. 32: 58-60.
Küpper, W. 1981. Immobilisierung von freilebenden Kuhantilopen und Schwarzfussmoorantilopen. Der Praktische Tierarzt. 3: 240-244.
Küpper, W., M. Wolters, and J. Gilbert. 1982. Immobilisierung von freilebenden Schwarzfussmoorantilopen. Der Praktische Tierarzt. 63: 994-996.
Kuruwita, V. Y. 1990. Capture and translocation. *In* Proceedings of the Seminar on Conservation Plan for Elephants of Sri Lanka. Department of Wildlife Conservation, Ministry of Lands and Irrigation and Mahaweli Development of Sri Lanka. Pp. 63-69.
Kusagaya, H., and K. Sato. 2001. A safe and practical inhalation anaesthesia for Weddell seals. Polar. Biol. 24: 549-552.

Kuttner, C., and H. Wiesner. 1987. Changes in blood values in Przewalski horses (*Equus przewalski przewalski*) and zebras (*Equus zebra hartmannae*) during chemical immobilization. J. Zoo An. Med. 18: 144-147.

Lacki, M. J., P. M. Smith, W. T. Peneston, and F. D. Vogt. 1989. Use of methoxyflurane to surgically implant transmitters in muskrats. J. Wildl. Manage. 53: 331-333.

Lafortune, M., M. A. Mitchell, and J. A. Smith. 2001. Evaluation of medetomdine, clove oil, and propofol for anesthesia in leopard frogs (*Rana pipiens*). J. Herp. Med. Surg. 11: 13-18.

Lafortune, M., C. Gunkel, A. Valverde, L. Klein, and S. B. Citino. 2005. Reversible anesthetic combination using medetomidine-butorphanol-midazolam (MBMZ) in cheetahs (*Acinonyx jubatus*). Proc. Am. Assoc. Zoo Vet. Pp. 270.

Laisher. 1972. Anesthesia of reindeer. Veterinariya. 5: 76-78.

Lamberski, N., A. Newell, and R. W. Radcliffe. 2004. Thirty immobilizations of captive giraffe (*Giraffa camelopardalis*) using a combination of medetomidine and ketamine. Proc. Am. Assoc. Zoo Vet. Pp. 118-120.

Lammintausta, R., O. Vaino, R. Virtanen, and T. Vähä-Vahe (eds.). 1989. Medetomidine, a novel alpha$_2$-agonist for veterinary sedative and analgesic use. Acta Vet. Scand. Suppl. 85. 202 pp.

Lance, W. R. 1991. New pharmaceutical tools for the 1990's. Proc. Am. Assoc. Zoo Vet. Pp. 354-359.

Lancia, R. A., R. P. Brooks, and M. W. Flemming. 1978. Ketamine hydrochloride as an immobilant and anesthetic for beaver. J. Wildl. Manage. 42: 946-948.

Landowska-Plazewska, E. 1970. Erfahrungen mit der Anwendung des Präparates Bay-Va-1470 bei Wildtieren im Zoo Warszawa. 12th Int. Symp. Dis. Zoo and Wild An. Budapest. Pp. 147-151.

Langan, J. N., J. Schumacher, C. Pollock, S. E. Orosz, M. P. Jones, and R. C. Harvey. 2000a. Cardiopulmonary and anesthetic effects of medetomidine-ketamine-butorphanol and antagonism with atipamezole in servals (*Felis serval*). J. Zoo Wildl. Med. 31: 329-334.

Langan, J. N., E. C. Ramsay, J. T. Blackford, and J. Schumacher. 2000b. Cardiopulmonary and sedative effects of intramuscular medetomidine- ketamine and intravenous propofol in ostriches (*Struthio camelus*). J. Avian Med. Surg. 14: 2-7.

Lange, R. E. 1982. Chemical immobilization of North American mule deer. *In* Nielsen, L., J. C. Haigh, and M. E. Fowler (eds.). Chemical Immobilization of North American Wildlife. Wisconsin Humane Society, Inc. Milwaukee, Wisconsin. Pp. 363-369.

Langenberg, J. A., N. K. Businga, and H. E. Nevill. 1998. Capture of wild sandhill cranes with alpha-chloralose: techniques and physiological effects. Proc. Joint Conf. Am. Assoc. Zoo Vet. and Am. Assoc. Wildl. Vet. Pp. 50-53.

Langman, V. A. 1973. The immobilization and capture of giraffe. So. Afr. J. Sci. 69: 200-203.

Langrehr, D., and R. Muller. 1967. Significence of CI-581 (ketamine) for anesthesiology in veterinary medicine with special attention to zoo animals. 9th Int. Symp. Dis. Zoo and Wild An., Prague.

Lanphear, P. R. 1963. Tranquilization and immobilization of wild animals. J. Am. Vet. Med. Assoc. 142: 1126-1129.

Lanthier, C., R. E. A. Stewart, and E. W. Born. 1999. Reversible anesthesia of Atlantic walruses (*Odobenus rosmarus rosmarus*) with carfentanil antagonized with naltrexone. Mar. Mamm. Sci. 15: 241-249.

Larivière, S. L. and F. Messier. 1996. Immobilization of striped skunks with Telazol®. Wildl. Soc. Bull. 24: 713-716.

Larivière, S. L. and F. Messier. 2000. Field anesthesia of striped skunks, *Mephitis mephitis*, using halothane. J. Wildl. Rehabil. 23: 10-12.

Larivière, S., L. R. Walton, and J. A. Virgl. 2000. Field anesthesia of American mink, *Mustela vison*, using halothane. Can. Field Natur. 114: 142-144.

Larivière, S., L. R. Walton, and J. A. Virgl. 2001. Field anesthesia of American mink (*Mustela vison*) using halothane. J. Wildl. Rehabil. 24: 18-20.

Larsen, R. S., A. Moresco, and K. E. Glander. 1999. Field anesthesia and capture techniques of free-ranging mantled howling monkeys (*Alouatta paliatta*) in Costa Rica. Proc. Am. Assoc. Zoo Vet. Pp. 243-247.

Larsen, R. S., M. R. Loomis, B. Kelly, A. B. Beyer, K. K. Sladky, M. K. Stoskopf, and W. A. Horne. 2001. Immobilization of red wolves (*Canis rufus*) using medetomidine and butorphanol. Proc. Am. Assoc. Zoo Vet. Pp. 171-175.

Larsen, R. S., M. R. Loomis, B. T. Kelly, K. K. Sladky, M. K. Stoskopf, and W. A. Horne. 2002. Cardiorespiratory effects of medetomidine-butorphanol, medetomidine-butorphanol-diazepam, and

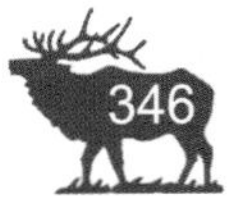

medetomidine-butorphanol-ketamine in captive red wolves (*Canis rufus*). J. Zoo Wildl. Med. 33: 101-107.

Larsen, L. H. 1963. Restraint and anesthesia of wild animals in captivity. Austral. Vet. J. 39: 73-80.

Larsen, T. 1966. The trapping and study of polar bears, Spitsbergen 1966. Polar Record. 13: 587-593.

Larsen, T. 1971. Capture, handling, and marking polar bears in Svalbard, Norway. J. Wildl. Manage. 35: 27-36.

Lateur, N., and P. Stolk. 1986. Repeated general anaesthesia in a male Indian elephant. Proc. Am. Assoc. Zoo Vet. Pp. 128-131.

Lawrence, K., and O. F. Jackson. 1983. Alphaxalone/alphadolone anaesthesia in reptiles. Vet. Rec. 112: 26-28.

Lawson, D., M. Hampton, and C. Morewood. 1987. A custom-built capture rifle for immobilizing small antelopes. Lammergeyer. 38: 8-11.

Lawson, D., M. Hampton, and C. Morewood. 1987. A modification of the Palmer Cap-chur gas-powered capture rifle. So. Afr. J. Wildl. Res. 17: 136-138.

Lawson, D. M., and D. Melton. 1989. A radio-tagged game capture dart. So. Afr. J. Wildl. Res. 19: 99-101.

LeBlanc, P. H., S. W. Eicker, M. Curtis, and B. Beehler. 1987. Hypertension following etorphine anesthesia in a rhinoceros (*Diceros simus*). J. Zoo An. Med. 18: 141-143.

Lee, A. F. 1981. Drugs, anesthetics and toxic conditions in alligators. Proc. Ann. Alligator Production Conf. 1: 52-57.

Lee, J., R. Schweinsburg, F. Kernan, and J. Haigh. 1981. Immobilization of polar bears (*Ursus maritimus*, Phipps) with ketamine hydrochloride and xylazine hydrochloride. J. Wildl. Dis. 17: 331-336.

Leege, T., and M. W. Schlegel. 1974. Study VI: Evaluation of long range immobilization equipment and new drugs on big game animals. Progress Report W-160-R. Idaho Fish and Game Pp. 21-22.

Lees, P., and C. J. Hillidge. 1976. Immobilon: some comments on its action. Vet. Rec. 99: 55-56.

Lemm, C. A. 1993. Evaluation of five anesthetics on striped bass. U. S. Fish & Wildl. Serv. Resource Pub. 196: 1-10.

Lentfer, J. W. 1968. A technique for immobilizing and marking polar bears. J. Wildl. Manage. 32: 317-321.

Lentz, W. M., R. L. Marchinton, L. B. Flynn, S, M. Shea, and P. J. Stuart. 1986. The immobilisation of sambar deer with succinylcholine chloride. Austrl. Deer 11: 3-11.

Letcher, J. D. 1992. Intracelomic use of tricaine methanesulfonate for anesthesia of bullfrogs (*Rana catesbeiana*) and leopard frogs (*Rana pipiens*). Zoo Biol. 11: 243-251.

Letcher, J. D., and S. Amsel. 1989. Practitioners guide to anesthesia in anurans. Compend. Anim. Pract. 19: 21-24.

Letcher, J., and R. Durante. 1995. Evaluation of use of tiletamine/zolazepam for anesthesia of bullfrogs and leopard frogs. J. Am. Vet. Med. Assoc. 207: 80-80-82.

Lewandowski, A. H., C. J. Bonar, and S. E. Evans. 2002. Tiletamine-zolazepam, ketamine, and xylazine anesthesia of captive cheetah (*Acinonyx jubatus*). J. Zoo Wildl. Med. 33: 332-336.

Lewis, J. C. M. 1991. Reversible immobilisation of Asian small-clawed otters with medetomidine and ketamine. Vet. Rec. 128: 86-87.

Lewis, J. C. M. 1993. Medetomidine-ketamine anaesthesia in the chimpanzee (*Pan troglodytes*). J. Vet. Anaesth. 20: 18-20.

Lewis, J. C. M. 2004. Field use of isoflurane and air anesthetic equipment in wildlife. J. Zoo Wildl. Med. 35: 303-311.

Lewis, J. W., K. W. Bentley, and A. Cowan. 1971. Narcotic analgesics and antagonists. Ann. Rev. Pharmacol. 11: 241-270.

Lewis, R. J., G. A. Chalmers, M. W. Barrett, and R. Bhatnagar. 1977. Capture myopathy in elk in Alberta, Canada: A report of three cases. J. Am. Vet. Med. Assoc. 171: 927-932.

Lietsch, C. D. 1969. L'immobilisation des elephants. Cahiers Bleus Veterinaries. 16: 35-39.

Lightfoote, W. E., and G. F. Molinari. 1978. Comparison of ketamine and pentobarbital anesthesia in the Mongolian gerbil. Am. J. Vet. Res. 39: 1061-1063.

Lin, H. C., and J. C. H. Ko. 1997. Anesthetic management of ratites. Compend. Cont. Educ. Pract. Vet. 19: S127.

Lin, H. C., J. C. Thurmon, G. J. Benson, and W. J. Tranquilli. 1993a. Immobilization and anesthesia of two hand-reared zebras. J. Am. Vet. Med. Assoc. 202: 988-990.

Lin, H. C., J. C. Thurmon, G. J. Benson, and W. J. Tranquilli. 1993b. Telazol - a review of its pharmacol-

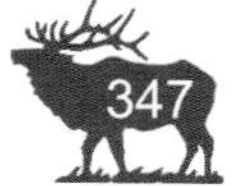

ogy and use in veterinary medicine. J. Vet. Pharmacol. Ther. 16: 383-418.

Lin, H. C., P. G. Todhunter, T. A. Powe, and D. C. Ruffin. 1997. Use of xylazine, butorphanol, tiletamine-zolazepam, and isoflurane for induction and maintenance of anesthesia in ratites. J. Am. Vet. Med. Assoc. 210: 244.

Lindau, K. H., and M. Gorgas. 1969. Versuche mit Bay VA 1470. Int. Symp. Dis. Zoo and Wild An. Zagreb. 11: 135-137.

Ling, J. K., and D. G. Nicholls. 1963. Immobilization of elephant seals using succinylcholine chloride. Nature 200: 1021-1022.

Ling, J. K., D. G. Nicholls, and C. D. B. Thomas. 1967. Immobilization of southern elephant seals with succinylcholine chloride. J. Wildl. Manage. 31: 468-479.

Linklater, W. L., E. Z. Cameron, K. J. Stafford, and T. Austin. 1998. Chemical immobilization and temporary confinement of two Kaimanawa feral stallions. N. Z. Vet. J. 46: 117-118.

Linn, K. 1986. Guidelines for avian anesthesia. Norden News. 61: 22-24.

Linnehan, R. M., and A. D. MacMillan. 1991. Propofol/isoflurane anesthesia and debridement of a corneal ulcer in an Atlantic bottlenosed dolphin (*Tursiops truncatus*). Proc. Am. Assoc. Zoo Vet. Pp. 290-291.

Liscinsky, S. A., G. P. Howard, and R. B. Waldeisen. 1969. A new device for injecting powdered drugs. J. Wildl. Manage. 33: 1037-1038.

Litchford, R. G., and R. M. Durham. 1977. Surgery on a red-tailed hawk (*Buteo jamaicensis gmelin*). J. Tennesee Acad. Sci. 52: 110-111.

Lloyd, M. L. 1999. Crocodilian anesthesia. *In* Fowler, M. E., and R. E. Miller (eds.). Zoo & Wild Animal Medicine. Current Therapy 4. W. B. Saunders Company, Philadelphia, Pennsylvania. Pp. 205-216.

Lloyd, M. L., T. Reichard, and R. A. Odum. 1994. Gallamine reversal in Cuban crocodiles (*Crocodylus rhombifer*) using neostigmine alone versus neostigmine with hyaluronidase. Proc. Joint Conf. Am. Assoc. Zoo Vet. Assoc. Reptil. Amphib. Vet. Pp. 117-120.

Lochmiller, R. L., and W. E. Grant. 1983. A sodium bicarbonate-acid powered blow-gun syringe for remote injection of wildlife. J. Wildl. Dis. 19: 48-51.

Lock, B. A., D. J. Heard, and P. Dennis. 1998. Preliminary evaluation of medetomidine/ketamine combinations for immobilization and reversal with atipamezole in three tortoise species. Bull. Assoc. Rept. Amphib. Vet. 8:6-9.

Lock, J. A., and A. M. Harthoorn. 1959a. A note on the use of suxamethonium chloride (succinylcholine chloride) for restraint of zebra. Vet. Rec. 71: 334.

Lock, J. A., and A. M. Harthoorn. 1959b. The use of succinylcholine chloride (suxamethonium chloride) for the control and management of wild animals. Vet. Rec. 71: 919-920.

Lockie, J. D., and M. G. Day. 1966. The use of anaesthesia in the handling of stoats and weasels. *In* Jones, O. G. (ed.). Symposium on Small Mammal Anesthesia. Pergamon Press, Oxford. Pp. 187-189.

Logan, K. A., E. T. Thorne, L. L. Irwin, and R. Skinner. 1986. Immobilizing wild mountain lions (*Felis concolor*) with ketamine hydrochloride and xylazine hydrochloride. J. Wildl. Dis. 22: 97-103.

Loibl, M. F., U. S. Clutton, B. D. Marx, and C. J. McGrath. 1988. Alpha-chloralose as a capture and restraint agent of birds: therapeutic index determination in the chicken. J. Wildl. Dis. 24: 684-687.

Loomis, M. R., and E. C. Ramsay. 1999. Anesthesia for captive Nile hippopotamus. *In* Fowler, M. E., and R. E. Miller (eds.). Zoo & Wild Animal Medicine. Current Therapy 4. W. B. Saunders Company, Philadelphia, Pennsylvania. Pp. 638-639.

López González, C. A., A. González-Romero, J. W. Laundré, L. Cantú Salazar, M. G. Hidalgo Mihart, A. De Villa Meza, E. Martínez Meyer, and Ma. Antonieta Casariego. 1998. Field immobilization of pygmy spotted skunks from Mexico. J. Wildl. Dis. 34: 186-189.

Loughlin, T. R., and T. Spraker. 1989. Use of Telazol to immobilize female northern sea lions (*Eumetopias jubatus*) in Alaska. J. Wildl. Dis. 25: 353-358.

Louw, A. J. 1957. The use of chlorpromazine hydrochloride (Largactil-Maybaker) in anesthesia of brown bear (*Ursus arctos*). J. So. Afr. Vet. Assoc. 28: 261-263.

Love, J. A. 1970. Use of fentanyl and droperidol in guinea pigs, lemmings, ground squirrels, and cats. J. Am. Vet. Med. Assoc. 157: 675-677.

Loveridge, J. P. 1979. The immobilization and anaesthesia of crocodilians. Int. Zoo Yb. 19: 103-112.

Loveridge, J. P., and D. K. Blake. 1972. Techniques in the immobilization and handling of the Nile crocodile, *Crocodylus niloticus*. Arnoldia (Rhod.). 40: 1-14.

Loveridge, J. P., and D. K. Blake. 1987. Crocodile immobilization and anaesthesia. *In* Webb, G. J. W., C.

Manolis, P. and J. Whitehead (eds.). Wildlife Management: Crocodiles and Alligators. Surrey Beatty & Sons Pty Ltd, Chipping Norton, NSW, Australia. Pp. 259-267.

Lovett, J. W., and E. P. Hill. 1977. A transmitter syringe for recovery of immobilized deer. J. Wildl. Manage. 41: 313-315.

Low, R. J. 1973. Immobilon in deer. Vet. Rec. 93: 86-87.

Lu, J., C. Yu, C. Liang, Y. Ding, and D. Sun. 1992. A study on immobilization of Pere David's deer with miannaining. Forest research 5: 601-605 (Chinese).

Ludders, J. W., and A. D. Ojerio. 1980. Brief observations on handling and chemical restraint of the rat kangaroo (*Potorous tridactylus*). J. Zoo An. Med. 11: 106-108.

Ludders, J. W., C. J. Sedgwick, S. V. Manley, and S. S. Haskins. 1982. Anesthesia for restraint and transportation of five lowland gorillas (*Gorilla gorilla*). J. Zoo An. Med. 13: 78-81.

Ludders, J. W., J. A. Rode, and G. S. Mitchell. 1987. The effective dose and cardiopulmonary effects of isoflurane in sandhill cranes (*Grus canadensis*) during spontaneous ventilation. Vet. Surg. 16: 322.

Lumeij, J. T. 1986. Anesthetic fatalities in goshawks. Conf. Avian Dis. 5: 201-207.

Lydersen, C., D. Griffiths, I. Gjertz, and Ø. Wiig. 1992. A tritiated water experiment on male Atlantic walrus (*Odobenus rosmarus rosmarus*). Mar. Mamm. Sci. 8: 418-420.

Lynch, G. M., and J. A. Hanson. 1981. Use of etorphine to immobilize moose. J. Wildl. Manage. 45: 981-985.

Lynch, G. M., W. Hall, B. Pelchat, and J. A. Hanson. 1982. Chemical immobilization of black bear with special reference to the use of ketamine-xylazine. *In* Nielsen, L., J. C. Haigh, and M. E. Fowler (eds.). Chemical Immobilization of North American Wildlife. Wisconsin Humane Society, Inc. Milwaukee, Wisconsin. Pp. 245-266.

Lynch, M. J., A. D. M. E. Oosterhaus, D. V. Cousins, P. Selleck, and P. Williams. 1999. Anesthesia, hematology and disease investigation of free-ranging crabeater seals (*Lobodon carcinophagus*). Proc. Am. Assoc. Zoo Vet. Pp. 41-42.

Lynch, M. J., M. A. Tahmindjis, and H. Gardner. 1999. Immobilisation of pinniped species. Aust. Vet. J. 77: 181-185.

Lynch, S., and S. Line. 1985. Failure of yohimbine to reverse ketamine anesthesia in rhesus monkeys. Lab. An. Sci. 35: 7-8.

Lyon, D. G., and D. C. Dinning. 1973. Veterinary laboratory - annual report 1973. North of England Zoological Society, Chester Zoological Gardens. Pp. 14-16.

Maas, A., and D. Brunson. 2002. Comparison of anesthetic potency and cardiopulmonary effects of isoflurane and sevoflurane in colubrid snakes. Proc. Am. Assoc. Zoo Vet. Pp. 306-308.

Mac Lentz, W., R. L. Marchinton, L. B. Flynn, S. M. Shea, and P. J. Stuart. 1986. The immobilization of sambar deer with succinylcholine chloride. Austral. Deer. 11: 3-9.

Macek, D. 1987. Immobilization of some species of big game animals. Trans. Congr. Int. Union Game Biol. 18: 108-109.

Machado, C. R., C. W. Furley, and H. Hood. 1983. Observations on the use of M99, immobilon and xylazine in the Arabian oryx (*Oryx leucoryx*). J. Zoo An. Med. 14: 107-110.

Machin, K. 2004. Waterfowl anesthesia. Semin. Avian Exotic Pet Med. 13: 206-212.

Machin, K. L., and N. A. Caulkett. 1996. The cardiopulmonary effects of propofol in mallard ducks. Proc. Am. Assoc. Zoo Vet. Pp. 149-153.

Machin, K. L., and N. A. Caulkett. 1998a. Cardiopulmonary effects of propofol and a combination of medetomidine-midazolam-ketamine in mallard ducks. Am. J. Vet. Res. 59:598-602.

Machin, K. L., and N. A. Caulkett. 1998b. Investigation of injectable anesthetics in mallard ducks (*Anas platyrhynchos*): a descriptive study. J. Avian Med. Surg. 12:255-262.

Machin, K. L., and N. A. Caulkett. 1999. Cardiopulmonary effects of propofol infusion in canvasback ducks (*Aythya valisineria*). J. Avian Med. Surg. 13:167-172.

Machin, K. L., and N. A. Caulkett. 2000. Evaluation of isoflurane and propofol anesthesia for intraabdominal transmitter placement in nesting female canvasback ducks. J. Wildl. Dis. 36:324-334.

MacKintosh, C. G. 1985. Potential antidote for Rompun (xylazine) in humans. N. Z. Med. J. 98: 714-715.

MacKintosh, C. G., and G. Van Reenen. 1984a. Yohimbine injection in deer. N. Z. Vet. J. 32: 217-218.

MacKintosh, C. G., and G. Van Reenen. 1984b. Comparison of yohimbine, 4-aminopyridine and doxapram antagonism of xylazine sedation in deer (*Cervus elaphus*). N. Z. Vet. J. 32: 181-184.

MacKintosh, C. G., J. A. MacArthur, T. W. A. Little, and P. Stuart. 1976. The immobilization of the badger (*Meles meles*). Br. Vet. J. 132: 609-614.

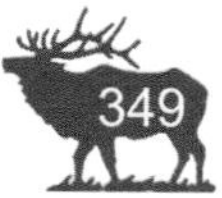

MacLean, R. A., C. A. Harms, and J. Braun-McNeill. 2005. Propofol anesthesia in loggerhead sea turtles (*Caretta caretta*). Proc. Am. Assoc. Zoo Vet. Pp. 296-297.

Maddock, A. H. 1989. Anaesthesia of four species of viverridae with ketamine. So. Afr. J. Wildl. Res. 19: 80-84.

Magonigle, R. A., E. H. Stauber, and H. W. Vaughn. 1977. The immobilization of wapiti with etorphine hydrochloride. J. Wildl. Dis. 13: 258-261.

Mainka, S. A., and T. He. 1993. Immobilization of healthy male giant pandas (*Ailuropoda melanoleuca*) at the Wolong nature reserve. J. Zoo Wildl. Med. 24: 430-433.

Majonica, I., and C. H. Bonath. 1993. Tiletamine-zolazepam immobilisation of East African oryx antelopes (*Oryx beisa callotis*). J. Vet. Anaesth. 20: 53.

Malmstrom, T., R. Salte, H. M. Gjoen, and A. Linseth. 1993. A practical evaluation of metomidate and MS-222 as anaesthetics for Atlantic halibut (*Hippoglossus hippoglossus* L.). Aquaculture 113: 331-338.

Mama, K. R., L. G. Phillips, and P. J. Pascoe. 1996. Use of propofol for induction and maintenance of anesthesia in a barn owl (*Tyto alba*) undergoing tracheal resection. J. Zoo Wildl. Med. 27: 397-401.

Mama, K. R., E. P. Steffey, and S. J. Withrow. 2000. Use of orally administered carfentanil prior to isoflurane-induced anesthesia in a Kodiak brown bear. J. Am. Vet. Med. Assoc. 217: 546-549.

Mandelker, L. 1993. The dosages and drawbacks of propofol. Vet. Forum (Nov.). P. 36.

Manton, V. J. A. 1964. Immobilisation of wild animals. Vet. Rec. 76: 707-708.

Manton, V. J. A., and D. M. Jones. 1974. Scientific report 1971-1973, Whipsnade Park. J. Zool., Lond. 173: 84-97.

Marini, R. P., L. R. Jackson, M. I. Esteves, K. A. Andrutis, C. M. Goslant, and J. G. Fox. 1994. Effect of isoflurane on hematologic values in ferrets. Am. J. Vet. Res. 55: 1479-1483.

Maritz, T. 1993. Chemical capture of the hippopotamus *Hippopotamus amphibius*. *In* McKenzie, A. A. (ed.). The Capture and Care Manual. Wildlife Decision Support Services and The South African Veterinary Foundation, Pretoria. Pp. 571-574.

Marlow, B. J. 1956. Chloral hydrate narcosis for the live capture of mammals. CSIRO Wildl. Res. 1: 63-65.

Marma, B. B. 1970. [Immobilizing roe deer for transportation]. Trans. Congr. Int. Union Game Biol. 9: 182-184.

Marsboom, R. 1969. On the pharmacology of azaperone, a neuroleptic for the restraint of wild animals. Acta Zool. Path. Antver. 48: 155-161.

Marsboom, R. 1985. Immobilization of wild animals with carfentanil - a review. Trans. Congr. Int. Union Game Biol. 17: 803-810.

Marsboom, R., J. Mortelmans, and J. Vercruysse. 1963. Neuroleptanalgesia in monkeys. Vet. Rec. 75: 132-133.

Marsboom, R., J. Mortelmans, and J. Vercruysse. 1964. A new hypnotic agent in birds. Int. Zoo Yb. 5: 200-201.

Marsboom, R., and J. Mortelmans. 1964. Some pharmacological aspects of analgesics and neuroleptiques and their use for neuroleptanalgesia in primates and lower monkeys. Sm. Anim. Anesth. Symp. London. Pp. 31-44.

Marsboom, R., J. Mortelmans, J. Vercruysse, and D. Thienpont. 1962. Effective sedation and anesthesia in gorillas and chimpanzee. Nord. Vet. Med. 14: 95-101.

Martin, L. L. 1967. Comparison of methoxymol, alpha-chloralose and two barbituates for capturing doves. Proc. Ann. Conf. Southeast. Assoc. Game Fish Comm. 21: 193-200.

Martyn, E. 1955. Pentobarbital sodium as an anesthetic for bears. J. Am. Vet. Med. Assoc. 127: 415.

Masangkay, J. S., T. Namikawa, V. G. Momongan, and R. Escalada. 1993. The use of xylazine for the restraint of captive tamaraw (*Bubalus mondorensis*). Phillipine J. Vet. Med. 30: 37-38.

Massolo, A., A. Sforzi, and S. Lovari. 2003. Chemical immobiliation of crested porcupines with tiletamine HCL and zolazepam HCL (Zoletil®) under field conditions. J. Wildl. Dis. 39: 727-731.

Mathews, F., P. Honess, and S. Wolfensohn. 2002. Use of inhalation anaesthesia for wild mammals in the field. Vet. Rec. 150: 785-787.

Mathieu-Nolf, M., M. A. Babe, V. Coquelle-Couplet, C. Billaut, P. Nisse, and D. Mathieu. 2001. Flumazenil use in an emergency department: A survey. J. Toxicol. Clin. Toxicol. 39: 15-20.

Matschke, G. H., and V. G. Henry. 1969a. Immobilizing European wild hogs with Cap-Chur gun. Proc. Ann. Conf. Southeast. Assoc. Game Fish Comm. 23: 185-188.

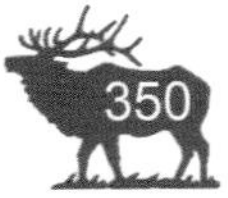

Matschke, G. H., and V. G. Henry. 1969b. Immobilizing European wild hogs with succinylcholine chloride. J. Wildl. Manage. 33: 1039-1041.

Matthews, M. 1971. The use of ketamine to immobilize a black leopard. J. Zoo An. Med. 2: 25.

Matthews, M. 1977. Capturing desert bighorn sheep in Baja California, Mexico. J. Zoo An. Med. 8: 9-10.

Matthews, N. S., and M. W. Meyers. 1993. The use of tiletamine-zolazepam for darting feral horses. J. Equine Vet. Sci. 13: 264-267.

Matthews, N. S., K. R. Petrini, and P. L. Wolff. 1995. Anesthesia of Przewalski's horses (*Equus przewalskii przewalskii*) with medetomidine-ketamine and antagonism with atipamezole. J. Zoo Wildl. Med. 26: 231-236.

Mattingly, B. E. 1972. Injectable anesthetic for raptors. Raptor Res. 6: 51-52.

Mautz, W. W., U. S. Seal, and C. B. Boardman. 1980. Blood serum analyses of chemically and physically restrained white-tailed deer. J. Wildl. Manage. 44: 343-351.

Mazzi, A. 1994. Sedation and anaesthesia in wild Artiodactyla, Cervidae, Camelidae, Bovidae. Obiettivi e Documenti Veterinari 15: 11-17.

McAllum, H. J. 1977. Some veterinary techniques used in New Zealand deer farming. N. Z. Vet. J. 25: 130-131.

McColl, C. J., and R. Boonstra. 1999. Physiological effects of three inhalant anesthetics on Arctic ground squirrels. Wildl. Soc. Bull. 27:946-951.

McCorquodale, S. M. Eberhardt, and S. E. Petron. 1988. Helicopter immobilization of elk in southcentral Washington. Northwest Sci. 62: 49-52.

McDonnel, W. 1972. Anesthesia of the harp seal. J. Wildl. Dis. 8: 287-295.

McFarland, W. N., and G. W. Klontz. 1969. Anaesthesia in fishes. Fed. Proc. 28: 1535-1540.

McGrath, C. J., R. J. Farnsworth, E. A. Usenik, M. Wise, P. N. Ogburn, A. J. Crimi, M. Wright, M. R. Raffe, and N. Burtnick. 1979. Anesthesia in a California sea lion using a bain breathing circuit. J. Zoo An. Med. 10: 129-135.

McJames, S. W., I. L. Smith, T. H. Stanley, and G. Painter. 1993. Elk immobilization with potent opioids: A-3080 vs. carfentanil. Proc. Am. Assoc. Zoo Vet. Pp. 418-419.

McJames, S. W., J. F. Kimball, and T. H. Stanley. 1994. Immobilization of moose with A-3080 and reversal with nalmefene HCL or naltrexone HCL. Alces 30: 21-24.

McKean, T. A., and B. Magonigle. 1978. The effect of immobilization with M-99 plus acepromazine on physiological parameters of domestic goats. J. Wildl. Manage. 42: 176-179. 113

McKelvey, W. A. C., and C. A. Simpson. 1985. Reversal of the effects of xylazine and xylazine/ketamine in red deer. Vet. Rec. 117: 362-363.

McKenzie, A. A. 1989. Increasing the rate of recovery of projectile syringes and of animals darted at night. So. Afr. J. Vet. Res. 19: 85-86.

McKenzie, A. A. (ed.). 1993. The Capture and Care Manual. Wildlife Decision Support Services and The South African Veterinary Foundation, Pretoria. 729 pp.

McKenzie, A. A., and R. E. J. Burroughs. 1993. Chemical capture of carnivores. *In* McKenzie, A. A. (ed.). The Capture and Care Manual. Wildlife Decision Support Services and The South African Veterinary Foundation, Pretoria. Pp. 224-243.

McKintosh, C. G., and G. Van Reenen. 1984. Comparison of yohimbine, 4-aminopyridine and doxapram antagonism of xylazine sedation in deer (*Cervus elaphus*). New Zealand Vet. J. 32: 181-184.

McLaren, G. W., P. D. Thornton, C. Newman, C. D. Buesching, S. E. Baker, F. Mathews, and D. W. MacDonald. 2005a. High rectal temperature indicates an increased risk of unexpected recovery in anaesthetized badgers. Vet. Anaesth. Analg. 32: 48-52.

McLaren, G. W., P. D. Thornton, C. Newman, C. D. Buesching, S. E. Baker, F. Mathews, and D. W. MacDonald. 2005b. The use and assessment of ketamine-medatomidine-butorphanol combinations for field anaesthsia in wild European badgers (*Meles meles*). Vet. Anaesth. Analg. 32: 367-372.

McLaughlin, C. R. 1993. Notes on the use of Telazol® on denned black bears. Int. Bear News. 2: 1.

McMahon, C. R., H. Burton, S. McLean, D. Slip, and M. Bester. 2000. Field immobilisation of southern elephant seals with intravenous tiletamine and zolazepam. Vet. Rec. 146: 251-254.

McMahon, C., J. vandenHoff, and H. Burton. 2005. Handling intensity and short- and long-term survival of elephant seals: addressing and quantifying research effects on wild animals. Ambio. 34: 426-429.

McNaught P. 1991. Husbandary hint – a tranquilizer dart puller. Animal Keepers' Forum, 18: 126-127.

McWade, D. H. 1982. An evaluation of ketamine and xylazine in combination as agents for the remote chemical immobilization of feral and stray dogs. *In* Nielsen, L., J. C. Haigh, and M. E. Fowler (eds.).

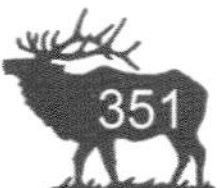

Chemical Immobilization of North American Wildlife. Wisconsin Humane Society, Inc. Milwaukee, Wisconsin. Pp. 175-187.

Mech, L. D. 1965. Sodium pentobarbital as an anesthetic for raccoons. J. Mammal. 46: 343-344.

Mech, L. D. 1974. Current techniques in the study of elusive wilderness carnivores. Trans. Congr. Int. Union Game Biol. 11: 315-322.

Mech, L. D., and E. M. Gese. 1992. Field testing the Wildlink capture collar on wolves. Wildl. Soc. Bull. 20: 221-223.

Mech, L. D., R. C. Chapman, W. W. Cochran, L. Simmons, and U. S. Seal. 1984. Radio-triggered anesthetic-dart collar for recapturing large mammals. Wildl. Soc. Bull. 12: 69-74.

Mech, L. D., G. D. Del Giudice, P. D. Karns, and U. S. Seal. 1985. Yohimbine hydrochloride as an antagonist to xylazine hydrochloride-ketamine hydrochloride immobilization of white-tailed deer. J. Wildl. Dis. 21: 405-410.

Mech, L. D., K. Kunkel, R. C. Chapman, and T. J. Kreeger. 1990. Field testing of a commercially manufactured capture collar on white-tailed deer. J. Wildl. Manage. 54: 297-299.

Medway, W., J. G. McCormick, S. H. Ridgway, and J. F. Crump. 1970. Effects of prolonged halothane anesthesia on some cetaceans. J. Am. Vet. Med. Assoc. 157: 576-582.

Meert, T. F. 1996. Pharmacotherapy of opioids: present and future developments. Pharm. World Sci. 18: 1-15.

Mehren, K. G., and W. A. Rapley. 1975. The use of Dopram to counteract the effects of Rompun-induced immobilization in captive ungulates. Proc. Am. Assoc. Zool. Parks Aquaria. Pp. 48-53.

Melby, E. C., and H. J. Baker. 1965. Phencyclidine and anesthesia in simian primates. J. Am. Vet. Med. Assoc. 147: 1068.

Melton, C. A. 1980. Baboon (*Papia ursinus*) capture using a blow-dart system. So. Afr. J. Wildl. Res. 10: 67-70.

Melton, D. A., and C. Melton. 1982. Immobilisation and blood analyses of baboons (*Papio ursinus*) in the Okavango swamp. Botswana Notes Rec. 13: 119-122.

Meltzer, D. G. A., R. Burroughs, F. G. Stegmann, A. R. Hargens, R. W. Millard, K. Johansen, D. H. Gershuni, K. Petterson, and W. Van Hoven. 1985. The capture and restraint of giraffe (*Giraffa camelopardalis*) for blood and interstitial fluid pressure studies. *In* Dawson, P. (ed.). Exotic Animals in Research. So. Afr. Assoc. Lab. Anim., Pretoria. Pp. 42-46.

Meritt, D. A. 1972. Edentate immobilisation at Lincoln Park Zoo, Chicago. Int. Zoo Yrbk. 12: 218-220.

Meritt, D. A. 1974. A further note on the immobilisation of sloths *Choloepus* spp. Int. Zoo Yrbk. 14: 160-161.

Merriam, H. 1962. Immobilisation technique of free-ranging sitka black-tail deer in southeast Alaska. Alaska Dept. Fish Game Infor. Leafl. 18.

Merwin, D. S., J. J. Millspaugh, G. C. Brundige, D. Schultz, and C. L. Tyner. 1999. Immobilization of free-ranging Rocky Mountain bighorn ewes with Telazol and xylazine hydrochloride. Trans. 2nd No. Am. Wild Sheep Conf. Pp. 263.

Merwin, D. S., J. J. Millspaugh, G. C. Brundige, D. Schultz, and C. L. Tyner. 2000. Immobilization of free-ranging Rocky Mountain bighorn sheep, *Ovis canadensis canadensis*, ewes with Telazol and xylazine hydrochloride. Can. Field Natur. 114: 471-475.

Meshcherskii, R. M., N. V. Menyailov, I. S. Shepeleva, I. I. Korenev, Y. A.Toporov, I. A. Gorelov, and I. S. Ivanov. 1978. Narcotization of the porpoises without blocking their own respiration. Zhurnal Evolyutsionnoi Biokhmii i Fiziologii. 14: 410-411.

Messel, H., and D. R. Stephens. 1980. Drug immobilization of crocodiles. J. Wildl. Manage. 44: 295-296.

Metcalfe, J., J. T. Parer, M. Rur, D. El-Yassin, J. Oufi, H. Bartels, K. Riegel, and E. Kleihauer. 1968. Cardiodynamics of the Dromedary camel (*Camelus dromedarius*) during phencyclidine analgesia. Am. J. Vet. Res. 29: 2063-2066.

Meuleman, T., J. D. Port, T. H. Stanley, K. F. Williard, and J. Kimball. 1984. Immobilization of elk and moose with carfentanil. J. Wildl. Manage. 48: 258-262.

Meyer, F. A. 1959. Use of tranquillizer drugs for moving bears at John Ball Zoo, U.S.A. Int. Zoo Yb. 2: 308-309.

Mikalsen, R., and J. M. Arnemo. 1993. Immobilization of elk with Rompun. Norsk Veterinaer. 105: 1230-1231.

Mikota, S., S. G. Kamerling, and S. A. Barker. 1999. Serum concentrations and behavioral effects of oral haloperidol in bongo antelope (*Tragelaphus eurycerus*). Proc. Am. Assoc. Zoo Vet. Pp. 364-366.

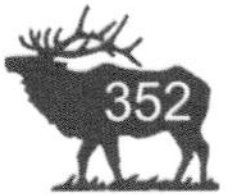

Miller, B. F., L. I. Muller, T. N. Storms, E. C. Ramsay, D. A. Osborn, R. J. Warren, K. V. Miller, and K. A. Adams. 2003. A comparison of carfentanil/xylazine and Telazol®/xylazine for immobilization of white-tailed deer. J. Wildl. Dis. 39: 851-858.

Miller, B. F., L. I. Muller, T. Doherty, D. A. Osborn, K. V. Miller, and R. J. Warren. 2004. Effectiveness of antagonists for tiletamine-zolazepam/xylazine immobilization in female white-tailed deer. J. Wildl. Dis. 40: 533-537.

Miller, F. L. 1968. Immobilization of free-ranging black-tailed deer with succinylcholine chloride. J. Wildl. Manage. 32: 195-197.

Miller, M., M. Weber, B. Mangold, and D. Neiffer. 2000. Use of oral detomidine and ketamine for anesthetic induction in nonhuman primates. Proc. Joint Conf. Am. Assoc. Zoo Vet. and Intl. Assoc. Aquatic An. Med. Pp. 179-180.

Miller, M., M. Weber, D. Neiffer, B. Mangold, D. Fontenot, and M. Stetter. 2003. Anesthetic induction of captive tigers (*Panthera tigris*) using medetomidine-ketamine combination. J. Zoo Wildl. Med. 34: 307-308.

Miller, M. W., M. A. Wild, and W. R. Lance. 1996. Efficacy and safety of naltrexone hydrochloride for antagonizing carfentanil citrate immobilization in captive Rocky Mountain elk (Cervus elaphus nelsoni). J. Wildl. Dis. 32: 234-239.

Miller, R. L., and G. B. Will. 1974. The use of M99 etorphine and antagonists to immobilize and handle black bears. Third Int. Conf. Black Bears. Pp. 225-234.

Miller, R. L., and G. B. Will. 1976. The use of M99 etorphine and antagonists to immobilize and handle black bears. *In* Pelton, M. R., J. W. Lentfer, and G. E. Folk Jr. (eds.). Bears - Their Biology and Management. IUCN Publ. New Ser. 40. Pp. 247-260.

Miller, R. L., E. R. McCaffrey, and G. B. Will. 1973. Recent capture and handling techniques for black bears in New York. Trans. Northeast Fish Wildl. Conf. 30: 117-137.

Miller, R. M. 1979. Exotic carnivores. Vet. Clin. North Am. [Sm. Anim. Pract.]. 9: 569-580.

Miller, S. M., M. A. Mitchell, J. J. Heatley, T. Wolf, F. Lapuz, M. Lafortune, J. A. Smith. 2005. Clinical and cardiorespiratory effects of propofol in the spotted bamboo shark (*Chylloscyllium plagiosum*). J. Zoo Wildl. Med. 36: 673-676.

Miller-Edge, M., and S. Amsel. 1994. Carfentanil, ketamine, xylazine combination (CKX) for immobilization of exotic ungulates; clinical experience in bongo (*Tragelaphus euryceros*) and mountain tapir (*Tapirus pinchaque*). Joint Conf. Am. Assoc. Zoo Vet. Assoc. Reptil. Amphib. Vet. Pp. 192-195.

Millspaugh, J. J., G. C. Brundige, J. A. Jenks, C. L. Tyner, and D. R. Hunstead. 1995. Immobilization of Rocky Mountain elk with Telazol® and xylazine hydrochloride, and antagonism by yohimbine hydrochloride. J. Wildl. Dis. 31: 259-262.

Millspaugh, J. J., B. E. Washburn, T. M. Meyer, J. Beringer, and L. P. Hansen. 2004. Immobilization of clover-trapped white-tailed deer, *Odocoileus virginianus*, with medetomidine and ketamine, and antagonism with atipamezole. an. Field Natur. 118: 185-190.

Mitchell, P. J., and H. R. Burton. 1991. Immobilization of southern elephant seals and leopard seals with cyclohexamine anaesthetics and xylazine. Vet. Rec. 129: 332-336.

Mitcheltree, D. H., T. L. Serfass, W. M. Tzilkowski, R. L. Peper, M. T. Whary, and R. P. Brooks. 1999. Physiological responses of fishers to immobilization with ketamine-xylazine, or Telazol®. Wildl. Soc. Bull. 27: 582-591.

Miyabe, T., R. Nishimura, M. Mochizuki, and S. Sasaki. 2001. Chemical restraint by medetomidine and medetomidine-midazolam and its reversal by atipamezole in Japanese macaques (*Macaca fuscata*). Vet. Anaesth. Analg. 28: 168-174.

Moller, H. 1983. An apparatus for anaesthetizing small mammals. J. Zool. London. 201: 579-581.

Monson, D. H., C. McCormick, and B. E. Ballachey. 2002. Chemical anesthesia of northern sea otters (*Enhydra lutra*): results of past field studies. J. Zoo Wildl. Med. 32: 181-189.

Montané, J., J. López-Olvera, D. Perpiñá, X. Manteca, and S. Lavín. 2003. Effects of acepromazine on capture stress in roe deer (*Capreolus capreolus*). J. Wildl. Dis. 39: 375-386.

Montgomery, G. G. 1961. A modification of the nicotine dart capture method. J. Wildl. Manage. 25: 101-102.

Montgomery, G. G, and R. E. Hawkins. 1967. Diazepam baiting for capture of white-tailed deer. J. Wildl. Manage. 31: 464-468.

Moon, P. F., and E. K. Stabenau. 1996. Anesthetic and postanesthetic management of sea turtles. J. Am.

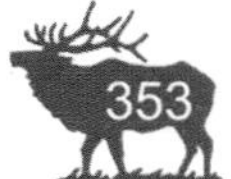

Vet. Med. Assoc. 208: 720-726.
Moran, J. F., F. Ballesteros, P. Quiros, and J. Benito. 1994. Immobilization of wild Spanish Cantabrian chamois (*Rupicapra rupicapra*). J. Vet. Anaesth. 21: abstract.
More, G. 1977. Immobilization of marten with sodium pentobarbital. J. Wildl. Manage. 41: 796-798.
Moreland, A. F., and C. Glaser. 1985. Evaluation of ketamine, ketamine-xylazine and ketamine-diazepam anesthesia in the ferret. Lab. An. Sci. 35: 287-290.
Moresco, A., R. S. Larsen, J. M. Sleeman, M. A. Wild, and J. S. Gaynor. 2000. Use of naloxone to reverse carfentanil citrate-induced hypoxemia and cardiopulmonary depression in Rocky Mountain wapiti (*Cervus elaphus nelsoni*). Proc. Joint Conf. Am. Assoc. Zoo Vet. and Intl. Assoc. Aquatic An. Med. Pp. 264-265.
Moresco, A., R. S. Larsen, J. M. Sleeman, M. A. Wild, and J. S. Gaynor. 2001. Use of naloxone to reverse carfentanil citrate-induced hypoxemia and cardiopulmonary depression in Rocky Mountain wapiti (*Cervus elaphus nelsoni*). J. Zoo Wildl. Med. 32: 81-89.
Moresco, A. 2002. Medetomidine-ketamine-butorphanol combinations in biturongs (*Arctictis binturong*). Proc. Am. Assoc. Zoo Vet. Pp. 426-427.
Morgan, R. J., L. B. Eddy, T. N. Solie, and C. C. Turbes. 1981. Ketamine-acepromazine as an anaesthetic agent for chinchillas (*Chinchilla laniger*). Lab. An. 15: 281-283.
Morgan-Davies, A. M. 1980. Immobilization of the Nile crocodile (*Crocodilus niloticus*) with gallamine triethiodine. J. Zoo An. Med. 11: 85-87.
Morin, P., and D. Berteaux. 2003. Immobilization of North American porcupines (*Erethizon dorsatum*) using ketamine and xylazine. J. Wildl. Dis. 39: 675-682.
Morkel, P. 1989. Drugs and dosages for capture and treatment of black rhinoceros *Diceros bicornis* in Namibia. Koedoe 10: 65-68.
Morkel, P. 1992a. Depot neuroleptics in roan antelope. *In* Ebedes, H. (ed.) The Use of Tranquillizers in Wildlife. Dept. Ag. Develop., Pretoria. Bull. No. 423. Pp. 38-39.
Morkel, P. 1992b. Giraffe capture with etorphine HCL (M-99) and hyalase - a new approach. *In* Ebedes, H. (ed.) The Use of Tranquillizers in Wildlife. Dept. Ag. Develop., Pretoria. Bull. No. 423. Pp. 58-59.
Morkel, P. 1993a. Prevention and management of capture drug accidents. *In* McKenzie, A. A. (ed.). The Capture and Care Manual. Wildlife Decision Support Services and The South African Veterinary Foundation, Pretoria. Pp. 100-115.
Morkel, P. 1993b. Chemical capture of the giraffe *Giraffa camelopardalis*. *In* McKenzie, A. A. (ed.). The Capture and Care Manual. Wildlife Decision Support Services and The South African Veterinary Foundation, Pretoria. Pp. 601-606.
Morley, J. E. 1981. The endocrinology of the opiates and opioid peptides. Metabolism. 30: 195-209.
Morris, M. A. 1986. Anesthesia of snakes (*Pituophis melanoleucus* and *Python regius*) fed ether-killed rats. Herpertol. Rev. 17: 88.
Morris, P. J. 1992. Evaluation of potential adjuncts for equine chemical immobilization. Proc. Joint Conf. Am. Assoc. Zoo Vet. and Am. Assoc. Wildl. Vet. Pp. 235-250.
Morris, P. J. 1996. Recent developments in anesthesia of exotic ungulates. Proc. No. Am. Vet. Conf. Pp. 901-902.
Morris, P. J., E. Bicknese, D. Janssen, M. Sutherland-Smith, A. Shima, L. Young, and J. Zuba. 2000. Chemical immobilization of takin (*Budorcas taxicolor*) at the San Diego Zoo. Proc. Joint Conf. Am. Assoc. Zoo Vet. and Intl. Assoc. Aquatic An. Med. Pp. 102-105.
Mortelmans, J. 1971. L'Anesthesie des animaux sauvages. Ann. Med. Vet. 5: 317-332.
Mortelmans, J. 1978. Anesthesia in okapis. Acta Zool. Pathol. Antverpiensia. 71: 41-44.
Mortelmans, J., and J. Vercruysse. 1971. Immobilization and analgesia in wild animals in captivity. Int. Symp. Dis. Zoo and Wild An. Pp. 203-204.
Mortelmans, J., J. Vercruysse, D. Thienpont, R. Marsboom, R. Van Brabant, and B. Van Puÿenbroeck. 1972. Immobilisation, analgésie et narcose chez ruminants sauvages en captivité. Verhandlungsber. XIII. Symp. Erkankungen Zootiere, Helsinki. Pp. 125-129.
Mortenson, J. 1994. Oral carfentanil citrate use in white-handed gibbons (*Hylobates lar*). Joint Conf. Am. Assoc. Zoo Vet. Assoc. Reptil. Amphib. Vet. P. 163.
Mortenson, J., and U. Bechert. 1996. Carfentanil citrate as an oral anesthetic agent for brown bears (*Ursus arctos*). Proc. Am. Assoc. Zoo Vet. Pp. 518-525.
Mortenson, J., and U. Bechert. 2002. Carfentanil citrate used as an oral anesthetic agent for brown bears

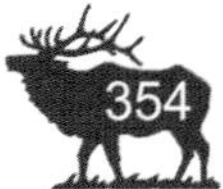

(*Ursus arctos*). J. Zoo Wildl. Med. 32: 217-221.
Morton, D. J., and M. D. Kock. 1991. Stability of hyaluronidase in solution with etorphine and xylazine. J. Zoo Wildl. Med. 22: 345-347.
Mosby, H. S., and D. E. Canter. 1956. The use of Avertin in capturing wild turkeys and as an oral-based anesthetic for other wild animals. Southwest. Vet. 9: 132-136.
Mosley, C. A., D. Dyson, and D. A. Smith. 2003a. Minimum alveolar concentration of isoflurane in gree iguanas and the effect of butorphanol on minimum alveolar concentration. J. Am. Vet. Med. Assoc. 222: 1559-1564.
Mosley, C. A., D. Dyson, and D. A. Smith. 2003b. The cardiac anesthetic index of isoflurane in green iguanas. J. Am. Vet. Med. Assoc. 222: 1565-1568.
Mosley, C. A., D. Dyson, and D. A. Smith. 2004. The cardiovascular dose-response effects of isoflurane alone and combined with butorphanol in the green iguana (*Iguana iguana*). Vet. Anaesth. Analg. 31: 64-72.
Mudappa, D., and R. Chellam. 2001. Capture and immobilization of wild brown palm civets in Western Ghats. J. Wildl. Dis. 37: 383-386.
Mugera, G. M., and J. G. Wandera. 1967. Degenerative polymyopathies in East African domestic and wild animals. Vet. Rec. 80: 410-413.
Muir, W. W., J. A. E. Hubbell, R. T. Skarda, and R. M.Bednarski. 2000. Handbook of veterinary anesthesia. Mosby, St. Louis, Mo. 574 pp.
Mulcahy, D. M., P. Tuomi, and R. S. Larsen. 2003. Differential mortality of male spectacled eiders (*Somateria fischeri*) and king eiders (*Somateria spectabilis*) subsequent to anesthesia with propofol, bupivacaine, and ketoprofen. J. Avian Med. Surg. 17: 117-123.
Mulder, J. B. 1978a. Anesthesia in the coyote using a combination of ketamine and xylazine. J. Wildl. Dis. 14: 501-502.
Mulder, J. B. 1978b. Anesthesia in the mouse using a combination of ketamine and promazine. Lab. An. Sci. 28: 70-71.
Mulder, J. B., and H. B. Johnson. 1978. Ketamine and promazine for anesthesia in the rat. J. Am. Vet. Med. Assoc. 173: 1152-1153.
Mulder, J. B., and J. J. Hauser. 1984. A device for anesthesia and restraint of snakes. Vet. Med. Small Anim. Clin. 79: 936-937.
Mulder, J. B., H. B. Johnson, G. S. McKee, and S. E. Sellers. 1979. Anesthesia with Ketaset Plus in guinea pigs and hamsters. Vet. Med. Sm. Anim. Clin. 1807-1808.
Muller, K., E. Schettler, K. Frolich, and L. Brunnberg. 2005. Development of body temperature under ketamine-xylazine-injection anaesethesia in combination with isoflurane in North American river otters (*Lutra canadensis*). Kleintierprax. 50: 429-434.
Mülling, M., and H. Henning. 1971. The use of Bay Va 1470 ("Rompun") for the capture of wild animals (Red, Fallow and Roe deer). Vet. Med. Rev. 1: 73-83.
Muraleedharan, K. N., K. Chandrasekharan, J. V. Cheeran, and K. Radhakrishnan. 1979. General anaesthesia in an elephant (*Elephas maximus*) - a clinical case report. Kerala J. Vet. Sci. 10: 197-200.
Murdoch, C. A. 1971. A history of the syringe weapon. Tussock Grassl. Mt. Lakes Inst. Rev. 21: 22-30.
Murray, M. G., A. R. Lewis, and A. M. Coetzee. 1981. An evaluation of capture techniques for research on impala populations. So. Afr. J. Wildl. Res. 11: 105-109.
Murray, S. S. L. Monfort, L. Ware, W. J. McShea, and M. Bush. 2000. Anesthesia in female white-tailed deer using Telazol® and xylazine. J. Wildl. Dis. 36: 670-675.
Murry, R. E. 1964. Tranquilized deer. Louisiana Conservationist 14: 8-9.
Murry, R. E. 1965. Tranquilizing techniques for capturing deer. Proc. Ann. Conf. Southeast. Assoc. Game Fish Comm. 19: 4-15.
Murry, R. E., and D. Dennett. 1963. A preliminary report on the use of tranquilizing compounds in capturing wildlife. Proc. Ann. Conf. Southeast. Assoc. Game Fish Comm. 17: 134-139.
Murton, R. K., A. J. Isaacson, and N. J. Westwood. 1963. The use of baits treated with α-chloralose to catch wood-pigeons. Ann. Appl. Biol. 52: 271-293.
Murton, R. K., A. J. Isaacson, and N. J. Westwood. 1965. Capturing columbids at the nest with stupefying baits. J. Wildl. Manage. 29: 647-649.
Mutlow, A., R. Isaza, J. W. Carpenter, D. E. Koch, and R. P. Hunter. 2004. Pharmacokinetics of carfentanil and naltrexone in domestic goats (*Capra hircus*). J. Zoo Wildl. Med. 35: 489-496.
Naccarato, E. F., and W. S. Hunter. 1979. Anaesthetic effects of various ratios of ketamine and xylazine in

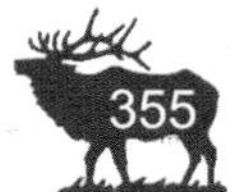

rhesus monkeys (*Macaca mulatta*). Lab. An. 13: 317-319.

Nagel, E. L., P. J. Morgane, and W. L. McFarland. 1964. Anesthesia for the bottlenose dolphin, *Tursiops truncatus*. Science 146: 1591.

Nair, N. R. 1977. The art of scientific immobilisation of animals. Indian Forester. 103: 64-79.

Neal, L. A., R. S. Custer, and M. Bush. 1981. Ketamine anesthesia in pigeons (*Columba livia*): Arterial blood gas and acid-base status. J. Zoo An. Med. 12: 48-51.

Neiffer, D. L., M. A. Miller, M. Weber, M. Stetter, D. K. Fontenot, P. K. Robbins, and G. W. Pye. 2005. Standing sedation in African elephants (*Loxodonta africana*) using detomidine-butorphanol combinations. J. Zoo Wildl. Med. 36: 250-256.

Nel, P. J., A. Taylor, D. G. A. Meltzer, and M. A. Haupt. 2000. Capture and immobilisation of aardvark (*Orycteropus afer*) using different drug combinations. J. S. Afr. Vet. Assoc. 71: 58-63.

Nesbitt, S. A. 1976. Capturing sandhill crane with oral tranquilizers. Proc. Int. Crane Workshop. 1: 296-298.

Nesbitt, S. A. 1984. Effects of an oral tranquilizer on survival of sandhill cranes. Wildl. Soc. Bull. 12: 387-388.

Nesterov, G. A. 1972. [Observations on survival periods of fur seals after ditilinum injection]. Izv. Tikhookean. Nauchno-Issled. Inst. Rybn. Khoz. Okeanogr. 70: 232-233.

Nevalainen, T., L. Pyhälä, H.-M. Voipio, and R. Virtanen. 1989. Evaluation of anesthetic potency of medetomidine-ketamine combination in rate, guinea pigs and rabbits. Acta Vet. Scand. Suppl. 85. Pp. 139-143.

Ngai, S. H., B. A. Berkowitz, J. C. Yang, J. Hempstead, and S. Spector. 1976. Pharmacokinetics of naloxone in rats and in man. Anesthesiology. 44: 398-401.

Nichols, D. K., and E. W. Lamirande. 1994. Use of methohexital sodium as an anesthetic in two species of colubrid snakes. Joint Conf. Am. Assoc. Zoo Vet. Assoc. Reptil. Amphib. Vet. Pp. 161-162.

Nicholls, P. K., T. A. Bailey, C. A. Baker, and K. Wilson. 1996. Anesthesia of the grey duiker (*Sylvicapra grimmia*) using a combination of ketamine and xylazine with reversal by atipamezole. J. Zoo Wldl. Med. 27: 49-53.

Nielsen, L. 1982a. Chemical Immobilization in Urban Animal Control Work. Wisconsin Humane Society, Inc. Milwaukee, Wisconsin. 93 pp.

Nielsen, L. 1982b. Electronic ground tracking of white-tailed deer chemically immobilized with a combination of etorphine and xylazine hydrochloride. *In* Nielsen, L., J. C. Haigh, and M. E. Fowler (eds.). Chemical Immobilization of North American Wildlife. Wisconsin Humane Society, Inc. Milwaukee, Wisconsin. Pp. 355-362.

Nielsen, L. 1982c. The use of chemical immobilization in urban animal control work. *In* Nielsen, L., J. C. Haigh, and M. E. Fowler (eds.). Chemical Immobilization of North American Wildlife. Wisconsin Humane Society, Inc. Milwaukee, Wisconsin. pp. 165-174.

Nielsen, L. 1984. Chemical capture of stray and feral animals, part II. Community Animal Control. Pp. 11-29.

Nielsen, L. 1999. Chemical immobilization of wild and exotic animals. Iowa State University Press. 342 p.

Nielsen, L., J. C. Haigh, and M. E. Fowler (eds). 1982. Chemical immobilization of North American Wildlife. Wisconsin Humane Society, Inc. Milwaukee, Wisconsin. 447 pp.

Nielson, A. E., and W. M. Shaw. 1967. A helicopter dart technique for capturing moose. Proc. Western Assoc. Game Fish Comm. 47: 182-199.

Nordan, H. C., A. J. Wood, and I. M. Cowan. 1962. Further studies on the immobilization of deer with succinylcholine. Can. J. Comp. Med. Vet. Sci. 26: 246-248.

Norment, J. L., C. L. Elliot, and P. S. Costello. 1994. Another look at chemical immobilization of raccoons (*Procyon lotor*) with ketamine hydrochloride. J. Wildl. Dis. 30: 541-544.

Norton, T. M., J. Spratt, J. Behler, and K. Hernandez. 1998. Medetomidine and ketamine anesthesia with atipamezole reversal in private free-ranging gopher tortoises, *Gopherus polyphemus*. Proc. Assoc. Reptil. Amphib. Vet. Pp. 25-27.

Nowak, R. M. 1999. Walker's Mammals of the World (6th ed.). The Johns Hopkins University Press, Baltimore. 1,936 pp.

Noyes, D. H., and D. M. Siekierski. 1975. Anesthesia of marmots with sodium pentobarbital, ketamine hydrochloride, and a combination of droperidol and fentanyl. Lab. An. Sci. 25: 557-562.

Nutter, F. B., M. Haulena, and S. A. Bai. 1998. Preliminary pharmacokinetics of single-dose intramuscular butorphanol in elephant seals (*Mirounga angustirostris*). Proc. Joint Conf. Am. Assoc. Zoo Vet

and Am. Assoc. Wildl. Vet. Pp. 372-373.
Øen, E. O. 1980. Drug immobilization and anaesthesia of a lynx in connection with a broken leg. Nord. Vet. Med. 32: 318-320.
Øen, E. O. 1982. A new darting gun for the capture of wild animals. Nord. Vet. Med. 34: 39-43.
Ofri, R., I. Horowitz, S. Jacobson, and P. H. Kass. 1998. The effects of anesthesia and gender in intraocular pressure in lions (*Panthera leo*). J. Zoo Wildl. Med. 29: 307-310.
O'Gara, B. W. 1987. A preliminary evaluation of carfentanil citrate and xylazine hydrochloride for immobilizing pronghorns. Wildl. Soc. Bull. 15: 549-551.
Ogunranti, J. O. 1987. Some physiological observation on ketamine hydrochloride anaesthesia in the agamid lizard. Lab. An. 21: 183-187.
Okaeme, A. N., E. A. Agbelusi, J. Mshelbwala, M. Wari, A. Ngulge, and M. Haliru. 1988. Effects of immobilon and revivon in the immobilization of Western kob (*Kobus kob kob*). Afr. J. Ecol. 26: 63-67.
Olsen, C. D., and L. A. Renecker. 1985. Xylazine immobilization of wapiti: antagonism with yohimbine and 4-aminopyridine. *In* Nelson, R. W. (ed.). Proc. 1984 Western States and Provinces Elk Workshop. P. 176.
Olson, M. E., and K. McCabe. 1986. Anesthesia in the Richardson's ground squirrel: comparison of ketamine, ketamine and xylazine, droperidol and fentanyl, and sodium pentobarbital. J. Am. Vet. Med. Assoc. 189: 1035-1037.
Onuma, M. 2003. Immobilization of sun bears (*Helarctos malayanus*) with medetomidine-zolazepam-tiletamine. J. Zoo Wildl. Med. 34: 202-205.
Oosterhuis, J. E. 1979. Immobilization of nondomestic equidae at the San Diego wild animal park (1975-1979). Proc. Am. Assoc. Zoo Vet. Pp. 118-119.
Oppenheim, Y. C., and P. F. Moon. 1995. Sedative effects of midazolam in red-eared slider turtles (*Trachemys scripta elegans*). J. Zoo Wildl. Med. 26: 409-413.
Orbanyi, I. 1972. Kiserletek nehany emlosfaj immobilizalasara. [Experiments for the immobilization of some mammal species]. Allattani Kozl. 59: 111-117.
Orr, C. M. 1977. Accidental self-injection. Vet. Rec. 100: 574.
Orr, D. J. C., and S. M. Moore-Gilbert. 1964. Field immobilisation of young wildebeest with succinylcholine chloride. East Africa Wildl. J. 2: 60-66.
Ortega, J. J. Z., and J. I. Otter. 1967. Phencyclidine for capture of stray dogs. J. Am. Vet. Med. Assoc. 150: 772-776.
Osen, H., J. M. Arnemo, and N. J. C. Tyler. 1994. Sedation with medetomidine and its reversal with atipamezole reduces voluntary food intake in reindeer. 3d Intl. Congr. Biol. Deer, Edinburgh, Scotland (Abstract).
Osofsky, S. A. 1995. Pulse oximetry monitoring of free-ranging African elephants (*Loxodonta africana*) immobilized with an etorphine/hyaluronidase combination antagonized with diprenorphine. Proc. Joint Conf. Am. Assoc. Zoo Vet., Wildl. Dis. Assoc., Am. Assoc. Wildl. Vet. East Lansing, Michigan. Pp. 273-277.
Osofsky, S. A. 1997. A practical anesthesia monitoring protocol for free-ranging adult African elephants (*Loxodonta africana*). J. Wildl. Dis. 33: 72-77.
Osofsky, S. A. and K. J. Hirsch. 2000. Chemical restraint of endangered mammals for conservation purposes: a practical primer. Oryx 34:27-33.
Osofsky, S. A., J. W. McNutt, and K. J. Hirsch. 1995. Immobilization and monitoring of free-ranging wild dogs (*Lycaon pictus*) using a ketamine/xylazine/atropine combination, yohimbine reversal and pulse oximetry. Proc. Joint Conf. Am. Assoc. Zoo Vet., Wildl. Dis. Assoc., Am. Assoc. Wildl. Vet. East Lansing, Michigan. Pp. 278-279.
Osofsky, S. A., J. W. McNutt, and K. J. Hirsch. 1996. Immobilization of free-ranging African wild dogs (*Lycaon pictus*) using a ketamine/xylazine/atropine combination. J. Zoo Wildl. Med. 27: 528-532.
Ostrowski, S. and M. Ancrenaz. 1995. Chemical immobilization of red-necked ostriches (*Struthio camelus*) under field conditions. Vet. Rec. 136: 145-147.
Pachaly, J. R., and P. R. Werner. 1998. Restraint of the paca (*Agouti paca*) with ketamine hydrochloride, acetylpromazine maleate, and atropine sulfate. J. Zoo Wildl. Med. 29: 303-306.
Pade, K. 1974. Ein Beitrag zur Immobilisation von Zootieren. Kleintierpraxis 19: 249-280.
Padilla, L. 2004. Immobilization of babirussa (*Babyroussa babyroussa*) using a butrophanol-tiletamine-zolazepam combination. Proc. Am. Assoc. Zoo Vet. Pp. 606-607.

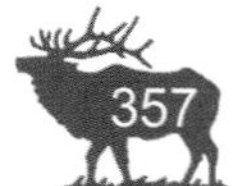

Page, C. D. 1986. Sloth bear immobilization with a ketamine-xylazine combination: reversal with yohimbine. J. Am. Vet. Med. Assoc. 189: 1050-1051.

Page, C. D. 1993. Current reptilian anesthesia procedures. *In* Fowler, M. E. (ed.). Zoo & Wild Animal Medicine: Current Therapy 3. W. B. Saunders Co., Philadelphia, Pennsylvania. Pp. 140-143.

Page, C. D. 1994. Anesthesia and chemical restraint. *In* Mikota, S. K., E. L. Sargent, and G. S. Ranglack (eds.). Medical Management of the Elephant. Indira Publishing House, West Bloomfield, Michigan. Pp. 41-49.

Palomares, F., and M. Delibes. 1992. Immobilization of Egyptian mongooses *Herpestes ichneumon* with a combination of ketamine and xylazine. Zeitschrift fuer Saeugetierkunde 57: 251-252.

Palomares, F. 1993. Immobilization of common genets, *Genetta genetta*, with a combination of ketamine and xylazine. J. Wildl. Dis. 29: 174-176.

Pang, D. S. J., Y. Rondenay, L. Measures, and S. Lair. 2006. The effects of two dosages of midazolam on short-duration anesthesia in the harp seal (*Phoca groenlandica*). J. Zoo Wildl. Med. 37: 27-32.

Paponov, V. A. 1978. Immobilization of sika deer (*Cervus nippon hortulorum* S.) by means of a ditillin (anectin) paste. Congr. Theriol. Int. 2: 305.

Páras, A., M. A. Benitez, D. M. Brousset., D. Aurioles, S. Luque, and C. Godinez. 1998. Anesthesia of California sea lions (*Zalophus californianus*) in eleven reproductive rookeries of the Gulf of California, Mexico. Proc. Joint Conf. Am. Assoc. Zoo Vet. and Am. Assoc. Wildl. Vet. Omaha, Nebraska. Pp. 425-429.

Páras, A., O. Martínez, and A. Hernández. 2002a. Alpha-2 agonist in combination with butorphanol and tiletamine-zolazepam for the immobilization of non-domestic hoofstock. Proc. Am. Assoc. Zoo Vet. Pp. 194-197.

Páras, A., D. M. Brousset, S. Salazar, and D. Aurioles. 2002b. Field anesthesia of two species of pinnipeds (*Arctocephalus galapagoensis* and *Zalophus wollebaeki*) found in the Galapagos islands. Proc. Am. Assoc. Zoo Vet. Pp. 431-433.

Paras-Garcia, A., C. R. Forester, S. M. Hernandez, and D. Leandro. 1996. Immobilization of free-ranging Baird's tapir (*Tapirus bairdii*). Proc. Am. Assoc. Zoo Vet. Pp. 12-15.

Parker, J. B. R., and J. C Haigh. 1982. Human exposure to immobilizing agents. *In* Nielsen, L., J. C. Haigh, and M. E. Fowler (eds.). Chemical Immobilization of North American Wildlife. Wisconsin Humane Society, Inc. Milwaukee, Wisconsin. Pp. 119-136.

Parry, K., S. S. Anderson, and M. A. Fedak. 1981. Chemical immobilization of gray seals. J. Wildl. Manage. 45: 986-990.

Patenaude, R. P. 1979. Evaluation of fentanyl citrate, etorphine hydrochloride, and naloxone hydrochloride in captive polar bears. J. Am. Vet. Med. Assoc. 175: 1006-1007.

Patenaude, R. P. 1982a. Chemical immobilization of North American caribou. *In* Nielsen, L., J. C. Haigh, and M. E. Fowler (eds.). Chemical Immobilization of North American Wildlife. Wisconsin Humane Society, Inc. Milwaukee, Wisconsin. pp. 370-379.

Patenaude, R. P. 1982b. Chemical immobilization of North American muskox. *In* Nielsen, L., J. C. Haigh, and M. E. Fowler (eds.). Chemical Immobilization of North American Wildlife. Wisconsin Humane Society, Inc. Milwaukee, Wisoconsin. pp. 439-447.

Paterson, J. M., N. A. Caulkett, and M. R. Woodbury. 2006. Comparative physiologic effects during carfentanil-xylazine anesthesia in North American elk (*Cervus elaphus*) supplemented with nasopharyngeal medical air or oxygen. Proc. Am. Assoc. Zoo Vet. Pp. 226-227.

Pathak, S. C., A. Mukit, J. Saikia, and J. Lekharu. 1985. Excision of a leiomyofibroma in a leopard (*Panthera pardus*) under ketamine anesthesia. J. Zoo An. Med. 16: 125-126.

Patrick, D. 1971. Immobilisation of topi. East African Wildl. J. 9: 152.

Payton, A. J., and J. R. Pick. 1989. Evaluation of a combination of tiletamine and zolazepam as an anesthetic for ferrets. Lab. An. Sci. 39: 243-246.

Peacock, A. 2005. Drug acquisition. *In* Cattet, M., T. Shury, and R. Patenaude (eds.). The chemical immobilization of wildlife, 2nd ed. Canadian Association of Zoo and Wildlife Veterinarians. pp. 4/1-4/13.

Pearce, P. C., C. Gustavo, F. Gulland, and J. Knight. 1985. Immobilization of pygmy hippopotamus (*Choeropsis liberiensis*). J. Zoo An. Med. 16: 104-106.

Pearce, P. C., L. Dorr, and R. Kock. 1985. "Anaesthetic death" in a black fallow deer. Vet. Rec. 116: 591-593.

Pearce, P. C., and R. Kock. 1989a. Physiological effects of etorphine, acepromazine and xylazine on black

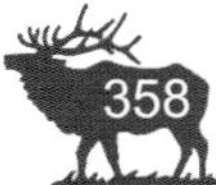

fallow deer (*Dama dama*). Res. Vet. Sci. 46: 380-386.

Pearce, P. C., and R. Kock. 1989b. Physiological effects of etorphine, acepromazine and xylazine on scimitar horned oryx (*Oryx dammaha*). Res. Vet. Sci. 47: 78-83.

Pearson, A. M., R. M. Bradley, and R. T. McLaughlin. 1968. Evaluation of phencyclidine hydrochloride and other drugs for immobilizing grizzly and black bears. J. Wildl. Manage. 32: 532-537.

Pearson, A. M., and D. W. Halloran.1972. Hematology of the brown bear (*Ursus arctos*) from southwestern Yukon Territory, Canada. Can. J. Zool. 50: 279-286.

Pearson, H. A., A. D. Smith, and P. J. Urness. 1963. Effects of succinylcholine chloride on mule deer. J. Wildl. Manage. 27: 297-299.

Pedersen, R. J., and J. W. Thomas. 1975. Immobilization of Rocky Mountain elk using powdered succinylcholine chloride. U.S. For. Ser. Res. Note. PNW 240: 4.

Pedersen, R. J., and A. A. Pedersen. 1975. Blood chemistry and haematology of elk. J. Wildl. Manage. 39: 617-620.

Pedersoli, W. M. 1970. The use of drugs in the capture and restraint of wild animals. Auburn Vet. Pp. 57-59, 84-85.

Peek, F. W. 1972. The effect of tranquilization upon territory maintenance in the male red-winged blackbird (*Agelaius phoeniceus*). An. Behav. 20: 119-122.

Peek, J. M. 1966. Chlordiazepoxide and pentobarbital as tranquilizers for cowbirds and coturnix quail. J. Am. Vet. Med. Assoc. 149: 950-952.

Peinado, V. I., A. Fernandez-Aria, G. Viscor, and A. Palomeque. 1993. Haematology of Spanish ibex (*Capra pyrenaica hispanica*) restrained by physical or chemical means. Vet. Rec. 132: 580-583.

Pemberton, D., and N. Gales. 1991. Field immobilization of Tasmanian devils (*Sarcophilus harrisii*) with ketamine hydrochloride and xylazine hydrochloride. Wildl. Res. 18: 695-698.

Perry, J. L. 1977. Remote immobilization of bears with Ketaset® and mixtures of Rompun® and Ketaset®. Border Grizzly Project Field Report. No. 35.

Pertz, C., and J. P. Sundberg. 1978. Malignant hyperthermia induced by etorphine and xylazine in a fallow deer. J. Am. Vet. Med. Assoc. 173: 1243.

Peshin, P. K., J. M. Nigam, S. C. Singh, and B. A. Robinson. 1980. Evaluation of xylazine in camels. J. Am. Vet. Med. Assoc. 177: 875-878.

Peshin, P. K., J. Singh, A. P. Singh, and D. B. Patil. 1992. Experimental and clinical evaluation of some sedatives and anaesthetic agents in dromedary camels (*Camelus dromedarius*). *In* Allen W. R., A. J. Higgins, I. G. Mayhew, D. H. Snow, and J. F. Wade. (eds.). Proc. First International Camel Conference, Dubai. Pp. 371-374.

Peterson, R. S. 1965. Drugs for handling fur seals. J. Wildl. Manage. 29: 688-693.

Petrini, K. 1992. The medical management and diseases of mustelids. Proc. Am. Assoc. Zoo Vet. Pp. 116-135.

Petrini, K. R., D. E. Keyler, L. Ling, and D. Borys. 1993. Immobilization agents – developing an urgent response protocol for human exposure. Proc. Am. Assoc. Zoo Vet. Pp. 147-154.

Phelan, J. R., and K. Green. 1992. Chemical restraint of Weddell seals (*Leptonychotes weddellii*) with a combination of tiletamine and zolazepam. J. Wildl. Dis. 28: 230-235.

Phillips, L. G., M. Bush, W. Lance, and J. P. Raath. 1998. Ketamine/medetomidine immobilization and atipamezole reversal of captive and free-ranging impala (*Aepyceros melampus*) in the Kruger National Park, South Africa. Proc. Joint Conf. Am. Assoc. Zoo Vet. and Am. Assoc. Wildl. Vet. Pp. 19-21.

Philo, L. M. 1978. Evaluation of xylazine for chemical restraint of captive Arctic wolves. J. Am. Vet. Med. Assoc. 173: 1163-1166.

Pienaar, U. de V. 1963. Elephant control in National Parks: a new approach. Oryx. 7: 35-38.

Pienaar, U. de V. 1967a. The field immobilization and capture of hippopotami (*Hippopotamus amphibius linnaeus*) in their aquatic elements. Koedoe. 10: 149-157.

Pienaar, U. de V. 1967b. Operation "Khomandlopfu" (capture the elephants). Koedoe 10: 158-164.

Pienaar, U. de V. 1968a. Recent advances in the field immobilization and restraint of wild ungulates in South African national parks. Acta Zool. Pathol. Antverp. 46: 17-38.

Pienaar, U. de V. 1968b. The use of the immobilizing drugs in conservation procedures for roan antelope. Acta Zool. Pathol. Antwerp. 46: 39-51.

Pienaar, U. de V. 1969a. The use of drugs in the field immobilization and restraint of large wild mammals in South African national parks. Acta Zool. Pathol. Antwerp. 48: 163-177.

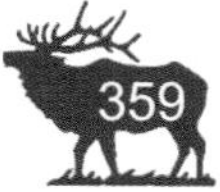

Pienaar, U. de V. 1969b. Capture and immobilization techniques currently employed in South African national parks and reserves. *In* Golley, F. B., and H. K. Buechner (eds.). A Practical Guide to the Study of the Productivity of Large Herbivores. Blackwell Scientific, Oxford. Pp. 132-144.

Pienaar, U. de V. 1970. The drug-immobilizing technique on the game farm or ranch. Game Owners Assoc. of So. Afr. and S.W. Afr. Information Sheet No. 1. 9 pp.

Pienaar, U. de V. 1973a. The drug immobilization of antelope species. *In* Young, E. (ed.). The Capture and Care of Wild Animals. Human and Rousseau, Cape Town, South Africa. Pp. 35-50.

Pienaar, U. de V. 1973b. Darting and injection equipment and techniques. *In* Young, E. (ed.). The Capture and Care of Wild Animals. Human and Rousseau, Cape Town, South Africa. Pp. 7-13.

Pienaar, U. de V., and J. W. Van Niekerk. 1963. The capture and translocation of three species of wild ungulates in the Eastern Transvall with special reference to R05-2807/B-SF (Roache) as a tranquillizer in game animals. Koedoe 6: 83-91.

Pienaar, U. de V., and N. Fairall. 1963. A preliminary note on the use of Quiloflex (Benzodioxane hydrochloride) in the immobilization of game. Koedoe 6: 109-115.

Pienaar, U. de V., J. W. Van Niekerk, E. Young, P. Van Wyk, and N. Fairall. 1966a. Neuroleptic narcosis of large wild herbivores in South African national parks with the new potent morphine analogues M.99 and M.183. J. So. Afr. Vet. Assoc. 37: 277-291.

Pienaar, U. de V., J. W. Van Niekerk, E. Young, P. Van Wyk, and N. Fairall. 1966b. The use of oripavine hydrochloride (M99) in the drug immobilization and marking of wild African elephant (*Loxodonta africana*) in the Kruger National Parks. Koedoe 9: 108-123.

Pienaar, U. de V., E. Le Riche, and C. S. Le Roux. 1969. The use of drugs in the management and control of large carnivorous mammals. Koedoe 12: 177-183.

Pietrak, M. 1992. Pharmacolgical restraint (immobilization) of reptiles. Magazyn Weterynaryjny 1: 42-43. (Polish)

Pietrak, M. 1994. Palmer's rifle - equipment for application of drugs to wild or zoo animals. Magazyn Weterynaryjny 3: 48-49. (Polish)

Pigozzi, G. 1987. Immobilization of crested porcupines with xylazine hydrochloride and ketamine hydrochloride. J. Wildl. Manage. 51: 120-123.

Pigozzi, G. 1988. The capture and immobilization of the European badger, *Meles meles* (L.), in its natural environment. Atti Soc. Ital. Sci. Nat. Mus. Civ. Stor. Nat. Milano. 129: 56-70.

Pimlott, D. G., and L. W. J. Carberry. 1958 North American moose transplantations and handling techniques. J. Wildl. Manage. 22: 51-62.

Pinchin, A. 1993. Zimbabwe's rhino dehorning programme. Intl. Zoo News 40: 9-13.

Pirhonin, J., and C. B. Schreck. 2003. Effects of anaesthesia with MS-222, clove oil and CO_2 on feed intake and plasma cortisol in steelhead trout (*Oncorhynchus mykiss*). Aquaculture 220: 507-514.

Pistey, W. R., and J. F Wright. 1959. Immobilization of captive wild animals. Vet. Med. 54: 446-449.

Pistey, W. R., and J. F. Wright. 1961. The immobilization of captive wild animals with succinylcholine. Can. J. Comp. Med. Vet. Sci.. 25: 59-68.

Piwowarczyk, S. 1967. Narcosis induced in European bison by means of chloral hydrate and ethyl alcohol. Acta Theriol. 32: 467-470.

Player, I. C. 1967. The translocation of the white rhinoceros: a success in wildlife conservation in South Africa. Oryx 60: 137-150.

Plotka, E. D., U. S. Seal, T. C. Eagle, C. S. Asa, J. R. Tester, and D. B. Siniff. 1987. Rapid reversible immobilizations of feral stallions using etorphine hydrochloride, xylazine hydrochloride and atropine sulfate. J. Wildl. Dis. 23: 471-478.

Poklis, A., M. A. Mackell, and M. E. S. Case. 1985. Xylazine in human tissues and fluids in a case of fatal drug abuse. J. Analyt. Toxicol. 9: 234-236.

Pokras, M. A., and C. J. Sedgwick. 1990. Wildlife emergencies: how to cope with them before they happen. *In* D. R. Ludwig (ed.). Wildlife Rehabilitation. Eighth Ann. Symp. Natl. Wildl. Rehabilitators Assoc. Ithaca, New York. Pp. 117-133.

Pollock, C. G., and E. C. Ramsay. 2003. Serial immobilization of Brazilian tapir (*Tapirus terrestrus*) with oral detomidine and oral carfentanil. J. Zoo Wildl. Med. 34: 408-410.

Pomeroy, D. E., and M. H. Woodford. 1976. Drug immobilization of marabou storks. J. Wildl. Manage. 40: 177-179.

Pond, D. B., and B. W. O'Gara. 1994. Chemical immobilization of large mammals. *In* Bookhout, T. A. (ed.). Research and Management Techniques for Wildlife and Habitats. The Wildlife Society, Bethesda,

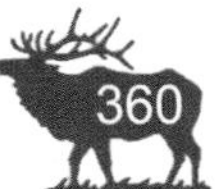

Md. Pp. 125-139.
Poole, K. G., G. Mowat, and B. G. Slough. 1993. Chemical immobilization of lynx. Wildl. Soc. Bull. 21: 136-140.
Portas, T. 2004. A review of drugs and techniques used for sedation and anaesthesia in a captive rhinoceros species. Aust. Vet. J. 82: 542-549.
Portas, T. J., M. J. Lynch, and L. Vogelnest. 2003. Comparison of etorphine-detomidine and medetomidine-ketamine anesthesia in captive addax (*Addax nasomaculatus*). J. Zoo Wildl. Med. 34: 269-273.
Porter, W. P. 1982a. Hematologic and other effects of ketamine and ketamine-acepromazine in rhesus monkeys (*Macaca mulatta*). Lab. An. Sci. 32: 373-375. 731
Porter, W. P. 1982b. A comparison of hematologic and other parameters while rhesus monkeys (*Macaca mulatta*) are immobilized with ketamine vs. ketamine combined with acepromazine. Lab. An. Sci. 32: 438. 379
Posner, L. P., J. B. Woodie, P. D. Curtis, H. N. Erb, R. Gilbert, W. A. Adams, and R. D. Gleed. 2005. Acid-base, blood gas, and physiologic parameters during laproscopy in the head-down position in white-tailed deer (*Odocoileus virginianus*). J. Zoo Wildl. Med. 36: 642-647.
Pospisil, J., F. Kase, and J. Vahala. 1989. Comparison of basic haematological values in grevy's zebra (*Equus grevyi*) during the summer and winter seasons. Comp. Biochem. Physiol. 92: 31-32.
Post, G. 1959. The use of curare and curare-like drugs on elk (wapiti). J. Wildl. Manage. 23: 365-366.
Pratap, K., Amarpal, P. Kinjavdekar, H. P. Aithal, and A. M. Pawde. 2006. Xylazine-ketamine anaesthesia in snakes (*Naja naja*) and its reversal with atipamezole. Indian J. Anim. Sci. 76: 580-581.
Presidente, P. J. A., and M. Draisma. 1978. The capture, sedation and immobilisation of wild ungulates, with special reference to deer. Part I. Post capture problems. Aust. Deer 3(2): 29-32.
Presidente, P. J. A., J. H. Lumsden, D. R. Presnell, W. A. Rapley, and B. M. McCraw. 1973. Combination of etorphine and xylazine in captive white-tailed deer: II. Effects on hematologic, serum biochemical and blood gas values. J. Wildl. Dis. 9: 342-348.
Presidente, P. J. A., P. G. Taylor, and M. Draisma. 1978a. The capture, sedation and immobilisation of wild ungulates, with special reference to deer. Part II. Mechanical means of capture. Aust. Deer 3(3): 27-32.
Presidente, P. J. A., R. Butler, R. Horsey, M. Draisma, P. G. Taylor, and P. Stuart. 1978b. The capture, sedation and immobilisation of wild ungulates, with special reference to deer. Part III. Drugs, projectile systems and their application. Aust. Deer 3(4): 27-40.
Presnell, K. R., P. J. S. Presidente, and W. A. Rapley. 1973. Combination of etorphine and xylazine in captive white-tailed deer: I. Sedative and immobilization properties. J. Wildl. Dis. 9: 236-341.
Prinsloo, M., and H. Ebedes. 1992. The use of some long-acting neuroleptics in wildlife captured with the "pop-up corral." *In* Ebedes, H. (ed.) The Use of Tranquillizers in Wildlife. Dept. Ag. Develop., Pretoria. Bull. No. 423. Pp. 49-51.
Pulley, A. C. S., J. A. Roberts, N. W. Lerche. 2004. Four preanesthetic oral sedation protocols for rhesus macaques (*Macaca mulatta*). J. Zoo Wildl. Med. 35: 497-502.
Puri, C. P., V. Puri, and T. C. Anand Kumar. 1981. Serum levels of testosterone, cortisol, prolactin and bioactive luteinizing hormone in adult male rhesus monkeys following cage-restraint or anaesthetizing with ketamine hydrochloride. Acta Endocrinol. 97: 118-124.
Pusateri, F. M., C. P. Hibler, and T. M. Pojar. 1982. Oral administration of diazepam and promazine hydrochloride to immobilize pronghorn. J. Wildl. Dis. 18: 9-16.
Pybus, M. J., and D. K. Onderka. 1992. On the proper use of succinycholine in elk. J. Wildl. Dis. 28: 685 (letter).
Pye, G. W., and R. J. Booth. 1998. Medetomidine-ketamine immobilization and atipamezole reversal of eastern grey kangaroos (*Macropus gaiganteus*). Proc. Joint Conf. Am. Assoc. Zoo Vet and Am. Assoc. Wildl. Vet. Pp. 306-309.
Pye, G. W., and J. W. Carpenter. 1998. Ketamine sedation followed by propofol anesthesia in a slider (*Trachemys scripta*) to facilitate removal of an esophageal foreign body. Bull. Assoc. Reptile Amphib. Vet. 8: 16-17.
Pye, G. W., S. B. Citino, M. Bush, L. Klein, and W. Lance. 2001. Anesthesia of eastern giant eland (*Taurotragus derbianus gigas*) at White Oak Conservation Center. Proc. Am. Assoc. Zoo Vet. Pp. 226-231.
Qiu, X. 1990. Anesthesia of the giant panda. J. Sichuan Teachers College 11: 114-117. (Chinese)
Quandt, J. E., and C. Greenacre. 1999. Sevoflurane anesthesia in psittacines. J. Zoo Wildl. 30: 308-309.

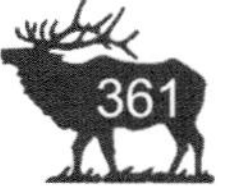

Quandt, S. K. F. 1992. The pharmacology of medetomidine in combination with ketamine hydrochloride in African lions (*Panthera leo*). MVM Thesis, University of Pretoria, 167 pp.

Quintana, F., C. Campagna, and R. Werner. 1992. Aspectos practicos de la anestesia de elefantes marinos en condiciones de campo. 5 Reunion de Trabajos de Especialistas en Mamiferos Acuaticos de America del Sur. Buenos Aires, Argentina.

Raath, J. P. 1993. Chemical capture of the African elephant *Loxodonta africana*. *In* McKenzie, A. A. (ed.). The Capture and Care Manual. Wildlife Decision Support Services and The South African Veterinary Foundation, Pretoria. Pp. 484-492.

Raath, J. P. 1994. Anaesthesia of the white rhino. *In* Penzhorn, B. L., and N. P. J. Kriek (eds.). Proc. Symp. Rhino Game Ranch Anim. Onderstepoort, Republic of South Africa. Pp. 119-127.

Raath, J. P. 1999. Relocation of African elephants. *In* Fowler, M. E., and R. E. Miller (eds.). Zoo & Wild Animal Medicine. Current Therapy 4. W. B. Saunders Company, Philadelphia, Pennsylvania. Pp. 525-533.

Raath, J. P. 1999. Anesthesia of white rhinoceroses. *In* Fowler, M. E., and R. E. Miller (eds.). Zoo & Wild Animal Medicine. Current Therapy 4. W. B. Saunders Company, Philadelphia, Pennsylvania. Pp. 556-561.

Raath, J. P., and C. M. Knox. 1989. The use of tranquilizers in confining newly captured impalas to bomas. Proc. Am. Assoc. Zoo Vet. P. 15.

Raath, J. P., S. K. F. Quandt, and J. H. Malan. 1992. Ostrich (*Struthio camelus*) immobilization using carfentanil and xylazine and reversal with yohimbine and naltrexone. J. So. Afr. Vet. Assoc. 63: 138-140.

Raath, J. P., J. Hattingh, and C. M. Knox. 1993. Physiological changes following wild dog (*Lycaon pictus*) immobilization with fentanyl and xylazine. Proc. Int. Symp. Capture, Care, Manage. Threatened Mammals. P. 80 (abstr.).

Raath, J. P., C. M. Knox, D. Kernes, D. F. Keet, and M. G. L. Mills. 1995. Anesthesia of free-ranging wild dogs (*Lycaon pictus*) with fentanyl and xylazine. Proc. Joint Conf. Am. Assoc. Zoo Vet., Wildl. Dis. Assoc., Am. Assoc. Wildl. Vet. East Lansing, Michigan. Pp. 287-289.

Radcliffe, R. W., S. T. Ferrell, and S. E. Childs. 2000. Butorphanol and azaperone as a safe alternative for repeated chemical restraint in captive white rhinoceros (*Ceratotherium simum*). J. Zoo Wildl. Med. 31: 196-200.

Ramdohr, S., H. Bornemann, J. Plotz, and M. N. Bester. 2001. Immobilization of free-ranging adult male southern elephant seals with Immobilon[tm] (etorphine/acepromazine) and ketamine. S. Afr. J. Wildl. Res. 31: 135-140.

Ramsay, E. 2000. Standing sedation and tranquilization in captive African elephants (*Loxodonta africana*). Proc. Joint Conf. Am. Assoc. Zoo Vet. and Intl. Assoc. Aquatic An. Med. Pp. 111-114.

Ramsay, E. C., D. Grove, M. Miller, and J. Schumacher. 1999. Immobilization of felids using oral detomidine and ketamine. Proc. Am. Assoc. Zoo Vet. Pp. 47-48.

Ramsay, E. C., J. M. Sleeman, V. L. Clyde, and D. Gieser. 1994. Immobilization of bears using orally administered carfentanil citrate. Joint Conf. Am. Assoc. Zoo Vet. Assoc. and Reptil. Amphib. Vet. P. 214.

Ramsay, E. C., J. M. Sleeman, and V. L. Clyde. 1995. Immobilization of black bears (*Ursus americanus*) with orally administered carfentanil citrate. J. Wildl. Dis. 31: 391-393.

Ramsay, E. C., M. R. Loomis, K. G. Mehren, W. S. J. Boardman, J. Jensen, and D. Geiser. 1998. Chemical restraint of the Nile hippopotamus (*Hippopotamus amphibius*) in captivity. J. Zoo Wildl. Med. 29: 45-49

Ramsay, E. C., D. Grove, M. Miller, and J. Schumacher. 1999. Immobilization of felids using oral detomidine and ketamine. Proc. Am. Assoc. Zoo Vet. Pp. 47-48.

Ramsay, M. A., and I. Stirling. 1986. Long-term effects of drugging and handling free-ranging polar bears. J. Wildl. Manage. 50: 619-626.

Ramsay, M. A., I. Stirling, L. Ø. Knutsen, and E. Broughton. 1985. Use of yohimbine hydrochloride to reverse immobilization of polar bears by ketamine hydrochloride and xylazine hydrochloride. J. Wildl. Dis. 21: 396-400.

Ramsden, R. O., P. F. Coppin, and D. H. Johnston. 1976. Clinical observations on the use of ketamine hydrochloride in wild carnivores. J. Wildl. Dis. 12: 221-225.

Ranheim, B. 1999. Pharmacology of medetomidine and atipamezole in cattle, sheep and reindeer. Ph.D. Dissert., Norwegian School Vet. Sci., Oslo, Norway.

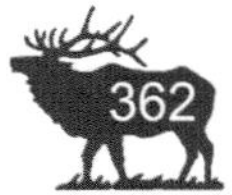

Ranheim, B., T. E. Horsberg, U. Nymoen, N. E. Søli, N. J. C. Tyler, and J. M. Arnemo. 1997. Reversal of medetomidine-induced sedation in reindeer (*Rangifer tarandus*) with atipamezole increases the medetomidine concentration in plasma. J. Vet. Pharmacol. Ther. 20: 350-354.

Ranheim, B., F. Rosell, H. A. Haga, and J. M. Arnemo. 2004. Field anaesthetic and surgical techniques for implantation of intraperitoneal radio transmitters in Eurasian beavers (*Castor fiber*). Wildl. Biol. 10: 11-15.

Raphael, B. L. 1999. Okapi medicine and surgery. *In* Fowler, M. E., and R. E. Miller (eds.). Zoo & Wild Animal Medicine. Current Therapy 4. W. B. Saunders Company, Philadelphia, Pennsylvania. Pp. 646-650.

Raphael, B. L., S. James, P. P. Calle, T. L. Clippinger, and R. A. Cook. 2001. The use of ketamine as a primary immobilizing agent in gorillas (*Gorilla gorilla*). Proc. Am. Assoc. Zoo Vet. Pp. 169-170.

Rapley, W. A., K. G. Mehren, C. J. Bonar, and G. B. Topolie. 1975. Repair of a fractured mandible in a giraffe using Rompun and M99 immobilization. Proc. Am. Assoc. Zoo Vet. Pp. 12-15.

Rapley, W. A., and K. G. Mehren. 1975. The clinical usage of Rompun (xylazine) in captive ungulates at the Metropolitan Toronto Zoo. Proc. Am. Assoc. Zoo Vet. Pp. 16-39.

Ratcliffe, H. L. 1962. Diazepam (tranimal) as a tranquilizer for zoo animals. Report of the Penrose Research Laboratory, Zoological Society of Philadelphia. Pp. 10-13.

Rathore, A. K. 1984. Use of alphachloralose in restraining dogs. Proc. Int. Conf. Wildl. Dis. Assoc. 4: 145-148.

Ratti, P., and K. Zeeb. 1972. Practical experience with Rompun® in the immobilization of game. Vet. Med. Rev. 3: 226-238.

Rausch, R. A., and R. W. Ritcey. 1961. Narcosis of moose with nicotine. J. Wildl. Manage. 25: 326-328.

Read, M. R. 2003. A review of $alpha_2$ adrenoreceptor agonists and the development of hypoxemia in domestic and wild ruminants. J. Zoo Wildl. Med. 34: 134-138.

Read, M. R. 2004. Evaluation of the use of anesthesia and analgesia in reptiles. J. Am. Vet. Med. Assoc. 224: 547-552.

Read, M. R., and R. B. McCorkell. 2002. Use of azaperone and zuclopenthixol acetate to facilitate translocation of white-tailed deer (*Odocoileus virginianus*). J. Zoo Wildl. Med. 33: 163-165.

Read, M., N. Caulkett, and M. McCallister. 2000a. Evaluation of zuclopenthixol acetate to decrease handling stress in wapiti. J. Zoo Wildl. Med. 36: 450-459.

Read, M. R., N. A. Caulkett, and M. McCallister. 2000b. Use of zuclopenthixol acetate to decrease handling stress in wapiti (*Cervus elaphus*). Proc. Joint Conf. Am. Assoc. Zoo Vet. and Intl. Assoc. Aquatic An. Med. Pp. 115-118.

Read, M. R., N. A. Caulkett, A. Symington, and T. K. Shury. 2001. Treatment of hypoxemia during xylazine-tiletamine-zolazepam immobilization of wapiti. Can. Vet. J. 42: 861-864.

Reddacliff, G. L. 1979. Home-made projectile syringes. N. Z. Vet. J. 27: 249-250.

Redman, S. D., J. R. Meinertz, and M. P. Gaikowski. 1998. Effects of immobilization by electricity and MS-222 on brown trout broodstock and their progeny. Progr. Fish. Cult. 60: 44-49.

Redig, P. T., A. A. Larson, and G. E. Duke. 1984. Response of great horned owls given the optical isomers of ketamine. Am. J. Vet. Res. 45: 125-127.

Redig, P. T., and G. E. Duke. 1976. Intravenously administered ketamine HCl and diazepam for anesthesia of raptors. J. Am. Vet. Med. Assoc. 169: 886-888.

Reed, G. T. 1978. Immobilization of two captive Nile hippo (*Hippopotamus amphibius*). Proc. Am. Assoc. Zoo Vet. Pp. 150-153.

Reich, D. L., and G. Silvay. 1989. Ketamine: an update on the first twenty-five years of clinical experience. Can. J. Anaes. 36: 186-197.

Renecker, L. A., and C. A. Olsen. 1985. Use of yohimbine and 4-aminopyridine to antagonize xylazine-induced immobilization in North American cervidae. J. Am. Vet. Med. Assoc. 187: 1199-1201.

Renecker, L. A., and C. A. Olsen. 1986. Antagonism of xylazine hydrochloride with yohimbine hydrochloride and 4-aminopyridine in captive wapiti. J. Wildl. Dis. 22: 91-96.

Renecker, L. A., J. Bertwistle, H. M. Kozak, R. J. Hudson, D. Chabot, and S. MacLean. 1992. R51163 as a sedative for handling and transporting plains bison and wapiti. J. Wildl. Dis. 28: 236-241.

Renner, M. S. 1998. Repeated immobilization of Grevy's zebra (*Equus grevyi*). Proc. Joint Conf. Am. Assoc. Zoo Vet and Am. Assoc. Wildl. Vet. Pp. 350-351.

Rerabek, J. 1954. The use of curare for capturing deer. Prace Vyskumaych Ustav Lesnickych 7: 199-212

Reuben, D. 1966. Valium as a tranquilizer in zoo animals. Int. Zoo Yb. 6: 270.

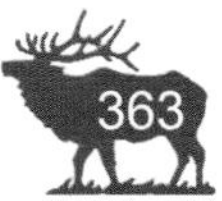

Reuss von, Prinz Heinrich III. 1966. Beitrag zum Immobilisierung von Rot- und Rehwild. Tierärtstl. Umsch. 21: 559-565.

Reuter, H.-O., and H. Winterbach. 1998. Current capture technique and drug dosage regime for the immobilization and tranquilization of free-ranging black rhinoceros (*Diceros bicornis bicornis*) in Namibia. Proc. Joint Conf. Am. Assoc. Zoo Vet and Am. Assoc. Wildl. Vet. Pp. 410-415.

Reuther, V. C. 1983. [Experiences with the immobilization of the European otter (*Lutra lutra*) with ketamine hydrochloride. Berl. Munch. Tierarztl. Wochenschr. 96: 401-405.

Reuther, V. C., and B. Brandes. 1984. [Occurrence of hyperthermia during the immobilisation of European otters (*Lutra lutra*) with ketamine hydrochloride]. Dtsch. Tierarztl. Wochenschr. 91: 66-68.

Reynolds, P. E., and G. W. Garner. 1983. Immobilizing and marking muskoxen in the Arctic National Wildlife Refuge, Alaska. Proc. Alaska Sci. Conf. 34: 71.

Reynolds, W. T. 1983. Unusual anaesthetic complication in a pelican. Vet. Rec. 113: 204.

Richardson, K. C., and L. K. Cullen. 1981. Anesthesia of small kangaroos. J. Am. Vet. Med. Assoc. 179: 1162-1165.

Reynolds, W. T. 1992. Anaesthesia of a bottle nose dolphin (*Tursiops truncatus*). J. Vet. Anaesth. 19.

Richardson, P. R. K., and M. D. Anderson. 1993. Chemical capture of the aardwolf *Proteles cristatus*. *In* McKenzie, A. A. (ed.). The Capture and Care Manual. Wildlife Decision Support Services and The South African Veterinary Foundation, Pretoria. Pp. 244-246.

Richardson, K. C., and L. K. Cullen. 1984. Physical and chemical restraint of small macropods. Int. Zoo Yb. 23: 215-218.

Richardson, P. R. K. 1983. An improved darting system for immobilizing smaller mammals in the wild. So. Afr. J. Wildl. Res. 13: 51-54.

Richter, A. G. 1977. Ketamine-xylazine immobilization of a mule deer. J. Am. Vet. Med. Assoc. 171: 987.

Richter, N. A. 1983. Lyophilization of ketamine hydrochloride to increase concentration. Proc. Am. Assoc. Zoo Vet. P. 4.

Ridgway, S. H., and J. G. McCormick. 1967. Anesthesia for major surgery in porpoises. Science 158: 510-512.

Ridgway, S. H., and J. G. Simpson. 1969. Anesthesia and restraint for the California sea lion. J. Am. Vet. Med. Assoc. 155: 1059-1063.

Ridgway, S. H., and J. G. McCormick. 1971. Anesthesia of the porpoise. *In* Soma, L. (ed.). Veterinary Anesthesia. Williams and Wilkins Co., Baltimore, Maryland. Pp. 394-402.

Ridgway, S. H., R. F. Green, and J. C. Sweeney. 1975. Mandibular anesthesia and tooth extraction in bottlenosed dolphin. J. Wildl. Dis. 11: 415-418.

Rie, I. P. 1973. Application of drugs to the skin of salamanders. Herpetologica. 29: 55-59.

Riebold, T. W., A. J. Kaneps, and W. B. Schmotzer. 1986. Reversal of xylazine-induced sedation in llamas, using doxapram or 4-aminopyridine and yohimbine. J. Am. Vet. Med. Assoc. 189: 1059-1061.

Riebold, T. W., W. B. Schmoltzer, and M. J. Huber. 1992a. Anaesthetic techniques in the llama. *In* Hall, L. W., J. S. M. M. van Dieten, P. van Dijk, L. J. Hellebrekers, and E. Lagerweij. (eds.). Proceedings of the 4th International Congress of Veterinary Anaesthesia. R & W Publications, Newmarket. Pp. 237-240.

Riebold, T. W., M. J. Huber, and W. B. Schmoltzer. 1992b. Monitoring techniques and supportive therapy in the anaesthetized llama. *In* Hall, L. W., J. S. M. M. van Dieten, P. van Dijk, L. J. Hellebrekers, and E. Lagerweij. (eds.). Proceedings of the 4th International Congress of Veterinary Anaesthesia. R & W Publications, Newmarket. Pp. 241-242.

Rietjkerk, F. E., and E. C. Delima. 1994. Clinical and haematological changes in gazelles during xylazine/ketamine anaesthesia and following reversal with RX-821002A. Vet. Rec. 134: 354-355.

Rietjkerk, F. E., E. C. Delima, and S. M. Mubarak. 1994. The hematological profile of the mountain gazelle (*Gazella gazella*): variations with sex, age, capture method, season and anesthesia. J. Wildl. Dis. 30: 69-76.

Rieu, M., and B. Gautheron. 1968. Preliminary observations concerning a method for introduction of a tube for anesthesia in small delphinids. Lab. d'Acoustique An. Lab. Publ. 78.

Right, J. M. 1983. Ketamine hydrochloride as a chemical restraint for selected small mammals. Wildl. Soc. Bull. 11: 76-79.

Ritchie, B. W., G. J. Harrison, and L. R. Harrison (eds.). 1994. Avian medicine: principles and applications. Wingers, Lake Worth, Florida. 1384 pp.

Robinson, M. E., and S. R. Scadding. 1983. The effect of pH on tricaine methanesulfonate induced anaes-

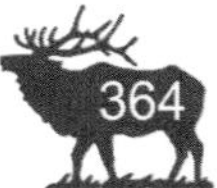

thesia of the newt *Notophthalmus viridescens*. Can. J. Zool. 61: 531-533.
Robinson, P. T. 1976. Immobilization of felidae with M99. J. Zoo An. Med. 7: 31.
Robinson, P. T. 1981. A review of thirty-three Queensland koala (*Phascolarctos cinereus adustus*) immobilization procedures. J. Zoo An. Med. 12: 121-123.
Robinson, P. T. 1983. The use of ketamine in restraint of a black-bellied pangolin (*Manis tetradactyla*). J. Zoo An. Med. 14: 19-23.
Robinson, P. T., and C. J. Sedgwick. 1973. Immobilization of a polar bear (*Thalarctos maritimus*) with ketamine HCl. J. Zoo An. Med. 4: 27-28.
Robinson, P. T., and C. J. Sedgwick. 1974. Comment on M99 insert's drug dosage information. J. Zoo An. Med. 6: 7.
Robinson, P. T., and J. Fairfield. 1974. Immobilization of an ostrich with ketamine HCI. J. Zoo An. Med. 5: 11.
Robinson, P. T., and D. Lambert. 1986. A review of 226 chemical restraint procedures in great apes at the San Diego Zoo. Proc. Am. Assoc. Zoo Vet. P. 183.
Roffe, T. J., K. Coffin, and J. Berger. 2001. Survival and immobilizing moose with carfentanil and xylazine. Wildl. Soc. Bull. 29: 1140-1146.
Rogers, L. L. 1970. An analysis of succinylcholine chloride immobilization of black bears. M.S. Thesis, University of Minnesota. 59 pp.
Rogers, L. L., C. M. Stowe, and A. W. Erickson. 1976. Succinylcholine chloride immobilization of black bears. *In* Pelton, M. R., J. W. Lentfer, and G. E. Folk Jr. (eds.). Bears - Their Biology and Management. IUCN Publ. New Ser. 40. Pp. 431-446.
Rogers, P. S. 1992. The immobilization of lions and leopards with Zoletil®. *In* Ebedes, H. (ed.) The Use of Tranquillizers in Wildlife. Dept. Ag. Develop., Pretoria. Bull. No. 423. Pp. 66-67.
Rogers, P. S. 1993a. The capture of large carnivores using orally administered drugs. *In* McKenzie, A. A. (ed.). The Capture and Care Manual. Wildlife Decision Support Services and The South African Veterinary Foundation, Pretoria. Pp. 251-254.
Rogers, P. S. 1993b. Chemical capture of the white rhinoceros *Ceratotherium simum*. *In* McKenzie, A. A. (ed.). The Capture and Care Manual. Wildlife Decision Support Services and The South African Veterinary Foundation, Pretoria. Pp. 512-528.
Rogers, P. S. 1993c. Chemical capture of the black rhinoceros *Diceros bicornis*. *In* McKenzie, A. A. (ed.). The Capture and Care Manual. Wildlife Decision Support Services and The South African Veterinary Foundation, Pretoria. Pp. 553-555.
Rogers, P. S. 1998. Chemical immobilization and anaesthesia of cheetahs. Proc. Symp. on Cheetahs as Game Ranch Animals. Onderstepoort, RSA. Wildlife Group, So, Afr. Vet. Assoc., Onderstepoort. pp. 100-102.
Rohr, F., and A. A. McKenzie. 1993. Remote injection equipment. *In* McKenzie, A. A. (ed.). The Capture and Care Manual. Wildlife Decision Support Services and The South African Veterinary Foundation, Pretoria. Pp. 116-130.
Röken, B. O. 1975. Chemical restraint and anaesthesia in African herbivores. Sonderdruck aus Verhandloungbericht des XVII Internationalen Symposiums uber die Erkrankungen der Zootiere Tunis. Berlin, Akademie-Verlag. Pp. 135-153.
Röken, B. O. 1985. Some medical observations on immobilizing free-ranging moose in Sweden. Proc. V Int. Conf. Wildl. Dis., Uppsala. Pp. 59.
Röken, B. O. 1987. Medetomidine in zoo animal anaesthesia. Proc. 1st Int. Conf. Zool. Avian Med. 1: 535-538.
Röken, B. O. 1975. Chemical restraints and anesthesia in African herbivores. *In* Sonderdruck aus Verhandlungsbericht des XVII Internationalen Symposiums uber die Erkrankungen der Zootiere. Berlin, Akademie-Verlag. Pp. 135-153.
Röken, B. O. 1997. Potent anesthetic combinations with low concentrated medetomidine in zoo animals. Proc. Am. Assoc. Zoo Vet. Pp. 134-136.
Rolfe, J. D., and J. C. Haigh. 1985. Yohimbine and physostigmine reversal of xylazine plus ketamine immobilizations in sheep, dogs and wapiti. Proc. Am. Assoc. Zoo Vet. Pp. 128-132.
Roney, E. E. 1971. Use of the blowgun to immobilize or medicate caged animals. J. Zoo An. Med. 2: 25.
Rooney, M. B., G. Levine, J. Gaynor, E. MacDonald, and J. Wimsatt. 1999. Sevoflurane anesthesia in desert tortoises (*Gopherus agassizii*). J. Zoo Wildl. Med. 30: 64-69.
Rosatte, R. C., and D. P. Hobson. 1983. Ketamine hydrochloride as an immobilizing agent for striped

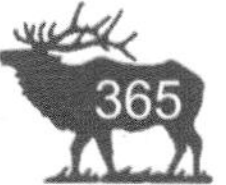

skunks. Can. Vet. J. 24: 134-135.
Rosborough, J. P., E. M. Bailey, L. A. Geddes, and W. A. Tacker. 1974. Experimental anesthetization of a dromedary camel. Zbl. Vet. Med. A. 21: 149-156.
Roslyn, J., J. E. Thompson, and L. Denbesten. 1979. Anesthesia for prairie dogs. Lab. An. Sci. 29: 542-544.
Ross, G. J. B., and G. S. Saayman. 1970. A young bull elephant seal immobilized. Afr. Wildl. 24: 331-336.
Ross, L. G., and B. Ross. 1999. Anaesthetic & sedative techniques for aquatic animals. Blackwell Science Ltd., London, U.K. 159 pp.
Ross, R. M., T. W. H. Backman, and R. M. Bennett. 1993. Evaluation of the anesthetic metomidate for the handling and transport of juvenile American shad. Progressive Fish-Culturist 55: 236-243.
Rotella, J. J., and J. T. Ratti. 1990. Use of methoxyflurane to reduce nest abandonment of mallards. J. Wildl. Manage. 57:696-703.
Roth, H. H., and B. Montemayor-Taca. 1971. Immobilization of tamaraw (*Anoa midorensis*). Philippine J. Vet. Med. 10: 45-48.
Roubach, R., L. C. Gomes, F. A. L. Fonseca, and A. L. Val. 2005. Eugenol as an efficacious anaesthetic for tambaqui, *Colossoma macropomum* (Cuvier). Aquac. Res. 36: 1056-1061.
Roughton, R. D. 1975. Xylazine as an immobilizing agent for captive white-tailed deer. J. Am. Vet. Med. Assoc. 167: 574-576.
Roussel, Y. E., and Patenaude. 1975. Some physiological effects of M99 etorphine on immobilized free-ranging moose. J. Wildl. Manage. 39: 634-636.
Roussel, Y. E., and C. Pichette. 1974. Comparison of techniques used to restrain and mark moose. J. Wildl. Manage. 38: 783-788.
Rowe-Rowe, D. T., and B. Green. 1980. Ketamine and acetylpromazine for black-backed jackal immobilization. So. Afr. J. Wildl. Res. 10: 153.
Rowe-Rowe, D. T., and P. B. Lowry. 1982. A note on the immobilization of serval, *Felis serval* , with ketamine and acetylpromazine. So. Afr. J. Wildl. Res. 12: 109.
Rubright, W. C., and C. B. Thayer. 1970. The use of Innovar-Vet® as a surgical anesthetic for the guinea pig. Lab. An. Care 20: 989-991.
Rudge, A. J. B. (ed.). 1983. The Capture and Handling of Deer. Nature Conservancy Council, Peterborough, United Kingdom. 135 pp.
Rudge, M. R., and R. J. Joblin. 1976. Comparison of some methods of capturing and marking feral goats (*Capra hircus*). N. Z. J. Zool. 3: 51-55.
Rüedi, D., and J. Voellm. 1976. The blow gun - an anesthetizing instrument for the immobilization of wild animals. Vet. Med. Rev. 1: 85-90.
Rüedi, D., and J. Voellm. 1977. The use of the blow-pipe in the Basel Zoological Garden. Proc. Am. Assoc. Zoo Vet. Pp. 1-6
Ryding, F. N. 1982. Ketamine immobilization of southern elephant seals by a remote injection method. Br. Antarct. Survey Bull. 57: 21-26.
Ryeng, K. A., J. M. Arnemo, and S. Larsen. 2001a. Determination of optimal immobilizing doses of medetomidine hydrochloride and ketamine hydrochloride combination in captive reindeer. Am. J. Vet. Res. 62: 119-126.
Ryeng, K. A., S. Larsen, B. Ranheim, G. Albertsen, and J. M. Arnemo. 2001b. Clinical evaluation of established optimal immobilizing doses of medetomidine-ketamine in captive *reindeer (Rangifer tarandus tarandus*). Amer. J. Vet. Res. 62: 406-413.
Ryeng, K. A., S. Larsen, and J. M. Arnemo. 2002. Medetomidine-ketamine in reindeer (*Rangifer tarandus tarandus*): Effective immobilization by hand- and dart-administered injection. J. Zoo Wildl. Med. 33: 397-400.
Ryser, A., M. Scholl, M. Zwahlen, M. Oetliker, M.-P. Ryser-Degiorgis, and U. Breitenmoser. 2005. A remote-controlled teleinjection system for the low-stress capture of large mammals. Wildl. Soc. Bull. 33: 721-730.
Sabapara, R. H. 1995. Chemical restraint and sedation of leopards (*Panthera pardus*). Indian Vet. J. 72: 655-657.
Sagner, G., and G. Haas. 1969. Bayer Va 1470 for the anesthesia and sedation of domestic and wild animals. 11th Int. Symp. Dis. Zoo and Wild An., Zagreb. Berlin, Akademie-Verlag Pp. 131-133.
Sahr, D. P., and F. F. Knowlton. 2000. Evaluation of tranquilizer trap devices (TTDs) for foothold traps used to capture gray wolves. Wildl. Soc. Bull. 28: 597-605.

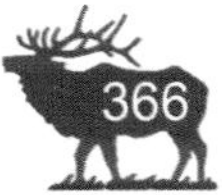

Saint John, B. E. 1992. Pulse oximetry: theory, technology, and clinical considerations. Proc. Joint Conf. Am. Assoc. Zoo Vet. and Am. Assoc. Wildl. Vet. Pp. 223-229.

Salas, L. A., S. A. Stephens. 2004. Capture and immobilisation of cuscuses and ringtail possums in Papua New Guinea. Wildl. Res. 31: 101-107.

Sale, J. B., V. Rishi, K. N. Singh, and V. K. Verma. 1986. Drug immobilization of the Indian elephant. J. Bombay Nat. Hist. Soc. 83: 49-56.

Salonen, J. S. 1989. Pharmacokinetics of medetomidine. Acta Vet. Scand. Suppl. 85: 49-54.

Samanta, A., C. Roffe, and K. L. Woods. 1990. Accidental self administration of xylazine in a veterinary nurse. Postgrad. Med. J. 66: 244-245.

Samelius, G., S. Larivière, and R. Alisauskas. 2003. Immobilization of arctic foxes with tiletamine hydrochloride and zolazepam hydrochloride (Zoletil®). Wildl. Soc. Bull. 31: 192-196.

Samour, J. H., D. M. Jones, J. A. Knight, and J. C. Howlett. 1984. Comparative studies of the use of some injectable anaesthetic agents in birds. Vet. Rec. 115: 6-11.

Samour, J. H., J. Irwin-Davies, and E. Faraj. 1990. Chemical immobilisation in ostriches (*Struthio camelus*) using etorphine hydrochloride. Vet. Rec. 127: 575-576.

Samuelson, J. 1983. Trapping methods for big game. N. D. Outdoors. 45: 20-21.

Sancken, U., and K. Fischer. 1988. [Biotelemetrically established daily profile of the core body temperature of the female fallow deer (*Dama dama* L.) following immobilization with the Hellabrunner mixture in various environmental temperatures]. Deutsche Tierärztliche Wochenschrift 95: 16-19.

Sandegren, F., L. Pettersson, P. Ahlqvist, and B. O. Röken. 1987. Immobilization of moose in Sweden. Swed. Wildl. Res. Viltrevy. 1: 785-791.

Sandelien, H. 1966. Oral administration of Valium® to restless and aggressive mink. Nord. Vet. Med. 18: 271-276.

Sandmeier, P. 2000. Evaluation of medetomidine for short-term immobilization of domestic pigeons (*Columba livia*) and Amazon parrots (*Amazona* species). J. Avian Med. Surg. 14: 8-14.

Sarma, B., S. C. Pathak, and K. K. Sarma. 2002. Medetomidine - a novel immobilizing agent for the elephant (*Elaphus maximus*). Res. Vet. Sci. 73: 315-317.

Sarma, K. K., M. Sarma, and D. K. Sarma. 2004. Safety of repeated xylazine hydrochloride administrations in elephants. Indian Vet. 81: 886-889.

Sarno, R. J., R. L. Hunter, and W. L. Franklin. 1996. Immobilization of guanacos by use of tiletamine/zolazepam. J. Am. Vet. Med. Assoc. 208: 408-409.

Sauer, B. W., H. A. Gorman, and R. J. Boyd. 1969. A new technique for restraining mule deer. J. Am. Vet. Med. Assoc. 155: 1080-1084.

Savage, B. 1985. Giraffe restraint. Proc. Am. Assoc. Zool. Parks Aquaria. Pp. 48-50.

Savarie, P. J. 1976. Pharmacological review of chemicals used for the capture of animals. Proc. Vertebrate Pest Control Conf. 7: 178-184.

Sawyer, D. C., and T. D. Williams. 1996. Chemical restraint and anesthesia of sea otters affected by the oil spill on Prince William Sound, Alaska. J. Am. Vet. Med. Assoc. 208:1831-1834.

Scanlon, J. J., and M. R. Vaughan. 1985. Relationship between injection point of succinylcholine chloride and time to immobilization for white-tailed deer. Trans. Northeast Sect. Wildl. Soc. 42: 219.

Scanlon, P. F. 1973. Observations on the immobilization of fallow deer with powdered succinylcholine chloride injected by dart. Vet. Rec. 93: 396-398.

Scanlon, P. F., and P. Brunjak. 1984. Drug immobilization methods. *In* Halls, L. K. (ed). White-tailed Deer Ecology and Management. Stackpole, Harrisburg, Pa. Pp. 677-686.

Scanlon, P. F., and R. E. Mirarchi. 1974. Variation in reaction of white-tailed deer to immobilization attempts using darts containing succinylcholine chloride. Proc. Ann. Conf. Southeast. Assoc. Game Fish Comm. 27: 296.

Scanlon, P. F., R. E. Mirarchi, and J. A. Wesson. 1977. Aggression toward immobilized white-tailed deer by other deer and elk. Wildl. Soc. Bull. 5: 193-194.

Schafer, E. W., and D. J. Cunningham. 1972. An evaluation of 148 compounds as avian immobilizing agents. U.S. Fish Wildl. Serv. Spec. Sci. Rep. Wildl. No. 150. 30 pp.

Schafer, E. W., R. I. Starr, D. J. Cunningham, and T. J. DeCino. 1967. Substituted phenyl N-methylcarbamates as temporary immobilizing agents for birds. J. Agr. Food Chem. 15: 287-289.

Schaller, G. B., J. Hu, W. Pan, and J. Zhu. 1985. The Giant Pandas of Wolong. U. Chicago Press, Chicago, Illinois. Pp. 109-100.

Scheepers, J. L., and K. A. E. Venzke. 1993. The use of a laser sight for the nocturnal immobilization of

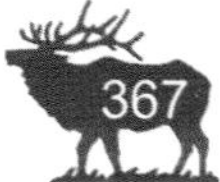

free-ranging lions. Madoqua 18: 181-182.
Scheinin, H., A. Kallio, M. Koulu, and M. Sceinin. 1989. Pharmacological effects of medetomidine in humans. Acta Vet. Scand. 85: 145-147.
Schels, H. F., and I. Nowrouzian. 1977. The effects of reversible narcotic immobilisation in the Iranian camel. Vet. Rec. 101: 388.
Schiappacasse Faundes, M. P. 1991. Characterization and evaluation of the sedation, immobilization and anesthesia with xylazine-ketamine, of vicunas (*Vicugna vicugna*) in captivity. Avances en Ciencias Veterinarias 6: 76-77 (abstract of thesis, Universidad de Chile).
Schildger, B. J., R. Baumgartner, W. Hafeli, A. Rubel, and E. Isenbugel. 1993. Anaesthesia and immobilization of reptiles. Tierarztliche Praxis 21: 361-376.
Schloeth, R., K. Klingler, and D. Burckhardt. 1960. Markierung von Rotwild in der Umgebung des Schweizerischen Nationalparkes. Revue Suisse de Zoologie 67: 281-286.
Schmidl, J. A. 1974. Experimental use of Rompun in the exotic species. J. Zoo An. Med. 5: 8-10.
Schmidt, M. J. 1975a. A preliminary report on the use of Rompun in captive Asian elephants. J. Zoo An. Med. 6: 13-21.
Schmidt, M. J. 1975b. The use of xylazine in captive Asian elephants. Proc. Am. Assoc. Zoo Vet. Pp. 1-11.
Schmidt, M. J. 1983. Antagonism of xylazine sedation by yohimbine and 4-aminopyridine in an adult Asian elephant (*Elephas maximus*). J. Zoo An. Med. 14: 94-97.
Schmitt, D. L., J. P. Bradford, and D. A. Hardy. 1996. Azaperone for standing sedation in Asian elephants (*Elephas maximus*). Proc. Am. Assoc. Zoo Vet. Pp. 48-51.
Schmitt, S. M., and R. W. Aho. 1988. Reintroduction of moose from Ontario to Michigan. *In* Nielsen, L., and R. D. Brown (eds.). Translocation of Wild Animals. Wisconsin Humane Society, Inc., and Cesar Kleberg Wildlife Research Institute, Milwaukee, Wisconsin. Pp. 258-274.
Schmitt, S. M., and W. J. Dalton. 1987. Immobilization of moose by carfentanil and xylazine and reversal by naltrexone, a long-acting antagonist. Alces. 23: 195-219.
Schobert, E. 1987. Telazol® use in wild and exotic animals. Vet. Med. Sm. An. Clin. Pp. 1080-1088.
Schöne, J., C. Hackenbroich, K. H. Bonath, K. Failing, and M. Böer. 2002. Medetomidine-ketamine-remote anaesthesia of the Eurasian lynx (*Lynx lynx*, Linne 1758) and its effects on anaesthetic depth, respiration, circulation and metabolism. Tierarztl. Prax. Aus. Klein. Heim. 30: 454-460.
Schultz, R. S., M. K. Johnson, and W. A. Forbes. 1991. Immobilization of captive white-tailed deer with mixtures of Telazol® and Rompun®. Proc. Ann. Conf. S.E. Assoc. Fish Wildlife Agencies. Pp. 29-36.
Schultze, H., J. Werner, and H. Breustedt. 1976. Unsatisfactory results with xylazine (Rompun) for the immobilization of a roe deer. Praktische Tierarzt. 57: 833-835.
Schulz, G., and W. Dingeldein. 1980. [Experiences in sedation and immobilisation of fenced fallow deer]. Z. Jagdwiss. 26: 153-158.
Schulz, T. A., and M. E. Fowler. 1974. The clinical effects of CI 744 in chinchillas, *Chinchilla villidera* (Laniger). Lab. An.Sci. 24: 810-812.
Schulz, T. A., and S. Silverman. 1973. Chemical restraint of two slow Lorises (*Nycticebus coucang*) with Vetalar (ketamine). J. Zoo An. Med. 4: 27-28.
Schumacher, J. 1999. Reptile anesthesia: update on drugs and monitoring techniques. Proc. Am. Assoc. Zoo Vet. Pp. 16-19.
Schumacher, J., H. B. Lillywhite, W. Norman, and E. R. Jacobson. 1992. The effects of ketamine on cardiopulmonary function in snakes. Proc. Joint Conf. Am. Assoc. Zoo Vet. and Am. Assoc. Wildl. Vet. P. 173.
Schumacher, J., D. J. Heard, R. Caligiuri, T. Norton, and E. R. Jacobson. 1996. Comparative effects of etorphine and carfentanil on cardiopulmonary parameters in juvenile elephants (*Loxodonta africana*). J. Zoo Wildl. Med. 26: 503-507.
Schumacher, J., D. J. Heard, and L. Young. 1995. Cardiopulmonary effects of carfentanil in dama gazelles (*Gazella dama*). Proc. Joint Conf. Am. Assoc. Zoo Vet., Wildl. Dis. Assoc., Am. Assoc. Wildl. Vet. East Lansing, Michigan. Pp. 296.
Schumacher, J., D. J. Heard, L. Young, and S. B. Citino. 1997a. Cardiopulmonary effects of carfentanil in dama gazelles (*Gazella dama*). J. Zoo Wildl. Med. 28: 166-170.
Schumacher, J., S. B. Citino, K. Hernandez, J. Hutt, and B. Dixon. 1997b. Cardiopulmonary and anesthetic effects of propofol in wild turkeys. J. Vet. Res. 58:1014-1017.
Schumacher, J., S. B. Citino, and R. Dawson. 1997c. Effects of carfentanil-xylazine combination on car-

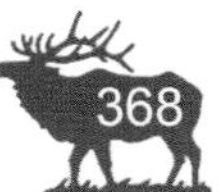

diopulmonary function and plasma catecholamine concentrations in female bongo antelopes. Am. J. Vet. Res. 58: 157-161.

Schumacher, J., J. Erdtmann, C. Pollock, and R. Harvey. 1999. Comparative cardiopulmonary and anesthetic effects of ketamine-medetomidine and ketamine-xylazine in cougars (*Felis concolor*). Proc. Am. Assoc. Zoo Vet. Pp. 45-46.

Schwab, F. E., S. W. Schwab, and M. D. Pitt. 1984. Moose immobilization program in Northcentral British Columbia. Alces. 20: 209-221.

Schwantje, H. M., R. Weir, and M. McAdie. 1998. Capture and immobilization of mustelids in British Columbia. Proc. Joint Conf. Am. Assoc. Zoo Vet. and Am. Assoc. Wildl. Vet. Omaha, Nebraska. P. 450.

Schwartz, C. C., K. J. Hundertmark, and W. R. Lance. 1991. Effects of R51163 on intake and metabolism in moose. J. Wildl. Dis. 27: 119-122.

Schwartz, C. C., T. R. Stephenson, and K. J. Hundertmark. 1997. Xylazine immobilization of moose with yohimbine or tolazoline as antagonist: a comparison to carfentanil and naltrexone. Alces 33: 33-42.

Schwartz, J. A., R. J. Warren, D. W. Henderson, D. A. Osborn, and D. J. Kesler. 1997. Captive and field tests of a method for immobilization and euthanasia of urban deer. Wildl. Soc. Bull. 25: 532-541.

Schweinsburg, R. E., L. J. Lee, and J. C. Haigh. 1982. Capturing and handling polar bears. *In* Nielsen, L., J. C. Haigh, and M. E. Fowler (eds.). Chemical Immobilization of North American Wildlife. Wisconsin Humane Society, Inc. Milwaukee, Wisconsin. Pp. 267-288.

Scott, H., and R. J. Kolata. 1982. Anesthesia for the North American opossum (*Didelphis virginiana*). Lab. An. Sci. 32: 433.

Seal, U. S. 1987. Phencyclidine immobilization of wild grizzly bears (*Ursus arctos*): analysis of possible persistent effects. Int. Conf. Bear Res. and Manage. 6.

Seal, U. S. 1990. Adverse reactions to Telazol® in tigers. Am. Assoc. Zool. Parks Aquar. Comm. 19.

Seal, U. S., and A. W. Erickson. 1969. Immobilization of carnivora and other mammals with phencyclidine and promazine. Fed. Proc. 28: 1410-1419.

Seal, U. S., and R. L. Hoskinson. 1978. Metabolic indicators of habitat condition and capture stress in pronghorns. J. Wildl. Manage. 42: 755-763.

Seal, U. S., and M. Bush. 1987. Capture and chemical immobilization of cervids. *In* Wemmer, C. M. (ed.). Biology and Management of the Cervidae. Smithsonian Institution Press, Washington D.C. Pp. 480-504.

Seal, U. S., and T. J. Kreeger. 1987. Chemical immobilization of furbearers. *In* Novak, M., J. A. Baker, M. E. Obbard, and B. Malloch (eds.). Wild Furbearer Management and Conservation in North America. Ontario Ministry of Natural Resources, Toronto. Pp. 191-215.

Seal, U. S., A. W. Erickson, and J. G. Mayo. 1970a. Drug immobilization of the Carnivora. Int. Zoo Yb. 10: 157-170.

Seal, U. S., J. Anderson, R. Farnsworth, and J. Fletcher. 1970b. Airborne transport of an uncaged, immobilized 260 kg (572 lb) lowland gorilla. Intl. Zoo Yb. 10: 134.

Seal, U. S., J. J. Ozoga, A. W. Erickson, and L. F. Verme. 1972. Effects of immobilization on blood analyses of white-tailed deer. J. Wildl. Manage. 36: 1034-1040.

Seal, U. S., D. B. Siniff, J. R. Tester, and T. D. Williams. 1985a. Chemical immobilization and blood analysis of feral horses (*Equus caballus*). J. Wildl. Dis. 21: 411-416.

Seal, U. S., S. M. Schmitt, and R. O. Peterson. 1985b. Carfentanil and xylazine for immobilization of moose (*Alces alces*) on Isle Royale. J. Wildl. Dis. 21: 48-51.

Seal, U. S., D. L. Armstrong, and L. G. Simmons. 1987. Yohimbine hydrochloride and xylazine hydrochloride immobilization of Bengal tigers and effects of hematology and serum chemistries. J. Wildl. Dis. 23: 296-300.

Sedgwick, C. J. 1979. Field anesthesia in stressed animals. Mod. Vet. Pract. 60: 531-537.

Sedgwick, C. J. 1980a. Issues in zoo animal anesthesia. Proc. Am. Assoc. Zoo Vet. Pp. 12-15.

Sedgwick, C. J. 1980b. Anesthesia of reptiles. *In* Kirk, R. W. (ed.). Current Veterinary Therapy VII. W. B. Saunders Co., Philadelphia, Pennsylvania. Pp. 618-620.

Sedgwick, C. J. 1986a. Chemical immobilization of wildlife. Seminars Vet. Med. Surg. (Small Anim.). 1: 215-223.

Sedgwick, C. J. 1986b. Inhalation anesthesia for captive wild mammals, birds, and reptiles. *In* Fowler, M. E. (ed.). Zoo and Animal Medicine (2nd ed.). W. B. Saunders Co., Philadelphia, Pennsylvania. Pp. 52-56.

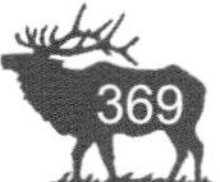

Sedgwick, C. J. 1991. Allometrically scaling the data base for vital sign assessment used in general anesthesia of zoological species. Proc. Am. Assoc. Zoo Vet. Pp. 360-369.

Sedgwick, C. J., and A. L. Acosta. 1969. Capture drugs. Mod. Vet. Pract. 12: 32-36.

Sedgwick, C. J., and J. C. Martin. 1994. Concepts of veterinary practice in wild mammals. Vet. Clin. No. Am. Sm. An. Pract. 24: 175-185.

Seidel, B. 1971. Erfahrungen mit Rompun (BAY Va 1470) bei Immobilisation und Anesthesia von Wildtieren. Verhandlungbericht des XIII. Proc. Int. Symp. Erkrankungen Zootiere, Helsinki, Finland. Pp. 219-225.

Seidel, B. 1979. Tierärztliche Gesichtspunkte der Gefangenschaftshaltung von Moschusochsen (*Ovibos moschatus*). Zool. Garten N. F. Jena 49: 131-160.

Seidel, B., and G. Strauss. 1984. [Observation on the clinical anesthesiology of cervidae]. Zool. Gart. 54: 49-100.

Seidensticker, J., M. G. Hornocker, R. R. Knight, and S. L. Judd. 1970. Techniques and equipment for radiotracking mountain lions and elk. Univ. Idaho For. Wildl. Range Exp. Sta. Bull. No. 6: 1-20.

Seidensticker, J., K. M. Tamang, and C. W. Gray. 1974. The use of CI-744 to immobilize free-ranging tigers and leopards. J. Zoo An. Med. 5: 22-25.

Selmi, A. L., G. M. Mendes, J. P. Figueiredo, F. B. Guimares, G. R. B. Selmi, F. E. Bernal, C. McMannus, and G. R. Paludo. 2003. Chemical restraint of peccaries with tiletamine/zolazepam and xylazine or tiletamine/zolazepam and butorphanol. Vet. Anaesth. Analg. 30: 24-29.

Selmi, A. L., J. P. Figueiredo, G. M. Mendes, and B. T. Lins. 2004a. Effects of tiletamine/zolazepam-romifidine-atropine in ocelots (*Leopardus pardalis*). Vet. Anaesth. Analg. 31: 222-226.

Selmi, A. L., G. M. Mendes, J. P. Figueiredo, G. R. BarbudoSelmi, and T. Bruno. 2004b. Comparison of medetomidine-ketamine and dexmedetomidine-ketamine anesthesia in golden-headed lion tamarins. Can. Vet. J. 45: 481-485.

Selmi, A. L., G. M. Mendes, V. Boere, L. A. S. Cozer, F. S. Filho, and C. A. Silva. 2004c. Assessment of dexmedetomidine/ketamine anesthesia in golden-headed lion tamarins (*Leontopithecus chrysomelas*). Vet. Anaesth. Analg. 31: 138-145.

Semple, H. A., D. K. J. Gorecki, S. D. Farley, and M. A. Ramsay. 2000. Pharmacokinetics and tissue residues of Telazol® in free-ranging polar bears. J. Wildl. Dis. 36: 653-662.

Sepúlveda, M. S., H. Ochoa-Acuña, and G. S. McLaughlin. 1994. Immobilization of Juan Fernandez fur seals, *Arctocephalus philippii*, with ketamine hydrochloride and diazepam. J. Wildl. Dis. 30: 536-540.

Servín, J., C. Huxley, and M. Vences. 1990. The combined use of ketamine hydrochloride and xylazine hydrochloride for immobilization of the wild coyote *Canis latrans*. Acta Zoologica Mexicana 36: 27-37.

Servín, J., and C. Huxley. 1992. Immobilization of wild carnivores with a mixture of ketamine and xylazine. Veterinaria Mexico 23: 135-139.

Severinghaus, C. W. 1950. Anesthetization of white-tailed deer. Cornell Vet. 40: 275-282.

Shafer, E. W., and D. J. Cunningham. 1972. An evaluation of 146 compounds as avian immobilizing agents. U. S. Dept. Interior Bur. Sport Fish. Wildl. Spec. Sci. Rep. 150: 1-21.

Sharma, S. K., J. M. Nigam, M. Singh, A. C. Varshney, and A. Kumar. 1998. Sedative and clinicobiochemical effects of medetomidine in yaks (*Bos grunniens*) and its reversal by atipamezole. Indian J. Anim Sci. 68: 236-237.

Sharma, S. K., J. M. Nigam, A. C. Varshney, M. Singh, and A. Kumar. 2001. Detomidine as a sedative in yaks. Indian J. Anim. Sci. 71: 691-692.

Shashidhar, M. K. 1981. Translocation of four horned antelope *Tetrecerus quadricornis* using ketamine anaesthesia. Tigerpaper. 8: 8.

Shaughnessy, P. D. 1991. Immobilisation of crabeater seals, *Lobodon carcinophagus*, with ketamine and diazepam. Wildl. Res. 18: 165-168.

Shaw, M. L., J. W. Carpenter, and D. E. Leith. 1995. Complications with the use of carfentanil citrate and xylazine hydrochloride to immobilize domestic horses. J. Amer. Vet. Med. Assn. 206: 833-836.

Shima, A. L. 1999. Sedationand anesthesia in marsupials. *In* Fowler, M. E., and R. E. Miller (eds.). Zoo & Wild Animal Medicine. Current Therapy 4. W. B. Saunders Company, Philadelphia, Pennsylvania. Pp. 333-336.

Shima, A., H. McCracken, R. Booth, and M. J. Lynch. 1993. Use of tiletamine-zolazepam in the immobilization of marsupials. Proc. Am. Assoc. Zoo Vet. Pp. 171-174.

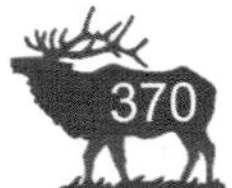

Shindle, D. B., and M. E. Tewes. 2000. Immobilization of wild oceolots with tiletamine and zolazepam in southern Texas. J. Wildl. Dis.. 36: 546-550.
Shmidl, J. A. 1974. Experimental use of rompun in the exotic species. J. Zoo An. Med. 5: 8-11.
Short, C. E. 1969. Anesthesia, sedation and chemical restraint in wild and domestic animals. J. Wildl. Dis. 5: 307-310.
Short, C. E., and J. M. King. 1963. The design of a crossbow for immobilization of wild animals. Vet. Rec. 76: 628-630.
Short, R. V. 1963. A syringe projectile for use with a bow and arrow. Vet. Rec. 75: 883-885.
Short, R. V., and J. M. King. 1964. The design of a crossbow and dart for the immobilization of wild animals. Vet. Rec. 76: 628-630.
Short, R. V., and C. A. Spinage. 1967. Drug immobilization of the Defassa waterbuck. Vet. Rec. 81: 336-340.
Shrestha, M. N., and S. Shrestha. 1981/1982. The use of xylazine and ketamine hydrochloride in combination in zoo animals. Bull. Vet. Sci. An Health, Nepal 10/11: 24-27.
Shryer, J. 1971. A new device for remote injection of liquid drugs. J. Wildl. Manage. 35: 180-181.
Shury, T. K. 1998. Use of azaperone with zuclopenthixol acetate for tranquilization of free ranging bison and immobilization with carfentanil and xylazine. Proc. Joint Conf. Am. Assoc. Zoo Vet and Am. Assoc. Wildl. Vet. Pp. 408-409.
Shury, T. K. and N. Caulkett. 2006. Chemical immobilization of free-ranging plains bison (*Bison bison*) and Rocky Mountain bighorn sheep (*Ovis canadensis canadensis*) with tiletamine-zolazepam-xylazine-hydromorphone combination. Proc. Am. Assoc. Zoo Vet. Pp. 220-223.
Siemon, A., H. Wiesner, and G. Von Hegel. 1992. Combination of tiletamine, zolazepam and romifidine for remote immobilization of wild pigs. Tierarztliche Praxis 20: 55-58.
Siglin, R. J. 1965. Movements and capture techniques. A literature review of mule deer. Colorado Dept. Game Fish Parks and Colorado Coop. Wildl. Res. Unit Spec. Rpt. No. 4. 39 pp.
Siemon, A. 1991. Pulse and respiration measurements in zoo and wild animals anaesthetized with ketamine and xylazine or with etorphine, acepromazine and xylazine, and the effect of narcotic antagonists. Inaugural Dissertation, Tierarztliche Fakultat, Ludwig-Maxmilians-Universitat, Munchen, Germany, 189 pp.
Sikarskie, J. G., T. Riebold, and J. Stick. 1981. Management of esophagotomy in an Asian elephant. Proc. Am. Assoc. Zoo Vet. Pp. 106-108.
Silberman, M. S. 1974. Restraint and handling of carnivores. Proc. Am. Assoc. Zoo Vet. P. 193.
Silberman, M. S. 1977. Tranquilization of the African Elephant (*Loxodonta africana*, Blumenbach) with the neuroleptic azaperone (R 1929). J. Zoo An. Med. 8: 7-8.
Silberman, M. S. 1982. Emergency medicine during drug immobilization. *In* Nielsen, L., J. C. Haigh, and M. E. Fowler (eds.). Chemical Immobilization of North American Wildlife. Wisconsin Humane Society, Inc. Milwaukee, Wisconsin. Pp. 72-82.
Silberman, M. S., and L. J. McWilliams. 1972. Notes on practical applications of Cap-Chur equipment in large animal medicine. Part I. Ga. Vet. 24: 14-15.
Sillero-Zubiri, C. 1996. Field immobilization of Ethiopian wolves (*Canis simensis*). J. Wildl. Dis. 32: 147-151.
Silva, I. D., and V. Y. Kuruwita. 1993. Hematology, plasma, and serum biochemistry values in free-ranging elephants (*Elephas maximus ceylonicus*) in Sri Lanka. J. Zoo Wildl. Med. 24: 434-439.
Silvestris, R., and H. Heck. 1984. Further experiments for immobilization at the Catskill Game Farm. Zool. Gart. 54: 46-48.
Simpson, A. M., J. M. Suttie, G. A. M. Sharman, and W. Corrigal. 1983. Influence of some sedative drugs on the appetite of red deer. Vet. Rec. 112: 385.
Singh, A. N., and A. Singh. 1982. Vetalar and Rompun, an ideal combination of immobilizing drugs for subhuman primates and ungulates. Indian For. 108: 676-677.
Singh, A. N., and A. Singh. 1985. Ketamine hydrochloride - an ideal chemical restraint for leopards. Tigerpaper. 12: 16-18.
Singh, L. A. K., B. T. Nayak, H. S. Upadhyaya, and B. C. Prusty. 1995. Chemical capture and translocation of a leopard from Baripada. Indian Forester 121: 965-967.
Singh, R., P. K. Peshin, D. B. Patil, R. Sharda, J. Singh, A. P. Singh, and D. Sharifi. 1994. Evaluation of halothane as an anaesthetic to camels (*Camelus dromedarius*). J. Vet. Med. (India). 41: 359-368.
Sinha, S. K. 1976. Drug immobilization trials on free-living Indian wild animals. Cheetal. 17: 29-54.

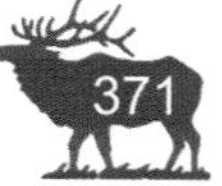

Sinnett, E. E., E. A. Wahrenbrock, and G. L. Kooyman. 1981. Cardiovascular depression and thermoregulatory disruption caused by pentothal/ holathane anesthesia in the harbor seal, *Phoca vitulina*. J. Wildl. Dis. 17: 121-130.

Skalka, P. 1979. The use of Immobilon preparat in *Equus zebra hartmannae*. Fauna Bohemiae Septentrionalis 4: 7-8.

Skjonsberg, T., and A. Westhaver. 1978. A study in the chemical immobilization of animals with suggestions for application in Canada's national parks. Unpublished Working Paper. 82 pp.

Sladky, K. K., C. R. Swanson, M. K. Stoskopf, and G. A. Lewbart. 1999a. Anesthesia of red pacu (*Piaractus brachypomus*): comparative efficacy of MS-222 and eugenol. Proc. Am. Assoc. Zoo Vet. Pp. 30-31.

Sladky, K. K., M. R. Loomis, B. Kelly, M. K. Stoskopf, and W. A. Horne. 1999b. Comparative anesthetic efficacy and cardiopulmonary effects of medetomidine-ketamine combinations and xylazine-ketamine in red wolves (*Canis rufus*). Proc. Am. Assoc. Zoo Vet. Pp. 49-52.

Sladky, K. K., B. T. Kelly, M. R. Loomis, M. K. Stoskopf, and W. A. Horne. 2000. Cardiorespiratory effects of four α_2-adrenoceptor agonist-ketamine combinations in captive red wolves. J. Am. Vet. Med. Assoc. 217: 1366-1371.

Sladky, K. K., C. R. Swanson, M. K. Stoskopf, M. R. Loomis, and G. A. Lewbart. 2001. Comparative efficacy of tricaine methanesulfonate and clove oil for use as anesthetics in red pacu (*Piaractus brachypomus*). Amer. J. Vet. Res. 62: 337-342.

Slee, F. W., and G. M. Walker. 1977. Immobilising exotic animals. Vet. Rec. 101: 312.

Sleeman, J., and E. Ramsay. 1995. Preliminary investigations in the use of orally administered carfentanil and detomidine to immobilize domestic goats (*Capra hircus*). Proc. Joint Conf. Am. Assoc. Zoo Vet., Wildl. Dis. Assoc., Am. Assoc. Wildl. Vet. East Lansing, Michigan. Pp. 271-272.

Sleeman, J. M., and J. Gaynor. 2000. Sedative and cardiopulmonary effects of medetomidine and reversal with atipamezole in desert tortoises (*Gopherus agassizii*). J. Zoo Wildl. Med. 31: 28-35.

Sleeman, J. M., W. Carter, T. Tobin, and E. C. Ramsay. 1997a. Immobilization of domestic goats (*Capra hircus*) using orally administered carfentanil citrate and detomidine hydrochloride. J. Zoo Wildl. Med. 28: 158-165.

Sleeman, J., R. Stevens, and E. Ramsay. 1997b. Field immobilization of muskrats (*Ondatra zibethicus*) for minor surgical procedures. J. Wildl. Dis. 33: 165-168.

Sleeman, J. M., K. Cameron, A. B. Mudakikwa, S. Anderson, J. E. Cooper, B. Hastings, J. W. Foster, E. J. Macfie, and H. M. Richardson. 1998. Field anesthesia of free-ranging mountain gorillas (*Gorilla gorilla beringei*) from the Virunga Volcano region, central Africa. Proc. Joint Conf. Am. Assoc. Zoo Vet. and Am. Assoc. Wildl. Vet. Pp. 1-4.

Sleeman, J. M., K. Cameron, A. B. Mudakikwa, J.-B. Nizeyi, S. Anderson, J. E. Cooper, H. M. Richardson, E. J. Macfie, B. Hastings, and J. W. Foster. 2000. Field anesthesia of free-living mountain gorillas (*Gorilla gorilla beringei*) from the Virunga Volcano region, central Africa. J. Zoo Wildl. Med. 31: 9-14.

Slip, D. J., and R. Woods. 1996. Intramuscular and intravenous immobilization of juvenile southern elephant seals. J. Wildl. Manage. 60: 802-807.

Small, B. C. 2003. Anesthetic efficacy of metomidate and comparison of plasma cortisol responses to tricaine methanesulfonate, quinaldine and clove oil anesthetized channel catfish, *Ictalurus punctatus*. Aquaculture 218: 177-185.

Smeller, J. M., M. Bush, and R. W. Custer. 1977. The immobilization of marsupials. J. Zoo An. Med. 8: 16-20.

Smeller, J., and M. Bush. 1976. A physiological study of immobilized cheetahs (*Acinonyx jubatus*). J. Zoo An. Med. 7: 5-7.

Smeller, J., M. Bush, and U. S. Seal. 1976. Observations on immobilization of Pére David's deer. J. Am. Vet. Med. Assoc. 169: 890-893.

Smit, G. L., J. Hattingh, and A. P. Burger. 1979. Haematological assessment of the effects of the anaesthetic MS 222 in natural and neutralized form in three freshwater fish species; interspecies differences. J. Fish Biol. 15: 633-643.

Smit, G. L., and J. Hattingh. Anaesthetic potency of MS 222 and neutralized MS 222 as studied in three freshwater fish species. Comp. Biochem. Physiol. 62C: 237-241.

Smith, C. A., and A. W. Franzmann. 1979. Productivity and physiology of Yakutat Forelands moose. Alaska Department of Fish and Game. Pittman-Robertson Final Report. W-17-10 and W-17-11. 18 pp.

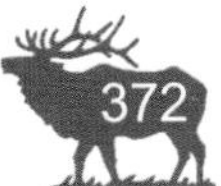

Smith, C. W., and D. C. Huse. 1980. Tranquilizer dart injury in a dog. J. Am. Vet. Med. Assoc. 176: 140-1.
Smith, I. L., S. W. McJames, R. Natte, T. H. Stanley, J. F. Kimball, T. Becker, B. Hague, and B. Barrus. 1993. A-3080 studies in elk: effective immobilizing doses by syringe and dart injection. Proc. Am. Assoc. Zoo Vet. Pp. 420-421.
Smith, J. A., M. A. Mitchell, and T. N. Tulley. 1997. Evaluation of sedative and cardiopulmonary effects of medetomidine and atipamezole in green iguanas (*Iguana iguana*): preliminary data. Proc. Assoc. Reptil. Amphib. Vet. Pp. 63.
Smith, J. A., M. A. Mitchell, K. A. Backues, T. N. Tulley, and R. F. Aguilar. 1998. Sedative and cardiopulmonary effects of medetomidine and atipamezole in American alligator (*Alligator mississippiensis*). Proc. Joint Conf. Am. Assoc. Zoo Vet and Am. Assoc. Wildl. Vet. Pp. 276-277.
Smith, J. C., S. A. Robertson, K. Springsteen, D. W. Agnew, A. E. Duncan, and B. Bolon. 2005. A dosing regimen for oral carfentanil immobilization with intranasal naltrexone reversal for restraint of lion-tailed macaques (*Macaca silensus*). Proc. Am. Assoc. Zoo Vet. Pp. 307.
Smith, J. L. D., M. W. Sunquist, K. M. Tamang, and P. B. Rai. 1983. A technique for capturing and immobilizing tigers. J. Wildl. Manage.. 47: 255-259.
Smith, K. M., B. L. Raphael, P. P. Calle, S. James, R. Moore, H. Zurawka, and S. Goscilo. 2005. Immobilization of axis deer (*Axis axis*): evaluation of thiafentanil, medetomidine, and ketamine vs. medetomidine and ketamine. Proc. Am. Assoc. Zoo Vet. Pp. 264-265.
Smith, K. M., D. M. Powell, S. B. James, P. P. Calle, R. P. Moore, H. S. Zurawka, S. Goscilo, and B. L. Raphael. 2006. Anesthesia of male axis deer (*Axis axis*): evaluation of thiafentanil, medetomidine, and ketamine versus medetomidine and ketamine. J. Zoo Wildl. Med. 37: 513-517.
Smith, L. M., J. W. Hupp, and J. T. Ratti. 1980. Reducing abandonment of nest-trapped gray partridge with methoxyflurane. J. Wildl. Manage. 44: 690-691.
Smith, N. G. 1967. Capturing seabirds with Avertin. J. Wildl. Manage. 31: 479-483.
Smith, R. H., J. Tatsuno, and R. L. Zouhar. 1967. Electroanesthesia: a review - 1966. Anesth. Anal. Curr. Res. 46: 109-125.
Smits, J. E. G., and J. C. Haigh. 1989. Yohimbine hydrochloride administration to reverse xylazine sedation in white-tailed deer and mule deer. J. Zoo Wildl. Med. 20: 170-172.
Smuts, G. L. 1973a. Xylazine hydrochloride (Rompun) and the new retractable-barbed dart ("drop-out" dart) for the capture of some nervous and aggressive antelope species. Koedoe. 16: 159-173.
Smuts, G. L. 1973b. Ketamine hydrochloride - a useful drug for the field immobilization of the spotted hyaena *Crocuta crocuta.* Koedoe 16: 175-180.
Smuts, G. L. 1975. An appraisal of naloxone hydrochloride as a narcotic antagonist in the capture and release of wild herbivores. J. Am. Vet. Med. Assoc. 167: 559-561.
Smuts, G. L., B. R. Bryden, V. De Vos, and E. Young. 1973. Some practical advantages of CI-581 (ketamine) for the field immobilization of larger wild felines, with comparative notes on baboons and impala. Lammergeyer. 18: 1-14.
Snyder, S. B., M. J. Richard, and W. R. Foster. 1992. Etorphine, ketamine, and xylazine in combination (M99KX) for immobilization of exotic ruminants: a significant additive effect. Proc. Joint Conf. Am. Assoc. Zoo Vet. and Am. Assoc. Wildl. Vet. Pp. 253-263.
Somers, G. F. 1965. Tranquillizers for elephants. "Ours" Magazine. 4: 8-12.
Sapolsky, R. M., and L. J. Share. 1998. Darting terrestrial primates in the wild: a primer. Am. J. Primatol. 44:155-167.
Soveri, T., S. Sankari, J. S. Salonen, and M. Nieminen. 1999. Effects of immobilization with medetomidine and reversal with atipamezole on blood chemistry of semi-domesticated reindeer (*Rangifer tarandus tarandus* L.) in autumn and late winter. Acta Vet. Scand. 40: 335-349.
Sowls, L. K., and R. E. Schweinsburg. 1967. An improved propulsion system for short-range projection of immobilization darts. J. Wildl. Manage. 31: 345-346.
Speckmann, G. 1975. Ketaset (ketamine HCI) anesthesia for orchiectomy on a raccon (*Procyon lotor*). J. Zoo An. Med. 6: 31-32.
Spellerberg, I. F. 1969. Capturing and immobilizing McCormick skuas. J. Am. Vet. Med. Assoc. 155: 1040-1043.
Spelman, L. H. 1999. Otter anesthesia. *In* Fowler, M. E., and R. E. Miller (eds.). Zoo & Wild Animal Medicine. Current Therapy 4. W. B. Saunders Company, Philadelphia, Pennsylvania. Pp. 436-443.
Spelman, L. H. 2004. Reversible anesthesia of captive California sea lions (*Zalophus californianus*) with

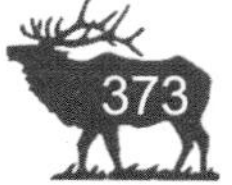

medetomidine, midazolam, butorphanol, and isoflurane. J. Zoo Wildl. Med. 35: 65-69.

Spelman, L. H., P. W. Sumner, J. F. Levine, and M. K. Stoskopf. 1993a. Field anesthesia in the North American river otter (*Lutra canadensis*). J. Zoo Wildl. Med. 24: 19-27.

Spelman, L. H., M. K. Stoskopf, J. F. Levine, and P. W. Sumner. 1993b. Immobilization of North American river otters (*Lutra canadensis*) with medetomidine-ketamine and reversal by atipamezole. Proc. Am. Assoc. Zoo Vet. Pp. 142-143.

Spelman, L. H., M. K. Stoskopf, and W. J. Jochem. 1994. Post anesthetic monitoring of core body temperature using telemetry. Joint Conf. Am. Assoc. Zoo Vet. Assoc. Reptil. Amphib. Vet. Pp. 211-213.

Spelman, L. H., P. W. Sumner, J. F. Levine, and M. K. Stoskopf. 1994. Anesthesia of North American river otters (*Lutra canadensis*) with medetomidine-ketamine and reversal by atipamezole. J. Zoo Wildl. Med. 25: 214-223.

Spelman, L. H., R. C. Cambre, T. Walsh, and R. Rosscoe. 1996. Anesthetic techniques in Komodo dragons (*Varanus komodoensis*). Proc. Am. Assoc. Zoo Vet. Pp. 247-250.

Spelman, L. H., W. J. Jochem, P. W. Sumner, D. P. Redmond, and M. K. Stoskopf. 1997a. Postanesthetic monitoring of core body temperature using telemetry in North American river otters (*Lutra canadensis*). J. Zoo Wildl. Med. 28: 413-417.

Spelman, L. H., P. W. Sumner, W. B. Karesh, and M. K. Stoskopf. 1997b. Tiletamine-zolazepam anesthesia in North American river otters (*Lutra canadensis*) and partial antagonism with flumazenil. J. Zoo Wildl. Med. 28:418-423.

Spiegel, R. A., R. E. Larsen, T. J. Lane, and P. T. Cardeilhac. 1984a. Chemical restraint in the American alligator (*Alligator mississippiensis*) using a combination of diazepam and succinylcholine chloride. Proc. Int. Assoc. Aquat. Anim. Med. 1: 13-16.

Spiegel, R. A., T. J. Lane, R. E. Larsen, and P. T. Cardeilhac. 1984b. Diazepam and succinylcholine chloride for restraint of the American alligator. J. Am. Vet. Med. Assoc. 185: 1335-1336.

Spraker, T. R. 1977. Capture myopathy of Rocky Mountain bighorn sheep. Desert Bighorn Council Trans. 21: 14-16.

Spraker, T. R. 1982. An overview of the pathophysiology of capture myopathy and related conditions that occur at the time of capture of wild animals. *In* Nielsen, L., J. C. Haigh, and M. E. Fowler (eds.). Chemical Immobilization of North American Wildlife. Wisconsin Humane Society, Inc. Milwaukee, Wisconsin. Pp. 83-118.

Spraker, T. R. 1986. Capture techniques in feral ruminants. Vet. Clin. North Am. [Food Anim. Pract.]. 2: 693-710.

Spraker, T. R. 1993. Stress and capture myopathy in artiodactylids. *In* Fowler, M. E. (ed.). Zoo & Wild Animal Medicine: Current Therapy 3. W. B. Saunders Co., Philadelphia, Pennsylvania. Pp. 481-488.

Spurlock, G. H., and S. L. Spurlock. 1988. Projectile dart foreign body in a horse. J. Am. Vet. Med. Assoc. 193: 565.

Stafford, S. K., and L. E. Williams Jr. 1968. Data on capturing black bears with alpha-chloralose. Proc. Ann. Conf. Southeast. Assoc. Game Fish Comm.

Stander, P. E., and P. V. B. Morkel. 1991. Field immobilization of lions using dissociative anaesthetics in combination with sedatives. Afr. J. Ecol. 29: 137-148.

Stander, P. E., and W. C. Gasaway. 1991. Spotted hyenas immobilized with ketamine/xylazine and antagonized with tolazoline. Afr. J. Ecol. 29: 168-169.

Stander, P., X. Ghau, and X. Tsisaba. 1996. A new method of darting: stepping back in time. Afr. J. Ecol. 34: 48-53.

Stanley, T. H. 2000. Immobilization of wild animals: both the two-legged and four-legged types. Proc. Joint Conf. Am. Assoc. Zoo Vet. and Intl. Assoc. Aquatic An. Med. P. 97.

Stanley, T. H., and S. McJames. 1986. Chemical immobilization using new high potency opioids and other drugs and drug combinations with high therapeutic indices. U.S. Department of Defense, Final Report, Contract DAAK11-84-K-0002, Washington, D.C., USA.

Stanley, T. H., J. D. Port, J. Kimball, J. E. Oosterhuis, and D. L. Janssen. 1984. New drugs for immobilization of non-domestic hoofstock. Proc. Am. Assoc. Zoo Vet. P. 56.

Stanley, T. H., J. D. Port, J. Van der Maaten, and J. Kimball. 1986. Treatment of stress hyperthermia in elk with ketanserin, a serotonin receptor blocker. Vet. Surg. 15: 214-217.

Stanley, T. H., S. McJames, J. Kimball, J. D. Port, and N. L. Pace. 1988. Immobilization of elk with A-3080. J. Wildl. Manage. 52: 577-581.

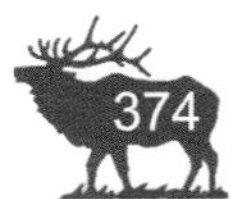

Stanley, T. H., S. McJames, and J. Kimball. 1989. Chemical immobilization for the capture and transportation of big game. Proc. Am. Assoc. Zoo Vet. Pp. 13-14.

Stanley, T. H., J. D. Port, N. L. Pace, J. Kimball, and S. McJames. 1988. Chemical immobilization using new high potency opioids and other drugs and drug combinations with high therapeutic indices. U. S. Dept. Defense Chemical Research Development & Engineering Center, CRDEC-CR-88077. 122 pp.

Starke, R. 1991. Observations on the use of xylazine in combination with other agents for the immobilization of wapiti. *In* Renecker, L.A., and R. J. Hudson (eds.). Wildlife Production: Conservation and Sustainable Development. University of Alaska, Fairbanks.

Stegmann, G. F. 2000. Observations on the use of midazolam-ketamine for induction of anaesthesia in four ostriches. S. Afr. J. Wildl. Res. 30: 58-61.

Stegman, G. F., L. Bester, and L. Venter. 2000. Halothane anaesthesia in African lion. So. Afr. J.f Wildl. Res. 30: 93-95.

Stelfox, J. G., and J. R. Robertson. 1976. Immobilizing bighorn sheep with succinylcholine chloride and phencyclidine hydrochloride. J. Wildl. Manage. 40: 174-176.

Stemmler, O., and A. Zingg. 1969. Das Betäuben von Schlangen (The anesthetizing of snakes). Der Zool. Gart. 37: 76-80.

Stetter, M. D., B. Raphael, F. Indiviglio, and R. A. Cook. 1996. Isoflurane anesthesia in amphibians: comparison of five application methods. Proc. Am. Assoc. Zoo. Vet. Pp. 255-257.

Stewart, G. R., J. M. Siperek, and V. R. Wheeler. 1980. Use of the cataleptoid anesthetic CI-744 for chemical restraint of black bears. Int. Conf. Bear Res. Manage. 4: 57-61.

Stewart, M. C., and A. W. English. 1990. The reversal of xylazine/ketamine immobilization of fallow deer with yohimbine. Austr. Vet. J. 67: 315-317.

Steyn, D. G. 1975. The effect of phencyclidine anaesthesia on the blood chemistry and haematology of the chacma baboon (*Papio ursinus*). J. So. Afr. Vet. Assoc. 46: 235-239.

Still, J. 1993. Etorphine-azaperone anaesthesia in an African elephant (*Loxodonta africana*). J. Vet. Anaesth. 20: 54-55.

Still, J., J. P. Raath, and L. Matzner. 1996. Respiratory and circulatory parameters of African elephants (*Loxodonta africana*) anesthetized with etorphine and azaperone. J. So. Afr. Vet. Assoc. 67: 123-127.

Stirling, I., and B. Sjare. 1988. Preliminary observations on the immobilization of male Atlantic walruses (*Odobenus rosmarus rosmarus*) with Telazol. Mar. Mammal Sci. 4: 163-168.

Stirling, I., E. Broughton, L. Ø. Knutsen, M. A. Ramsay, and D. S. Andriashek. 1985. Immobilization of polar bears with Telazol® on the western coast of Hudson Bay during summer, 1984. Can. Wildl. Serv. Prog. Notes. 157: 1-7.

Stirling, I., C. Spencer, and D. S. Andriashek. 1989. Immobilization of polar bears (*Ursus maritimus*) with Telazol® in the Canadian Arctic. J. Wildl. Dis. 25: 159-168.

Stirrat, S. C. 1997. Behavioral responses of agile wallabies (*Macropus agilis*) to darting and immobilization with tiletamine hydrochloride and zolazepam hydrochloride. Wildl. Res. 24: 89-95.

Storms, T. N., J. Schumacher, N. Zagaya, D. A. Osborn, K. V. Miller, and E. C. Ramsay. 2004. Determination and evaluation of an optimal dosage of carfentanil and xylazine for the immobilization of white-tailed deer (*Odocoileus virginianus*). Proc. Am. Assoc. Zoo Vet. Pp. 517-518.

Storms, T. N., J. Schumacher, N. Zagaya, D. A. Osborn, K. V. Miller, and E. C. Ramsay. 2005. Determination and evaluation of an optimal dosage of carfentanil and xylazine for the immobilization of white-tailed deer (*Odocoileus virginianus*). J. Wildl. Dis. 41: 559-568.

Storms, T. N., J. Schumacher, D. A. Osborn, K. V. Miller, and E. C. Ramsay. 2006. Effects of ketamine on carfentanil and xylazine immobilization of white-tailed deer (*Odocoileus virginianus*). J. Zoo Wildl. Med. 37: 347-353.

Stoskopf, M. K. 1979. Anesthesia of zoo rodents. Proc. Am. Assoc. Zoo Vet. Pp. 68-69.

Stoskopf, M. K. 1986. Immobilization of captive sharks. Proc. Am. Assoc. Zoo Vet. Pp. 106-108.

Stoskopf, M. K. 1993. Shark pharmacology and toxicology. *In* Stoskopf, M. K. (ed.). Fish Medicine. Saunders, Philadelphia. Pp. 809-816.

Stoskopf, M. K., and L. Bishop. 1978. Immobilization of two captive adult Nile hippo (*Hippopotamus amphibius*). J. Zoo An. Med. 9: 103-107.

Stoskopf, M. K., F. B. Beall, P. K. Ensley, and E. Neely. 1982. Immobilization of large ratites: blue necked

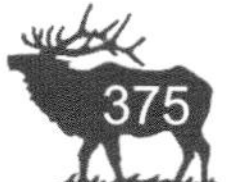

ostrich (*Struthio camelus austrealis*) and double wattled cassowary (*Casuarius casuarius*) — with hematologic and serum chemistry data. J. Zoo An. Med. 13: 160-168.

Stoskopf, M. K., R. E. Meyer, M. Jones, and D. O. Baumbarger. 1999. Field immobilization and euthanasia of American opossum. J. Wildl. Dis. 35: 145-149.

Stouffer, P. C., D. F. Caccamise. 1991. Capturing American crows using alpha-chloralose. J. Field Ornithol. 62: 450-453.

Strauss, G. 1987. Zum Einsatz von Tolazolin bei der Xylazin/Ketamin Immobilisation. 29th Int. Symp. Dis. Zoo and Wild An. Pp 151-155.

Strauss, G. 1992. Erfahrungen bei der Immobilisation verschneidener Equidenarten im Tierpark Berlin-Friedrichsfelde. Erkr Zootiere 34: 163-169.

Strond, W. L., and S. D. Baxter. 1980. The use of ketaset (ketamine hydrochloride) as a rapid acting anesthetic agent in two species of sympatric rattlesnakes. Proc. Neb. Acad. Sci. Affil. Soc. 90: 21.

Stullken, D. E., and C. M. Kirkpatrick. 1955. Physiological investigation of captivity mortality in the sea otter (*Enhydra lutris*). Trans. No. Am. Wildl. Conf. 20: 476-494.

Stunkard, J. A., and J. C. Miller. 1974. An outline guide to general anesthesia in exotic species. Vet. Med. Sm. An. Clin. 69: 1181-1186.

Summerhays, G. 1976. Overdosage with nalorphine hydrobromide following self-inflicted injury with Immobilon. Vet. Rec. 99: 36.

Sutherland, C., and J. Hodgkin. 1974. Tranquilizing deer. Vet. Rec. 95: 71.

Sutherland-Smith, M., J. M. Campos, C. Cramer, C. Thorstadt, W. Toone, and P. J. Morris. 2004. Immobilization of Chacoan peccaries (*Catagonus wagneri*) using medetomidine, Telazol®, and ketamine. J. Wildl. Dis. 40: 731-736.

Suzuki, M., Y. Nakamura, M. Onuma, J. Tanaka, H. Takahashi, K. Kaji, and N. Ohtaishi. 2001. Acid-base status and blood gas arterial values in free-ranging sika deer hinds immobilized with medetomidine and ketamine. J. Wildl. Dis. 37: 366-369.

Swan, G. E. 1993. Drugs used for the immobilization, capture, and translocation of wild animals. *In* McKenzie, A. A. (ed.). The Capture and Care Manual. Wildlife Decision Support Services and The South African Veterinary Foundation, Pretoria. Pp. 2-64.

Sweitzer, R. A., G. S. Ghneim, I. A. Gardner, D. Van Vuren, B. J. Gonzales, and W. M. Boyce. 1997. Immobilization and physiological parameters associated with chemical restraint of wild pigs with Telazol® and xylazine hydrochloride. J. Wildl. Dis. 33: 198-205.

Sylvester, J. R. 1975. Factors influencing the efficacy of MS-222 to striped mullet (*Mugil cephalus*). Aquaculture 6: 163-169.

Sylvia, P., S. Belle, R. Cooper, and H. Krum. 1994. Handling, restraint, anesthesia and surgery in the bluefin tuna (*Thunnus thynnus*). Proc. Am. Assoc. Zoo Vet. P. 189.

Szabuniewicz, M., L. Sanches, A. Sosa, And M. De Gomez. 1978. Sedatión y anestesia del chiguire (*Hydrochoerus hydrochoeris*, Linné). Revista de la Facultad de Ciencias veterinarias de la Universidad Central de Venezuela 8: 61-78.

Taber, R. D., and I. M. Cowan. 1969. Capturing and marking wild animals. *In* Giles, R. H. (ed.). Wildlife Management Techniques. The Wildlife Society. Washington, D. C. Pp. 277-318.

Tahmindjis, M. A., D. P. Higgins, M. L. Lynch, J. A. Barnes, and C. J. Southwell. 2003. Use of pethidine and midazolam combination for the reversible sedation of crabeater seals (*Lobodon carcinophagus*). Mar. Mamm. Sci. 19: 581-589.

Talbot, L. M. 1960. Field immobilization of some East African wild animals and cattle. East Afr. Agric. For. J. 26: 92-102.

Talbot, L. M., and H. F. Lamprey. 1961. Immobilization of free-ranging East African ungulates with succinylcholine chloride. J. Wildl. Manage. 25: 303-310.

Talbot, L. M., and M. H. Talbot. 1962. Flaxedil and other drugs in field immobilization and translocation of large mammals in East Africa. J. Mammal. 43: 76-88.

Tamas, P. M., and D. R. Geiser. 1983. Etorphine analgesia supplemented by halothane anesthesia in an adult African elephant. J. Am. Vet. Med. Assoc. 183: 1312-1314.

Taulman, J. F., and J. H. Williamson. 1993. A simple apparatus and technique for anesthetizing raccoons. Am. Mid. Naturalist. 129: 210-214.

Taylor, D. C., and N. Chandler. 1971. Cesarean section in a zebra. Vet. Rec. 89: 388-389.

Taylor, M. 1987. Avian anesthesia - a clinical update. Proc. Int. Conf. Zool. Avian Med. 1: 519-524.

Taylor, M. K., D. P. Demaster, S. P. Sheldon, and R. E. Sorensen. 1982. Use of M50-50 as a therapeutic

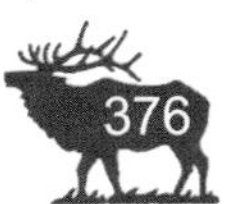

drug for M99-induced trauma. J. Wildl. Manage. 46: 252-253.

Taylor, R. H., and W. B. Magnussen. 1965. Preliminary note on capture and marking of wild ungulates in New Zealand. N. Z. J. Sci. 8: 205-213.

Taylor, S. K., E. D. Land, M. E. Roelke-Parker, S. B. Citino, and D. Rotstein. 1998. Anesthesia of free-ranging Florida panthers (*Puma concolor coryi*), 1981-1998. Proc. Joint Conf. Am. Assoc. Zoo Vet. and Am. Assoc. Wildl. Vet. Pp. 26-29.

Taylor, W. P., H. V. Reynolds, and W. B. Ballard. 1989. Immobilization of grizzly bears with tiletamine hydrochloride and zolazepam hydrochloride. J. Wildl. Manage. 53: 978-981.

Teare, J. A. 1987. Antagonism of xylazine hydrochloride-ketamine hydrochloride immobilization in guineafowl (*Numida meleagris*) by yohimbine hydrochloride. J. Wildl. Dis. 23: 301-305.

Teferra, Z. 1992. Chemical immobilisation of wildlife. Walia 14: 9-15.

Telesco, R., and M. A. Sovada. 2002. Immobilization of swift foxes with ketamine hydrochloride-xylazine hydrochloride. J. Wildl. Dis. 38: 764-768.

Terpin, K. M., P. Dodson, and J. R. Spotila. 1978. Observations on ketamine hydrochloride as an anaesthetic for alligators. Copeia. 1978: 147-148.

Thil, M. A., and R. Groscolas. 2002. Field immobilization of king penguins with tiletamine-zolazepam. J. Field Ornithol. 73: 308-317.

Thomas, J. W., and R. G. Marburger. 1964. Mortality in deer shot in the thoracic area with the Cap-Chur gun. J. Wildl. Manage. 28: 173-175.

Thomas, J. W., R. M. Robinson, and R. G. Marburger. 1967. Use of diazepam in the capture and handling of cervids. J. Wildl. Manage. 31: 686-692.

Thomas, W. D. 1961. Chemical immobilization of wild animals. J. Am. Vet. Med. Assoc. 138: 263-265.

Thomson, P. C., K. Rose, and N. E. Kok. 1992. Dingoes in northwestern Australia. Wildl. Res. 19: 509-603.

Thorne, E. T. 1971. The use of M-99 etorphine and acetylpromazine in the immobilization and capture of free ranging Rocky Mountain bighorn sheep. Trans. No. Amer. Wild Sheep Conf. 127-134.

Thorne, E. T. 1980. Immobilization of wild ungulates: considerations and drugs. Biotelem. Patient Monitg. 7: 178-187.

Thorne, E. T. 1982. Agents used in North American ruminant immobilization. *In* Nielsen, L., J. C. Haigh, and M. E. Fowler (eds.). Chemical Immobilization of North American Wildlife. Wisconsin Humane Society, Inc. Milwaukee, Wisconsin. Pp. 304-334.

Thorne, E. T., M. H. Schroeder, S. C. Forest, T. M. Cambell, L. Richardson, D. Biggins, L. R. Hanebury, D. Belitsky, and E. S. Williams. 1985. Capture, immobilization, and care of black-footed ferrets for research. *In* Anderson, S. H., and D. B. Inkley (eds.). Proceedings of the Black-footed Ferret Workshop. Laramie, Wyoming. Pp. 9.1-9.8.

Thornton, P. D., C. Newman, P. J. Johnson, C. D. Buesching, S. E Baker, D. D. P. Johnson, and D. W. MacDonald. 2005. Preliminary comparison of four anaesthetic techniques in badgers (*Meles meles*). Vet. Anaesth. Analg. 32: 40-47.

Throckmorton, G. S. 1981. Ketamine hydrochloride as an anesthetic agent for lizard surgery. Copeia 1981: 241-243.

Thurman, G. D., S. J. T. Downes, and S. Barrow. 1982. Anaesthetization of a cape fur seal (*Arctocephalus pusillus*) for the treatment of a chronic eye infection and amputation of a metatarsal bone. J. So. Afr. Vet. Assoc. 53: 255-257.

Thurmon, J. C., D. R. Nelson, and J. O. Mozier. 1972. A preliminary report on the sedative effect of Bay Va 1470 in elk (*Cervus c. canadensis*). J. Zoo An. Med. 3: 9-14.

Thurmon, J. C., W. J. Tranquilli, and G. J. Benson. 1992. α_2-antagonists: use in domestic and wild animal species. *In* Short, C. E., and A. Van Poznak (eds). Animal Pain. Churchill Livingstone, New York. Pp. 237-247.

Tobey, R. W., and W. B. Ballard. 1985. Increased mortality in gray wolves captured with acepromazine and etorphine hydrochloride in combination. J. Wildl. Dis. 21: 188-190.

Tolo, D., and D. Keyler. 1998. Field management of inadvertent carfentanil (Wildnil™)/etorphine (M99™) human exposure. Proc. Joint Conf. Am. Assoc. Zoo Vet. and Am. Assoc. Wildl. Vet. Omaha, Nebraska. P. 501.

Tomizawa, N., T. Tsujimoto, K. Itoh, T. Ogino, K. Nakamura, and S. Hara. 1997. Chemical restraint of African lions (*Panthero leo*) with medetomidine-ketamine. J. Vet. Med. Sci. 59: 307-310.

Tomkiewicz, S. M. 1982. Advances in capture technology. *In* Nielsen, L., J. C. Haigh, and M. E. Fowler

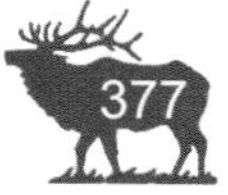

(eds.). Chemical Immobilization of North American Wildlife. Wisconsin Humane Society, Inc. Milwaukee, Wisconsin. Pp. 1-17.

Torgerson, R. W. 1990. Polar bear biology and medicine. *In* Dierauf, L. A. (ed.). CRC Handbook of Marine Mammal Medicine: Health, Disease, and Rehabilitation. CRC Press, Boca Raton. Pp. 649-657.

Tranquilli, W. J. 1993a. Injectable anesthesia. Proc. No. Am. Vet. Conf. Orlando, Florida. Pp. 14-15.

Tranquilli, W. J. 1993b. New anesthetic agents. Proc. No. Am. Vet. Conf. Orlando, Florida. Pp. 16-17.

Travaini, A., and M. Delibes. 1994. Immobilization of free-ranging red foxes (*Vulpes vulpes*) with tiletamine hydrochloride and zolazepam. J. Wildl. Dis. 30: 589-591.

Travaini, A., P. Ferreras, M. Delibes, and J. J. Aldama. 1992. Xylazine hydrochloride-ketamine hydrochloride immobilization of free-living red foxes (*Vulpes vulpes*) in Spain. J. Wildl. Dis. 28: 507-509.

Travaini, A., P. Ferreras, J. J. Aldama, J. M. Fedriani, and M. Delibes. 1994. Chemical immobilization of wild badgers (*Meles meles*). Revue de Médicine Véterinaire 145: 577-580.

Treimo, T. 1971. Immobilisering av isbjorn (*Thalarctos maritimus*). [Immobilization of polar bears (*Thalarctos maritimus*)]. Nor. Vet. Tidsskr. 82: 169-174.

Trembath, P. R. 1985. Restraint of baby elephants with Rompun. Vet. Med. Rev. 2: 169-170.

Trillmich, F. 1983. Ketamine xylazine combination for the immobilization of Galapagos seal lions and fur seals. Vet. Rec. 112: 279-280.

Trillmich, F., and H. Wiesner. 1979. Immobilisation of free-ranging Galapagos sea lions (*Zalophus californianus wollebaeki*). Vet. Rec. 105: 465-466.

Trim, C. M., N. Lamberski, D. Kissel, and J. E. Quandt. 1998. Anesthesia in Baird's tapir (*Tapirus bairdii*). J. Zoo Wildl. Med. 29:195-198.

Trindle, B. D., and L. D. Lewis. 1978. Methoxyflurane anesthesia in mule deer (*Odocoileus hemionus*) fawns. J. Wildl. Dis. 14: 519-522.

Troy, S., D. Middleton, and J. Phelan. 1997. On capture, anesthesia and branding of adult male New-Zealand fur seals *Arctocephalus forsteri*. *In:* Hindell, M., and C. Kemper (eds.). Marine Mammal Research in the Southern Hemisphere, Vol 1. Chipping Norton NSW: Surrey Beatty & Sons. Pp. 179-183.

Troyer, W. A., R. J. Hensel, and K. E. Durley. 1961. Live-trapping and handling of brown bears. J. Wildl. Manage. 25: 330-331.

Tsubota, T., K. Yamamoto, T. Mano, M. Yamanaka, and H. Kanagawa. 1991. Immobilization of the free-ranging Hokkaido brown bear, *Ursus arctos yesoensis*, with ketamine hydrochloride and xylazine hydrochloride. J. Vet. Med. Sci. 53: 321-322.

Tsuruga, H., M. Susuki, H. Takahashi, K. Jinma, and K. Kaji. 1999. Immobilization of sika deer with medetomidine and ketamine, and antagonism by atipamezole. J. Wildl. Dis. 35: 774-778.

Tung, K. C., J. S. Wang, C. L. Shyu, C. L. Yang, and C. H. Shih. 1993. Studies on the clinical choice and application of chemical immobilization drugs in deer in Taiwan. Taiwan J. Vet. Med. An. Husbandry. 61: 9-18.

Tuomi, P. A., D. M. Mulcahy, and G. W. Garner. 1996. Immobilization of Pacific walrus (*Odobenus rosmarus divergens*) with carfentanil, naltrexone reversal and isoflurane anesthesia. Proc. Intl. Assoc. Aquatic Anim. Med. Pp. 121-123.

Tuomi, P., M. Grey, and D. Christen. 2000. Butorphanol and butorphanol/diazepam administration for analgesia and sedation of harbor seals (*Phoca vitulina*). Proc. Joint Conf. Am. Assoc. Zoo Vet. and Intl. Assoc. Aquatic An. Med. Pp. 382-383.

Tyler, N. J., R. Hotvedt, A. S. Blix, and D. R. SØrensen. 1990. Immobilization of Norwegian reindeer (*Rangifer tarandus tarandus*) and Svalblad reindeer (*R. t. platyrhynchus*) with medetomidine and medetomidine-ketamine and reversal of immobilization by atipamezole. Acta Vet. Scand. 31: 479-488.

Umbreit, N. 1980. Chemical restraint of reptiles, amphibians, fish, birds, small mammals and selected marine mammals in North America. An annotated bibliography. U. S. Bur. Land Manage. Tech. Note. TN-340. 181 pp.

Vahala, J. 1993. Clinical experience and comparison of ketamine-medetomidine with ketamine-xylazine anesthesia in the African wild dog (*Lycaon pictus*) in captivity. Vet. Med. Czech. 38: 569-578.

Vahala, J. 1994. Field experience from immobilization of captive impala (*Aepyceros melamphus*) Internationales Symposium ueber die Erkrankungen der Zootiere (ISEZ): Verhandlungsberichte 36: 325-331.

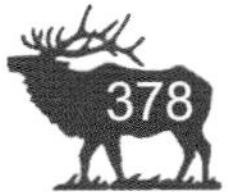

Valerio, F. L. Brugnola, F. Rocconi, V. Varasano, C. Civitella, and C. Guglielmini. 2005. Evaluation of the cardiovascular effects of an anesthetic protocol for immobilization and anaesthesia in grey wolves (*Canis lupus* L, 1978). Vet. Res. Commun. 29: 315-318.

Valkenburg, P., R. D. Boertje, and J. L. Davis. 1983. Effects of darting and netting caribou in Alaska. J. Wildl. Manage. 47: 1233-1237.

Valkenburg, P., R. W. Tobey, and D. Kirk. 1999. Velocity of tranquilizer darts and capture mortality of caribou calves. Wildl. Soc. Bull. 27: 894-896.

Valkenburg, P., and R. W. Tobey. 2001. Reducing capture-related mortality and dart injury: reply to Jessup. Wildl. Soc. Bull. 29: 752-753.

Van Aarde, R. J. 1985. Husbandry and immobilization of captive porcupines *Hystrix africaeaustralis*. So. Afr. J. Wildl. Res. 15: 77-79.

Van Bever, W. F., C. J. Niemegeers, K. H. Schellekens, and P. A. Janssen. 1976. N-4-substituted 1-(2-arylethyl)-4-piperidinyl-N-phenylpropanamides, a novel series of extremely potent analgesics with unusually high safety margin. Arzneimittelforschung. 26: 1548-1551.

Van Der Eems, K., and R. D. Brown. 1986. Effect of caffeine sodium benzoate, ketamine hydrochloride, and yohimbine hydrochloride on xylazine hydrochloride-induced anorexia in white-tailed deer. J. Wildl. Dis. 22: 403-406.

Van Der Merwe, J. N., D. B. Du Bruyn, W. H. Van Der Walt, and M. R. Sly. 1987. Effects of certain anaesthetics on plasma metabolite concentrations in the baboon (*Papio ursinus*). J. So. Afr. Vet. Assoc. 58: 125-128.

Van Foreest, A. 1980. Use of ketamine/xylazine combination for the tail amputation in nutria (*Myocaster coypus*). J. Zoo An. Med. 11: 19-20.

Van Heerden, J. 1984. Capture and immobilization of the Cape ground squirrel *Xerus inauris* with ketamine hydrochloride. So. Afr. J. Wildl. Res. 14: 127-128.

Van Heerden, J. 1993. Chemical capture of the wild dog *Lycaon pictus*. *In* McKenzie, A. A. (ed.). Capture and Care Manual. Wildlife Decision Support Services and The South African Veterinary Foundation, Pretoria. Pp. 247-250.

Van Heerden, J., and V. de Vos. 1981. Immobilization of the hunting dog *Lycaon pictus* with ketamine hydrochloride and a fentanyl/ droperidol combination. So. Afr. J. Wildl. Res. 11: 112-113.

Van Heerden, J., and J. Dauth. 1985. Serum potassium and sodium concentrations in dead and hypoxic dogs, shot mountain zebra *Equus zebra zebra*, and chemically immobilized laboratory rats and ground squirrels *Xerus inauris*. So. Afr. J. Wildl. Res. 15: 32-36.

Van Heerden, J. and R. H. Keffen. 1991. A preliminary investigation into the immobilising potential of a tiletamine/zolazepam mixture, metomidate, a metomidate and azaperone combination and medetomidine on ostriches (*Struthio camelus*). J. So. Afr. Vet. Assoc. 62: 114-117.

Van Heerden, J., J. Komen, and E. Myer. 1987. The use of ketamine hydrochloride in the immobilisation of the cape vulture *Gyps coprotheres*. J. So. Afr. Vet. Assoc. 58: 143-144.

Van Heerden, J., G. E. Swan, J. Dauth, R. E. J. Burroughs, and M. J. Dreyer. 1991a. Sedation and immobilization of wild dogs *Lycaon pictus* using medetomidine-ketamine hydrochloride combination. So. Afr. J. Wildl. Res. 21: 88-93.

Van Heerden, J., R. E. J. Burroughs, J. Dauth, and M. J. Dreyer. 1991b. Immobilization of wild dogs (*Lycaon pictus*) with a tiletamine hydrochloride/zolazepam hydrochloride combination and subsequent evaluation of selected blood chemistry parameters. J. Wildl. Dis. 27: 225-229.

Van Jaarsveld, A. S. 1988. The use of Zoletil® for the immobilization of spotted hyaenas. So. Afr. J. Wildl. Res. 18: 65-66.

Van Jaarsveld, A. S., and J. D. Skinner. 1992. Adrenocorticol responsiveness to immobilization stress in spotted hyenas (*Crocuta crocuta*). Comp. Biochem. Physiol. Pt. A. Compar. Physiol. 103: 73-79.

Van Jaarsveld, A. S., A. A. McKenzie, and D. G. A. Meltzer. 1984. Immobilization and anaesthesia of spotted hyaenas, *Crocuta crocuta*. So. Afr. J. Wildl. Res. 14: 120-122.

Van Mourik, S., and T. Stelmasiak. 1984. The effect of immobilizing drugs on adrenal responsiveness to ACTH in Rusa deer. Comp. Biochem. Physiol. 78: 467-471.

Van Mourik, S., and T. Stelmasiak. 1984. The use of Rompun® for immobilization of mature rusa deer (*Cervus rusa timorensis*) – first report. Vet. Med. Rev. 1984: 163-166.

Van Mourik, S., T. Stelmasiak, and L. Murray 1988. Immobilization of sambar, rusa, red, fallow and chital deer with Fentaz®/Rompun® and reversal with Narcan®/tolazoline. Vet. Med. Rev. 59: 167-170.

Van Niekerk, J. W., and U. De V. Pienaar. 1962. Adaptions of the immobilizing technique to the capture,

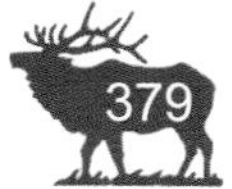

marking and translocation of game animals in the Kruger National Park. Koedoe 5: 137-143.
Van Niekerk, J. W., and U. De V. Pienaar. 1963a. A report on some immobilizing drugs used in the capture of wild animals in the Kruger National Park. Koedoe 6: 126-133.
Van Niekerk, J. W., and U. De V. Pienaar. 1963b. Adaptation of the immobilizing techniques to the capture, marking and translocation of game animals in the Kruger National Park. Koedoe 5: 137-143.
Van Niekerk, J. W., and U. De V. Pienaar. 1963c. A report on some immobilizing drugs used in the capture of wild animals in the Kruger National Park. Koedoe 6: 126-133.
Van Niekerk, J. W., U. De V. Pienaar, and N. Fairall. 1963a. Immobilizing drugs used in the capture of wild animals in the Kruger Park National. J. So. Afr. Vet. Assoc. 34: 403-411.
Van Niekerk, J. W., U. De V. Pienaar, and N. Fairall. 1963b. A preliminary note on the use of Quiloflex (benzodioxane hydrochloride) in the immobilization of game. Koedoe 6: 109-114.
Van Ouwerkerk, M. T. 1986. Effect of etorphine hydrochloride and xylazine hydrochloride on various physiological parameters of the goat *Capra hircus*. M.S. Thesis, University of Pretoria (South Africa).
Van Reenen, G. 1982. Field experiences in the capture of red deer by helicopter in New Zealand with reference to post-capture sequela and management. *In* Nielsen, L., J. C. Haigh, and M. E. Fowler (eds.). Chemical Immobilization of North American Wildlife. Wisconsin Humane Society, Inc. Milwaukee, Wisconsin. Pp. 408-421.
Van Rensburg, P. J. J. 1993. Chemical capture of the bushpig, *Potamochoerus larvatus*. *In* McKenzie, A. A. (ed.). The Capture and Care Manual. Wildlife Decision Support Services and The South African Veterinary Foundation, Pretoria. Pp. 615-616.
Van Rooyen, G. L., and P. J. De Beer. 1973. A retractable barb needle for drug darts. Koedoe 16: 155-158.
Van Wyk, T. C., and H. H. Berry. 1986. Tolazoline as an antagonist in free-living lions immobilised with a ketamine-xylazine combination. J. So. Afr. Vet. Assoc. 57: 221-224.
Varland, K. L. 1976. Techniques for elk immobilization with succinylcholine chloride. Proc. Iowa Acad. 82: 194-197.
Velisek, J., Z. Svobodova, and V. Piackova. 2005. Effects of clove oil anaesthesia on rainbow trout (*Oncorhynchus mykiss*). Acta Vet. Brno. 74: 139-146.
Vercruysse, J., and J. Mortelmans. 1978. The chemical restraint of apes and monkeys by means of phencyclidine or ketamine. Acta. Zool. Pathol. Antverpiensia. 70: 211-220.
Vergani, D. F., H. J. Spainrani, and C. A. Aguirre. 1986. Immobilization of crabeater seals, *Lobodon carcinophagus*, with the use of xylazine hydrochloride at 25 De Mayo Island (Antarctica) and identification of polymorphism in transferrins. Contribution No. 317, Direccion Nacional Del Antartico, Instituto Antartico Argentino.
Vertessen, K. 1970. Immobilizatie van everzwijnen door middel van azaperone en fentanyl (Immobilization of wild pigs by means of azaperone and fentanyl). Tijdschr. Diergeneesk. 10: 541-543
Verts, B. J. 1960. A device for anesthetizing skunks. J. Wildl. Manage. 24: 335-336.
Vethamany-Globus, S., M. Globus, and I. Fraser. Effects of tricaine methane sulphonate (M.S. 222) on the blood glucose levels in adult slamanders (*Diemictylus viridescens*). Experientia 33: 1027.
Vice, T. E., L. D. Claborn, and R. A. Ratner. 1965. Anesthetic technics in the baboon with some observations on other primates. *In* Sawyer, D. C. (ed.). Symposium on Experimental Animal Anesthesiology. Brooks Air Force Base, Texas.
Vie, J.-C., and B. de Thoisy. 1996. Anesthesia of wild red howler monkeys (*Alouatta seniculus*) with medetomidine-ketamine and reversal by atipamezole. Proc. Am. Assoc. Zoo Vet. P. 208.
Vie, J.-C., B. de Thoisy, P. Fournier, C. Fournier-Chambrillon, C. Gentry, and J. Keravec. 1998. Anesthesia of wild red howler monkeys (*Alouatta seniculus*) with medetomidine-ketamine and reversal by atipamezole. Am. J. Primatol. 45:399-410.
Vienet, V. 2001. Anaesthesia in green iguanas (*Iguana iguana*). Point. Vet. 32: 26.
Viggers, K. L., and D. B. Lindenmayer. 1995. The use of tiletamine hydrochloride and zolazepam hydrochloride for sedation of the mountain brushtail possum *Trichosurus caninus*. Austral. Vet. 72:215-216.
Vilà, C., and J. Castroviejo. 1994. Use of tiletamine and zolazepam to immobilize captive Iberian wolves (*Canis lupus*). J. Wildl. Dis. 30: 119-122.
Viljoen, P. C. 1981. Fentanyl citrate for the field immobilization of oribi. So. Afr. J. Wildl. Res. 11: 56-58.
Virtanen, R., and E., MacDonald. 1987. Reversal of the sedative/analgesic and other effects of detomidine and medetomidine by MPV-1248, a novel alpha$_2$-antagonist. Pharmacol. Toxicol. 60: 73.

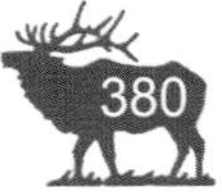

Vitaud, C. 1993. *Equus burchelli boehmi*, sedation- anaesthesia, use of tiletamine/zolazepam comibination and detomidine. Erkrankungen der Zootiere 35: 277-280.

Vodicka, R. 2004. Chemical immobilization of captive aardvark (*Orycteropus afer*). J. Zoo Wildl. Med. 35: 544-545.

Vogel, I., B. de Thoisy, and J.-C. Vie. 1998. Comparison of injectable anesthetic combinations in free-ranging two-toed sloths in French Guiana. J. Wildl. Dis. 34: 555-566.

Vogelnest, L. 1998. Transport of ten western lowland gorillas (*Gorilla gorilla gorilla*) from the Netherlands to Australia, and their subsequent anaesthesia and health assessment. Proc. Joint Conf. Am. Assoc. Zoo Vet. and Am. Assoc. Wildl. Vet. Pp. 30-37.

Vogelnest, L. 1999. Tiger anaesthesia. Austr. Vet. J. 77: 378.

Vogelnest, L. and H. K. Ralph. 1997. Chemical Immobilization of giraffe to facilitate short procedures. Austr. Vet. J. 75: 180-182.

Volkers, J., T. Wensing, and G. W. T. A. Bruinderink. 1994. Sedation of wild boar (*Sus scrofa*) and red deer (*Cervus elaphus*) with medetomidine and the influence on some haematological and serum biochemical variables. Vet. Quart. 16: 7-9.

Volmer, K., and A. Herzog. 1986. [Mineral content of the blood of immobilised red deer of various origins]. Z. Jagdwiss. 32: 22-29.

VonDegerfeld, M. M. 2004. Personal experiences in the use of association tiletamine/zolazepam for anaesthesia of the green iguana (*Iguana iguana*). Res. Vet. Commun. 28: 351-353.

VonDegerfeld, M. M. 2005. Personal experiences in the use of Zoletil for anaesthesia of the red-necked wallaby (*Macropus rufogriseus*). Res. Vet. Commun. 29: 297-300.

Vondruska, J. F. 1965. Phencyclidine anesthesia in baboons. J. Am. Vet. Med. Assoc. 147: 1073-1074.

Waldridge, B. M., H. C. Lin, F. J. Degraves, and D. G. Pugh. 1997. Sedative effects of medetomidine and its reversal by atipamezole in llamas. J. Am. Vet. Med. Assoc. 211: 1562.

Wallace, R. S., and M. Bush. 1987. Exertional myopathy complicated by a ruptured bladder in a dama gazelle (*Gazella dama*). J. Zoo An. Med. 18: 111-114.

Wallach, G. D., A. R. Fodor, and L. H. Barton. 1960. Restraint of chimpanzees with perphenazine. J. Am. Vet. Med. Assoc. 136: 222-224.

Wallach, J. D. 1966. Immobilization and translocation of the white (Square-lipped) rhinoceros. J. Am. Vet. Med. Assoc. 149: 871-874.

Wallach, J. D. 1968. Wild animal immobilization with the oripavine M-99. Missouri Vet. 19: 12-15.

Wallach, J. D. 1969. Etorphine (M99), a new analgesic immobilizing agent and its antagonists. Vet. Med. Sm. An. Clin. 64: 53-58.

Wallach, J. D. 1977. Anesthesia of reptiles. *In* Kirk, R. W. (ed.). Current Veterinary Therapy VI. W. B. Saunders Co., Philadelphia, Pennsylvania. Pp. 807-808.

Wallach, J. D., and J. L. Anderson. 1968. Oripavine (M99) combinations and solvents for immobilization of the African elephant. J. Am. Vet. Med. Assoc. 153: 793-797.

Wallach, J. D., and C. Hoessle. 1970. M-99 as an immobilizing agent in poikilothermes. Vet. Med. Sm. An. Clin. 65: 163-167.

Wallach, J. D., R. Frueh, and M. Lentz. 1967. The use of M99 as an immobilizing and analgesic agent in captive wild animals. J. Am. Vet. Med. Assoc. 151: 870-876.

Wallingford, B. D., R. A. Lancia, and E. C. Soutiere. 1996. Antagonism of xylazine in white-tailed deer with intramuscular injection of yohimbine. J. Wildl. Dis. 32: 399-402.

Walsh, M. T., and G. D. Bossart. 1999. Manatee medicine. *In* Fowler, M. E., and R. E. Miller (eds.). Zoo & Wild Animal Medicine. Current Therapy 4. W. B. Saunders Company, Philadelphia, Pennsylvania. Pp. 507-516.

Walsh, M. T., A. I. Webb, D. O. Beusse, D. A. Brock, S. A. Robertson, N. Abou-Madi, R. A. Cook, and L. Klein. 1988. Sedation and general anesthesia of four arctic walrus (*Odobenus rosmaru*). Abstract, 19th Ann. Intl. Assoc. Aquatic An. Med. Orlando, Florida.

Walsh, V. P., and P. R. Wilson. 2002. Sedation and chemical restraint of deer. N. Z. Vet. J. 50: 228-236.

Walter, W. D., D. M. Leslie, J. H. Herner-Thogmartin, K. G. Smith, and M. E. Cartwright. 2005. Efficacy of immobilizing free-ranging elk with Telazol® and xylazine hydrochloride using transmitter-equipped darts. J. Wildl. Dis. 41: 395-400.

Walzer, C. 1995. Beitrag zur Immobilisation von Wildschweinen mit Tiletamin-Zolazepam (Immobilization of wild boar with tiletamine-zolazepam). Wien. Tierärztl. Mschr. 82: 29-31.

Walzer, C., and C. Huber. 1999. Comparison of two benzodiazepine antagonists: flumazenil and sarmazenil

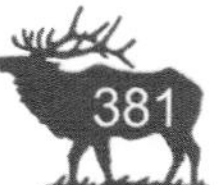

in cheetah (*Acinonyx jubatus*). Erkrankungen Der Zootiere 39: 377-382.

Walzer, C., and C. Huber. 2002. Partial antagonism of tiletamine-zolazepam anesthesia in cheetah. J. Wildl. Dis. 38: 468-472.

Walzer, C., R. Bogel, and C. Walzerwagner. 1996. Medetomidine-ketamine-hyaluronidase-atipamezole anesthesia in chamois (*Rupicapra rupicapra*). Wien. Tierarztl. Monatsschr. 83: 297-301.

Walzer, C., F. Gsritz, H. Pucher, R. Hermes, T. Hildebrandt, and F. Schwarzenberger. 2000. Chemical restraint and anesthesia in white rhinoceros (*Ceratotherium simum*) for reproductive evaluation, semen collection and artificial insemination. Proc. Joint Conf. Am. Assoc. Zoo Vet. and Intl. Assoc. Aquatic An. Med. Pp. 98-101.

Wang, R., J. L. Kubie, and M. Halpern. 1977. Brevital sodium: an effective anesthetic agent for performing surgery on small reptiles. Copeia 1977: 738-743.

Wang, T., W. Fernandes, and A. S. Abe. 1993. Blood pH and O_2 homeostasis upon CO_2 anesthesia in the rattlesnake (*Crotalus durissus*). Snake 25: 21-26.

Wanzie, C. 1986. Buffon's kob (*Kobus kob kob* Erxleben) immobilisation in Waza National Park, Cameroon. Mammalia. 50: 253-262.

Ward, D. G., D. Blyde, J. Lemon, and S. Johnston. 2006. Anesthesia of captive African wild dogs (*Lycaon pictus*) using medetomidine-ketamine-atropine combination. J. Zoo Wildl. Med. 37: 160-164.

Ward, G. S., D. O. Johnson, and C. R. Roberts. 1974. The use of CI 744 as an anesthetic for laboratory animals. Lab. An. Sci. 24: 737-742.

Warren, R. J., N. L. Schauer, J. T. Jones, P. F. Scanlon, and R. L. Kirkpatrick. 1979. A modified blow-gun syringe for remote injection of captive wildlife. J. Wildl. Dis. 15: 537-541.

Warren, R. J., R. L. Kirkpatrick, D. F. Gibson, and P. F. Scanlon. 1984. Xylazine hydrochloride-induced anorexia in white-tailed deer. J. Wildl. Dis. 20: 66-68.

Wass, J. A., and H. M. Kaplan. 1974. Methoxyflurane anesthesia for *Rana pipiens*. Lab. An. Sci. 24: 669-671.

Watson, C. R. R., and J. S. Way. 1972. The unusual tolerance of marsupials to barbiturate anaesthetics. Int. Zoo Yb. 12: 208-211.

Watson, C. R. R., and J. S. Way. 1973. Anaesthetics for kangaroos. Int. Zoo Yb. 11: 12-13.

Webster, D. M., and V. D. Hollard. 1973. A safe and simple injection anesthetic for birds. Physiol. Behav. 10: 831.

Wedemeyer, G. 1970. Stress of anesthesia with M.S. 222 and benzocaine in rainbow trout (*Salmo gairdneri*). J. Fish. Res. Bd. Canada. 27: 909-914.

Weilenmann, P. 1971. Einige Angaben über die im Zoologischen Garten Zürich und im Wildpark Langenberg verwendeten Sedativa, Tranquilizer und Narkotika. Verhandlungbericht des XIII. Proc. Int. Symp. Erkrankungen Zootiere, Helsinki, Finland. Pp. 207-211.

Weisbroth, S. H., and J. H. Fudens. 1972. Use of ketamine hydrochloride in laboratory rabbits, rats, mice, and guinea pigs. Lab. An. Sci. 22: 904-906.

Wellington, B. J. 1972. Effective sedation and anesthesia of two kangaroos. Austral. Vet. J. 48: 127.

Welsch, D. M. D., E. R. Jacobson, G. V. Kollias, L. Kramer, H. Gardner, and D. Page. 1989. Tusk extraction in the African elephant (*Loxodonta africana*). J. Zoo Wildl. Med. 20: 446-453.

Wentges, H. 1975. Medicine administration by blowpipe. Vet. Rec. 97: 281.

Wesson, J. A., P. F. Scanlon, and R. E. Mirarchi. 1974. Immobilization of white-tailed deer with succinylcholine chloride: success rate, reactions of deer and some physiological effects. Proc. Ann. Conf. Southeast. Assoc. Game Fish Comm. 28: 500-506.

Wesson, J. A., P. F. Scanlon, and R. L. Kirkpatrick. 1976. Increase in progestin and estrone levels in white-tailed deer following drug restraint. Va. J. Sci. 27: 52.

Wesson, J. A., P. F. Scanlon, R. L. Kirkpatrick, and H. S. Mosby. 1977. Influence of immobilizing drugs on blood characteristics of cottontail rabbits. Va. J. Sci. 28: 69.

Wesson, J. A., P. F. Scanlon, R. L. Kirkpatrick, and H. S. Mosby. 1979a. Influence of chemical immobilization and physical restraint on packed cell volume, total protein, glucose, and blood urea nitrogen in blood of white-tailed deer. Can. J. Zool. 57: 756-767.

Wesson, J. A., P. F. Scanlon, R. L. Kirkpatrick, H. S. Mosby, and R. L. Butcher. 1979b. Influence of chemical immobilization and physical restraint on steroid hormone levels in blood of white-tailed deer. Can. J. Zool. 57: 768-776.

Westcott, D. A., and K. E. Reid. 2002. Use of medetomidine for capture and restraint of cassowaries (*Casuarius casuarius*). Aust. Vet. J. 80: 150-153.

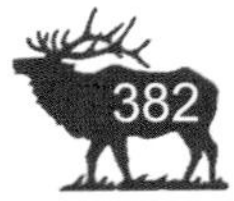

Weston, H. S., A, M. Fagella, L. Burt, K. Crowley, and T. Moore. 1996. Immobilization of a pygmy hippopotamus (*Choeropsis liberiensis*) for the removal of an oral mass. Proc. Am. Assoc. Zoo Vet. Pp. 576-581.

Whateley, A. 1979. Selective capture of spotted hyaenas using orally administered sernylan. Lammergeyer. 27: 25-27.

Wheler, C. 1993. Avian anesthesia, analgesics, and tranquilizers. Seminars in Avian Exotic Pet Med. 2: 7-12.

Whitaker, R., and H. Andrews. 1989. Chemical immobilization of the mugger crocodile (*Crocodylus palustris*) with gallamine triethiodide. Indian-Forester 115: 355-356.

White, G. L., and D. D. Holmes. 1976. A comparison of ketamine and the combination ketamine-xylazine for effective surgical anesthesia in the rabbit. Lab. An. Sci. 26: 804-806.

White, G. L., and J. F. Cummings. 1976. A comparison of ketamine and ketamine-xylazine in the baboon. Vet. Med. Sm. An. Clin. 74: 392-396.

White, P. F., W. L. Way, and A. J. Trevor. 1982. Ketamine – Its pharmacology and therapeutic uses. Anesthesiology. 56: 119-136.

White, P. J., T. J. Kreeger, U. S. Seal, and J. R. Tester. 1990. Pathological responses of red foxes to box traps. J. Wildl. Manage. 55: 75-80.

White, R. J. 1986. Anesthetic management of the camel. *In:* Higgins, A. J. (ed.). The Camel in Health and Disease. Balliere Tindall, London. Pp. 136-148.

White, R. J., P. H. Cribb, G. Glover, and J. Rowell. 1985. Halothane anesthesia in a muskox (*Ovibos moschatus*). J. Zoo An. Med. 16: 58-61.

White, T. H., M. K. Oli, B. D. Leopold, H. A. Jacobson, and J. W. Kasbohm. 1996. Field evaluation of Telazol® and ketamine-xylazine for immobilizing black bears. Wildl. Soc. Bull. 24: 521-527.

Wiesner, H. 1975. Zur Neuroleptanalgesie bei Zootieren und Gatterwild unter Anwendung des Telinject-Systems. Kleintier-Praxis 20: 18-24.

Wiesner, H. 1977. Tranquilization by the "blowgun rifle" method. Kleintier-Praxis 22: 327-330.

Wiesner, H. 1993. Chemical immobilization of wild equids. *In* Fowler, M. E. (ed.). Zoo & Wild Animal Medicine: Current Therapy 3. W. B. Saunders Co., Philadelphia, Pennsylvania. Pp. 475-476.

Wiesner, H. 1998. Tierschutzrelevante Neuentwicklungen zur Optimierung der Distanzimmobilisation (Developments in the field of distance immobilization with regard to animal welfare). Tieraerztliche Praxis 26(G): 225-233.

Wiesner, H., and G. von Hegel. 1985. Praktische Hinweise zur Immobilization von Wild und Zootieren [Practical advice concerning immobilization of wild and zoo animals]. Tierärtzliche Praxis 13: 113-127.

Wiesner, H., and G. Von Hegel. 1989. Zur Immobilisation von Giraffen. Tierärtzliche Praxis 17: 97-100.

Wiesner, H., W. Rietschel, and T. Gatesman. 1982. [Practical experiences with the combination on "Immobilon" and "Rompun" in zoo animals]. Z. Koeln. Zoo. 25: 47-55.

Wiesner, H., W. Rietschel, and T. J. Gatesman. 1984. The use of the morphine-like analgesic carfentanil in captive wild mammals at Tierpark Hellebraun. J. Zoo An. Med. 15: 18-23.

Wiesner, H., and G. Von Hegel. 1990. Zur Immobilisation von Wildequiden mit STH 2130 und Tiletamin/Zolazepam. Tierärtzliche Praxis 18: 151-154.

Wildt, D. E. S. J. O'Brien, and J. A. M. Graves. 1988. Anesthesia and reproductive characteristics of free-ranging male koalas (*Phascolarctos cinereus*). Proc. Am. Assoc. Zoo Vet. Toronto, Ont. Pp. 109-111.

Williams, C. V., K. M. Glenn, J. F. Levine, and W. A. Horne. 2003. Comparison of the efficacy and cardio-respiratory effects of medetomidine-based anesthetic protocols in ring-tailed lemurs (*Lemur catta*). J. Zoo Wildl. Med. 34: 163-170.

Williams, D. E., and D. H. Riedesel. 1987. Chemical immobilization of wild ruminants. Iowa State Univ. Vet. 49: 26-32.

Williams, K. D. 1979. Trapping and immobilization of the malayan tapir in West Malaysia. Malay. Nat. J. 33: 117-122.

Williams, L. E. 1966. Capturing wild turkeys with alpha-chloralose. J. Wildl. Manage. 30: 50-56.

Williams, L. E. 1967. Preliminary report on methoxymol to capture turkeys. Proc. Ann. Conf. Southeast. Assoc. Game Fish Comm. 21: 189-193.

Williams, L. E., D. H. Austin, and T. E. Peoples. 1966. Progress in capturing turkeys with drugs applied to baits. Proc. Ann. Conf. Southeast. Assoc. Game Fish Comm. 20: 219-226.

Williams, L. E., and R. W. Phillips. 1972. Tests of oral anesthetics to capture mourning doves and bobwhites. J. Wildl. Manage. 36: 968-971.

Williams, L. E., and R. W. Phillips. 1973. Capturing sandhill cranes with alpha-chloralose. J. Wildl. Manage. 37: 94-97.

Williams, L. E., D. H. Austin, T. E. Peoples, and R. W. Phillips. 1973a. Capturing turkeys with oral drugs. *In* Sanderson, G. C., and H. C. Schultz (eds.). Wild Turkey Management: Current Problems and Programs. Univ. Missouri Press, Columbia.

Williams, L. E., D. H. Austin, T. E. Peoples, and R. W. Phillips. 1973b. Capturing turkeys with oral drugs. Proc. Natl. Wild Turkey Symp. 2: 219-227.

Williams, T. D. 1978. Chemical immobilization, baseline hematological parameters and oil contamination in the sea otter. PB-283-969, National Technical Information Service, Washington, D. C.

Williams, T. D. 1990. Sea otter biology and medicine. *In* Dierauf, L. A. (ed.). CRC Handbook of Marine Mammal Medicine: Health, Disease, and Rehabilitation. CRC Press, Boca Raton. Pp. 625-648.

Williams, T. D., and F. H. Kocher. 1978. Comparison of anesthetic agents in the sea otter. J. Am. Vet. Med. Assoc. 173: 1127-1130.

Williams, T. D., A. L. Williams, and D. B. Siniff. 1981. Fentanyl and azaperone produced neuroleptanalgesia in the sea otter (*Enhydra lutris*). J. Wildl. Dis. 17: 337-342.

Williams, T. D., A. L. Williams, and M. Stoskopf. 1990a. Marine mammal anesthesia. *In* Dierauf, L. A. (ed.). CRC Handbook of Marine Mammal Medicine: Health, Disease, and Rehabilitation. CRC Press, Boca Raton. Pp. 175-191.

Williams, T. D., D. M. Baylis, S. H. Downey, and R. O. Clark. 1990b. A physical restraint device for sea otters. J. Zoo Wildl. Med. 21: 105-107.

Williams, T. D., A. H. Rebar, R. F. Teclaw, and P. E. Yews. 1992. Influence of age, sex, capture technique, and restraint on hematologic measurements and serum chemistries of wild California sea otters. Vet. Clin. Path. 21: 106-110.

Williams, T. D., J. Christiansen, and S. Nygren. 1993. A comparison of intramuscular anesthetics in teleosts and elasmobranchs. Proc. Int. Assoc. Aquatic Anim. Med. 24:6.

Williams, T. D., M. Rollins, and B. A. Block. 2004. Intramuscular anesthesia of bonito and Pacific mackerel with ketamine and medetomidine and reversal of anesthesia with atipamezole. J. Am. Vet. Med. Assoc. 225: 417-421.

Williamson, W. V., and J. D. Wallach. 1968. M.99 induced recumbency and analgesia in a giraffe. J. Am. Vet. Med. Assoc. 153: 816-817.

Wilson, D. E. 1988. Maintaining bats for captive studies. Kunz, T. H. (ed.). Ecological and Behavioral Methods for the Study of Bats. Smithsonian, Washington, D.C. Pp. 247-264.

Wilson, G. R. 1974. The restraint of red kangaroos using etorphine-methotrimprazine mixtures. Austr. Vet. J. 50: 454-458.

Wilson, G. R. 1976. Intramuscular anaesthesia in the red kangaroo. Aust. Vet. Pract. 6: 51-62.

Wilson, P., and P. J. Warner. 1976. Chemical restraint in the pine marten. Vet. Rec. 98: 302-303.

Wilson, S. C., D. L. Armstrong, L. G. Simmons, D. J. Morris, and T. S. Gross. 1993. A clinical trial using three regimens for immobilizing gaur (*Bos gaurus*). J. Zoo Wildl. Med. 24: 93-101.

Wilson, V. J. 1967. The use of oripavine hydrochloride (M.99) in the drug immobilization of duiker (*Sylvicapra grimmia*). Arnoldia, National Museums of Southern Rhodesia. 3: 1-6.

Wimsatt, J., T J. O'Shea, L. E. Ellison, R. D. Pearce, and V. R. Price. 2005. Anesthesia and blood sampling of wild big brown bats (*Eptesicus fuscus*) with an assessment of impacts on survival. J. Wildl. Dis. 41: 87-95.

Winegardner, S. C., L. B. Dalton, and J. W. Bates. 1977. Capture and transplant of desert bighorn sheep with M-99. Trans. Desert Bighorn Council. Pp. 18-20.

Wisnicky, W. 1940. Anesthesia of fur-bearing animals. No. Am. Vet. 21: 277-279.

Wobeser, G., J. E. C. Bellamy, B. G. Boysen, P. S. MacWilliams, and W. Runge. 1976. Myopathy and myoglobinuria in a wild white-tailed deer. J. Am. Vet. Med. Assoc. 169: 971-974.

Wolfensohn, S. E. 1992. Use of medetomidine-fentanyl-fluanisone combinations in the badger. Vet. Rec. 130: 34-36.

Wolfe, L. L., and M. W. Miller. 2005. Suspected secondary thiafentanil intoxication in a captive mountain lion (*Puma concolor*). J. Wildl. Dis. 41: 829-833.

Wolfe, L. L., W. R. Lance, and M. W. Miller. 2004. Immobilization of mule deer with thiafentanil (A-3080) or thiafentanil plus xylazine. J. Wildl. Dis. 40: 282-287.

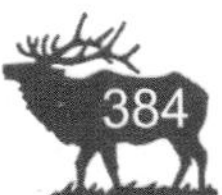

Wolff, W. A., R. W. Davis, and W. V. Lumb. 1965. Chloral hydrate-halothane-nitrous oxide anesthesia in deer. J. Am. Vet. Med. Assoc. 147: 1099-1101.

Wolkers, J., T. Wensing, and G. W. T. A. GrootBruinderink. 1994. Sedation of wild boar (*Sus scrofa*) and red deer (*Cervus elaphus*) with medetomidine and the influence of some haematological and serum biochemical variables. Vet. Quart. 16: 7-9.

Wood, F. E., K. H. Critchley, and J. R. Wood. 1982. Anesthesia in the green sea turtle, *Chelonia mydas*. Am. J. Vet. Res. 43: 1882-1883.

Wood, G. W., E. E. Johnson, and R. E. Brenneman. 1977. Observations on the use of succinylcholine chloride to immobilize feral hogs. J. Wildl. Manage. 41: 798-800.

Woodbury, M. R., N. A. Caulkett, C. B. Johnson, and P. R. Wilson. 2005. Comparison of analgesic techniques for antler removal in halothane-anaesthetized red deer (*Cervus elaphus*): cardiovascular and somatic responses. Vet. Anaesth. Analg. 32: 72-82.

Woods, R., M. Hindell, and D. J. Slip. 1989. Effects of physiological state on duration of sedation in southern elephant seals. J. Wildl. Dis. 25: 586-590.

Woods, R., S. McLean, S. Nicol, and H. Burton. 1994. Use of midazolam, pethidine, ketamine and thiopentone for the restraint of southern elephant seals (*Mirounga leonina*). Vet. Rec. 135: 572-577.

Woods, R., S. McLean, S. Nicol, and H. Burton. 1996. Chemical restraint of southern elephant seals (*Mirounga leonina*); use of medetomidine, ketamine and atipamezole and comparison with other cyclohexamine-based combinations. Brit. Vet. J. 152:213-224.

Woodford, M. H. 1972. The use of gallamine triethiodide as a chemical immobilizing agent for the Nile crocodile (*Crocodilus niloticus*). E. Afr. Wildl. J. 10: 67-70.

Woodford, M. H., S. K. Eltringham, and J. R. Wyatt. 1972. An analysis of mechanical failure of darts and costs involved in drug immobilization of elephant and buffalo. E. Afr. Wildl. J. 10: 279-285.

Woodring, M. W. 1978. A low-cost capture system. Mod. Vet. Prac. 59: 837-838.

Woodroffe, R. 2001. Assessing the risks of intervention: immobilization, radio-collaring and vaccination of African wild dogs. Oryx 35: 234-244.

Woods, R., M. Hindell, and D. J. Slip. 1989. Effects of physiological state on duration of sedation in southern elephant seals. J. Wildl. Dis. 25: 586-590.

Woods, R., S. McLean, S. Nicol, and H. Burton. 1994a. Use of midazolam, pethidine, ketamine and thiopentone for the restraint of southern elephant seals (*Mirounga leonina*). Vet. Rec. 135: 572-577.

Woods, R., S. McLean, S. Nicol, and H. Burton. 1994b. A comparison of some cyclohexamine based drug combinations for chemical restraint of southern elephant seals (*Mirounga leonina*). Mar. Mammal. Sci. 10: 412-429.

Woods, R., S. McLean, S. Nicol, and H. Burton. 1995. Antagonism of some cyclohexamine-based drug combinations used for chemical restraint of southern elephant seals (*Mirounga leonina*). Austr. Vet. J. 72: 165-171.

Woods, R., S. McLean, S. Nicol, and H. Burton. 1996a. Chemical restraint of southern elephant seals (*Mirounga leonina*); use of medetomidine, ketamine and atipamezole and comparison with other cyclohexane-based combinations. Br. Vet. J. 152: 231-234.

Woods, R., S. McLean, S. Nicol, D. J. Slip, and H. R. Burton. 1996b. Use of the respiratory stimulant doxapram in southern elephant seals (*Mirounga leonina*). Vet. Rec. 138: 514-517.

Woolf, A. 1970. Immobilization of captive and free-ranging white-tailed deer (*Odocoileus virginianus*) with etorphine hydrochloride. J. Am. Vet. Med. Assoc. 157: 636-640.

Woolf, A. 1974. Recovery of M99 immobilized white-tailed deer and wapiti using low dosages of M50-50. J. Zoo An. Med. 5: 18.

Woolf, A. 1984. Inanition following implantation of a radiotelemetry device in a river otter. J. Am. Vet. Med. Assoc. 185: 15-16.

Woolf, A., and J. H. Swart. 1970. Etorphine hydrochloride: anesthetic for surgery on an elk (*Cervus canadensis canadensis*). J. Am. Vet. Med. Assoc. 157: 641-642.

Woolf, A., H. R. Hays, W. B. Allen, and J. Swart. 1973. Immobilization of wild ungulates with etorphine HCL. J. Zoo An. Med. 4: 16-19.

Woolfson, M. W., J. A. Foran, H. M. Freedman, P. A. Moore, L. B. Shulman, and P. A. Schnitman. 1980. Immobilization of baboons (*Papio anubis*) using ketamine and diazepam. Lab. An. Care. 30: 902-904.

Work, T. M., R. L. DeLong, S. R. Melin, and T. R. Spraker. 1992. The use of halothane anesthesia as a method of immobilizing free-ranging California sea lions (*Zalophus californianus*). Proc. Joint Conf.

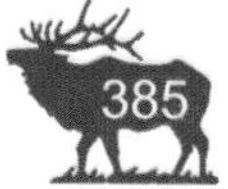

Am. Assoc. Zoo Vet. and Am. Assoc. Wildl. Vet. Pp. 57.

Work, T. M., R. L. DeLong, T. R. Spraker, and S. R. Melin. 1993. Halothane anesthesia as a method for immobilizing free-ranging California sea lions (*Zalophus californianus*). J. Zoo Wildl. Med. 24: 482-487.

Woronecki, P. P., R. A. Dolbeer, and T. W. Seamans. 1990. Use of alpha-chloralose to remove waterfowl from nuisance and damage situations. Proc. Vert. Pest Conf. 14: 343-349.

Wright, F. H. 1981. Use of diazepam as an adjunctive agent in Przewalski horse immobilization. Proc. Am. Assoc. Zoo Vet. Pp. 109-112.

Wright, J. F. 1959. Treatment of captive wild animals using an automatic projectile type syringe. Vet. Med. 54: 32-33.

Wright, J. F. 1962. Immobilization of wild animals. Vet. Med. 57: 331-332.

Wright, J. F. 1963. Chemical restraint of exotic animals in a disease regulatory program. Can. J. Comp. Med. Vet. Sci. 27: 13-16.

Wright, J. M. 1983. Ketamine hydrochloride as a chemical restraint for selected small mammals. Wildl. Soc. Bull. 11: 76-79.

Wright, M. 1982. Pharmacologic effects of ketamine and its use in veterinary medicine. J. Am. Vet. Med. Assoc. 180: 1462-1471.

Yamaya, Y., S. Ohba, H. Koie, T. Watari, M. Tokuriki, and S. Tanaka. 2006. Isolfurane anaesthesia in four sea lions (*Otaria byronia* and *Zalophus californianus*). Vet. Anaesth. Analg. 33: 302-306.

Yaralioglu-Gurgoze, S., N. Sindak, T. Sahin, and O. Cen. 2005. Levels of glutathione peroxidase, lipoperoxidase and some biochemical and haematological parameters in gazelles anaesthetised with tiletamine-zolazepam-xylazine combination. Vet. J. 169: 126-128.

York, W. 1973a. Pharmacological restraint of felids. World's Cats. 1: 213-216.

York, W. 1973b. Immobilization of a hippo. Proc. Am. Assoc. Zoo Vet.

York, W. 1975. Fentanyl citrate for wild animal capture. J. Zoo An. Med. 6: 14-15.

York, W., and C. Kidder. 1971. Chemical restraint and castration of an adult giraffe. J. Zoo An. Med. 4: 17-21.

York, W., and K. Huggins. 1972. Rompun (Bay VA 1470). J. Zoo An. Med. 3: 15-17.

Youatt, W. G., and A. W. Erickson. 1959. Some effects of sodium pentobarbital anesthesia on juvenile black bears. J. Wildl. Manage. 23: 243-244.

Young, E. 1966a. The use of tranquillizers, muscle relaxants and anesthetics, as an aid in the management of wild carnivors in captivity. Twenty-five case reports. J. So. Afr. Vet. Assoc. 37: 293-296.

Young, E. 1966b. Use of anaesthesics in the transport of animals. Intl. Zoo Yb. 6: 273.

Young, E. 1972. Notes on the chemical immobilization and restraint of the Addo elephant (*Loxodonta africana*). Koedoe 15: 97-99.

Young, E. (ed.). 1975. The Capture and Care of Wild Animals. Ralph Curtis Books, Hollywood, Florida. 224 pp.

Young, E., and B. L. Penzhorn. 1972. The reaction of the Cape mountain zebra (*Equus zebra zebra*) to certain chemical immobilization drugs. Koedoe 15: 95-96.

Young, E., and I. J. Whyte. 1973. Experiences with xylazine hydrochloride (Rompun, Bayer) in the capture, control and treatment of some African wildlife species. J. So. Afr. Vet. Assoc. 44: 177-184.

Young, E., P. J. Burger, and I. J. Whyte. 1972. The use of doxapram hydrochloride on newly-captured wild animals. Vet. Clin. 11: 11-13.

Young, R., and H. M. Kaplan. 1960. Anesthesia of turtles with chlorpromazine and sodium pentobarbital. Proc. An. Care Panel. 10: 57-62.

Young, R. A., and E. A. H. Sims. 1979. The woodchuck, *Marmota monax*, as a laboratory animal. Lab. An. Sci. 29: 770-780.

Yu, B., and Z. Yu. 1987. Anesthetic treatments of the giant panda. *In* Proceedings of Therapeutics of the Giant Panda. China Forestry Publishing House. Pp. 51-53. (Chinese)

Zabarain, C. 1985. [Chemical immobilization of *Odocoileus virginianus* and *Cervus nippon* with xylazine]. Veterinaria (Mexico City). 16: 70.

Zaniewski, L. 1967. The immobilization of European bison x cattle hybrid with suxamethonium. Acta Theriol. 12: 471-474.

Zatzman, M. L. , and G. V. Thornhill. 1988. Effects of anesthetics on cardiovascular responses of the marmot, *Marmota flaviventris*. Cryobiology. 25: 212-226.

Zhu, B. R., and J. Wang. 1992. Comparative studies on anaesthesia of giant panda using ketamine and its

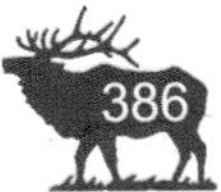

combination. Acta Zool. Sin. 38: 230-232.

Zinn, R. S., A. A. Gabel, and R. B. Heath. 1970. Effects of succinylcholine and promazine on the cardiovascular and respiratory systems of horses. J. Am. Vet. Med. Assoc. 157: 1495-1499.

Zomborszky, Z., J. Hafner, and T. Feher. 1993. Values of serum cortisol concentration studies on the stress-sensibility and adaption ability of red deer with intensive keeping. Magy Allatorv Lapja (Hung.) 48: 91-95.

Zuba, J. R., and J. L. Allen. 1992. Affordable, portable, noninvasive monitoring equipment and its place in zoo and wildlife anesthesia. Proc. Joint Conf. Am. Assoc. Zoo Vet. and Am. Assoc. Wildl. Vet. Pp. 230-234.

Zuba, J. R., and R. P. Burns. 1998. The use of supplemental propofol in narcotic anesthetized non-domestic equids. Proc. Joint Conf. Am. Assoc. Zoo Vet. and Am. Assoc. Wildl. Vet. Pp. 11-16.

Zurowski, W., and M. Sakowicz. 1965. Effects of succinylcholine chloride on wild boars. J. Wildl. Manage. 29: 626-629.

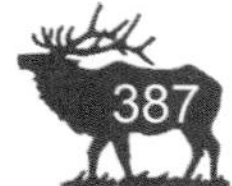

Glossary

Adjuvant - Pharmacological agent added to a drug to increase or aid its effect
Agonist - Drug capable of combining with receptors to initiate drug actions
Akinesia - Loss of motor response due to paralysis of motor nerves
Alpha-adrenergic - Drugs that mimic the actions of the sympathetic nervous system that employ norepinephrine as their neurotransmitter
Amnestic - Agent causing amnesia
Analgesia - Loss of sensitivity to pain
Anesthesia, General - Loss of ability to perceive pain associated with loss of consciousness
Antagonist - Drugs that neutralize or impede the action or effect of others
Apnea - Absence of breathing
Apneic - Related to or suffering from apnea
Arrhythmia - Loss of rhythm, especially an irregularity of the heart beat
Auscultation - Listening to the sounds made by the various body structures
Benzodiazepine - Compounds with sedative, antianxiety, anticonvulsant, and muscle relaxant properties
BP - Blood pressure
Bradycardia - Slowness of the heart beat
Bronchospasm - Contraction of the smooth muscles of the walls of the bronchi and bronchioles causing narrowing of the lumen
BT - Body temperature
Catalepsy - State of malleable rigidity of the limbs.
Cerebration - Activity of the mental processes
CNS - Central nervous system
Congener - A member of the same class or group
Contralateral - Relating to the opposite side
CRT - Capillary refill time
Cyanosis - A dark bluish or purplish coloration of the skin and mucous membranes due to deficient oxygenation of the blood
Cyclohexane - Dissociative anesthetic
Cycloplegia - Loss of power in the ciliary muscle of the eye
Distal - Situated away from the center of the body
Dosage - Amount of drug given on a per weight basis, usually expressed as mg/kg
Dose - Total amount of drug given to an animal, usually expressed in mg
ED_{50} - Dosage causing desired effect in 50% of the sample population
Endogenous - Originating or produced within the organism
Exogenous - Originating or produced outside of the organism
GABA - Gamma-aminobutyric acid; a neurotransmitter in the CNS
Gm - Gram
Hepatotoxic - Relating to an agent that damages the liver

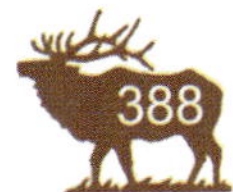

HR - Heart rate

Hyperglycemia - Abnormally high concentration of glucose in the circulating blood

Hyperkalemia - Abnormally high concentration of potassium ions in the circulating blood

Hyperthermia - Unusually high body temperature

Hyperventilation - Abnormally fast or deep respiration

Hypnosis - Artificially induced sleep or state resembling sleep.

Hypocalcemia - Abnormally low concentration of calcium in the circulating blood

Hypoglycemia - Abnormally low concentration of glucose in the circulating blood

Hypokalemia -Abnormally low concentration of potassium ions in the circulating blood

Hypotension - Low blood pressure

Hypothermia - Unusually low body temperature

Hypoxia - Decrease below normal levels of oxygen in the blood or tissue

IC - Intracardiac; within the chambers of the heart

IM - Intramuscular; within the substance of the muscle

IP - Intraperitoneal; within the peritoneal cavity

IV - Intravascular; within the lumen of blood vessels

Kg - Kilogram

Lateral - On the side away from the median plane

Lb - Pound

LD_{50} - Dosage lethal to 50% of the sample population

Medial - Relating to the middle or center

Mg - Milligram

Ml - Milliliter

Mydriasis - Dilation of the pupil

Myoglobinuria - Excretion of myoglobin in the urine

Narcosis - Sedation in which the animal is oblivious to pain with or without hypnosis

Nephrotoxic - Relating to an agent that damages the kidney

Neuroleptanalgesia - Amnesia and analgesia produced by a combination of a neuroleptic drug and a narcotic analgesic drug.

Neuroleptic - Antipsychotic drug causing suppression of spontaneous movements with retention of spinal reflexes and pain-avoidance behavior

Neuropathy - Any disorder affecting any segment of the nervous system

Nociceptive - Capable of appreciation or transmission of pain

Opioid - Drug that has opium- or morphine-like properties

Paresis - Partial or incomplete paralysis

Patent - Open, exposed

Peritonitis - Inflammation of the peritoneum

Phenothiazine - Antipsychotic drug

PO - Per os; orally

Polyuria - Excessive urination

Proximal - Nearest the trunk or point of origin

RR - Respiratory rate

SC - Subcutaneous

Safety Margin - The ratio of the drug dose that causes death in 1% of the sample population (LD_1) to the drug dose that causes the desired effect in 99% of the sample population (ED_{99}); a small safety factor implies that the effective dose is close to the lethal dose

Sedation - See tranquilization.

$T_{1/2}$ - Half-life; the period of time during which the concentration of a substance in the blood is reduced to one-half of its initial concentration

Tachycardia - Rapid beating of the heart

Thypnea - Rapid breathing

Therapeutic Index - The ratio of the drug dose that causes death in one-half of the sample population (LD_{50}) to the drug dose that causes the desired effect in one-half of the sample population (ED_{50})

Tidal Volume - The volume of air that is inspired and expired in a single breath during regular breathing

Tranquilization - State of calmness in which the animal is relaxed, awake and unconcerned about its surroundings and may be indifferent to minor pain

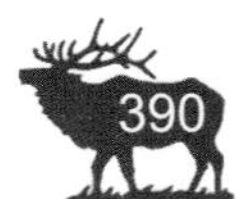

Index

A

B

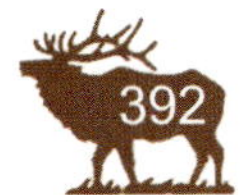

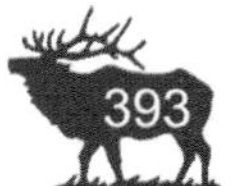

C

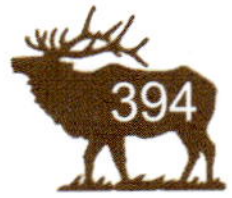

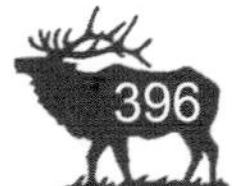

D

E

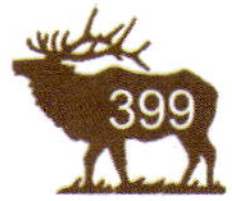

F

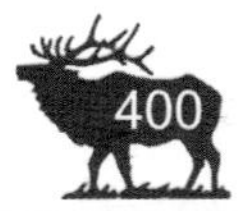

G

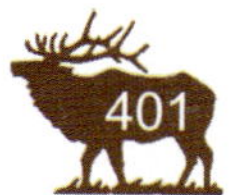

H

I

J

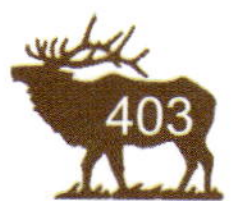

K

L

M

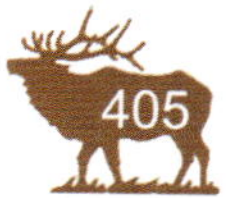

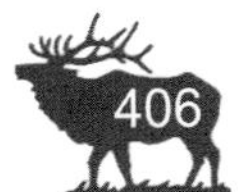

N

O

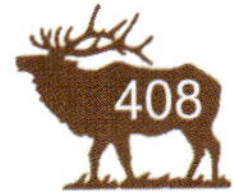

P

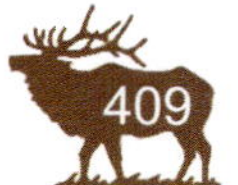

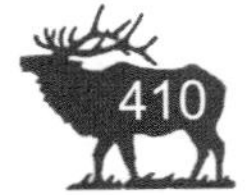

Q

R

S

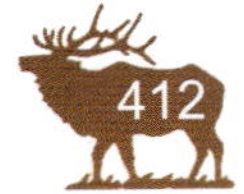

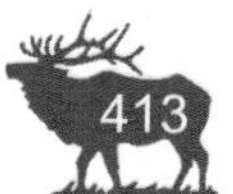

T

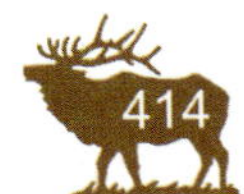

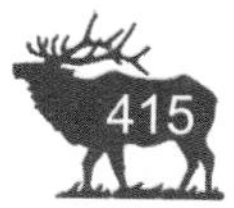

U

V

W

X

Y

Z

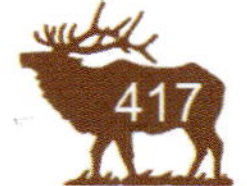

English-Metric Conversion

Kilogram-Pounds

The dosages in this handbook are presented on a body weight basis, expressed in the metric system (grams, kilograms). For those not familiar with the metric system, following are two methods for converting pounds to kilograms without the use of a calculator.

For those of you who just have to use a calculator: 1 pound (lb) = 0.454 kilograms or 1 kilogram (kg) = 2.205 pounds. You can use the following scales to convert back and forth between pounds and kilograms.

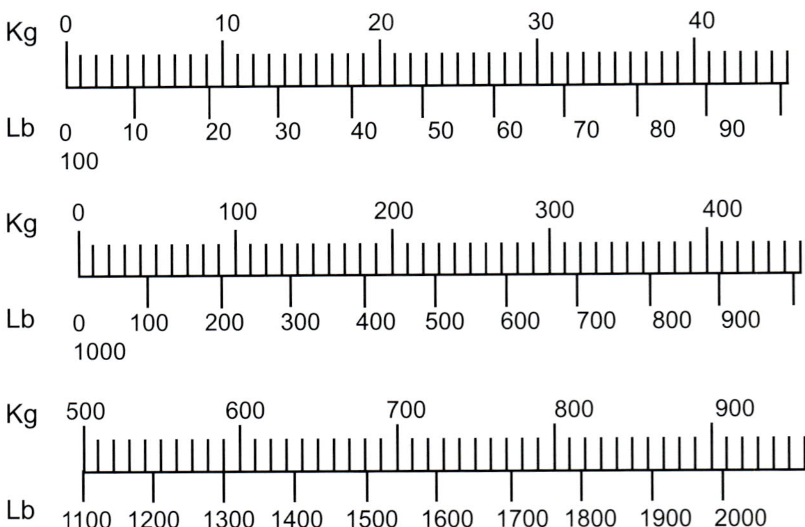

Celsius-Fahrenheit

Temperatures in this handbook are given in degrees Celsius with the equivalent Fahrenheit temperature given in parentheses. If you have a need to convert other temperatures, the conversions are as follows:

To convert Celcius to Fahrenheit:
Multiply the Celcius temperature by 9, divide by 5, add 32. For example: 25 °C x 9 = 225; 225/5 = 45; 45 + 32 = 77 °F.

To convert Fahrenheit to Celcius:
Subtract 32 from the Fahrenheit temperature, multiply by 5, divide by 9. For example: 77 °F - 32 = 45; 45 x 5 = 225; 225/9 = 25 °C.

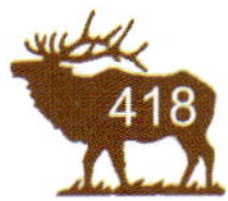

Notes

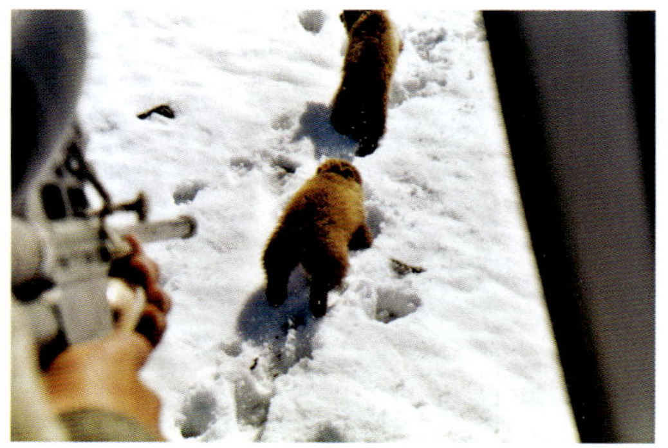

Notes

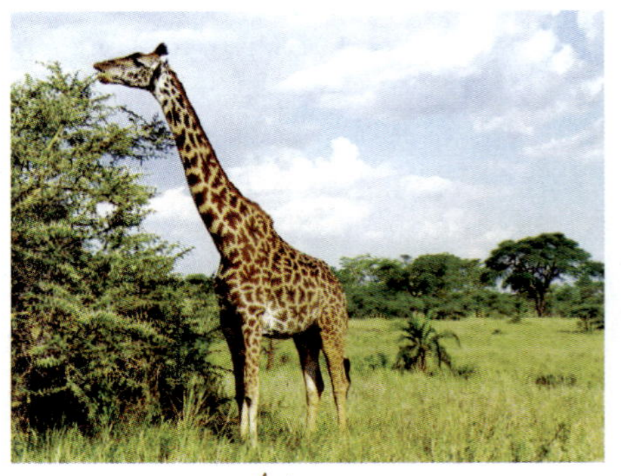

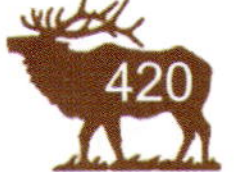

Notes

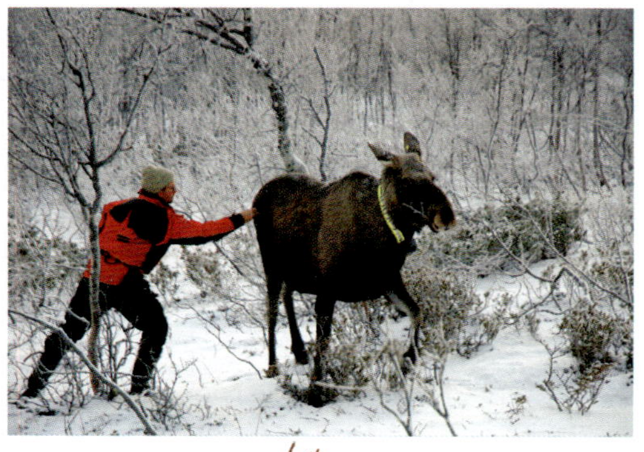

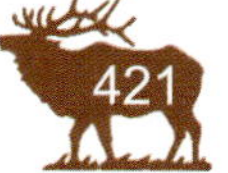

Notes

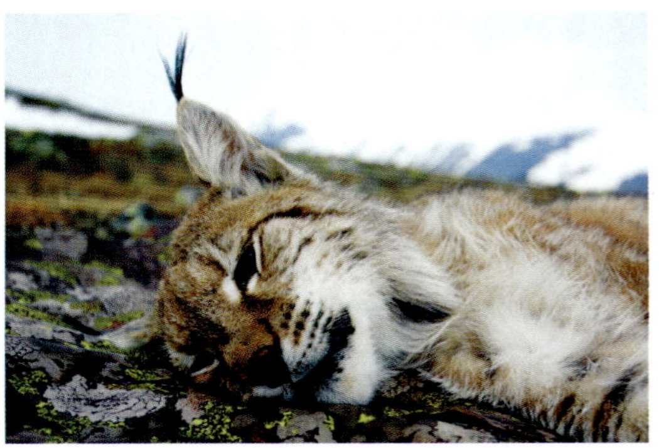

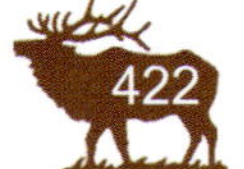

Notes

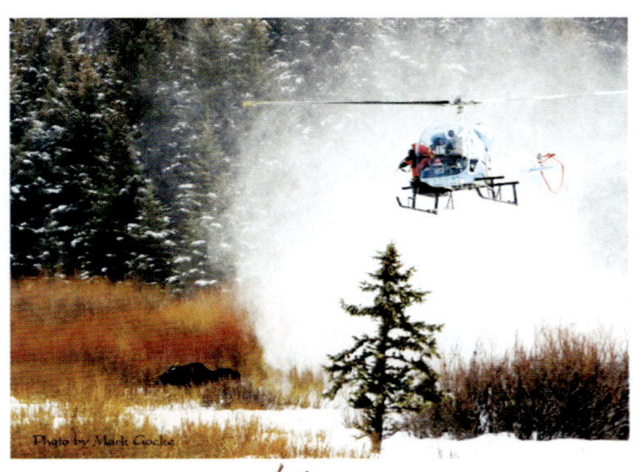

Photo by Mark Gocke

Notes

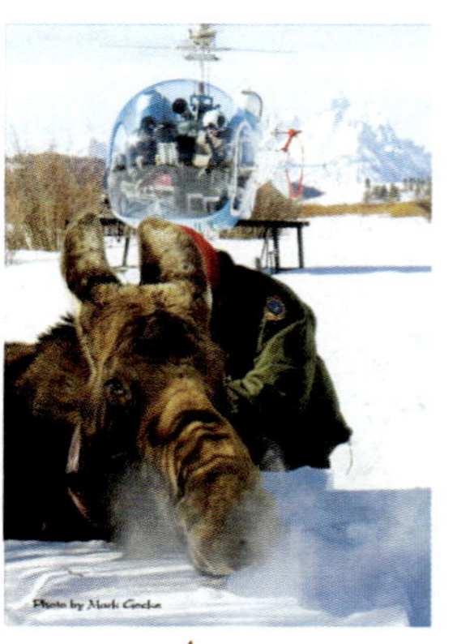
Photo by Mark Gocke

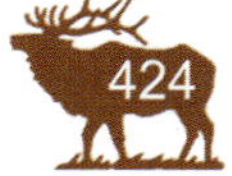

Notes

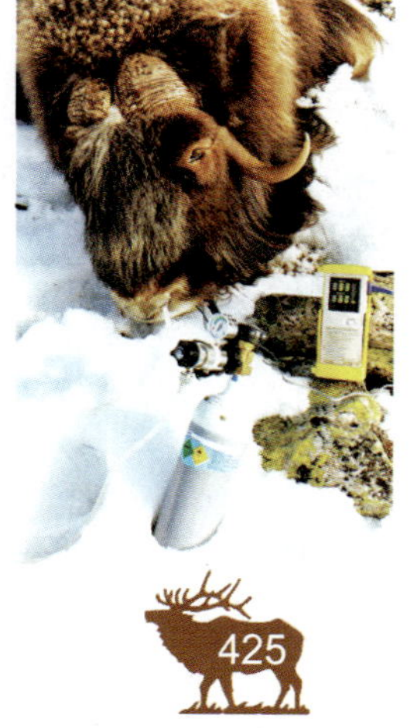

Notes

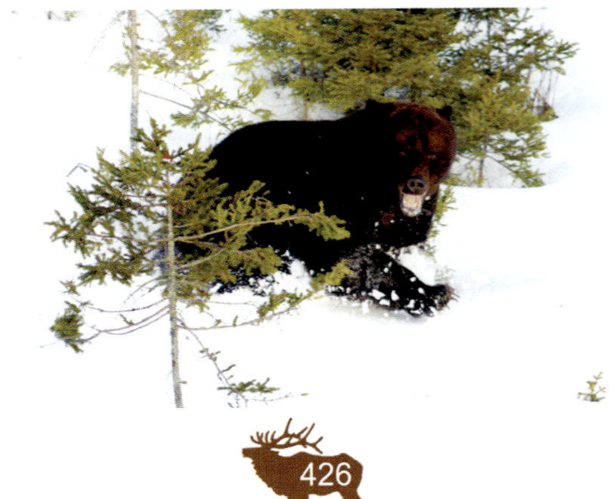

Notes

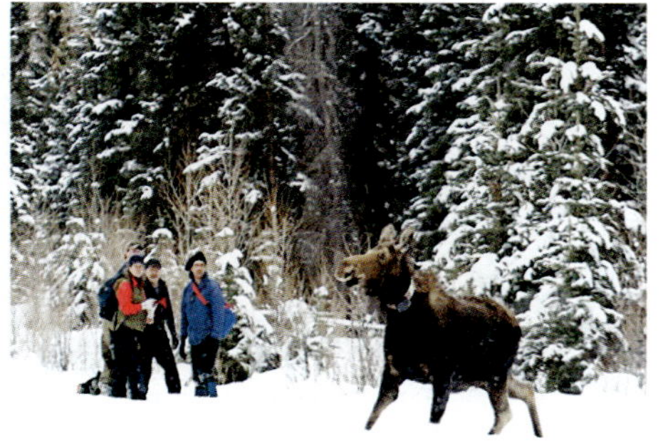

Photo by Mark Gocke

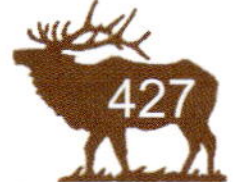

Notes

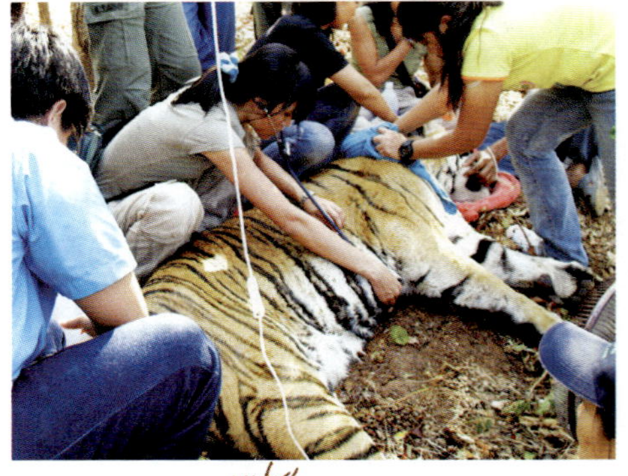

Notes

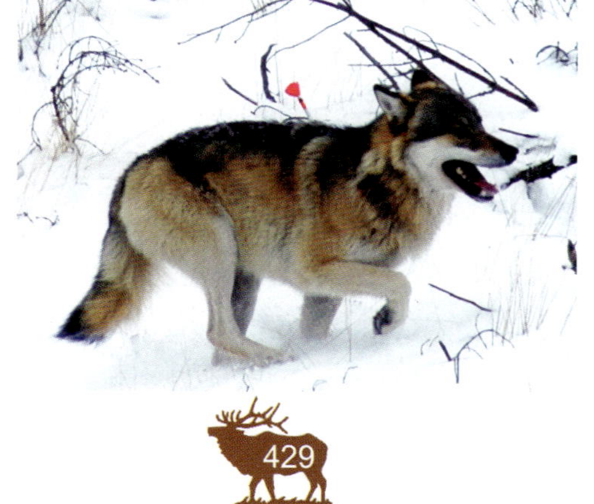

Notes

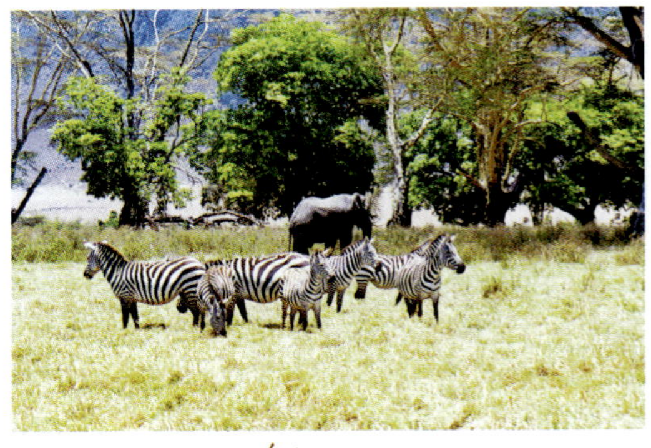

Notes

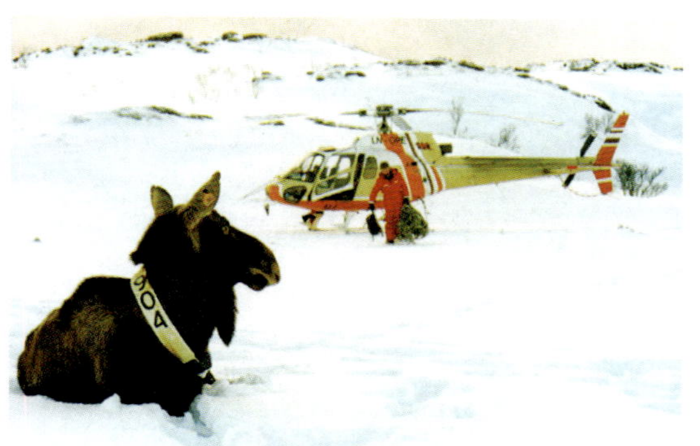

Notes

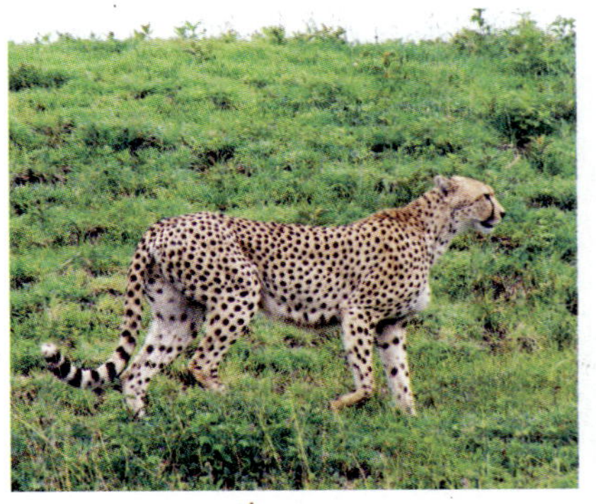